TEXTBOOK OF
URGENT CARE MANAGEMENT

TEXTBOOK OF URGENT CARE MANAGEMENT

JOHN SHUFELDT, MD, JD, MBA, FACEP

Urgent Care Textbooks • Scottsdale • 2014

© 2014 by Urgent Care Textbooks, 7332 Butherus Hangar One, Scottsdale, AZ 85260.

All rights reserved. No part of this book may be reproduced or transmitted in any form or by any means, electronic or mechanical, including photocopying, recording, or by any information storage or retrieval system, without permission in writing from the copyright holder, except for brief quotations embodied in critical articles and reviews.

To purchase additional copies, call 480-339-5345 or fax orders to 480-247-6482. To order print or electronic copies online, go to www.urgentcaretextbooks.com.

ISBN: 978-0-9914795-3-5 Trade paperback
ISBN: 978-0-9914795-4-2 Electronic book

Care has been taken to confirm the accuracy of the information presented and to describe generally accepted practices. However, the authors, editors, and publisher are not responsible for errors or omissions or for any consequences from application of the information in this book and make no warranty, expressed or implied, with respect to the currency, completeness, or accuracy of the contents of the publication. Application of the information in a particular situation remains the professional responsibility of the practitioner. The authors, editors, and publisher have exerted every effort to ensure that the information set forth in this text is in accordance with current recommendations and practice at the time of publication. The information in this book is provided for informational purposes only and does not represent legal or financial advice on any subject matter. The contents of this book should not be relied upon or used as a substitute for consultation with professional advisors. You should contact your attorney, accountant, or other appropriate professional to obtain advice with respect to any particular issue or problem.

Editor: John Shufeldt, MD, JD, MBA, FACEP

Chief copyeditor: Katharine O'Moore-Klopf, ELS, www.kokedit.com

Team copyeditors: Dick Margulis, www.dmargulis.com;
  Frédérique Courard-Hauri, www.fchcomm.com;
  and Renee Pessin, www.rdpeditorial.com

Indexer: Marilyn Augst, www.prairiemoonindexing.com

Proofreaders: Mary L. Tod, ELS, www.drtodediting.com;
  and Katharine R. Wiencke, kwiencke@verizon.net

Cover design: Fabrizio Romano, theforzadesign@gmail.com

Design and composition: Dick Margulis, www.dmargulis.com

Second printing, October 2014

MANUFACTURED IN THE REPUBLIC OF KOREA

To my colleagues in urgent care medicine who have fought the good fight for the betterment of our industry.

John Shufeldt, MD, JD, MBA, FACEP

Contents

Contributors ix

Preface xiii

1	Introduction to Urgent Care Management • *John Shufeldt*	3
2	Developing the Business Plan • *John Shufeldt*	11
3	Site Selection • *Mike Zelnik and Jim Garrett*	23
4	Building Out Your Urgent Care Center • *Tracy Altemus*	49
5	Design of the Floor Plan in an Urgent Care Center • *Rajiv Kapadia*	63
6	Business Formation and Entity Structuring • *Adam Winger*	77
7	Exit Transactions: The Process of Selling an Urgent Care Company • *Adam Winger*	87
8	Corporate Practice of Medicine and Other Legal Impediments to Nonphysician Ownership • *Adam Winger*	105
9	Insurance Requirements for the Urgent Care Center • *David Wood*	115
10	Equipment and Supply Vendor Selection • *Sybil Yeaman*	127
11	Urgent Care Accreditation • *Michael Kulczycki, Laurel Stoimenoff, and John Shufeldt*	145
12	Pro Forma Financial Statements: Creating Income, Balance Sheet, and Cash-Flow Forecasts • *Glenn Dean*	157
13	Financial Management: Internal Control, Performance Measurement, and Evaluation • *Glenn Dean*	183
14	Physician Leadership • *DeVry C. Anderson*	203
15	Human Resources Overview: Key Labor and Employment Issues • *Laura Schiesl*	217
16	Urgent Care Duties, Staffing Mix, and Ratios • *John Shufeldt*	233
17	Physician Extenders in the Urgent Care Center • *John Shufeldt and Adam Winger*	247
18	Provider Compensation • *John Shufeldt*	253
19	Hiring and Managing Medical Providers • *John Shufeldt*	263
20	Strategic Talent Management: Talent Makes All the Difference • *Marty Martin*	275
21	Employment Contracts and Compensation • *Adam Winger*	289
22	Health Plan Contracting • *Sybil Yeaman*	305
23	Choosing the Electronic Health Record • *John Shufeldt*	319
24	Revenue Cycle Management and Partnership • *Sybil Yeaman*	339
25	Marketing Overview • *Megan Lamy*	351
26	Consumer Engagement Using Social Media • *Lisa Cintron*	365
27	Public Relations: A Tool for Success • *Erin Terjesen*	377
28	Crisis Communications Management • *Erin Terjesen*	385
29	Developing Your Brand • *Kat Smith*	393
30	Metric-Driven Management: Harnessing Information in the Urgent Care Organization • *Laurel Stoimenoff*	403

31	Laboratory Overview • *Tracy Patterson*	415
32	Implementation of a Moderate-Complexity Clinical Laboratory • *Lynn R. Glass*	427
33	EMTALA in Urgent Care Medicine • *Rachel A. Lindor*	451
34	Engaging Accountable Care Organizations in Urgent Care Centers • *John Harris*	463
35	Urgent Care Imaging and Interpretation • *Tim Hogan*	475
36	Virtual Care • *Ian Vasquez*	485
37	Setting Up a Health-Care Compliance Program • *Tracy Patterson*	499
38	Audits by Managed-Care Organizations and Regulatory Agencies • *Damaris L. Medina*	511
39	Ensuring Patient Safety • *John Shufeldt*	521
40	Implementing Occupational Medicine • *Laurel Stoimenoff*	535
41	Measuring and Improving Patient Satisfaction • *Sybil Yeaman*	547
42	Evaluation and Management of Coding and Documentation • *Sybil Yeaman*	561
43	Additional Services in Urgent Care • *Natasha N. Deonarain*	575
44	Integrative Medicine • *Marty Martin*	587
45	Pediatric Urgent Care • *Gary Gerlacher*	599
46	Urgent Care Center Financing • *Glenn Dean*	611
47	The Future of Urgent Care • *John Shufeldt*	625
Index		629

Contributors

Tracy Altemus, CCIM
Executive Vice President
Healthcare Brokerage Services
Phoenix, AZ, USA

DeVry C. Anderson, MD, FS
Chief
Department of Deployment Medicine
Fort Hood, TX, USA
Owner
Quick Care Walk In Clinic
Austin, TX, USA

Lisa Cintron, BS
Chief Executive Officer
iMoxie Digital Marketing, LLC
Winston-Salem, NC, USA

Glenn Dean, MBA, CPA
MeMD, Inc.
Scottsdale, AZ, USA

Natasha N. Deonarain, MD, MBA
Founder and Chief Executive Officer
Conscious Health Systems
Chandler, AZ, USA

Jim Garrett, BS
Real Estate Consultant
National UC Realty
Tampa, FL, USA

Gary Gerlacher, MD, MBA, FAAP
Founder
Texas Children's Urgent Care
Houston, TX, USA

Lynn R. Glass, BS, MT (ASCP)
Senior Director
MedSol Laboratory Consulting
Jacksonville, FL, USA

Contributors

John Harris, MBA
Principal
DGA Partners
Bala Cynwyd, PA, USA

Tim Hogan, BA
Executive Director
UrgentRad Teleradiology
Scottsdale, AZ, USA

Rajiv Kapadia, MS, B.ARCH., RA, LEED AP
President and Owner
SPG Studios
Chandler, AZ, USA

Michael Kulczycki, MBA
Executive Director, Ambulatory Care Accreditation Program
Joint Commission
Oakbrook Terrace, IL, USA

Megan Lamy, MBA
Marketing and Branding Consultant
Tempe, AZ, USA

Rachel A. Lindor, MD, JD
Mayo Clinic
Rochester, MN, USA

Marty Martin, PSY.D., MPH, MA, MS
Director and Associate Professor, Health Sector Management
DePaul University
Chicago, IL, USA

Damaris L. Medina, ESQ.
Health-Care Attorney
Michelman & Robinson, LLP
Los Angeles, CA, USA

Tracy Patterson, MBA, MHSA, CHC
Principal
Continuum Health Solutions, LLC
Mesa, AZ, USA

Laura Schiesl, ESQ.
Farhang & Medcoff
Phoenix, AZ, USA

John Shufeldt, MD, JD, MBA, FACEP
Chief Executive Officer
MeMD, LLC
Scottsdale, AZ, USA

Kat Smith, BS
Marketing Communications Manager
MeMD, Inc.
Scottsdale, AZ, USA

Laurel Stoimenoff, PT, CHC
Principal
Continuum Health Solutions, LLC
Chandler, AZ, USA

Erin Terjesen, BA
Principal, Public Relations and Marketing
Propel Communications
Scottsdale, AZ, USA

Ian Vasquez, MBA
Health-Care Consultant
Phoenix, AZ, USA

Adam Winger, JD, CPA, LLM
Attorney
Baker, Donelson, Bearman, Caldwell & Berkowitz, PC
Birmingham, AL, USA

David Wood, BA
Managing Director of Health Care
The Wood Insurance Group
Scottsdale, AZ, USA

Sybil Yeaman, BA
Chief Operating Officer
Urgent Care Integrated Network
Scottsdale, AZ, USA

Mike Zelnik, CCIM, SIOR
President
Zelnik Realty Group
Tampa, FL, USA

Preface

THE FIELD OF URGENT care medicine is dynamic, quality-driven, and highly rigorous. Opening a center is not for the faint of heart or weak-willed. Using this book will help make opening and operating a center a more profitable and enjoyable experience for you.

I went to great lengths to search out the best minds in our industry to bring you the latest knowledge from their various fields of expertise. This textbook has been a labor of love for me and the authors involved in its creation. All of us saw the need to further our industry by distilling the best practices of our industry into actionable information.

Use this information as you would a consultant. It represents state-of-the-art thinking for urgent care medicine and care-on-demand delivery. The principles in every chapter are time- and battle-tested.

As new information comes to light, we will update both our website and future editions of this book.

John Shufeldt, MD, JD, MBA, FACEP
www.urgentcaretextbooks.com

TEXTBOOK OF URGENT CARE MANAGEMENT

CHAPTER 1

Introduction to Urgent Care Management

John Shufeldt

DEFINITION
The Urgent Care Association of America defines urgent care as "the delivery of ambulatory medical care outside of a hospital emergency department on a walk-in basis, without a scheduled appointment." Urgent care centers treat many problems that can be seen in a primary-care physician's office, but urgent care centers offer some services that are generally not available in primary-care physicians' offices, such as x-ray and minor trauma treatment.

This definition paints the urgent care industry with a broad, all-inclusive brush. Many centers have personnel trained in advanced cardiovascular life support and have a crash cart, defibrillator or automated external defibrillator, cardiac medications, and intravenous narcotics. The level of care provided in an urgent care center depends on the owner–operator and is typically determined by the training or background of the physician–founder.

INDUSTRY LIFE CYCLE
The initial urgent care centers opened in the late 1980s. Soon after, a *Harvard Business Review* article described this new trend as an innovative alternative (a precursor to *disruptive innovation*) that could render emergency departments (EDs) vulnerable to replacement.[1] Around the same time, *US News & World Report* ascribed the urgent care phenomenon to an oversupply of physicians who were opting for a new delivery model. Since then, after a decline in the mid-1980s, this sector of the health-care industry has expanded to approximately 6,000 centers. Many of these centers were started by emergency medicine and family practice physicians in response to consumer demand for convenient, affordable access to unscheduled medical care.

Much of the growth of these centers has been fueled by the significant savings that urgent care centers provide over the cost of care delivered in a hospital ED.

---

1 Goldsmith JC. The health care market: can hospitals survive? *Harvard Business Review*. 1980 September/October;100–12. Available from: www.healthfuture.net/pdf/w-chs.pdf. Accessed February 19, 2014.

Many managed-care organizations now encourage their customers to use the urgent care option.² This encouragement comes in the form of member education and differential co-pays.

The urgent care center industry began to accelerate rapidly beginning in the mid-1990s. Consumers' acceptance and use of urgent care centers has also been on the rise, even during the economic recession that began at the end of 2007. According to the results of the 2010 Urgent Care Benchmarking Survey³ produced by the Urgent Care Association of America, per-center visits increased each month by 28 per center between 2008 and 2012.

According to an IBISWorld report, the urgent care industry is in the growth phase of its industry life cycle, evidenced by expanding industry added value, strong company growth rates, greater employment opportunities, and rising per capita use of urgent care facilities.⁴ From 2007 through 2017, the urgent care industry is expected to grow at an average annual rate of 4.3%. By way of benchmarking, during the same 10-year time frame, US gross domestic product is expected to rise at an average annual rate of 1.9%. This indicates that the urgent care center industry is making up an increasing share of the national economy.

Furthermore, the size of the industry continues to expand, particularly in underserved rural areas of the United States. From 2007 through 2017, the number of urgent care facilities is expected to rise at an average annual rate of 4.4%, reaching more than 10,000 centers by the end of 2017. Employment is expected to increase steadily as well, growing in line with the number of urgent care centers.⁵ This growth, fueled by the lack of new-patient capacity of primary-care providers, is expected to continue through 2019.

URGENT CARE OVERVIEW

Urgent care medicine remains one of the fastest-growing segments in the healthcare system. At the time of publication, we found 5,190 facilities in the United States that define themselves as urgent care centers.

According to the IBISWorld report, urgent care revenue grew between 2007 and 2012 at an average annualized rate of 6.3% and is expected continue to grow at 5.6% through 2017, reaching a total revenue for the industry of $17.9 billion.⁶

These factors affect the growth of the urgent care industry:

- ► ED overcrowding and closures
- ► Cost of emergency care

---

2   Blue Cross of GA uses Google maps to encourage use of urgent care. *Urgent Care News*. 2011 June. Available from: http://www.urgentcarenews.com/June2011/bcbs.php. Accessed February 19, 2014.
3   Urgent Care Association of America. 2012 urgent care benchmarking report. Available from: http://www.ucaoa.org/orderreports.php. Accessed February 19, 2014.
4   IBISWorld. IBISWorld industry report OD5458, urgent care centers in the US, February 2012. Available from: http://www.ibisworld.com/industry/urgent-care-centers.html. Accessed February 19, 2014.
5   IBISWorld industry report OD5458.
6   IBISWorld industry report OD5458.

- Lack of insurance coverage
- More informed consumers
- Lack of primary-care availability
- Extended hours of urgent care centers
- Virtual care delivery integration

EMERGENCY DEPARTMENT OVERCROWDING AND CLOSURES

Every year EDs see 1 in every 5 Americans at least once.[7] Although many people depend on EDs, obtaining acute medical care is becoming a significant financial burden as total charges for ED services continue to rise.[8] According to a 2002 national survey, more than 90% of large US hospitals report EDs operating at or over capacity. The rate of closure of nonrural EDs exceeded 27%, dropping the absolute number of EDs from 2,446 in 1999 to 1,799 in 2009.[9]

This trend in ED overcrowding has been partially responsible for driving the growth in the urgent care industry. According to the Centers for Disease Control and Prevention, emergency visits in the United States reached an all-time high of nearly 124 million in 2008. Moreover, the rate of ED visits increased at twice the growth rate of the US population between 1997 and 2007. As a result, average wait times for ED visits have increased, prompting a greater number of hospitals to begin referring low-acuity patients to urgent care facilities to reduce overcrowding.[10]

COST OF EMERGENCY CARE

Caldwell et al studied 8,303 ED encounters, representing 76.6 million visits. Median charges for ED visits ranged from $740 (95% confidence interval [CI], $651–$817) for an upper respiratory infection to $3437 (95% CI, $2917–$3877) for a kidney stone. The median charge for all 10 outpatient conditions in the ED was $1233 (95% CI, $1199–$1268), with a high degree of charge variability.[11]

---

7   National Center for Health Statistics. *Health, United States, 2006, with Chartbook on Trends in the Health of Americans.* Hyattsville, MD: National Center for Health Statistics; 2006. Available from: http://www.ncbi.nlm.nih.gov/books/NBK21002/. Accessed February 19, 2014.
8   Hsia RY, MacIsaac D, Baker L. Decreasing reimbursements for outpatient emergency department visits across payer groups from 1996 to 2004. *Ann Emerg Med.* 2008;51:265–74.
9   Brophy MB. 2011 study: third of hospital ERs have closed over past 20 years. *USA Today.* May 18, 2011. Available from: http://usatoday30.usatoday.com/yourlife/health/healthcare/hospitals/2011-05-17-ERs-closing-US_n.htm. Accessed June 23, 2013.
10 IBISWorld industry report OD5458.
11 Caldwell N, Srebotnjak T, Wang T, Hsia R. "How much will I get charged for this?" Patient charges for top ten diagnoses in the emergency department. PLoS One 2013;8:e55491. Available from: http://dx.plos.org/10.1371/journal.pone.0055491. Accessed February 19, 2014.

Medica Choice has provided fee estimates for common ailments treated in an urgent care center[12]:

- Allergies: $97
- Acute bronchitis: $127
- Earache: $110
- Sore throat: $94
- Pinkeye: $102
- Sinusitis: $112
- Strep throat: $111
- Upper respiratory infection: $111
- Urinary tract infection: $110

Compare those figures with Medica Choice's estimates for the same ailments treated in an ED:

- Allergies: $345
- Acute bronchitis: $595
- Earache: $400
- Sore throat: $525
- Pinkeye: $370
- Sinusitis: $617
- Strep throat: $531
- Upper respiratory infection: $486
- Urinary tract infection: $665

LACK OF INSURANCE COVERAGE

Medicine is currently undergoing a sea change because of the adoption of the Affordable Care Act (ACA). The necessity for the adoption of the ACA was in part predicated on the lack of affordable coverage for a segment of the US population. According to the US Census Bureau, in 2009 there were 48.6 million people in the United States (15.7% of the population) who were without health insurance.[13]

---

12 Fay B. Emergency rooms vs. urgent care: differences in services and costs. Wilmington, DE: Debt.org; © 2014. Available from: http://www.debt.org/medical/emergency-room-urgent-care-costs/. Accessed February 19, 2014.

13 US Census Bureau. Income, poverty, and health insurance coverage in the United States: 2009. Issued September 2010. Washington DC. US Census Bureau. p. 22. Available from: http://www.census.gov/prod/2010pubs/p60-238.pdf. Accessed February 19, 2014.

More troubling are the results of a study published in the *American Journal of Public Health* in 2009, which found that lack of health insurance is associated with about 45,000 excess preventable deaths per year.[14]

The factors contributing to this rate of uninsurance have fueled public and political debate, culminating in the passing of the ACA. Rising insurance costs have contributed to a trend in which fewer employers are offering health insurance as part of their compensation package. Many employers are managing costs by requiring higher employee contributions or differential payment schemes designed to encourage healthy lifestyles.

Many of the uninsured are the working poor, are self-employed, or are unemployed.[15] Others are healthy—often young—and make the conscious decision to go without insurance. Others have been rejected by insurance companies because of past health issues and are considered uninsurable. Some are without health insurance only temporarily. A minority choose faith-based alternatives to health insurance.

The Affordable Care Act of 2010 was designed to extend health coverage to those without it by expanding Medicaid, creating financial incentives for employers to offer coverage, and requiring those without employer or public coverage to purchase insurance in newly created state-run health insurance exchanges. The Congressional Budget Office has estimated that by 2022, roughly 33 million Americans who would otherwise have been uninsured will receive coverage because of the act.[16]

MORE-INFORMED CONSUMERS

Consumers are becoming more informed about the disparities in cost between various avenues of care. Financial concerns have been cited as the number one reason individuals with nonurgent medical issues delay treatment until an urgent or emergency condition develops.[17] Efforts to inform consumers of expected charges for common outpatient ED treatments have been stymied by the unavailability of this data in most administrative datasets. In my experience, most emergency physicians do not know the actual cost of the care they deliver or prescribe.

---

14 Cecere D. New study finds 45,000 deaths annually linked to lack of health coverage. *Harvard Gazette*. September 17, 2009. Available from: http://news.harvard.edu/gazette/story/2009/09/new-study-finds-45000-deaths-annually-linked-to-lack-of-health-coverage/. Accessed February 19, 2014.

15 Henry J. Kaiser Family Foundation. Key facts about the uninsured population. September 26, 2013. Menlo Park: CA: Henry J. Kaiser Family Foundation. Available from: http://kff.org/uninsured/fact-sheet/key-facts-about-the-uninsured-population/. Accessed February 19, 2014.

16 Congressional Budget Office. CBO and JCT's estimates of the effects of the Affordable Care Act on the number of people obtaining employment-based health insurance. March 2012. Available from http://www.cbo.gov/sites/default/files/cbofiles/attachments/03-15-ACA_and_Insurance_2.pdf. Accessed February 19, 2014.

17 Cunningham PJ, Felland LE. Falling behind: Americans' access to medical care deteriorates, 2003–2007. Washington DC: Center for Studying Health System Change. June 2008. Available from: http://hschange.org/CONTENT/993/993.pdf. Accessed February 19, 2014.

Patients also are unaware of the potential costs of using the ED. Patients in the ED underestimate their financial responsibility and are often shocked at their bill.[18] The median charge for outpatient conditions in the ED in 2013 was $499.[19] Efforts to increase price transparency have been proposed in over 30 states and are being pursued by the public and private sector as the next phase in medical care.[20]

While the American College of Emergency Physicians reports that 92 percent of emergency visits are from "very sick people who need care within 1 minute to 2 hours," the National Hospital Ambulatory Medical Care Survey estimates that only one-third to one-half of all ED visits are for non-urgent care. In fact, the top three reasons for ER visits in 2007 were for superficial injuries and contusions, sprains and strains, and upper respiratory infections.[21]

My personal experience practicing emergency medicine in both large tertiary-care centers and rural EDs parallels the findings from the National Hospital Ambulatory Medical Care Survey that less than half of the patients presenting to the ED have an issue or illness that requires ED-level care.

LACK OF PRIMARY-CARE AVAILABILITY

The US Centers for Disease Control and Prevention estimates that each year in the United States there are more than 500 million primary-care office visits. One of the main reasons for increased patient volume in urgent care is the lack of timely primary-care intervention. The critical shortage in primary-care physicians and clinics affects approximately 66 million Americans, or about 1 in every 5 people. The primary-care shortage and inadequate access to proper and prompt care probably contributes to a higher incidence of more serious health conditions. The United States likely will need almost 52,000 additional primary-care physicians by 2025 to meet the country's health-care needs.[22]

The US graduate medical education system is producing primary-care physicians at an abysmally low rate.[23] Unless something drastic is done soon, the shortfall will get desperately worse. As the ACA pushes up demand for prima-

---

18   Caldwell et al. "How much will I get charged for this?"
19   PricewaterhouseCoopers. 2013 Health and Well-Being Touchstone Survey. Available from: http://www.pwc.com/us/en/hr-management/publications/health-well-being-touchstone-survey.jhtml and http://www.pwc.com/us/en/health-industries/behind-the-numbers/infographics.jhtml. Accessed February 19, 2014.
20   Richmond R. Lifting the veil on medical costs. *Wall Street Journal*. 2008. Available from: http://online.wsj.com/article/SB10001424052748704893604576200780982549822.html. Accessed July 5, 2013.
21   Fay B. Emergency rooms vs. urgent care.
22   Petterson S. Projecting US primary care physicians workforce needs: 2010–2025 *Ann Fam Med*. 2012;10:503–9.
23   Chen C, Petterson S, Phillips RL, et al. Toward graduate medical education (GME) accountability: measuring the outcomes of GME institutions. *J Assoc Am Med Coll*. 2013;88:1267–80. Available from: http://journals.lww.com/academicmedicine/Citation/2013/09000/Toward_Graduate_Medical_Education__GME_.31.aspx. Accessed February 19, 2014.

ry-care services (millions of newly insured patients), large parts of America are set for a serious health-care crisis. A study conducted by the Mongan Institute for Health Policy at Massachusetts General Hospital showed that a high percentage of primary-care doctors "probably won't care for the newly insured "patients."[24]

The states with the lowest per capita rate of active primary-care physicians are Nevada, Mississippi, Utah, Texas, and Idaho, according to the Association of American Medical Colleges. The problem will become more acute nationally when about 30 million uninsured people eventually gain coverage under the ACA. Roughly half of those who will gain coverage under the ACA are expected to go into Medicaid, the federal–state program for the poor and disabled. States can opt to expand Medicaid, and at least 24 states and the District of Columbia plan to.

Of equal concern is the graying of the current physician population. According to a 2012 Physicians Foundation survey, nearly half of the 830,000 doctors in the United States are over 50 and approaching retirement. They are also seeing fewer patients than they did in 2008. The patient pool is getting older, as well, with some 8 million people reaching retirement age every day.[25]

Older people need more health services, and some 15 million will be eligible for Medicare in the coming years. Entering the system in 2014 will be the 30 million additional people with access to services through the ACA. Massachusetts patients experienced significant delays seeking care because of shortages of primary-care providers when the state's version of the ACA was enacted.

EXTENDED HOURS OF URGENT CARE CENTERS WITH WALK-IN AVAILABILITY

At present, the only facilities or venues offering on-demand care are urgent care facilities, retail clinics, virtual care providers, and EDs. There appears to be a growing trend of extending the hours of primary-care practices, particularly if they are affiliated with or owned by accountable care organizations (ACOs).

Expansion of primary-care office hours and active direction toward an ACO's primary-care providers may result in a change in the landscape of on-demand health care and patients' increasing use of on-demand services. At one large ACO on the East Coast, members were economically disincented from using urgent care centers, inasmuch as the ACO deemed all urgent care centers "out of network."

---

24 Nordqvist C. Primary care doctor shortage set to get worse, USA. *Medical News Today*. June 17, 2013. Available from: http://www.medicalnewstoday.com/articles/262033.php. Accessed February 19, 2014.

25 Physicians Foundation. A survey of America's physicians: practice patterns and perspectives. September 2012. Available from: http://www.physiciansfoundation.org/uploads/default/Physicians_Foundation_2012_Biennial_Survey.pdf. Accessed February 19, 2014.

VIRTUAL CARE DELIVERY INTEGRATION

A number of virtual care providers have now entered the on-demand health-care marketplace. Previously, the majority of the virtual providers catered only to large, self-insured employers and associations. Today, most such providers have either entered the direct-to-consumer market or plan to enter it.

Virtual care (using video technology that is compliant with the Health Insurance Portability and Accountability Act to connect patients with health-care providers) has evolved from the nurse triage phone lines popular from the mid-1980s. Those call centers, staffed by registered nurses, offered algorithm-based triage protocols to assist patients in making the appropriate choice based on their complaint and symptoms. Today virtual providers not only offer the same direction but can often treat the patient's illness.

At present there are at least 16 states that have enacted legislation mandating telemedicine services to be reimbursed at parity if those same services are covered face-to-face. This trend will likely continue as the need for an affordable, convenient alternatives for low-acuity care grows.

CONCLUSION

The urgent care space is going through an exciting time as it continues to adapt to the changing needs of on-demand health care. The key to our collective success is to continue to practice great customer service and great care at an affordable price. With this delivery model, we will continue to react and lead the new normal of patient-centric health care.

CHAPTER 2

Developing the Business Plan

John Shufeldt

WHETHER YOUR CLINIC IS already up and running or you are still in the stages of pulling everything together for the grand opening, writing a business plan is an invaluable process that can mean the difference between success and failure for your facility. Although you likely already know that writing a business plan is important, it is essential to also understand why you are doing it, so that you can leverage this iterative process to your fullest advantage.

Many entrepreneurs think of creating a business plan almost like a homework assignment that they have to do. In reality, a business plan is more a process than a physical document. Writing a business plan is a way to get you thinking critically and in detail about the dynamics of your clinic. It helps you ask questions that you would not have asked otherwise, and it helps you not only to think proactively about how you will build revenue but also to understand all of the interrelationships between the different facets of your organization by asking some of the right questions:

- How quickly will my revenue grow?
- How many patients can my staff realistically handle?
- How should I allocate facility space to maximize efficiency?
- What impact will economic instability have on the number of patients and hence my revenue?
- What additional services should I offer to maximize revenue and profit margins?

A business plan can help both an operation that is still in the planning stages and one that is already running. Even if your practice has been in business for many years, if you have never written a business plan for it you could be foregoing significant return on investment (ROI) without realizing it.

BEFORE YOU START: LEVERAGING AVAILABLE INFORMATIONAL RESOURCES

You don't have to start writing your business plan from scratch. Many valuable resources are available either free of charge or for a nominal fee. The websites http://business.usa.gov and www.sba.gov (the website of the US Small Business Administration) have great information, including business plan templates that can help you save valuable time. The Small Business Administration website gives you access to a free, interactive template for a business plan after you register for an account. The website also provides a self-assessment tool for new business owners and a highly informational online training section that has a wealth of tips and training videos specifically designed for owners of small business.

Another good resource is SCORE, formerly known as the Service Corps Of Retired Executives, whose website (www.score.org) has great downloadable templates that you can use as a guide. These templates don't just provide a layout of what your business plan should look like. They also help you to start thinking about your business in more detail by giving you numerous questions to answer about it. These questions are general, but they are a good way to start drilling down into your operations and especially to look for potential pitfalls in your strategy.

THE BASIC LAYOUT

A typical business plan has the following sections:

- Cover page
- Executive summary
- Company description
- Industry analysis
- Market analysis
- Competitor analysis
- Description of products and services
- Marketing strategy
- Implementation strategy
- Management plan
- Financial plan

Each section plays a specific role in helping you understand your clinic operations. As you complete each of them and do your research, you will begin to have a better grasp of the various issues that may affect your clinic. From understanding your target consumer and figuring out how to market more effectively to building a certain image in the minds of the patients to planning your cash flow, all of the sections are designed to give you a complete picture of your business.

Cover Page

The cover page contains all the basic information identifying the company—the name of your company and your facility, the address, and any other pertinent identifying information. This section is an important formality, particularly if you are preparing a business plan that will also be used for raising capital or obtaining a loan and that is therefore going to be reviewed by a lender or a potential partner or investor. On the other hand, if your venture is fully self-funded, you don't really need to fill this out. A business plan is all about gaining an in-depth understanding of your clinic—not formalities.

Executive Summary

In the executive summary, you lay out the bare-bones concept of your clinic. It should be one to two pages long at the most, and should contain a condensed yet comprehensive overview of your business. This section aims to condense your business model into just a few paragraphs, without any frills or details, so that anyone reading it can quickly understand the basic operating strategy of your facility. If your urgent care facility specializes in a service that most clinics do not, has specialized equipment, or includes some other factor that differentiates your clinic from other clinics (even if it is seemingly insignificant), mention it here.

Although it appears in the beginning of the business plan, the executive summary should be one of the last sections you write. After you have compiled, analyzed, and synthesized the operational model of your facility, you can summarize your findings and strategies in the executive summary.

Company Description

The company description is similar to the executive summary, except that here you should include a more detailed overview of your practice. Go into more detail about any specialized staff training and how your center functions. Describe any special attributes of your center that differentiate it from others in the area, especially if those attributes address the specific concerns of your immediate community.

Industry Analysis

In the industry analysis section, take a look at the overall industry and at how other urgent care centers operate. You want to show that you have a clear understanding of the latest trends in the industry and of potential changes in insurance reimbursement policies, and that you have a clear strategy for adjusting to any changes in the near future and midterm.

Market Analysis

The analysis of your target market is one of the most important sections of the business plan. This section, the content of which is largely dependent on the geography where you operate, is where you really get to know your consumer—the average person who will walk through the door seeking medical services. Of course, you won't cover every type of person, but this is the section in which you take a bird's-eye view of the neighborhood where you operate or plan to operate and try to understand the average person who will need your practice's services. Average age, average income, family type and marital status, insurance type, and the most common health concerns should all play a significant role in shaping your clinic. Pitney Bowes is a great resource for gathering this type of demographic data. You can learn anything from the average age to the average household income of your consumers by using this service. You can also use US Census Bureau data for this analysis.

Understanding your average consumer is the only way to tailor your services to maximize your profit margins and your ROI. If you complete this section properly, with adequate effort and attention, it will give you insight that helps you determine everything from the services you offer to the languages you require your staff members to speak; this section should be one of the first things you research. Unless you understand your consumer better than you understand yourself, there is absolutely no way you will be able to structure your clinic to maximize profitability.

This is also the time to analyze the health insurance dynamics of your target consumer. Having a thorough understanding of the common insurance coverages your patients are likely to have, coupled with the understanding of their average household earnings and other demographic data, can help you create an out-of-pocket pricing structure to maximize your profit margins. This will be a useful piece of information for structuring your marketing efforts (see the section "Marketing Strategy" in this chapter).

Competitor Analysis

Once you have a clear understanding of industry patterns and developments and of your target market's demographics, it is time to assess your immediate competitors. Take a look at other clinics that operate within the area and try to understand their strengths and weaknesses. Visit their offices, and pretend to be a patient if you have to. If you can gain insight into their operations from a patient's perspective, you will be able to compare the service offering of your competitors with the needs of your target market. This type of comparison can uncover great service opportunities that you may not have thought about before. For example, you may realize that your competitors do not offer extended laboratory hours or maybe do not operate on Sundays. This could be a great opportunity to structure your operations in a way that will provide your community with access to medical services when other clinics do not. Or you may notice a large immigrant population in your area and see that your competitors do not make it easy for that population to get past a language barrier. This could be yet another opportunity to address—a need for bilingual staff members who will not only speak the immigrants' language but will also understand their culture and can help create a more inviting atmosphere.

Certainly, other centers could copy your efforts later on if they see that you are successful. However, being the first to make your community feel welcome and cared for and providing them with more access to services during more convenient times for them could set you apart from your competition early on. Once people use and like your clinic, it will help you continuously grow more revenue and build out your service offering.

Description of Products and Services

The section describing your products and services is a direct outgrowth of your consumer market research. By understanding your geographic location and your target consumer, you will have a better idea about which services you should offer. Beyond the basics that every urgent care clinic must cover, you may need to place more focus on certain types of services. For example, if you establish a clinic that has a large proportion of children and adolescents, you may want to ensure that your services are geared toward their needs. Parents will be bringing in their children with sports injuries as well as illnesses prevalent in young adults. If you operate in a community that is dominated by seniors, you will want to tailor your services in a way that is geared toward that age group.

List your urgent care center's services in great detail. This is the section where you have a lot of freedom and where you should place significant focus, especially if your clinic does things differently from others. A medical facility is rarely *just* about providing urgent care services. When someone comes to your clinic, you are servicing not just their medical needs but their emotional needs as well. If they are brought to your clinic by family members, you are implicitly taking care of those family members' emotional needs. Ask yourself how you will deliver above-average care. How will you not only make the patient comfortable but also take care of the emotional needs of the family members, so that they rave to all of their friends and neighbors about how great your clinic is? Any medically trained professional can provide medical services, but how will *your* clinic be different? How will *your* clinic mesmerize your patients and their families so that they want to send you thank-you letters and holiday cards? This is the section of your business plan that lets you address all of these factors and brainstorm all of the different ways to take care of your patients beyond the ordinary and differentiate your facility from your local competitors' facilities.

Marketing Strategy

Don't develop the marketing strategy section until after you have completed the description of your products and services and have a comprehensive understanding of your target market. The marketing strategy section is one of the most enjoyable parts of writing a business plan. This is where you get to be creative.

When you truly understand your target market's demographics, you will gain an amazing advantage over your competitors. Many businesses do not take the time to understand who their consumer is and therefore do not market effectively. Business owners tend to exhibit an "if I build it, they will come" hubris, without taking the time to build a relationship with their potential customers.

Here is what you have to understand: Yes, your consumer will often visit your clinic because they have an emergency and limited options for where to go for treatment. But if you build a relationship with that consumer, if you advertise to them in a way that builds rapport, and if you truly connect with their emotional needs and build trust, then they will eventually *choose* to come to your facility. They will do so not just because they need help and yours is the closest facility. They will do so because your clinic is the place where they feel safe and where they know they will always be taken care of with professionalism and respect.

The consumer always has a choice, and no matter how bad their situation is, the fact that they don't know about your clinic—or have heard negative things about it—will influence whether they decide to set foot on your premises. If your clinic has a good reputation, consumers will choose to go to your facility even if it's farther away from their house than comparable clinics because they feel that your staff will do a much better job.

Implementation Strategy

Once you have a clear understanding of your target market and the services your clinic will offer, you can address your implementation strategy. This strategy has two components: specific steps to achieve your goals and timelines for achieving them. It's one thing to build a clinic in your neighborhood, open its doors, and wait for people to start coming in, and quite another to have a clear, step-by-step strategy for bringing your facility to its desired goals. Building clear timelines is a crucial component of devising a sound implementation strategy. A strategy without timetables and clear, measurable goals will pretty much doom your plan to failure.

Everything from logistical build-out steps to the laddering of marketing efforts should go in this section. This is your road map to going from concept to physical and operational reality. One plague for many business owners is *operational paralysis*. This is that deer-in-the-headlights moment when you have no idea of what steps to take and where to go next. It is usually brought about by being overwhelmed by a new business or a new strategy and not being able to make any meaningful decisions because you simply have no idea what the right answer is. A way to address this issue is to have a clear implementation plan ahead of time. Your plan may not be perfect and it may have some gaps, but if you have at least a decent understanding of the major steps you must take to turn your concept into reality, then you will be more apt to stay on course to build out your facility, rather than drifting along at the mercy of the current.

This section of the plan is also a good place to review your strengths and weaknesses. Every medical facility will have its own set of unique dynamics. If you clearly identify your strengths and weaknesses ahead of time, you will be able to roll out your implementation strategy more effectively. If you are not great at hiring staff members, then instead of trying to do the job yourself, you could simply outsource the process to an experienced staffing firm that can get you prescreened, top-quality personnel. On the other hand, you may find that your experience with laboratory services is above average, and you could therefore devote more of your time to building out this aspect of your operations yourself.

Looking at strengths and weaknesses is about figuring out the most efficient ways to implement your strategy.

Your implementation strategy does not have to be perfect. No matter how much you plan ahead of time, you will likely have to change some of your steps along the way to accommodate reality. But the purpose of a road map is not to give you specific step-by-step instructions for what to do but to give you a good idea of what goals should be achieved—the way that you achieve those goals may change.

Management Plan

The management section is an integral part of your business plan. Just because you set up operations, that doesn't mean that your staff members will flawlessly follow all of the rules and procedures that you set forth. To ensure productivity and, most importantly, to prevent errors, strict operational controls have to be developed for your clinic.

Operational controls are systems that allow you and your management team to catch errors when they occur rather than allowing them to compound into major problems. These controls are mechanisms that keep your staff members on track and provide you with valuable insights as to which of your staff members need more training and, ultimately, which of them may be the wrong fit for your facility.

At the heart of every solid control is a good manager. Whether you run a small operation where you oversee every staff member or a larger facility where duties and responsibilities are segmented across different managerial levels, having clear guidelines for oversight and chain of command are absolutely essential. Without a clear chain of command, your facility will quickly break down. Staff members will not understand who is responsible for what, and this decreases accountability. This can be a huge problem for clinics because accountability is absolutely essential for delivering quality patient care. The only way to set clear guidelines for your staff and to develop a clear chain of command is to first understand it yourself. Once you have developed this, you can adequately train your staff, and you can develop a clear policies manual or ask your managerial staff to do this. Without a clear chain of command, an organization chart, and a reporting procedure for issues, your urgent care center is bound to fail—not from financial issues but instead from lack of proper patient care and possible malpractice lawsuits that could eventually cause a shutdown of the entire operation.

Do not skip this step. If you have never managed an urgent care clinic, take some time to write down hypothetical scenarios of possible issues and how those issues would be resolved by your frontline and supervisory staff members. If you do this, you will realize that solving everyday issues and operational abnormalities can be difficult without a clear chain of command, strict guidelines regarding staff and manager responsibilities, and clear instructions for how staff members must handle various situations.

Financial Plan

The financial plan for your business is the last major part of your business plan. It does two important things:

- ▶ It lays out your budgeting over time—how much you will need to spend, and on what.
- ▶ It helps you clearly understand your cash-flow needs so that you don't end up unpleasantly surprised when your operation needs cash the most.

Many operators of medical facilities make the mistake of focusing so much on their strategy that they forget to think about their financing needs. Finance is so far removed from providing medical care that many operators view it as some sort of a chore that must be handled, something that can be pushed off on the medical billers and bookkeepers. Delegating these tasks to your staff is obviously acceptable, but only if you realize that your staff will never understand the clinic budgeting and cash-flow needs the way that you do. No matter how great your clinic is, it will not function if you run out of money. That is why it is essential that you plan your cash flow in advance and have at least some sort of a timeline for your expenditures.

One way to do this is to use an Excel spreadsheet. You can create monthly or quarterly budgets and estimate your expenditures as well as your receivables. If you cannot do this yourself, hire an accountant or a firm that specializes in financial models. Whatever you do, don't just operate on a whim, hoping that everything will work out. Nothing destroys employee morale like late payroll. Undermining employee morale in turn destroys customer service, your revenue, and your reputation. It is a slippery slope, one that can spell disaster for your facility if you do not take the proper precautions.

BIGGEST MISTAKES

There are two mistakes concerning a business plan that many operators make and that are almost guaranteed to spell disaster:

- ▶ Focusing too much on creation of the business plan and not enough on its execution
- ▶ Shoving the business plan into obscurity after it is written

Business owners can become so enamored of their idea that instead of using their business plan to bring their vision into reality, they focus too much on making the business plan perfect, to the point that they forget to take action. They spend countless hours researching and get sucked into this cycle of "if I just plan this right, everything will be okay," without devoting enough time to implementing their plan to make it a reality. Whether you are considering opening a clinic or are working to reposition your current facility, make sure that you don't get so hung up on making your plan perfect that you never get around to actually implementing it. Implementation can sometimes be scary, especially if you are venturing into new territory, but you can't romanticize the business plan to the point that it becomes the final product rather than a stepping-stone to something bigger.

But don't go in the opposite direction and finish your business plan only to leave it in a drawer, unconsulted. Remember, your business plan is not your final product. It is a manual. If it is accurately compiled with enough care and effort, it can be a valuable road map for your operation. Therefore, you should consult it regularly to ensure that your clinic is on track with its original vision. Review it often, look at the original timelines that you set, and gauge the actual performance against the expectations laid out in the plan. Doing this is absolutely essential for one major reason: Most of your daily business decisions will be based on your gut feelings. The only way to bring those gut feelings in line with reality is to look at your original expectations, compare them with actual results, and learn from those experiences.

I FOUND AN URGENT CARE FACILITY BUSINESS PLAN ONLINE—CAN I USE IT?

Can you adapt someone else's business plan for an urgent care center? Yes and no. Many facility operators and new entrepreneurs resort to finding business plans online and just tweaking them to match their own situation. This strategy is acceptable only if you realize that these premade plans should only serve as a guide to writing your own plan, not replace it.

Your business plan is meant to be a unique assessment of your specific situation. It is meant to be a study that takes into account the geography within which you operate or plan to operate and the specific challenges you may face. Even though all urgent care facilities will have general similarities, your geography and client base will dictate the unique needs that your center must address to maximize revenue and ROI. Consequently, premade business plans should only serve as a guide and a source of valuable questions to ask yourself in preparation for helping your facility achieve its maximum potential. As with many aspects of running an urgent care facility, cutting corners in the planning phase could prove disastrous and could cost you tens of thousands—if not hundreds of thousands—of dollars. Remember, a business plan is not a document but is rather a process by which you gain detailed knowledge of the specific needs of your community and the unique challenges that you will face because of your distinctive situation.

CONCLUSION

Building an urgent care center from scratch or bringing an existing one to its full potential is not an easy task. A big part of the process is developing a solid business plan that can serve as a guide. Writing a business plan is a process designed to help you ask the right questions about your operations and plan for the various contingencies that you are likely to encounter. More than anything, a business plan is a way for you to understand all of the intricacies of your business and to develop a thorough feel for the interrelations between the various aspects. From hiring to operations to billing to internal controls and financing, a well-written plan that has been nurtured can serve as a priceless tool that will help you think through problems *before* they occur.

It is easy to get caught up in the excitement of writing a business plan and all the things you plan to achieve, to the point of forgetting to implement it. But it is a plan for action, not the action itself. Your business plan should serve as a constant guide to your operations. You should regularly review it to see if you are on track, if your original assumptions were correct, and if you must make any adjustments. Without it, you are likely to tread along without catching small problems until they become big issues.

KEY POINTS

1. A business plan is a process that is meant to give you, the owner, an understanding of your clinic's operations. Whether you write it all on your own or hire someone to write it, be as involved as possible in the process.

2. Use free tools and templates available online via websites such as www.sba.gov and www.score.org.

3. Make sure to have a thorough understanding of your target consumer and their demographics. This will help define everything from the services you offer to your pricing structure.

4. Build your marketing in a way that appeals to your target consumer. Identify their wants, needs, and pain points, and address those in your marketing. The patient's health concerns are rarely the only needs that must be resolved.

5. Design your services around your target market. Once you understand your target market demographics, you will be able to better anticipate your patients' needs and maybe even create upsell opportunities.

6. Develop a clear management structure and chain of command from the start. This will decrease misunderstandings and lower the frequency of situations in which no one addresses a problem because no one is sure whose responsibility it is.

7. Develop a thorough financial plan for your business. Having a clear anticipation of your future cash flow, and therefore possible funding problems, will eliminate many unpleasant surprises down the line. This is essential.

8. If you decide to use an already-completed business plan from another urgent care center, make sure that it serves only as a guide and doesn't

actually replace your plan for your unique center. Urgent care clinics are similar in nature, but no two will be completely alike. You will short-change yourself if you don't take the time to develop your own plan.

9. Once your business plan is written, make sure to use it. Don't set it aside to collect dust on the shelf. You've put time into it; now use it to your benefit.

10. Don't get so bogged down in writing your plan that it becomes a never-ending project, and don't avoid the uncertainty of taking action by hiding behind the safety of planning. The plan is meant to facilitate the growth of your business, not to be the final result of your efforts.

CHAPTER 3

Site Selection

Mike Zelnik and Jim Garrett

Finding the right location for your urgent care center is paramount to its success. The selection process should include the following steps:

- Define a general market area.
- Inventory the competition.
- Locate strong retail markets with good traffic flow.
- Profile the local population.
- Identify the ideal property.
- Compare potential sites.

To make the process easier, study the section "General Real Estate Terminology" that appears toward the end of this chapter.

DEFINE A GENERAL MARKET AREA

Gather Population Statistics

Because mapping is an effective tool that aids in site evaluation, your site search should start by defining a general market area, the region that can support your first location and provide suitable opportunities for future expansion. One search method is to select a county or city and use its boundaries to define the general market area. Information used in your analysis is readily available on the basis of county, city, and ZIP code.

As an illustration of this method, consider Franklin County in central Ohio. A review of the area determines that the total population is 1,148,954 and that there are 32 existing urgent care centers (Figure 1). By dividing the population by the number of existing centers (our competition), we can calculate the population per urgent care center: roughly 32,905 people. The national median population per urgent care center is 25,144 people. Therefore, if we base our analysis on the national median population per urgent care center, this general market area has the potential to add approximately 13.7 new locations.

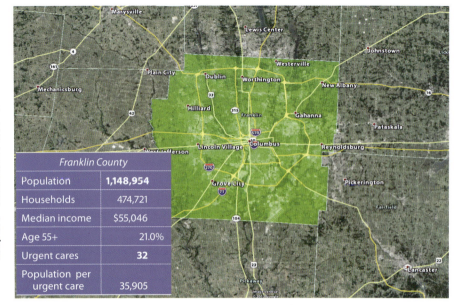

Figure 1. View of the population for Franklin County, Ohio. (Satellite image © 2013 Google.)

From a national perspective, there is 1 urgent care center for every 25,144 people. In our example market in Franklin County, there is 1 center for every 32,905 people. If you were using the national statistics as a benchmark, you could set up additional locations in this market and still be above the national median.

On the other hand, if we define our general market using the outer belt as the boundary, the population is 690,795 with 19 urgent care centers, for a population per urgent care center of 36,356. Compared with the national median population per center, this general market area could support 8.4 new urgent care centers (Figure 2).

Within this general trade area, the goal would be to find an underserved target market. The target market illustrated in Figure 3 has a population of 101,760 and 3 urgent care centers, with a population per center of 33,920. This suggests that the proposed target market has the potential of supporting a new urgent care location while maintaining a population of 25,440, which meets the national median requirement.

The comparison that we just worked through was based on national statistics for existing urgent care centers. It is generally beneficial to compare your proposed locations at the state or county level so that you can examine the numbers on an apples-to-apples basis. Note that the number of urgent care locations and the populations per urgent care center are constantly changing, so when you are researching in preparation for starting your own centers, you should not rely on the numbers used in the examples in this chapter.

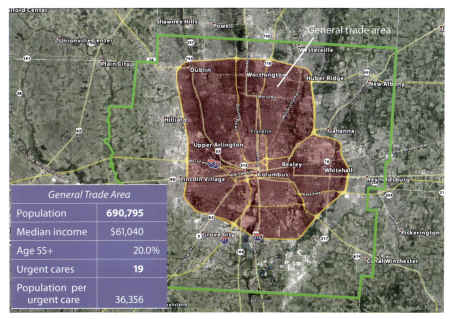

Figure 2. View of the general trade area for Franklin County, Ohio. (Satellite image © 2013 Google.)

Consider Market Barriers

Market barriers, artificial or natural, may limit access to a desired market. Artificial barriers include highways, railroads, and large industrial and retail shopping areas. Natural barriers include rivers, lakes, mountains, and inferior land-development sites, like marshlands, swamps, and wetlands. These barriers can have a positive or negative impact on your location, depending on the circumstances, so you must answer this question: How will a specific barrier increase or decrease the access or desirability for my proposed property?

Figure 4 shows a river dividing Franklin County's trade area into an east market and a west market. In this particular instance, consumer shopping habits are altered because of the division of the market. For example, despite the short distance across the river from a neighborhood on the west bank to a particular grocery store on the east bank, consumers on the west bank have to travel to out-of-their-way bridges to get to that grocery store. Will this inconvenience mean that they patronize a different grocery store on the west bank instead? Knowing barriers in the market and consumer behavior may help you identify obstacles or inducements to patronage of your urgent care center by potential patients. The trade area you want to explore may appear as a concentric ring or an outlined polygon on a map, shapes that may or may not represent barriers to your desired patient population. Therefore, it is important to remember that you may have to modify your trade area.

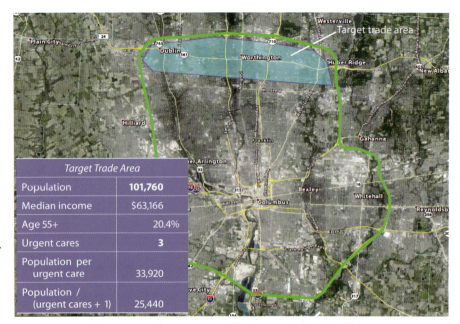

Figure 3. View of a target trade area in Franklin County, Ohio. (Satellite image © 2013 Google.)

INVENTORY THE COMPETITION

Locating the competition can be as simple as doing an online search to identify providers and their locations. Key search terms might be *urgent care*, *immediate care*, *minor medical*, and *walk-in clinic*. When using the Internet to uncover local competition, you will find that websites often do not differentiate general medical practices or hospitals from medical clinics. Recognizing this fact will help you eliminate search results that do not meet your criteria. Additional sources for locating competitors include database subscriptions and calls to local clinics.

Once you have compiled a list of surrounding competitors, plot the locations on a map (Figure 5). Mapping the competition provides a good overview of underserved areas and the impact of market barriers, which can help you identify the gaps in the market. In general, the distance between competitors should at least be 3 to 4 miles simply to avoid cannibalizing a competitor's market.

Qualify the Competition

According to the Urgent Care Association of America (UCAOA), *urgent care* is defined as "the delivery of ambulatory medical care outside of a hospital emergency department on a walk-in basis without a scheduled appointment." This definition further delineates urgent care sites as required to include onsite x-ray capability and an excess of 3,000 hours of operation annually.

No matter whether you use UCAOA's criteria or your own, it is important to classify competitors in the market. By qualifying the scope of service and annual

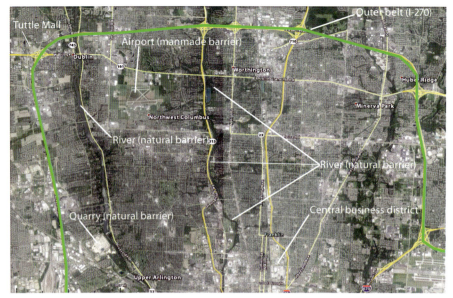

Figure 4. View of market barriers in Franklin County, Ohio, including a river down the middle of the trade area. (Satellite image © 2013 Google.)

hours of local operators, you will be able to gauge the competitiveness of the clinics and the threat they may or may not pose to your future location.

Figure 6 shows that for our proposed urgent care center in Franklin County, there appear to be three competitors in the area. On further investigation, however, we find that only one of them is a true urgent care center, one is a limited urgent care center (on the basis of its annual hours), and the other is not a true

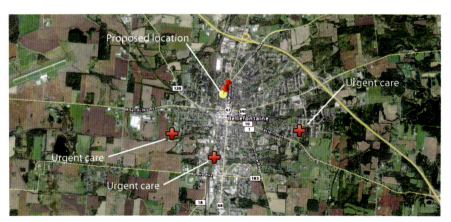

Figure 5. View of a proposed new location in Franklin County, Ohio, along with competitors' locations. (Satellite image © 2013 Google.)

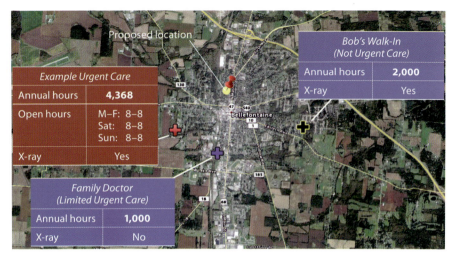

Figure 6. View of the competition in Franklin County, Ohio. (Satellite image © 2013 Google.)

competitor (because of its scope of service and hours of operation). You may want to classify your competitors differently, but labeling them allows you to understand the alternative medical providers in your area. Depending on your company's model, you may want to include pediatric urgent care centers and occupational health centers in your consideration of competitors, on the basis of the services they provide, their location, and their hours of operation.

Profile the Competition

After your competition has been qualified, search the Internet for the individual websites. Clinic websites help define the number of locations currently operated and the type of organization providing the service. Look for additional information about your competitors:

- Do they have multiple locations?
- Who operates them—local providers, national organizations, or hospital-based institutions?
- What are their hours of operation?
- Do they provide x-ray services?
- Where is the clinic located—in a shopping, office, or industrial area?
- How many seats are in their waiting rooms?
- How many parking stalls are available for their sites?
- What type of signage do they use?

Figure 7 shows an example of the home page of an urgent care website. As you can see, many pieces of information can be gathered here that may help you gauge the level of competition in the market that this center represents to you. Profiling your competition often gives you the opportunity to uncover information about an organization's proposed expansions or clinics that may be closing.

LOCATE STRONG RETAIL MARKETS WITH GOOD TRAFFIC FLOW

The urgent care industry has evolved into retail medicine. The goal is to locate in areas that have large amounts of flow-to traffic, not flow-through traffic. Ideally, the traffic flow should expose your center to consumers who visit the same shopping areas multiple times per week. Studies show that the average family travels to the grocery store 2.5 times a week. Such consistent travel helps increase awareness of an urgent care center located near the grocery store, which should decrease the time required for the center to achieve a stabilized patient count. The types of retailers servicing an area will help provide insight regarding the current population mix.

Figure 8 shows the spacing in Columbus, Ohio, between outlets owned by one major grocery chain. This retailer chose to space its outlets roughly 3 miles apart from each other, allowing each to operate in its own trade area of 1.5 to 2 miles in radius. Each location is evenly spaced, with exceptions occurring in areas of high population density or areas with natural or artificial barriers.

Grocery stores are not just an example of destination shopping places with consistent and repeat traffic. In addition, because chains of these stores often do extensive studies of market trends and population demographics, locating next

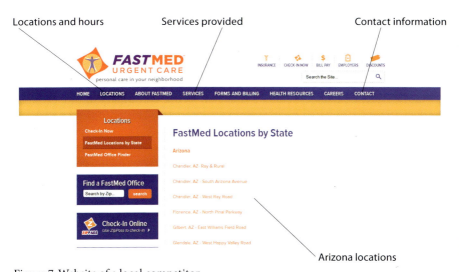

Figure 7. Website of a local competitor.

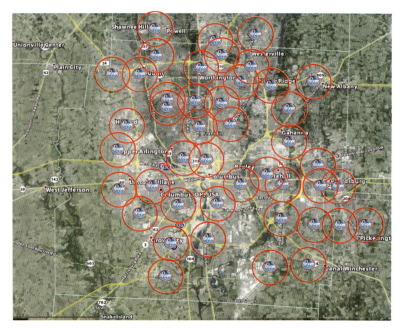

Figure 8. The spacing in Columbus, Ohio, between outlets owned by one major grocery chain. (Satellite image © 2013 Google.)

to a grocery store and following the example of proper spacing set by the grocery industry increases the probability that you will develop a strong urgent care location. In metropolitan markets across the United States, grocery stores often operate in trade areas with a radius of 1.5 to 2 miles.

Additional categories of retailers that generate regular weekly visits from consumers include drugstores, banks, gas stations, coffee shops, fast-food restaurants, day-care centers, fitness clubs, and dry cleaners.

Figure 9 identifies local retailers that may bring consumers to our example market. There is a diverse yet core group of stores. This cluster indicated the presence of destination shopping in the area.

Examples of retailers that draw consumers to an area are referred to as anchors. Depending on the market, anchors can be grocery stores, malls, or other retail stores. An additional anchor that is often overlooked is the pharmacy. A 2006 study by Boston University indicated that more than 82% of adults in the United States take at least one medication during a given week. Additionally, there is a pharmacy within 5 miles of virtually every household in America. Not only do pharmacies support the role of your practice by offering prescriptions to your patients but they also serve as a destination shopping center that brings consumers to your area and can be a source of referrals.

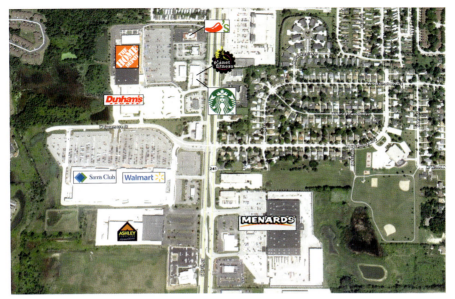

Figure 9. Retail store cluster. (Satellite image © 2013 Google.)

Finding the right retailer as a draw for flow-to traffic depends on the market as well as the retailer's commitment to the area. You don't want to be in the position of having identified a grocery store and selected your nearby site only to find out that the store is closing. It is important to notice trends in neighboring retail areas and consider how the particular market will look in 5 years. The goal is to develop an urgent care practice that has longevity and resilience in the market.

PROFILE THE LOCAL POPULATION

Now that you have defined your general market area, identified the competition, and located a strong retail area with limited competition, it is time to profile the people who live in the area. You need information from these four key categories:

- *The median income of the population*   Nationally the median income within a 3-mile radius is $57,923. That value varies by location, however, and a median income of $60,000 in Los Angeles is not the same as $60,000 in Columbus, Ohio.

- *The total population in a 3-mile radius of the proposed site*   The 3-mile radius should be evaluated to determine whether there are any barriers that would limit access to the potential site. For more than 4,000 urgent care centers across the United States, the median population within 3 miles is 62,911.

▶ *The percentage of the market's population over 55 years of age*   If a large percentage of the population of your hypothetical site is older than 55, that could limit your potential pool of patients. Many people in that age group prefer waiting for their primary-care provider, who has their complete medical history, over using an urgent care center. Nationally the median percentage of the population over age 55 is 24%.

▶ *The population per urgent care center within the 3-mile radius*   If there are multiple competitors in your target area, is there a sufficient population for each urgent care center to compete? Nationally the average population per urgent care center is 25,114.

These four categories are all important to consider, but equally important is to compare them against the proper benchmarks. The importance of benchmarking is illustrated in Table 1 in a comparison of three states.

Table 1. Comparison of Three States Relative to Population

	Texas (N = 479)		Massachusetts (N = 55)		Tennessee (N = 202)	
Population	77,059		79,962		22,057	
Median income	$59,904		$54,076		$44,371	
Traffic count	20,000		20,000		20,000	
Age 55+	19.7%		25.8%		27.0%	
Medical Options						
	#[a]	Pop. Per[b]	#	Pop. Per	#	Pop. Per
Hospitals	1.7	45,382	2.2	36,346	1.3	17,310
Existing urgent cares + 1	3.6	21,392	2.1	38,106	2.0	11,176
Family practice	11.6	6,644	4.8	16,717	1.5	14,878
Internal medicine	6.4	12,072	19.2	4,164	1.4	15,465
General practice	1.5	52,119	3.7	21,859	1.1	20,161
Pediatricians	3.3	23,478	5.0	16,034	1.3	17,456
Total medical options	27.5	2,807	36.6	2,185	6.0	3,637
% Within One Mile						
Grocery	69.10%		78.18%		82.67%	
Pharmacy	89.77%		96.35%		90.59%	
Walmart	25.47%		5.45%		30.20%	

[a] Average number.
[b] Population served by each, on average.

For example, Massachusetts is significantly smaller than Texas by surface area, but when the median 3-mile populations are compared, Massachusetts is much more dense. When compared with Tennessee, a state that is also larger by surface area, Massachusetts is almost four times as dense regarding the median population within 3 miles. Analyzing locations on a national basis is important, but not at the expense of homing in on your proposed trade area.

Sometimes it is better to select a smaller target zone. Morris County, New Jersey, has a sample size of eight urgent care competitors. The median population for this sample is 51,279, the percentage of the population over age 55 is 27.2%, and the median income is $91,741. As you can see, median values can vary widely, so it is best to compare your location with other competitors in your general area for the most detailed illustration. Table 2 illustrates the median values from national, state, and local perspectives.

With hundreds of sources and reports to choose from, identifying a reputable source with current information is key. Figure 10 is an example of a demographic report taken from the center point of a proposed location and examined on a 3-mile basis. The demographic report shown there is a community summary page from Esri, a company that offers demographic data with a wide range of report types (http://www.esri.com). Figure 10 highlights categories that may be useful during your site selection phase, but other reports can be created to fit your particular need.

IDENTIFY THE IDEAL PROPERTY

Identifying the ideal property involves analysis of many factors. After you have inventoried the competition and profiled the local population, the main areas to focus on are traffic counts, rental cost, and visibility. Imbalance in these areas decreases the probability of your success at a particular location. For example, you could end up with an expensive new building in an area with poor visibility, or with an inexpensive building that is old and out of date.

Figure 11 is an example of a map highlighting local competition as well as prominent traffic-generating retailers. In this particular example, the rings, which represent trade areas, have a radius of 3 miles. Holes or gaps in the market can be easily identified with the use of maps. Not all of the green circles in Figure 11 represent opportunities that will turn into an urgent care operation; instead, they represent areas that should be explored further.

Determine Traffic Counts

Retail businesses need traffic to succeed. Retail shopping areas typically see daily traffic counts of 20,000 to 30,000 cars per day. The traffic information concerning a potential site can be found from a variety of sources, such as Google Maps Engine Pro,[1] the US Census Bureau,[2] and Site To Do Business.[3] When evaluating

---
1   http://www.google.com/intl/en/enterprise/mapsearth/.
2   http://www.census.gov.
3   http://stdbinc.com.

Table 2. Three-Mile National, State, County, and Site Statistics

	Example Site in DuPage County, Illinois		National (N = 4,253)		State (N = 172)		County (N = 20)	
		Pop. Per[b]	#	Pop. Per	#	Pop. Per	#	Pop. Per
Population	86,200		62,911		72,760		88,847	
Median income	$82,986		$57,923		$68,033		$89,562	
Traffic count	46,000		20,000		20,000		20,000	
Age 55+	30.3%		23.7%		23.5%		24.1%	

	Medical Options							
	#[a]	Pop. Per[b]	#	Pop. Per	#	Pop. Per	#	Pop. Per
Hospitals	0	86,200		44,028		44,150		87,168
Existing urgent cares + 1	3	28,733		25,114		27,345		30,347
Family practice	3	28,733		9,426		13,850		13,103
Internal medicine	4	21,550		10,414		18,162		22,173
General practice	0	86,200		36,882		63,373		88,847
Pediatricians	2	43,100		24,297		26,463		27,243
Total medical options	12	7,183	21.7	2,902	16.7	4,359	17.0	5,226

	Within One Mile?	% Within One Mile		
Grocery	Yes	71.61%	75.00%	85.00%
Pharmacy	Yes	82.13%	91.28%	90.00%
Walmart	No	18.72%	27.33%	20.00%

[a] Average number.
[b] Population served by each, on average.

Ring: 3 miles radius

Summary	2000	2010	2015
Population	30,693	36,927	40,839
Households	12,348	15,149	16,798
Families	8,198	9,832	10,837
Average Household Size	2.44	2.40	2.40
Owner Occupied HUs	7,830	9,339	10,331
Renter Occupied HUs	4,517	5,809	6,467
Median Age	36.4	39.1	39.4
Total Housing Units	13,093	16,304	17,922
Vacant Housing Units	746	1,156	1,124
Average Home Value	$150,643	$182,871	$210,764
Median Household Income	$47,401	$62,080	$67,677
Average Household Income	$55,816	$68,258	$74,582
Per Capita Income	$23,103	$28,468	$31,162

Callouts:
- Population is projected to grow 33% in 15 years
- Income is projected to grow 43% in 15 years
- Median income is $6,000 less than mean income
- 26.8% of the 3-mile population is over the age of 55

Population by Age	2000 Number	Percent	2010 Number	Percent	2015 Number	Percent
0 - 4	1,978	6.4%	2,291	6.2%	2,506	6.1%
5 - 14	4,305	14.0%	4,742	12.8%	5,236	12.8%
15 - 19	1,768	5.8%	2,321	6.3%	2,365	5.8%
20 - 24	1,783	5.8%	2,523	6.8%	2,710	6.6%
25 - 34	4,831	15.7%	4,660	12.6%	5,605	13.7%
35 - 44	4,848	15.8%	4,932	13.4%	4,783	11.7%
45 - 54	4,587	14.9%	5,572	15.1%	5,805	14.2%
55 - 64	2,612	8.5%	4,710	12.8%	5,380	13.2%
65 - 74	1,885	6.1%	2,485	6.7%	3,532	8.6%
75 - 84	1,543	5.0%	1,792	4.9%	1,944	4.8%
85+	551	1.8%	900	2.4%	973	2.4%

Race and Ethnicity	2000 Number	Percent	2010 Number	Percent	2015 Number	Percent
White Alone	17,814	58.0%	19,458	52.7%	20,935	51.3%
Black Alone	11,100	36.2%	14,197	38.4%	15,857	38.8%
American Indian Alone	60	0.2%	82	0.2%	95	0.2%
Asian Alone	577	1.9%	890	2.4%	1,102	2.7%
Pacific Islander Alone	13	0.0%	25	0.1%	27	0.1%
Some Other Race Alone	643	2.1%	1,498	4.1%	1,873	4.6%
Two or More Races	485	1.6%	776	2.1%	950	2.3%
Hispanic Origin (Any Race)	1,104	3.6%	2,675	7.2%	3,515	8.6%

Data Note: Income is expressed in current dollars.
Source: U.S. Bureau of the Census, 2000 Census of Population and Housing. Esri forecasts for 2010 and 2015 were effective as of July 1, 2010. Copyright 2010, all rights reserved.

Figure 10. Community summary page from a demographic report. (Source: Esri.)

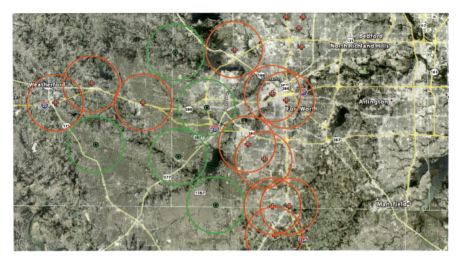

Figure 11. Map of local competition and prominent retailers. Red rings show the trade areas for existing urgent care centers; green rings show potential trade areas for centers considering an expansion in the market. (Satellite image © 2013 Google.)

sites for potential urgent care centers in the United States, use a 20,000-cars-per day equation. When examining traffic patterns of surrounding thoroughfares, be sure to make a distinction between "drive-through traffic" and "drive-to traffic." Examples of drive-through traffic are traffic patterns in which consumers are traveling to work or a large regional mall. Because many of these consumers are not located within your target market area and live outside your target market area, a competitor located closer to their home is in the position to intercept these potential patients. Drive-to traffic is typically within the boundaries of your proposed market area and is made up of consumers who are in the area on a weekly basis to take care of their personal shopping needs. A target number for traffic counts is more than 20,000 vehicles per day.

Despite the fact that every day more than 70,000 vehicles pass the site shown in Figure 12, the lack of visibility this location has from the highway is a serious drawback not illustrated in the aerial view. Although 73,880 vehicles per day pass this location, they should not be ranked the same as vehicles passing by on the road in front of the grocery store. Also, highways are often considered drive-through roads because when motorists travel them, they pass locations at upward of 60 miles per hour. Unless the proposed urgent care center has great signage and visibility from the road, the people in those vehicles may not even be aware of its existence. In Figure 12 you can also see that the two roads passing the grocery store have traffic counts of more than 20,000. Although this count is not as high as the count for the freeway that passes this location, the retail business at this location is viewable by many consumers. Traffic counts are calculated by tallying the total volume of vehicle traffic of a highway or road for a year and dividing it by 365, for the number of days in a year.

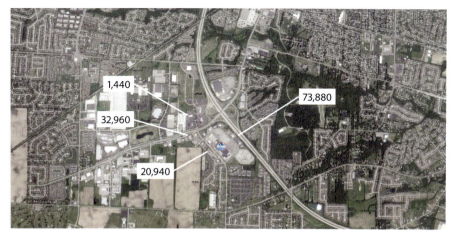

Figure 12. Drive-by visibility factors. (Satellite image © 2013 Google.)

Analyze and Understand Rental Rates

Rental rates vary from market to market, so a good way to pinpoint trends in pricing is to collect comparable rates from similar properties in the area. Having a baseline of the local pricing allows you to negotiate more effectively.

Normally, endcaps and outparcels are more costly than in-line space. (See the section "Choose a Location Within a Site That Provides the Best Visibility" in this chapter for definitions of these types of spaces for your urgent care center.) The visibility and sign potential on the fascia of the endcaps and outparcels make them more desirable and their price reflects desirability. Although the rental rate may be higher, the potential to capture a larger audience is also higher. The goal is to offset the cost of an outparcel or endcap by increasing the patients you see per day as a result of your superior location.

Many urgent care center operators and retailers have difficulty understanding the cost of their rent. In most markets, rental rates are quoted per square foot annually. In some markets such as California, rental rates are typically quoted per square foot monthly. Also, most rental rates are on a "triple net, or NNN" basis. The price per square foot represents the base rent, and the NNN expenses represent taxes, insurance, and common area maintenance. Together, base rent and NNN expense equal your total rent obligation (Figure 13).

Choose a Location Within a Site That Provides the Best Visibility

Your urgent care center's particular location within a site—such as an outparcel retail building, a retail center endcap, or a retail center in-line space—is just as crucial as the overall decision to locate at that site. Similar to other types of retail, urgent care practices rely on visibility and signage to establish a presence in the market. Unlike clothing stores and dining locations, urgent care centers are not necessarily top of mind to most consumers until there is an illness or injury that needs to be addressed. For this reason, outparcels and endcaps should be chosen

Area:	2,000 square feet
Base rent:	$12/square foot
Operating expenses:	$3/square foot
Base rent:	2,000 × $12 = $24,000/year
Operating expenses:	2,000 × $3 = $ 6,000/year
Total rent per year:	$30,000
Rent per month:	$ 2,500
Rent per day (based on 365 days):	$ 82.19

Figure 13. Example of calculation of the cost of rent.

before in-line spaces. Outparcels and endcaps allow passing traffic to see your practice from the road. It is the first and last thing consumers see when entering and exiting a center (Figure 14).

Outparcel or Pad Site

An *outparcel*, also called a *pad site,* is a freestanding building generally located on the periphery or in front of a shopping center. Popular tenants of outparcel spaces include banks, restaurants, gas stations, and pharmacies.

Endcap

Similar to book ends on a book shelf, *endcaps* are located at the ends of shopping centers or buildings. Endcaps typically have two or more sides of visibility;

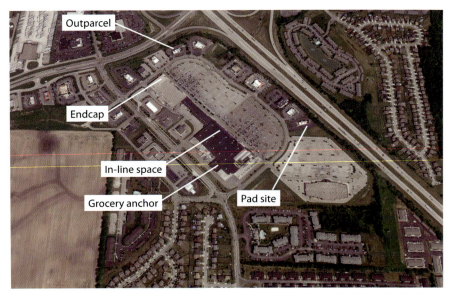

Figure 14. This retail encompasses several types of spaces: outparcels (also called pad sites), endcaps, in-line spaces, and anchors. See the text for descriptions of these. (Satellite image © 2013 Google.)

compare *in-line space*. Endcaps are often desired more than in-line space because of their increased visibility in the center.

In-line Space
Named for its location in the center, *in-line spaces* are typically retailers joined together as a row of businesses. In-line spaces are adjacent to other retailers in the center but are typically accessed through use of their own entrances. In-line spaces have only one side of visibility.

Choose Signage That Provides the Best Visibility
Signage allows consumers to notice your presence in the market and helps develop brand recognition of your services. Signage styles and prices vary, and may be limited by the landlord's stipulations or the city codes. If possible, obtain as much signage as possible. Common types of signs include the following.

Freestanding Signs
Freestanding signs are usually the business's main identification by the road (Figure 15). Typically internally illuminated, these are often found in shopping centers and other retail environments. The most common trait is the use of individual covered support poles underneath the main cabinet, giving the sign the

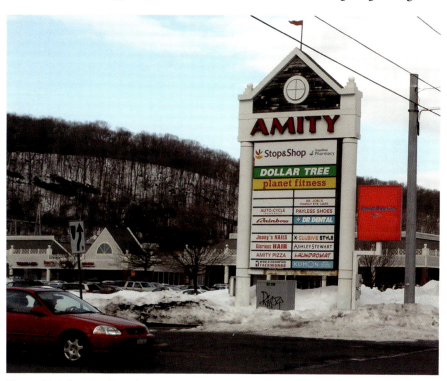

Figure 15. A freestanding sign.

appearance of having legs. Depending on individual municipalities' sign codes, freestanding signs can be as tall as 20 feet.

Monument Signs

Commonly found in single business centers, the monument sign is constructed very similar to freestanding signs, except for the area that contains the support poles are covered as one unit (Figure 16). These signs tend to be shorter in height, and are typically illuminated.

Pylon Signs

Compared with freestanding and monument signage, pylon signs are the least expensive. Construction consists of an illuminated cabinet atop a single support pole (Figure 17). The support pole is not covered with any kind of embellishment.

LED Message Unit Signs

Large, computer-controlled, illuminated electronic signs that have animated displays are called *LED (light-emitting diode) message units* (Figure 18). These displays are made up of hundreds of LED lights, either in a monochrome color such as amber or red or in full-color RGB (the red-green-blue color model). LED message units come in a variety of shapes and are priced according to cabinet size, pixel size, and color capabilities.

Wall Signs

A wall sign is an internally illuminated box sign with acrylic faces mounted to a wall. Signs are constructed from extruded aluminum and contain high-output fluorescent lamps. The sign face is covered with translucent vinyl graphics (Figure 19).

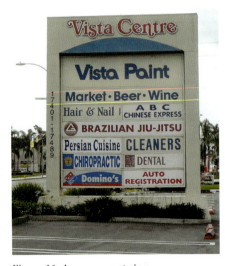

Figure 16. A monument sign.

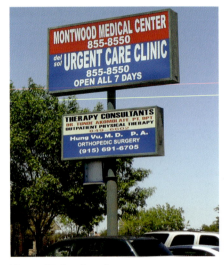

Figure 17. A pylon sign.

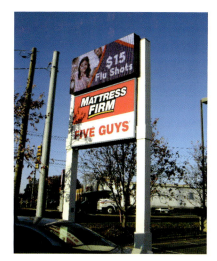
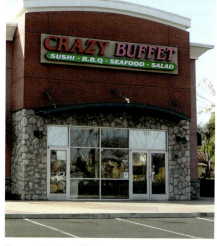

Figure 18. An LED message unit sign.   Figure 19. A wall sign.

COMPARE POTENTIAL SITES

Now that you have identified a list of potential properties, it is important to compare those opportunities to pinpoint the location that has the highest probability for success. The ways in which you choose to compile and organize the data can help you compare potential sites.

Choose Your Perspective for Compiling the Data

As far as the cost or price of the transaction is concerned, it is often more effective to examine the cost from a patients-per-day or patients-per-week perspective than from the perspective of monthly or annual cost. Table 3 highlights multiple prospective properties and the cost associated with each. Because property size and price may vary depending on the market or location, examining the patients per day that it would take to support your real estate cost allows you to play on a level. You can alter the expected reimbursement cost per patient to conform this model to your specific practice.

Reducing the information to a manageable amount allows you to conceptualize how many patients you would need to see daily to justify a space. In the example discussed throughout this chapter, the difference between a $96,000 location and a $125,000 location is less than 1 patient per day. In fact, the two locations would be the same because you cannot treat a portion of a person. For each location, you would need to see 3 patients per day.

Choose How to Organize Your Data

How should you organize the information you have collected? The old-school approach is to use *handwritten notes*. This is an easy choice for quick notes when

Table 3. Comparing Costs for Several Properties

Item	National Average (N = 32)	Potential Sites Within Target Area			
		Property 15	Property 16	Property 17	Property 18
Area leased (square feet)	4,008	1,422	5,500	5,000	4,070
Base rent ($)	23.49	14.00	14.00	25.00	17.00
Operating expense ($)	3.87	—	3.50	—	3.50
Total rent per square foot ($)	26.38	14.00	17.50	25.00	20.50
Landlord tenant improvements allowance ($)	23.60	—	—	—	15.00
Annual cost ($)	102,519	19,908	96,250	125,000	83,435
Monthly cost ($)	8,543	1,659	8,021	10,417	6,953
Daily cost ($)	280.87	54.54	263.70	342.47	228.59
Hourly cost ($)[a]	28.09	5.45	26.37	34.25	22.86
Daily patient visits to cover real estate cost[b]	2.25	0.44	2.11	2.74	1.83

[a] Based on 10 hours a day, 365 days a year.
[b] Based on $125 revenue per patient visit.

you are out in the field, but stacks of handwritten notes cannot be sorted and compared quickly.

Spreadsheets (Table 4) are another way to track information regarding your competition and the population. Spreadsheets allow you to rank and organize data effectively. But they limit the number of variables that can be used to analyze a potential site.

Databases are one of the most efficient ways to compile a variety of data. Databases allow you to organize using multiple variables (Figure 20), which will make possible a more in-depth analysis of the information. When you change the query criteria in using a database, you will get results that allow you to identify additional opportunities. As seen in Figure 21, changing the population and income criteria allows the database to uncover 38 additional opportunities that meet our numbers. The database whose query results are seen in Table 4 can compare the user's query against thousands of records simultaneously. This tool allows you to customize your search without creating a complex equation in Excel for every variation.

Table 4. Comparing Demographics for Several Properties

Item	National Benchmark	Property 15	Property 16	Property 17	Property 18
Population	50,000	116,304	122,704	138,596	131,325
Median income	$50,000	$53,902	$53,909	$53,141	$54,631
Traffic count	20,000	54,010	133,000	20,890	20,460
Adults 55+	24.0%	17.1%	17.3%	16.9%	17.5%

Medical Options

	#	Pop. Per[a]	#	Pop. Per	#	Pop. Per	#	Pop. Per
Hospitals	1	116,304	1	122,704	1	138,596	1	131,325
Urgent cares	0	116,304	0	122,704	0	138,596	0	131,325
Family practice	21	5,538	21	5,843	23	6,026	24	5,472
Internal medicine	7	16,615	7	17,529	7	19,799	9	14,592
General practice	5	23,261	5	24,541	5	27,719	4	32,831
Pediatricians	1	116,304	1	122,704	1	138,596	1	131,325
Total medical options	35	3,323	35	3,506	37	3,746	39	3,367

Area Retail Services

Grocery (major) within 1 mile	Yes	Yes	Yes	Yes
Drug store (major) within 1 mile	Yes	Yes	Yes	Yes
Walmart within 1 mile	Yes	No	No	No
Score	13.3	15.0	11.3	11.1

[a] Population served by each, on average.

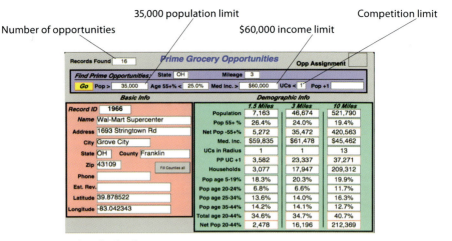

Figure 20. Results of a database query.

GENERAL REAL ESTATE TERMINOLOGY

Here are some of the terms you will encounter when assessing properties for your urgent care center:

- *Anchor tenant*   The anchor tenant is typically the largest and leading tenant in a shopping center. The brand recognition provided by the anchor attracts other tenants and shoppers to the center. Examples include major grocery chains, Walmart, and Target.

- *Strip center*   A strip center is an attached row of stores or service outlets managed as one retail center. Canopies may connect storefronts to create a contiguous covered sidewalk.

- *Neighborhood center*   A neighborhood center is intended to serve the day-to-day shopping needs of the consumers who live in the neighborhoods in close proximity to the center. Supermarkets anchor most neighborhood centers, but sometimes pharmacies or drugstores serve as anchors. Neighborhood centers are typically configured as straight-line strip centers with exterior walkways between stores.

- *Community center*   A community center typically offers a larger range of products and services than a neighborhood center does. In addition to supermarkets and drugstores, retailers such as home-improvement stores, sporting goods stores, and department stores are common anchors of community centers.

- *Regional center*   A regional center provides general merchandise (a large percentage of which is apparel) and services in full depth and variety. Its main attractions are its anchors: traditional mass merchants, discount

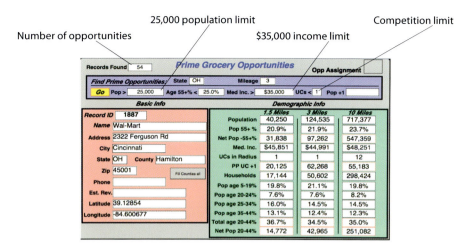

Figure 21. Database query using different criteria from those used to obtain the query results shown in Figure 20, providing additional information.

department stores, and fashion specialty stores. A typical regional center is usually enclosed and has inward-oriented stores connected by a common walkway; parking surrounds the outside perimeter.

▶ *Power center*   A power center is dominated by several large anchors, including discount department stores, off-price stores, warehouse clubs, and "category killers" (i.e., stores that offer tremendous selection in a particular merchandise category at low prices). The center typically consists of several freestanding (unconnected) anchors and only a minimum amount of small specialty tenants.

▶ *Lifestyle center*   A lifestyle center is a mixed-used commercial development that combines the traditional retail functions of a shopping mall with leisure amenities oriented to upscale consumers. Retailers that can be found in lifestyle centers include bookstores, coffee shops, restaurants, and clothing retailers.

▶ *Shadow center*   A shadow center is a nearby shopping center that may experience consumer traffic as a result of an another center close by. An example would be a sporting goods store across the street from a grocery store. Although the sporting goods store is not anchored by the grocery store, the presence of the grocery across the street is of direct benefit to the sporting center.

▶ *Dark center*   A dark center is either completely vacant or is missing a large anchor because of a vacancy. A center that has gone dark is usually not an optimal location for an urgent care center because of the absence of a major traffic-generating retailer. However, rental spaces do not always remain vacant and thus such centers may not stay dark indefinitely.

- *Single-tenant center*   Single-tenant centers are occupied by one user. These spaces can be outparcels or freestanding buildings. The term *single-tenant center* is used to describe pad locations or individual single-use buildings.

- *Multitenant center*   A multitenant center is one where there is more than one tenant in the same building. Strip centers and office buildings are good examples of multitenant buildings because they usually have more than one tenant or company located within them.

- *Base rent*   Base rent is the amount of rent assessed before inclusion of additional expenses or other factors that increase the amount of rent to be paid. Base rent is typically advertised as dollars per square foot per year ($/SF). If the base rent was $20/SF for 1,000 square feet, this would be your calculation of the annual total: $20 \times 1,000 = \$20,000$. Base rent is usually quoted on an annual basis, but in some parts of the country, such as California, rental rates are often quoted on a monthly basis.

- *Operating expenses*   Operating expenses are the costs of maintaining property; they do not include depreciation, the cost of financing, or income taxes. Examples include taxes, insurance, and common area maintenance, or CAM; the three items together are often referred to as CAMIT.

- *Common area maintenance*   Common area maintenance is rent charged to the tenant in addition to the base rent to maintain the common areas of the property that benefit all tenants. Most often, this does not include any capital improvements that are made to the property. Examples include
  - Snow removal
  - Outdoor lighting
  - Parking lot repair
  - Lawn care

- *Net lease*   A net lease has a provision for the tenant to pay certain costs in addition to rent that are associated with the operation of the property. These costs may include property taxes, insurance, repairs, utilities, and maintenance. There are also "NN" (double net) and "NNN" (triple net) leases. The difference between the three is the degree to which the tenant is responsible for operating costs.

- *Gross lease*   Under a gross lease, the tenant pays a flat sum for rent, out of which the landlord must pay all expenses such as taxes, insurance, maintenance, and utilities.

- *Pass-through*   A pass-through is the tenant's pro rata share of operating expenses (e.g., taxes, utilities, repairs) paid in addition to the base rent.
- *Pro rata share*   For a tenant, a pro rata share is the tenant's proportionate share of expenses for the maintenance and operation of the property. For example, if you were examining an available property that was 1,000 square feet of a building's total 10,000 square feet, the pro rata share of your property would be 1,000 SF/10,000 = .10, or 10%. This means that you would pay a rate directly related to the size of your space.
- *Tenant improvements*   Improvements that are made to the leased premises by or for a tenant are called tenant improvements. Generally, especially in a new space, negotiations will include in some detail the improvements to be made to the leased premises by the landlord.
- *Rent abatement*   Rent abatement is often referred to as "free rent" or "early occupancy" and may occur outside of or in addition to the primary term of the lease.
- *Rent commencement*   The date on which a tenant begins paying rent is called rent commencement. The dynamics of a marketplace will dictate whether this date coincides with the lease commencement date or whether it instead commences months later (i.e., in a weak market, the tenant may be granted several months' free rent). Rent commencement will never be before the lease commencement date.
- *Letter of intent*   A preliminary agreement stating the proposed terms for a final contract is called a letter of intent. It can be considered either binding or nonbinding. After identification of a desired property or parcel of land, submission of a letter of intent to the landlord or owner is typically the first step in the offer-and-acceptance process. Once the general terms are established, parties begin the lease-review process.
- *Mean*   The quotient of the sum of several quantities and their number is called the mean, or average. Using means is common when analyzing population statistics. Means are often used to generalize or summarize multiple data points. It is important to recognize how the computed average can be skewed by outliers (points that fall outside the norm). This can be seen in the second example here, where the number 45 is drastically larger than the other numbers in the set.

    The mean of 1, 2, 3, 4, 5, 6, and 7 = 4

    The mean of 5, 5, 5, 6, 6, 2, 9, 9, and 45 = 10.2222

- *Median*   The median is the middle value of a range of values. When analyzing population income, it is important that you examine the median value, so as to mitigate the effect of outliers in your sample set. When you are presented with an even number of data entries (thus making it difficult to determine the middle value), average the two middle numbers. When you are examining population income, the average household income may be $50,000, but the median may be $30,000. If you rely on the median value, you can say that half of your population earns more than $30,000.

The median of 1, 2, 3, 4, 5, 6, 7 = 4

The median of 1, 5, 7, 8, 9, 31, 33 = 8

The median of 1, 2, 3, 4, 5, 6, 7, 8 = 4.5

CONCLUSION

There are many factors to consider when identifying the best location for your urgent care center, all of equal importance. It is not simply a matter of identifying local competition and potential trade areas; it is the classification and understanding of those factors that allow you to enter the market confidently. Thorough research and analysis will help you identify the location with the highest probability of success.

KEY POINTS

1. Define a general market area. Use mapping to define a region that can support your first location and that allows for future expansion.

2. Inventory the competition. Gather enough data to determine who your competitors are and what they have to offer the population you want to reach.

3. Locate strong retail markets with good traffic flow. If your desired population doesn't naturally spend a lot of time in your proposed location but rather just passes through it, you won't be able to build a large enough client base.

4. Profile the local population. Learn how much your ideal clientele earns, what its largest age groups are, and if the population is large enough to support multiple competitors.

5. Identify the ideal property. To thrive, your urgent care center location must have good traffic flow, have an affordable rent but not a rent that is very low only because the building is outdated, and have good visibility.

6. Compare potential sites. Compile and organize your data in a way that allows you to easily determine which site will work best for you.

CHAPTER 4

Building Out Your Urgent Care Center

Tracy Altemus

BUILDING OUT YOUR URGENT care center requires the coordination of many moving pieces. Selecting the right design and choosing the right construction team are just two of the essential elements that will make the process as seamless as possible. A team with specific experience in urgent care centers, including issues related to permitting and construction, is a benefit to you as the owner because it will navigate the building process in the most cost-efficient and cost-effective way.

CONSTRUCTION MANAGER...OR YOU?

Managing the construction of an urgent care center is something you can choose to undertake yourself or assign to a general manager who works on your behalf. There is no doubt that hiring a construction manager will add to the cost of your project up front, but considerable savings can also be realized through the manager's expertise and know-how. When searching for such an expert, make sure you do due diligence: conduct extensive research and reference checks. Ask your colleagues and others in the construction industry for referrals. Negotiating a flat fee for services rather than a percentage of construction costs tends to reduce risk.

HOW LONG DOES IT TAKE TO OPEN A CENTER?

The time elapsed from conception to occupancy of an urgent care facility can vary widely and depends on a number of factors, including whether the building is already standing, the type of licensing required, the length of time required to hire the physicians and staff, and how strict the city and state regulations are. In general, if you find an existing building and face fairly normal requirements, the entire process will typically take 6 to 8 months (Figure 1).

Once you have selected and secured your site, either through ownership or a lease, the design and construction phases can begin in earnest. Usually the floor plan is approved during the site-procurement stage. Production of construction documents or working drawings, which require fine-tuning by the architect and by the mechanical engineer, plumbing engineer, electrical engineer, and

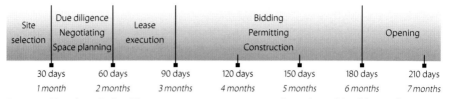

Figure 1. Timeline for building an urgent care center within a leased building. If you are constructing the building too, add 4 to 6 months.

sometimes structural engineer, takes 2 to 4 weeks. If there is an x-ray component, a physicist will need to review the drawings and specify the lead-shielding requirements, a task that takes several days.

When the plans are completed, they are ready to submit to the city or county for a permit. Permitting times can range from 1 day to 120 days and average 45 days. During that time, the architect and engineers may have to revise and resubmit the plans to deal with any redlines made to the drawings by the governing authority. While the plans are in the permitting process, they can be bid, and qualification of those bids and any value engineering required can be performed. This process allows you to be construction-ready by the time the permit is issued. Construction normally takes 6 to 10 weeks, including installation of x-ray equipment, phones, security, and computer lines. Occupancy typically occurs after construction.

DESIGN AND SPECIFICATION APPROVALS

A communication plan should be established to enable your team to understand the approval process, such as who approves your design and construction plans and at what junctures. Your real estate agent, architect, and contractor are invaluable resources to help you determine these requirements.

Municipalities and counties are typical resources for approving design and construction plans for permitting, but state approval and licensing may also be required. For instance, the states of Arizona, Colorado, and Florida have special licensing requirements from their respective departments of health services. Massachusetts has its own set of design requirements as well. In some cases, individual cities require special licensing or zoning, so check with the appropriate governing authority before you purchase a building or sign a lease. All states require written policies and a radiation survey to license any equipment using radiation in your center. For detailed information regarding the requirements of your state visit see www.radiationsafety.net/gov/statelist.html. Once you meet the zoning and licensing requirements, you may also need approvals from a franchisor, lender, and landlord if you are leasing the space.

DESIGN-BUILD OR DESIGN-BID-BUILD?

There are two ways an architect will deliver the project: design-build or design-bid-build. The differences between the two approaches will affect not only the cost of architectural and engineering work but also the fee that a general contractor (GC) assigns to the job.

In the *design-build approach*, the architect is responsible only for providing architectural design services; it is the GC who hires subcontractors and provides the more specific design services for their respective disciplines, such as mechanical, electrical, plumbing, and structural. Therefore, fees paid to the architect will be lower because of the work's more confined scope and the fact that construction management will be left to an outside party chosen by the center's owner. Design-build can result in cost savings in some areas but can also result in inconsistent heating, ventilation, and air-conditioning (HVAC) and electrical design when an architect is not available to oversee and coordinate the implementation of the various drawings. GCs usually have their own preferred subcontractors for HVAC as well, which means that from GC to GC the design can vary. When deciding whether you want to go with design-build or design-bid-build, it is important to find out in advance if the landlord has established subcontractors for HVAC and electrical. Many landlords prefer that all of their tenant improvements be handled by their established subcontractors to ensure consistency and efficiency.

In the *design-bid-build approach*, the architect is responsible for completing a full set of construction documents, including mechanical, plumbing, and electrical. The architect hires their own subcontractors for these respective disciplines. In addition, it's a good idea to have the architect undertake construction management to ensure that the completed facility is consistent with the drawings they have provided. Although you or your construction manager can perform this function, a better outcome is generally achieved by involving the architect in the process because it is often a question of interpreting the architect's drawings. The architect and project manager should also be responsible for reviewing and approving all submittals for the project. This manner of project delivery does result in higher fees, but design-bid-build also eliminates a lot of work for the owner because there is one person controlling all aspects of the project.

Once you've decided how to design the project, and assuming you have the right design team in place, selecting the right GC is your next crucial step.

GENERAL CONTRACTORS

In most cases it is a good idea to select a GC who has experience building medical facilities or offices. There are nuances to medical facilities not usually seen in office or retail build-outs, such as heavy electrical, plumbing, and possible lead-shielding requirements. There can be special licensing compliance issues that must be coordinated by the GC.

To Bid or Not to Bid

Negotiating your fee with a trusted contractor can work well if you want a seasoned contractor to provide design input. GCs typically charge a fee for their profit and overhead and for general conditions, which can include project supervision, cleanup, a construction waste container, and, if applicable, toilet facilities. You can negotiate the fee and general conditions up front with your contractor and request that they bid out the remaining work to the subcontractors. Because 70% to 90% of the work is completed by subcontractors and is competitively bid, you can get the advice of the GC as well as the benefit of a bid situation. Always request at least three bids in the major categories of mechanical, plumbing, electrical, and millwork.

Bidding out work is standard process if you don't have a favored contractor or if you are part of a franchise system and need to maintain the same specifications from center to center. Because the architect will do all of the design and specifications and there isn't room for variations, you don't need the contractor's input along the way.

Qualifying the General Contractor

Beyond obtaining professional recommendations for GCs, you should request that each candidate provide a Document A305 from the American Institute of Architects (AIA), the Contractor's Qualification Statement. The qualification statement asks detailed information about the GC's business to determine its financial ability to complete the project. A GC should not be selected to complete a project before submitting this form to you or the construction manager for verification. The verification process should include obtaining the GC's articles of incorporation and confirming that the GC has a contractor's license in the state where the work will be completed. Pending claims or lawsuits against the GC for unfinished work should be viewed as immediate disqualifications for bidding. Verification of each principal of the company should be completed to ensure that they have not done business under a different trade name of a company that ultimately failed. You must be very comfortable with the GC's background because the contractor will be subcontracting for all trades and will take on a substantial financial obligation. Always perform due diligence to confirm that the GC's business is financially sound.

Requesting a portfolio of completed projects is also recommended, so that you can verify that the quality of the GC's work runs parallel with your expectations. Look for evidence of extensive commercial experience with a focus on medical build-outs. Take the extra time to check references and obtain owners' names and the names of completed projects. Verify the names of the architects involved, the contract amount, the scheduled completion date, and the date that the certificate of occupancy was received. GCs with a successful portfolio should have no hesitation in providing any of this information for you. Ask about the percentage of their projects that were completed within budget and without change orders, and then verify their response. Some contractors provide extremely low bids in order to be awarded the project, only to submit change orders throughout the project to bring their overall price in line with the prices of other contractors who are possibly better-qualified GCs. Verifying details of past projects, including original contract amount and ending overall project cost, will prove to be invaluable during the qualification process.

Most landlords require the GC to hold a surety bond equal to the value of the contracted work. A *surety bond* is a promise to pay the owner of the project a certain amount if the bondholder fails to fulfill the terms of the contract. Surety bonds are expensive to obtain and will increase the cost of your project, so verify with your landlord whether one is required before your project is bid.

Bidding the Work

Once your drawings are complete and approved by all parties, they can be submitted to the municipality for permit. While these are in for permit, it's a good idea to bid the plans out (whether it's to one GC with multiple subcontractors or to multiple GCs) to establish a firm construction budget. For an accurate bid comparison, you should provide the bidders with a standard bidding form and require that they use it (Figure 2).

When the bids come in, you can compare the standard bid forms side by side (Figure 3) and see whether there are discrepancies. If there are widely varying numbers in any category, you should question the contractors to determine if they are simply employing a different way to categorize something (such as door frames in carpentry versus in the number of doors) or if they are missing something entirely.

If you have the flexibility to change specifications, then it's a good practice to request that contractors provide cost-saving alternatives, also known as *value engineering*, with their completed bids. The subcontractors can offer cost-saving options because of their previous experience and their supplier base. It is very important to review these choices with your construction manager and architect, because some changes can affect quality or aesthetics.

Once you have qualified the bids, the next step is to select your contractor and enter into the contract.

Contracting with the General Contractor

The AIA offers a variety of construction contracts for both design-build and design-bid-build projects. It is advisable to have an attorney review any contract because each particular circumstance dictates whether any changes must be made. Document AIA A107-2007, the Standard Form of Agreement Between Owner and Contractor for a Project of Limited Scope, is best suited to this type of build-out. It is imperative that any architectural drawings as well as any deviations from those drawings be specified in the contract. Here is a sample of items you should make clear in any contract language:

▶ *Determine the construction schedule and any penalties for schedule delays.* Penalties should be added to the contract for construction that is completed later than 30 days after the date specified if you incur costs, such as the commencement of rent before completion. With the inclusion of

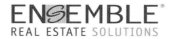

Tenant Improvement Final Bid Form

Bldg/Project Name: _____**Suite #:** _____

Bidder:_____Contact Name: _____

Telephone: _____Fax: _____Date: _____

BID BREAKDOWN : The following line items make up the TOTAL LUMP SUM BASE BID PRICE :

CSI	DESCRIPTION	COST
02050	Demolition	
02070	Final cleanup	
03000	Concrete	
03300	Concrete patch, core, and x-ray	
05500	Miscellaneous metals	
06200	Rough carpentry	
06400	Cabinetry/millwork	
07100	Waterproofing	
07200	Insulation	
07900	Sealants	
08100	Doors, frames, and hardware	
08710	Finish hardware	
08800	Glass and glazing, mirrors	
09100	Lath, plaster, drywall	
09500	Acoustical ceiling	
09660	VCT/sheet vinyl	
09660	Carpet	
09660	Ceramic tile	
09900	Painting	
10800	Toilet accessories and partitions	
10900	Special construction	
15400	Plumbing	
15300	Fire protection/fire extinguishers	
15500	HVAC	
15500	HVAC controls	
16000	Electrical	
16700	Fire alarm	
	Subtotal direct costs	
	Insurance and bonding	
	General conditions	
	Supervision	
	General contractor overhead and fee	
	Sales tax	
	Subtotal indirect costs	
	TOTAL ALL COSTS	
	ESTIMATED TIME TO COMPLETE (WEEKS)	

Figure 2. A standard bidding form.

Bid Comparison

Building Name _____
Contractors Name _____ **Suite #** _____

Avg Price $ —

Line Item	Contractor #1 Date Here			Contractor #2 Date Here		
	Bid	%	/SF	Bid	%	/SF
Demolition						
Final cleanup						
Concrete						
Concrete, patch, core, and x-ray						
Miscellaneous metals						
Rough carpentry						
Cabinetry/millwork						
Waterproofing						
Insulation						
Sealant						
Doors, frames, and hardware						
Finish hardware						
Glass and glazing, mirrors						
Lath, plaster, drywall						
VCT/sheet vinyl/carpet						
Acoustical ceiling						
Painting						
Toilet accessories/partitions						
Special construction						
Plumbing						
Fire protection/extinguishers						
HVAC						
Electrical						
Fire alarm						
Subtotal direct costs	$ —	0%		$ —	0%	
Insurance and bonding						
General condition						
Supervision						
Overhead and fee						
Subtotal indirect costs	$ —					
Sales Tax						
Contractor's total						
Plan check/permit fee						
Architectural and engineering						
Contingency						
GRAND TOTAL						

Grand total with ALL OPTION

Landlord allowance/tenant contribution

Suite USF	—	—
Allowance / USF _____		
Allowance _____		_____
Tenant overage		

Figure 3. Sample bid comparison form.

penalties, a contractor will want to be very specific regarding what is and what isn't in their control, and will require that the time frame for approvals is very tight.

▶ *Clarify insurance and bonding requirements.* Generally you should request that the contractor provide course of construction insurance. It is possible that your insurance company can provide this; however, the contractor can often include it at a lower cost. Your lender or landlord may also require a bond, and this should be identified in the contract.

- *Require 10% retention from the contractor.* The contract should withhold 10% of the total amount due until the end of the contract. This allows you to obtain the required lien waivers and ensure that any punch-list items (see the section "Punch Lists" in this chapter) are completed before you make the final payment.

- *Clarify that payments are made only on the basis of completed work and only after the appropriate lien waivers are received.* With each pay application (see the section "Pay Applications" in this chapter), you should request a conditional lien waiver or release for the work that was completed on the current pay application and an unconditional lien release for work that was completed on the prior pay application.

- *Include any lender requirements in the contract document.*

- *If materials purchased are included in pay applications, be sure that you include language documenting that the materials have been delivered to the site or otherwise can be verified.*

- *Require that the GC cooperate and coordinate with subcontractors that you hire, including phone and data, x-ray, and signage contractors.*

It is important to document your requirements as well as to include the contract with your bid package. This ensures that a contractor can't increase costs because there are unknown requirements in the contract.

LENDERS

If you are working with a lender to fund your construction, you should research the lender's requirements for including your equity and the lender's process for reviewing construction and process pay applications. A lender may require special forms, timing specifications, or documentation requirements for the GC, construction manager, or architect.

PERMITTING

The project's permitting requirements should be researched as soon as you procure your location. The selected architect and construction manager can typically assist with these requirements. The application forms and fees vary with governing body and space design. Separate permits are usually necessary for fire sprinklers and alarms. The architect should confirm those requirements. These permits can occasionally be submitted at a later time (called *deferred submittal*) in order for the specified subcontractor to design and submit those plans.

The method for submitting the forms depends on the municipality. Some allow you to submit the plans electronically, and others require originals with the architect's stamp and multiple copies. Some cities require that the contractor submit the plans for permit, but generally you are allowed to change contractors at any time. If you haven't selected a contractor because you are in the bidding process, you can request that the contractor submit the plans on your behalf with an understanding that the plans could be substituted if the GC doesn't win the bid. An *expediter* can also be retained to assist with this process. An expediter is beneficial if there are numerous submittals required, if there is a lot of interaction necessary with the governing body, or if you are simply too busy or too far away. An expediter is well versed in permitting and so can save you a lot of frustration.

THE CONSTRUCTION PROCESS

Construction Meetings

Once construction begins, you should schedule at a minimum a weekly meeting with your team to review progress and discuss any concerns as well as review the schedule to ensure that the project is on track. You should plan to designate time when you will be available throughout the construction process in case unforeseen circumstances occur and a decision must be made about how to accommodate any issues. Your construction manager and architect are key resources to help you analyze your choices in these circumstances. It is helpful to have someone on the team take minutes of these discussions to track progress.

Pay Applications

Most often the contractor submits monthly pay applications based on the work completed during the prior month—including any materials purchased. A thorough review of the pay applications should be completed to ensure that all work has been done. It's best to do this throughout the month and to require photographs of the work at various stages to ensure that it has been done in accordance with the plans. Photos of the stud installation can be beneficial, for instance, because once the drywall is installed, it's not possible to review the completed work.

A lender will most likely have a third-party inspector investigate and confirm the application. You or your construction manager, in conjunction with your architect, should do this as well. You should confirm that you have appropriate lien waivers to protect yourself and to ensure compliance with loan and lease documents. It is important that your contract allows you enough time to fund an approved application if you have a loan.

The final pay application, including any retention, should be paid only after you have received final unconditional lien waivers or releases and after the punch-list items have been completed.

Punch Lists

After completion of construction, you, your construction manager, your architect, the contractor, and sometimes the landlord will walk through the completed suite and make sure everything has been done to specifications. Any incomplete items or items requiring repair are put on a list called a *punch list*; the contractor completes these items over the next 7 to 15 days. It is possible to move in once you've received your certificate of occupancy or completion, even if the punch-list items have not been completed yet. However, the final payment should never be made until the punch-list items are complete.

Substantial Completion

Substantial completion means that the suite is complete, with the exception of any minor punch-list items and any tenant fixtures or equipment to be installed by the operator. This date is often used by a contractor to determine the contract completion date.

Certificate of Occupancy or Completion

The governing authority that issues the permit will issue a certificate of occupancy or completion when the suite is complete in accordance with the approved plans. This certificate is required before an operator can move furnishings or freestanding equipment into the center. The certificate is absolutely required before you can begin seeing patients.

As-Builts

Some landlords require that you provide them an as-built drawing, sometimes required in CAD (computer-aided design, or electronic) format. It is important to understand the desired format so that you can require the GC to provide what you need. An *as-built drawing* is a set of drawings with markups of any changes made during construction. This is necessary for any future maintenance; for instance, if the air-conditioning unit was moved to a different location or the plumbing line was found in a different location, this is information you would need.

Closeouts

The contractor should provide you with a closeout package that includes the as-builts, a listing of all subcontractors with a copy of the warranties, the original permit, a copy of the certificate of occupancy, a finish schedule, and copies of all submittals, including but not limited to door hardware, electrical components and heating, ventilation, air-conditioning, and a balancing report for your heating and cooling system. You will want all of this information at your fingertips should you have any issues with your equipment or want to order additional material for your center. The warranties for construction are generally for 1 to 2 years, depending on the construction documents' requirements, but many components carry material warranties insuring against failure. Your contractor must outline any material warranties outside the construction warranty time in the event that there are equipment failures, to prevent you from absorbing costs for warrantied components. A heating and cooling balance report is crucial to ensure your system has been properly installed and is working efficiently. In addition to providing a copy of the report to the landlord, a copy should be given to the company who will be contracted to maintain the equipment. The report will verify to the contractor that it was working efficiently at the time it was turned over to them for maintenance. The closeout book, if prepared completely, is your go-to reference for anything related to the construction of your center. These items should be included:

- A floor plan and a full set of as-built drawings
- An original building permit
- A certificate of occupancy
- GC contact information
- List of subcontractors, complete with their respective contact information and trades
- A finish schedule
- All submittals

Tenant Improvement Reimbursement

Often the landlord offers a monetary allowance contributable to the cost of the build-out. In most cases the landlord reimburses the owner after receiving the certificate of occupancy for the space, but in some cases reimbursement may occur as the project progresses. It is important that you, as an owner, read the lease agreement carefully to fully understand what documentation the landlord will require to release the funds. The usual documents required are unconditional lien waivers, a certificate of insurance, and a notarized affidavit showing that all materials and services associated with the project have been fully paid for.

Noncontractor Items

Some items aren't provided by the contractor but often must be coordinated with them:

- *Signage* The drawings of the space usually include only whatever signage is needed to comply with the Americans with Disabilities Act (restrooms, for example) or safety (exit signs, for example) requirements. Your landlord may provide some of the signage, so you should clarify what you need to provide in order to meet the lease agreement. Any other signage you wish to include must be contracted for through a signage vendor. In most cases, you provide your own monument or exterior signage, but it must comply with the landlord's specifications. Normally, you can install any signs that you need within your suite without the landlord's approval. However, it is important to always consult your lease and the property manager to determine if there are any requirements. Signage vendors can assist with design, obtain necessary permits, and install the signage. They must coordinate any interior signage installation with your contractor.

    It is advisable to begin any signage requirements as soon as you sign your lease and you have completed your floor plan. Timing on signage can vary because of signage complexity and local requirements. It is important to stay ahead of this issue so there are no delays in your opening.

- ▶ *Data and phone lines*   The architect works with you to identify where phone and data lines should be located. The GC provides the conduit for the lines, but you must contract with your own providers to install phone and data lines.

- ▶ *Artwork and furnishings*   Any finishing touches such as artwork and furniture are your personal choice. There are many options, and it might be worthwhile to work with an interior designer to help specify these items. An interior designer can save you money in the long run because they often receive trade discounts on purchases, and their specifications take durability into account.

CONCLUSION

Building out an urgent care center involves the careful coordination of several different entities, including a landlord, lender, architect, and contractor; city, state, and/or county licensing and permitting departments; signage, equipment, and furniture vendors; an insurance company; and an attorney. It can be very beneficial to hire an experienced construction manager to help you navigate the process, especially if you have no prior experience in opening an urgent care center.

Plan for at least 6 to 8 months from start to finish if you have selected an existing building, and always build in enough time to accommodate any unexpected issues when scheduling your grand opening.

KEY POINTS

1. If you are financing your project, meet with your lender before choosing a construction manager and contractor. Once you choose a construction manager and contractor, meet to outline loan draw procedures. Your lender will have certain procedures the construction manager and contractor will have to follow to comply with your loan documents. Find out if your lender has any qualifying policies you should be aware of before the project is bid out.

2. Choose a contractor with medical build-out experience and require that each contractor complete Document AIA A305, the Contractor's Qualification Statement. The build-out of a medical office has nuances and requirements that contractors experienced in general office build-outs or residential developments are not accustomed to dealing with.

3. Arm yourself with information regarding the types of permits, licenses, and inspections you will need for your center, and share the information with your contractor at the beginning of the project. Acquiring

information from all governing bodies in advance will tie in to your completion time.

4. Include monetary fines in your construction contract for failure to complete on time. Money motivates. Ensure that your contractor understands that they will be required to cover your out-of-pocket expenses should your project not be delivered on time.

5. When doing value engineering for your project, confirm with your contractor (and respective subcontractors) whether the savings up front could result in increased maintenance costs in the future.

6. Many times owners are so focused on saving cost on the build-out that they fail to realize installing high-quality components saves them maintenance costs in the future. Never compromise quality or efficiency. Understand the difference between price and cost and ask yourself, "Will the price now cost me later?"

7. Establish realistic goals with your contractor for completion time. Avoid creating an environment that could lead to contractors' paying less attention to quality simply to deliver your project on time.

8. Never pay your contractor without receiving unconditional lien waivers for the work previously compensated for. This will ensure that no mechanic liens will be filed against your project.

9. Hold weekly meetings and work off a 3-week look-ahead for the duration of the project. Regular meetings keep your contractor accountable to you and the schedule. Every 3 weeks, a new 3-week look-ahead meeting should be scheduled to ensure that timelines are being met.

10. If you are leasing your center, then once the project is completed, forward the certificate of occupancy to your landlord. Many leases have drop-dead dates for obtaining the allowance; review your lease closely and communicate with your contractor to hit those dates.

11. Require that your contractor prepare a warranty and operations manual for your project. This should include everything related to your project and will serve as a reference for years to come.

CHAPTER 5

Design of the Floor Plan in an Urgent Care Center

Rajiv Kapadia

Many urgent care centers are located in an existing building, either new or previously occupied by another tenant. In such a *shell* space, a building interior that is left unfinished, you will need to make *tenant improvements* (TIs), or customizations of the space to suit your center's needs.

SITE-SELECTION CHECKLIST

In the majority of cases, an architect is brought on board after site selection is complete, and often after the lease has been signed. However, it is still a good idea to cross the following items off your checklist of issues to resolve before embarking on the design phase:

- ► Site zoning and building use
- ► Parking
- ► Available utilities

Putting off dealing with some of them could mean the difference between an on-time opening and a months-long delay—or even abandoning a particular site altogether.

Site Zoning and Building Use

Real property in incorporated localities is usually subject to a land-use plan, approved and adopted by the governing jurisdiction. In most instances this is the city or county in which the property is located. The land-use plan is divided into various zones, usually designated by a letter code, a number code, or both, and is described in the zoning ordinance or a similar instrument. Check the zoning for your proposed site against the list of approved uses for that zone to verify that urgent care centers are allowed.

In some instances, an urgent care center may not be an allowed use of a zone, but this may sometimes be remedied by securing a special-use permit, waiver, or similar instrument. This usually entails a separate application process with the city and could take anywhere from a few hours to a few weeks or even months. If that process is not successful, the property may need to be rezoned, which is usually a fairly involved process requiring the services of other professionals such as attorneys, surveyors, and civil engineers, as well as a substantial time investment. If this is not a viable option, then it may be time to consider an alternative site for the center.

If the project site is part of a group of commercial establishments and subject to the conditions, covenants, and [deed] restrictions administered by the equivalent of an owner's association or property management agency, then the proposed urgent care center should be verified as allowable, or approvable after due process.

Parking

Many jurisdictions will not allow a particular use, even though it is otherwise allowed by the zoning ordinance, unless proof of adequate available parking can be demonstrated. Although many cities do not even question this, others will not budge on this requirement. The required minimum, and in some cases maximum, allowable parking for each type of use is usually described in the zoning ordinance, parking regulations, or other similar adopted instruments. In some existing (previously tenanted) spaces, the city may agree to limited waivers or creative agreements such as cross-parking easements or time-shared parking agreements in lieu of actual on-site parking count. Certain cities do not review for parking adequacy until after building plans have been approved by other departments, by which time the applicant may have already devoted substantial resources to a location, thus resulting in undue hardship.

Available Utilities

Utilities primarily encompass heating, ventilation, and air-conditioning (HVAC), water for domestic use, water for fire-protection use, sewer, electricity, and gas. It is critical to verify the available capacity for each of these for the proposed use before space-planning begins.

Heating, Ventilation and Air-Conditioning

Of all utilities, the HVAC system is usually the easiest to deal with if a deficiency must be remedied, which is not to say that resolution is painless. Most building shells are usually designed in some form to accommodate HVAC sources. This may be in the form of packaged units, gas furnaces, split systems, boilers, or evaporative coolers. The heating or cooling reaches the usable space through some form of distribution, usually ductwork. Although ductwork is modified as part of TIs and therefore is not as critical on a predesign checklist, the capacity of the source is highly relevant. Depending on the geographic location of the site and the orientation and exposure of the actual project suite, HVAC requirements can vary. However, on average, a capacity of 1 ton per 250 square feet will usually provide adequate capacity, with adjustments for extreme heat and cold conditions in the range of plus or minus 50 square feet. Bear in mind that the capacity of the power source for the required HVAC source also must be verified, whether it is gas, electricity, or water.

Many new buildings will not be equipped with HVAC sources but may instead be designed so that the shell can accommodate new units to be installed by the tenant. For example, the roof may have been built with curbs to facilitate the installation of rooftop packaged units. If new units have to be installed as part of TIs, then many cities will require evidence of the capacity of the existing roof to bear the additional load. This will require the services of a structural engineer. Some cities also have additional requirements such as visual screening of all mechanical equipment, which should be dealt with as early on as possible because they can have a substantial impact on TI costs.

Water for Domestic Use

Domestic use of water, in this context, refers to any use other than for fire protection (i.e., fire-sprinkler use). Urgent care centers tend to use more water than a nonmedical office or retail facility uses but less water than a restaurant uses. In a mixed-use building, with multiple kinds of tenants sharing the same water source, this could present a problem because buildings generally tend to be serviced by a single water meter with branches to individual tenants. The size of the water meter, the size of the succeeding water main, and its run relative to the project suite will usually give the engineer sufficient information to determine if there is enough water and pressure to service the urgent care center. Usually a 1-inch-diameter water meter, assuming it is not located too far from the project suite, will suffice to service only a six-exam-room urgent care center. Note that this does not mean that it is sufficient to service the entire building; that determination is predicated on the number and types of other tenants. A single restaurant, for example, could easily use all the water from a 1-inch-diameter water meter for itself, leaving no spare capacity for other tenants.

Water for Fire-Protection Use

Most cities require that water for fire sprinklers be tapped from the city main independently from the water for domestic use. The fire-protection (sprinkler) system itself is usually installed as part of the shell, and its distribution has to be modified as part of the TI. Because medical offices do not present a significantly higher hazard than other types of offices, this is usually not a problem. However, it is worth noting that under newer building codes most commercial spaces must have sprinkler systems. In older buildings not currently equipped with such a system, a change in use could potentially trigger a requirement for upgrading to current codes, which could easily add tens of thousands of dollars to the cost of TIs. Although most cities are usually cognizant of this hardship and will work with tenants to grant relief, it is worth investigating up front.

Sewer

The size, location, and invert of the sewer main should be adequate to support the urgent care center's needs. Most urgent care centers need to tap into a waste line that has a minimum diameter of 4 inches, and as long as the location of the waste main is at sufficient depth to allow for the farthest fixture in the suite to slope at the rate prescribed by building codes, there shouldn't be a problem. Modifications to the site sewer system tend to be an expensive affair, so the details of the waste main are therefore best verified beforehand.

Electricity

Power supply can sometimes be a deal breaker on an otherwise good location. The electrical requirements for an urgent care center will vary with overall size and equipment, and existing and expansion electrical capacity should be determined at the outset, preferably with the assistance of an electrical engineer. For perspective, most spaces of up to 2500 square feet in newer multitenant commercial buildings tend to be powered with one 200-ampere meter at 208/120 volts. This is very likely to not be enough for an urgent care center with at least five exam rooms plus an x-ray room because the x-ray machine alone may require a 100-ampere disconnect. A safer power requirement for this scenario, with some leftover capacity, might be to have 400 amperes instead. If the service-entrance switchboard has spare meters or empty slots for future meters, or if the landlord can make additional power available, then the electrical engineer can design an appropriate power distribution system. Otherwise, bringing in additional power from the utility company's off-site location can easily rack up construction dollars.

ARCHITECTURAL PROGRAM

Although the scope of a true architectural program is quite substantial and usually requires the services of an architect or other qualified professionals, a simplified version is nevertheless extremely beneficial in developing the design for an urgent care center. An *architectural program* is a document that defines the needs and goals of the center while identifying limiting parameters.

The section "Functions and Spaces to Accommodate" in this chapter presents a typical space program for an urgent care center. As a general note, the terms *architect* and *designer* are used somewhat interchangeably in this chapter and do not necessarily imply two separate professionals.

Caveats

In addition, when working on an architectural program, it is wise to be guided by the following three caveats:

Start With a Wish List

Compromises are inevitable as you work your way through the design, but often features that you think are out of reach can be incorporated relatively easily when handled by an experienced architect. Therefore, include everything at the start that you would like to incorporate, and then pare down your list of features after getting professional feedback.

Don't Try to Solve the Problem Yourself
Owners of urgent care centers are generally physicians or businesspeople, well versed in their chosen profession. When an owner takes on a design issue, this may take too much time away from other important considerations, the issue may appear unsolvable, and the desired design feature may perhaps be abandoned altogether as impossible. Instead, state the goal and let the designer either come up with a solution or advise that a compromise must be made.

Plan for Future Growth
Start-up costs are significant, and owners may start out with a limited staff until the center really takes off. But when your center's growth does take off, you do not want to be limited from expanding because of a lack of space. However, if a certain patient volume is reached, then an expansion of the entire center is likely in order.

To illustrate, you may be able to have the front-desk receptionist do double duty as the billing person at start-up, but once your center is well established, you will need the receptionist to be dedicated to reception duty, and you may perhaps even need to add a second biller once a particular milestone has been reached. However, if patient volume eventually requires a third biller, then perhaps the numbers of exam rooms, physicians, and assistants should be increased, which translates to a physical expansion of the center.

Functions and Spaces to Accommodate
The architectural program outlined in this section can serve as a guideline when you are planning the various functions and spaces that the center will likely have to accommodate. Each space should take into account the number of occupants likely to be in it, the tangible items required to be housed within, and the intangibles that will allow the space to fulfill its required function.

Front Lobby and Waiting Area
A good starting point in helping to define the size of the front lobby is to establish a chair count. For an urgent care center, depending on how the center is staffed and run, two chairs per exam room is generally a minimum. Three chairs are preferred, and in some cases even four. Bear in mind that patients are often accompanied by family members or friends and that patients can also wait in the exam rooms.

Identify other amenities that must be accessible from the front lobby, such as restrooms, sources of drinking water, vending machines, a play area for kids, televisions, games, coffee and tea counter, storage, reading material, and advertising materials.

Reception

Establish a head count for personnel likely to work at the front desk, in whatever capacity, and list what they will need in order to effectively perform their duties. These items might include computer workstations, a fax, a copier, a scanner, a printer, a filing system, storage, and forms, in addition to intangibles such as visual privacy in which to conduct financial transactions and document patient information, or acoustical privacy in which to speak with patients and with insurance carriers.

Triage

Triage may be an area for obtaining patients' vital signs, but it can also be many more things, such as a private area that is compliant with the Health Insurance Portability and Accountability Act (HIPAA) to obtain patient information, a blood-draw area, or even the exam room itself. Establish a list of equipment that will permanently stay in the room, along with items that may be brought in on an as-needed basis. This list should not be limited to medical equipment alone but should also include items such as chairs, a countertop area, a supply storage space, and a television.

Exam Rooms

The number of exam rooms should be established at the start of the program and should generally be the last aspect on which compromises are made during the evolution of the design. The number of exam rooms dictates the maximum possible patient volume and therefore revenue. It is generally a function of on-site caregiver head count and the business model for operating the center.

The exam room is the heart of the center, and the layout and design of each exam room must be worked out in great detail (Figure 1). The design should take into account not only the physical equipment but also the individual needs of the medical personnel who will use the space. For example, are the caregivers right-handed or left-handed, and will they need to approach the exam table or certain medical equipment a certain way?

Besides an exam table and required medical equipment and supplies, all other desired amenities should be clearly defined. These may include chairs for patients' companions, reading material, television, computer workstation, writing surface, sink, storage, trash can, disposal containers for biohazardous waste and sharps, and enough room for items that may be brought in only occasionally, such as surgical carts. Their relative placement should be worked out for efficient flow. Generally, most caregivers prefer that all exam rooms within a center have the same layout and therefore identical flow. Typical exam room sizes range from 8×10 feet up to approximately 120 square feet. Any exam room smaller than 80 square feet usually involves some form of compromise, with cramped quarters or elimination of a sink or writing surface being the most common modification. In rare instances, exam rooms may be as large as 140 square feet, but that is usually

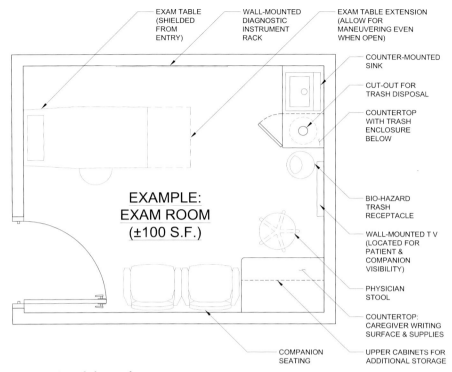

Figure 1. Sample layout for an exam room.

to meet a specific need. A size of 100 square feet is quite sufficient for an urgent care center, with the room preferably set up as a rectangle.

Ceiling heights of between 8 and 10 feet above a finished floor tend to work well, with a height of 9 feet striking a good balance between spatial perception and construction cost. A lower ceiling may make the room appear to close in on occupants who must wait there for more than a few minutes, whereas ceilings 10 feet or higher may just be wasted space. Bear in mind that building codes prohibit a ceiling height of less than 7 feet 6 inches for occupiable spaces.

Procedure Room

Some owners of urgent care centers prefer that their procedure room be a separate, larger room equipped with appropriate supplies and additional lighting. This room may be occupied by multiple caregivers during treatments, and they need access to additional medical equipment such as surgical carts or portable examination lights. Procedure rooms in urgent care centers range in size from 100 square feet to approximately 140 square feet, with some being larger to meet a specific need. A size of 120 square feet allows for good functionality in a small urgent care center.

X-Ray Room

If the center will be providing on-site x-ray services, the selection of x-ray equipment early on in the process will be beneficial for smooth flow of the design and engineering phases of the project. The size of the room is typically dictated by the selected equipment, but in general, a minimum room width of 9 feet is preferred, although many vendors will work with smaller widths, whereas caregivers often prefer a slightly larger width. The room length is a function not only of the size of the actual x-ray equipment but also of the adjacent electrical equipment required to support it.

A shielded control area either within the room or immediately adjacent to it, with direct visual access, will be required for technicians to operate the x-ray equipment. This usually consists of a counter area for accommodating a workstation and control equipment and there generally is no seating.

Lead shielding will be required around the x-ray equipment and is often provided in the form of lead-lined gypsum-board walls and lead-lined doors, windows, and frames. The actual shielding requirements are determined by a physicist, who will generate recommendations that are based on the actual equipment selected, the room layout, surrounding construction, and neighboring occupancies.

Laboratory

The placement of the laboratory within the center varies with the desired workflow, with most owners opting for a somewhat central location. It is worth noting that this is probably either a room that patients should never need to enter or one in which they are escorted at all times. The laboratory will likely have testing and sterilization equipment, patients' biologic samples, forms with patient or chain of custody information, and the like, all of which should be inaccessible to accidental visibility or tampering. Owners of some urgent care centers therefore prefer that the laboratory be located toward the back of the center, past all patient areas. However, some others, such as those with centers with a large volume of patients needing drug testing, prefer that it be positioned at the very front to allow for quick flow in and out of the clinic without disrupting any other processes. In all cases, it is usually beneficial to have the laboratory positioned relatively close to a restroom to allow for easy collection and transportation of samples. An immediately adjacent placement will allow for a pass-through cabinet in the common wall between the two.

The laboratory will usually require at least one sink and possibly two or more, depending on local requirements and desired activities. For example, some states mandate a separate sink for hand washing within the laboratory, whereas some owners of centers prefer a separate dumping sink for disposing of samples immediately after a drug test.

Take an inventory of all laboratory equipment at maximum capacity to establish utility requirements. Is special ventilation or exhausting required for the performed functions, or for the chemicals being used and stored? Some states will not grant a license without these requirements being met. Is any special plumbing required? For example, an urgent care center that caters to a higher volume of sports injuries may need ice available at all times, in which case a dedicated water line for an ice maker may be in order. The total and special electrical requirements should be identified up front so that the engineer can provide adequate power outlets, some of which may perhaps have to be serviced by a dedicated circuit. Multiple refrigerators may be required because most jurisdictions prohibit storing prescription drugs and laboratory samples together.

Lastly, the laboratory works best with adequate counter and storage space. Ensure that there is enough free length for workflow, in addition to the required space for equipment. Identifying storage needs within the laboratory, in detail, will go a long way in expediting patient turnaround times. If forms must be easily accessible, then slotted cabinets might perhaps work better than drawers, and strategically positioned cup storage for sample collection might mean that it is unnecessary to walk across the laboratory twice for every collection activity.

Offices

The definition of an *office* can be broadened to include working spaces, not necessarily defined by walls, for team members. Therefore, offices might include spaces for physicians, nurses, medical assistants, a center manager, billing personnel, administrative staff members, and so forth. Establish whether they need private or open spaces to perform their roles and what amenities they require. If staff members are performing multiple functions in a smaller center, then be sure to address the space needs for each of their roles. For example, a nurse might need a high-visibility position, easily accessible from the exam rooms, but if they are also the billing person or bookkeeper, then that role might require a private area for HIPAA compliance.

Nurse Station

A nurse station can be considered a special type of office space (Figure 2). Although some owners of urgent care centers elect not to provide a dedicated nurse station, most will provide at least some form of a workstation for nurses, physician assistants, medical assistants, and physicians that is somewhat central to the exam rooms, where they can perform administrative functions related to patient care. A well-designed nurse station can function as the nerve center of the urgent care center, allowing health-care providers to maintain visual and physical control over the center and ensure smooth patient flow. Most times it is an open desk, strategically located to maintain some form of monitoring over exam rooms, with easy access to any patient-care related amenities. Such amenities might include items as diverse as medical supplies, prescription drugs, equipment, instruments, autoclaves, crutches, computer workstations, printers, and fax machines. The nurse station should be within easy reach of patients in need, should allow physicians and staff members to make quick standing stops

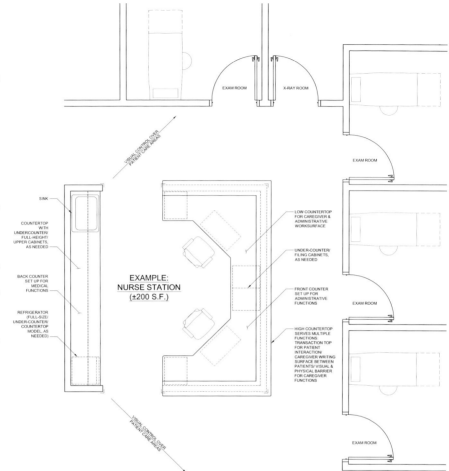

Figure 2. Sample layout incorporating a nurse station.

between patients, and should be designed such that seated working still allows for HIPAA-compliant private discussion of patient information.

Restrooms

Building codes usually mandate a minimum number of restrooms based on the area and use of each facility. The urgent care center might have specific needs in addition to the prescribed ratios, and these should be identified at the outset. Most owners of urgent care centers, given the option, prefer a restroom directly accessible from the front lobby for patients' use while waiting, in addition to at least one other on the "interior" side for use during examination or for urine sample collection. Where space restrictions allow for only a single restroom, its position should be optimized relative to its desired functionality. In centers conducting high volumes of drug testing, it is sometimes preferable to dedicate one restroom specifically for this function, for easier monitoring and control, leading to more efficient workflow.

Desired accessories within the restroom should be identified and should include required items such as grab bars, toilet-tissue dispensers, and trash receptacles, along with optional items such as seat-cover dispensers. If used for drug testing, the restroom should have some provision for locking away of personal effects prior to sample collection, as well as a pass-through cabinet for easy sample transfer. For centers with frequent sampling activities, the position or operation of the water shutoff valve may have to be modified for easier and quicker access.

Bear in mind that in the urgent care center setting, current building code interpretations will likely require all restrooms to be wheelchair accessible, even when the number of restrooms provided is in excess of the minimum code-mandated number.

Storage and Supplies

Storage should be considered in all of its many uses: storage of records, supplies, samples, drugs, equipment, personal effects, regular waste, biohazardous waste, and so on, and provisions should made for easy access, removal, use, and disposition. Storage can take the form of dedicated storage rooms, built-in cabinetry, or movable containers. Although some owners elect to have supplies stored directly at points of use and therefore not have any real estate dedicated exclusively to storage, most prefer to have at least a closet or room from which stocked items are distributed on an established schedule. Many jurisdictions have some form of restriction on certain types of storage, such as for prescription drugs and biohazardous waste. Conditioned environments for sample storage and the like should be taken into account too. Finally, secure storage for employee personal effects never goes unappreciated.

Utilities

Utilities don't take up much room within a center, but they are, of course, indispensable to its working. Some of them require physical floor space in some form, whereas others may require wall or ceiling space, and yet others may not even be within the space itself but will nevertheless have to be accounted for and tied into. Their positioning can also impact the construction budget, especially when located without consideration to their entry point into the building or space. Even though the actual placement, design, and engineering of these systems is fairly technical, for purposes of the architectural program one should, at a minimum, identify spaces for electrical panels, telephone board, computer server space, water heater, and mop sink.

Break Room

A break room is usually for employee use only, generally immediately before and after work as well as during breaks and lunchtime. Some owners opt to provide a larger break room that doubles as a weekly meeting room and occasionally as a training room. However, these options should be evaluated on a return-on-investment basis, in light of usage frequency versus cost of the dedicated real estate.

Amenities within the break room should be identified, along with the desired seating capacity, bearing in mind that most centers prefer that not all employees take a break at the same time. A sink, countertop, cabinets, microwave, coffee maker, and refrigerator are fairly standard to all break rooms. In addition, some employers elect to provide such items as a dishwasher, additional appliances, and lockers. The break room is a good location for an employee notice board. In space-challenged centers, a galley-style break room that is a long, narrow space with a standing counter only, may be an option for avoiding complete elimination.

Conference and Training Rooms

Larger urgent care centers, especially those operating in multiple locations within a given geographic area, may need a dedicated conference or training room when such activities occur on a regular basis. Required amenities within such rooms should be itemized for incorporation and may include videoconferencing capability, dimmable lighting, white boards, floor outlets for power, voice and data, and so forth.

Finally, there may be special needs unique to a specific location or operation. These should be identified up front and listed with their tangible and intangible requirements. It is exponentially more challenging to fit a forgotten function into an otherwise complete and approved space layout than it is to plan for it at the outset.

AESTHETICS

The appearance of a clinic can affect patient volumes to a surprising extent, and especially so in an optional and consumer-choice-driven health-care setting such as an urgent care center. Even large, established hospitals have undertaken extensive remodels to enhance the overall patient experience in recognition of this. A patient who feels comfortable and well taken care of is more likely to return and more likely to refer others than is one who remembers a stay in a cramped, dreary space.

From a design perspective, everything that the patient encounters during the visit, including accessories, amenities, colors, lighting, finishes, furniture, and even the flow of spaces, provides visual cues that together add up to the final perception of the center. An appropriate design goal, then, might be to translate the reassurance and professionalism of a physician's bedside manner into the spatial experience of the visit.

In terms of style, the design of the center can successfully traverse many different directions, from classic to contemporary. Be wary of choosing too eclectic a theme. Controversy in design works well to engage an audience, but an unwell patient is likely more in need of relaxation than stimulation. Colors and lighting should therefore convey comfort more than striking effects, yet still communicate a clean and professional setting.

Similarly, accessories can take many forms, conveying a personal touch, striking a bond with something uniquely local, presenting a professional theme, providing educational visuals, and many more. Finishes should be suitable for a health-care setting, easily cleanable or easily replaceable. For example, many owners of urgent care centers have a strong preference for using carpet in waiting areas and even corridors, to communicate a more homelike setting. Although carpet is not the best material in an area where there are open wounds and upset stomachs, a preference for carpet could be accommodated with a carpet tile rated for health-care use that is easily replaceable, assuming, of course, that carpet is an approvable material choice under the governing body's rules.

On a final note: Although budget is obviously a significant determinant in design choices and the final fit-out of the center, an experienced architect or designer can often deliver the desired look with alternative lower-cost materials and strategic splurging, such as through thoughtful use of paint, creative drywall work, and deliberate positioning of a few high-dollar items.

CONCLUSION

The success of an urgent care center is predicated on many factors, but a good design can do much to attract customers, facilitate efficient operation, and enhance the overall patient experience. A strong site with adequate utility support and regulatory approvability is the starting raw material, a well-formulated architectural program provides the necessary framework, and the creative process synthesizes these to yield a final product capable of meeting its diverse objectives.

KEY POINTS

1. Verify that an urgent care clinic is a permissible use for the project site.

2. Ensure that regulatory requirements are achievable with available resources.

3. Confirm that available infrastructure is capable of supporting an urgent care center. This should include, at a minimum, mechanical, plumbing, and electrical systems.

4. Formulate an architectural program to outline the needs and goals of the center, keeping limiting parameters in mind.

5. Define the spaces to be housed within the center. Quantify the head count, identify the supporting equipment, and describe the nonphysical aspects that will allow each space to fulfill its function.

6. The business model will set the minimum and maximum number of exam rooms required to make the center viable, serviceable, and profitable, which in turn will dictate the relative size of the remainder of the facility.

7. The size, the amenities, the equipment, and the optimal workflow within each exam room should be carefully worked out. Accommodate caregiver preferences to the extent feasible.

8. Compliance with various building codes and regulatory codes—Occupational Safety and Health Administration, Americans with Disabilities Act, and HIPAA—should be factored into the design. This may include additional governmental and nongovernmental regulations such as those of the state health department and the conditions, covenants, and [deed] restrictions of the office complex, compliance with which may be voluntary, for optional certification, or mandatory.

9. The sequencing of spaces should enhance patient workflow and simultaneously facilitate smooth and efficient staff workflow.

10. Materials and finishes should be rated for health-care use, as applicable, and easily cleanable or replaceable. Fixtures, furnishings, and accessories should complement the design concept and enhance the overall patient experience.

CHAPTER 6

Business Formation and Entity Structuring

Adam Winger

ENTITY TYPES

One of the most important decisions in the life cycle of an urgent care business is made before the first patient is treated. Choices relating to entity structuring and formation can and often do have a direct and dramatic impact on the tax and operational aspects of the urgent care business. This chapter addresses many of the basic issues an owner of an urgent care company must confront before opening its doors for business.

Common Entity Issues

Business entities are creations of, and are governed by, state law. As a result, the challenges faced by owners of urgent care companies in one state could differ materially from that of another. Most state statutes, however, allow for business to be conducted by or through any of the following entities: general partnerships, limited partnerships, corporations, limited liability companies (LLCs), and certain professional organizations such as professional corporations and professional LLCs. Because of the relative frequencies that each type of entity is used in the urgent care industry, this chapter focuses predominantly on corporations, LLCs, and professional organizations.

General Entity Characteristics

Corporations and LLCs (including professional corporations and professional LLCs) are the most common entity choices used in the urgent care industry. Although a complete explanation of the unique attributes of each of these entities is beyond the scope of this chapter, the following material should provide enough context for you to engage in a meaningful conversation with your attorney and accountant.

Among the differences between corporations and LLCs is the terminology used. Owners of corporations are referred to as *shareholders* or *stockholders*, whereas those of LLCs are referred to as *members*. Corporations are managed by a board of directors who delegate operational authority to officers, whereas in most states LLCs are managed either by one or more managers or directly by the members.[1]

LLCs are universally considered the more flexible choice of entity. For example, a number of formalities must be followed if owners of an urgent care company decide to operate as a corporation. Among other things, corporations in most states are required to hold an annual meeting, prepare and maintain corporate minutes, and maintain stock books with share certificates. LLC statutes, on the other hand, generally impose none of these requirements. Many state statutes also provide for corporate *dissenters' rights*, which entitle a minority shareholder to demand fair value for their shares when a majority approves certain extraordinary actions to which the minority shareholder objects. Although certain LLC statutes may provide for similar rights as a default measure, the majority of states permit LLC members to waive such rights in a written agreement.

Formation Mechanics

Although the terminology for the required documentation may vary from state to state, the process for forming a business entity is fairly consistent. States generally require that owners file a single document with the applicable state filing agent (usually the Secretary of State). The document typically to be filed for LLCs is the "Certificate of Formation," or the "Articles of Organization," and for corporations is the "Certificate of Incorporation," the "Charter," or the "Articles of Incorporation." The specific information required to be included in the formation documentation varies from state to state, but all such documents require that a *registered agent* be named, along with an address to which official state mail may be delivered. The registered agent is the person or entity that the company designates as the point person for all official contact with the state of formation. This includes receiving correspondence from applicable taxing authorities and also receiving any information pertaining to lawsuits against the company. Urgent care companies operating outside of their state of formation may choose to hire a company located within the state (normally for a nominal fee) to serve as their registered agent.

Governance Issues

Regardless of what entity type is chosen, owners must enter into one or more agreements to govern the relationship between the owners.

In the corporate context, *bylaws* are adopted by the board of directors. Bylaws establish certain operational mechanics of the corporation. This may include procedures relating to voting, appointment of officers, and conducting of board and shareholder meetings. Shareholders of a corporation typically also enter into a *shareholders' agreement* or *stockholders' agreement*, to more formally addresses the details of the owners' business relationship. This agreement is discussed in detail later in the chapter.

---

1   Note that although they are not required to, LLCs are free to appoint and delegate responsibility to officers or their state law equivalent.

LLCs address all relevant concepts in a single agreement generally referred to as the *operating agreement* or *LLC agreement*.

For the sake of convenience, the bylaws and shareholders' agreement for the corporation and the operating agreement for the LLC are referred to as the *equityholders' agreement* in the remainder of this chapter.

The equityholders' agreement sets forth the rights and obligations of the owners of the company. At a minimum, the agreement sets forth the owners' financial and governance rights. Financial rights are those entitling an owner to participate in the profits, losses, and distributions of the company. This includes a shareholder's right to receive dividends from a corporation and a member's right to receive distributions from an LLC.

Governance rights, on the other hand, refer to the owners' right to vote on specific matters. These rights may differ depending on the issue at hand. For example, the agreement may provide that though certain parties are entitled to make decisions regarding the day-to-day affairs of the company, all of the owners must consent to major transactions such as a merger or sale of all or substantially all the assets of the company.

The equityholders' agreement also addresses the various obligations of the owners. For example, the agreement will set forth the process to be followed if the company requires additional capital. Although this may involve a preliminary attempt to secure outside financing, of more interest to owners will be each owner's obligation to contribute additional funds in such a situation (a "capital call"). A complete discussion of capital calls and their effect on the relevant organization is beyond the scope of this chapter, but owners of urgent care centers should confirm that the concept is adequately addressed by their attorney in the equityholders' agreement to avoid unexpected ownership dilution or substantial financial liability.

The agreement will also address specific topics such as transferability of the owners' equity interest and the effect of certain events such as death, disability, or loss of a provider's medical license on ownership rights. Equityholders' agreements are frequently the subject of extensive negotiations, and urgent care owners should engage competent counsel to ensure the owners' arrangement is properly recorded in compliance with applicable state law.

Overall, the equityholders' agreement may be the single most important document to the owners of an entity. Before entering into the agreement, however, it must be determined which entity type will be used. In the urgent care context, this decision generally involves an analysis of three core aspects—health-care regulatory requirements, legal liability, and federal and state tax consequences. Entity structuring for urgent care businesses that are subject to health-care regulatory requirements such as a state prohibition against fee splitting, the corporate practice of medicine doctrine, or other similar legal limitations is addressed in Chapter 8 ("Corporate Practice of Medicine and Other Legal Impediments to Nonphysician Ownership"). The remainder of this chapter focuses on the legal liability and the federal income tax aspects of the choice of entity analysis.

CHOICE OF ENTITY: LIABILITY AND TAX CONSIDERATIONS

Corporations

Legal Liability

Corporations have existed in their modern form for years. Consequently, they enjoy a rich history of case law, making the legal risks of nearly every business decision somewhat predictable by competent counsel. With an understanding of the relevant legal risks, shareholders are better able to formulate and execute business strategies to reduce or limit overall organizational risk. By virtue of state statutes, shareholders of a corporation also enjoy substantive protection from the liabilities of the corporation.

In general, a shareholder is only at risk for the property that he or she contributed in exchange for his or her stock in the corporation. For example, assume that at an urgent care company formed as a corporation, a patient slips in an exam room and suffers serious (and costly) head injuries. Because of the liability limitation provided under state law and assuming no personal negligence on the part of the shareholders, only the amount of money initially contributed by the shareholders will be at risk to claims of the injured patient (now plaintiff). As is discussed below, this liability limitation differs from that of both a limited partnership and a general partnership.

Tax Considerations

Corporations are subject to tax under Subchapter C or Subchapter S of the Internal Revenue Code. Not surprisingly, corporations taxed under Subchapter C are called *C corporations* and those taxed under Subchapter S are called *S corporations*.

C corporations are subject to two layers of federal income tax: one at the corporate level when the income is earned and another at the shareholder level when dividends are paid. For example, assuming an urgent care company taxed as a C corporation earns $1,000,000 in profit, the corporation would pay approximately $350,000 (35%) in tax. Upon payment of the remaining $650,000 to the shareholders, up to an additional $130,000 (20%) would be payable by the shareholder's owner as a dividend tax.[2] Consequently, without even considering state tax obligations, approximately $480,000 ($350,000 + $130,000), or 48%, of the corporation's earnings will be paid in tax to the federal government.

Unlike the double-tax regimen applicable to C corporations, S corporations are subject to only one level of tax. For example, assume the same $1,000,000 in profit is earned by an S corporation that is owned in equal parts by two individuals. At the end of the year, each shareholder will report $500,000 of income

---

2   Note that only highly compensated individuals are taxed at the 20% dividend rate; others are currently subject to a maximum dividend rate of 15%.

on his or her personal income tax return. Assuming the shareholders are both subject to the highest rate of tax, which as of the date of this book is 39.6%, each will pay up to $198,000 for a total tax of $396,000.[3] When the earnings are paid to the shareholders, no additional tax will be owed. Consequently, by electing to be taxed as an S corporation, the urgent care company will save almost 10% in taxes.[4]

Although electing to be taxed as an S corporation has the potential to create significant tax benefits, not all entities are eligible to elect S status. Subchapter S imposes restrictions on the number and type of shareholders that may own an S corporation. The restrictions most applicable to an urgent care company are as follows:

- The owners of the S corporation may only be individuals.[5]
- The entity must have only one class of stock.
- The entity must have 100 or fewer owners.

Of the three restrictions, the first two pose the largest challenge for urgent care arrangements. For example, because (except in rare circumstances) only individuals are permitted to own an interest in an S corporation, an urgent care company that elects to be taxed as an S corporation will be limited in its ability to attract investors that desire to invest through an entity. This will almost entirely limit the entity's ability to sell an equity interest to a hospital or other sophisticated investors such as private equity companies.[6]

The second restriction, prohibiting the entity from issuing more than one class of stock, also limits an urgent care company's ability to attract investors. For example, assume an investor desires to receive an 8% return prior to the repayment of any other investor in exchange for a contribution of 90% of the necessary capital for the urgent care venture. Because of the varying financial rights of the owners, the Internal Revenue Service views such an arrangement as creating multiple classes of stock. Consequently, to retain one's status as an S corporation, cash must be distributed proportionately, and this could make it extremely difficult to attract investment capital.

An S corporation's failure to comply with the applicable requirements leads to a revocation of the entity's status as an S corporation, and the entity immediately defaults into the double-tax regime applicable to C corporations. Therefore, if an urgent care company taxed as an S corporation permits an entity as a shareholder or agrees to pay a preferred rate of return to an investor, the entity

---

3   Note that for purpose of illustration, the progressive nature of the federal income tax brackets is ignored.
4   Additional tax benefits currently apply with respect to federal payroll taxes. These are briefly addressed in the remainder of the chapter.
5   Note that certain exceptions exist for single-member LLCs, trusts, and certain other entities that are all beyond the scope of this chapter.
6   Note that certain structuring alternatives may be used to achieve a similar result.

will be left paying almost 10% more of all earnings retained by the company as federal tax.

General and Limited Partnerships

Although preferable tax treatment is enjoyed by general and limited partnerships, owners will be exposed to additional legal liability.

Legal Liability

A general partnership is owned by two or more partners, and there is no limit to the liability to which they are exposed. For example, if the urgent care company were sued for the slip and fall described above, all of the assets of each of the general partners (including their house, cars, bank accounts, and so forth) would be at risk to the claims of the injured plaintiff. A limited partnership, on the other hand, is owned by at least one general partner and at least one limited partner. Unlike the general partnership, only the personal assets of the general partner are exposed to unlimited legal liability.[7]

Tax Consequences

General and limited partnerships enjoy the same single-level tax as S corporations, but are not subject to the various ownership restrictions. As a result, although all partners in a general partnership and the general partner in a limited partnership remain subject to unlimited legal liability, they avoid both the second layer of tax of the C corporation and the ownership restrictions of the S corporation. Although the federal income tax consequences make the partnership an attractive entity choice, few choose to operate as a partnership because of the vast liability exposure involved.

Limited Liability Company

The limited liability company provides the best of both worlds. It affords investors the same legal protections as corporate shareholders and provides the single-level tax advantages of a partnership without the S corporation restrictions on ownership. The first state laws allowing for the creation of LLCs were enacted in the late 1970s. Since then, all 50 states have enacted such statutes, and because of its attractive features, the LLC has quickly become one of the most popular choices for business operators. Although the LLC solves many of the issues associated with the other entity choices, the relatively recent creation of the entity does create some uncertainty from a legal perspective. Unlike corporations, LLCs do not enjoy the same rich history of case law. Consequently, owners of urgent care companies are less able to predict the legal outcome of their business decisions. Most observers, however, view this as a minor drawback given the case law applicable to corporations, and it is therefore not surprising that the LLC has become the entity of choice for most private companies.

---

7   Although an entity form known as the limited liability limited partnership provided for complete liability protection to its owners, the development of the limited liability company essentially rendered that entity obsolete.

Governance of the Limited Liability Company

Much as with the shareholders of a corporation, decision-making power generally rests with the members of an LLC. Although the relationship of LLC members is largely governed by an operating agreement, state statutes do establish the fundamental framework for the entity's governance. Such statutes allow for an LLC to be either member-managed or manager-managed.

Member-Managed Structure   A member-managed LLC typically allows for the company's members to take an active role in the management of the company's affairs. Retaining a high degree of control and authority can prove useful in the event of a dispute among the members; however, giving too many members the opportunity to participate in low-level business decisions can result in the entity's inability to make ordinary day-to-day management decisions. As a result, in a member-managed structure, the operating agreement generally sets forth certain decisions that may be made by a select group of members (or delegate such decisions to officers of the company), with only the most important decisions requiring the consent of a percentage of the members.

Manager-Managed Structure   A manager-managed governance structure resembles that of a corporation. As its name indicates, one or more managers are appointed to oversee the operations of the company. The extent of the manager's authority is delineated in the operating agreement, which generally affords the manager control over all of the day-to-day affairs of the company. All decisions that are not properly approved by the manager generally require the consent of the members.

Following are examples of actions that a manager of a manager-managed LLC frequently will be required to submit to the members for approval:

- ► Merger of the LLC with or into another company
- ► Sale of all or substantially all of the assets of the LLC
- ► Material amendment of the LLC operating agreement
- ► Issuance of additional equity and admission of new members
- ► Compensation of the manager
- ► Dissolution of the LLC

Legal Liability

In most states, investors in an LLC enjoy the same limited liability as that of corporate shareholders. As a result, each investor is only at risk for the amount of money or property that he, she, or it invests. Although this limitation does not apply to an owner's personal negligence (such as for medical malpractice), it provides comfort to investors that may not be intimately involved in the day-to-day operations of the urgent care business.

Tax Consequences

LLCs have the option to be taxed as a corporation or a partnership. Given the double-tax structure applicable to C corporations, most LLCs elect to retain the default tax status as a partnership. Consequently, for most LLCs, profits are taxed only at the member level (not the LLC level), and no additional income tax is owed when profits are distributed to the members. Although it is generally not advisable for an urgent care company to do so, there may be limited situations where an LLC could be taxed as a corporation. In those circumstances, it almost always makes sense for the entity also to make an election to be taxed as an S corporation where possible.

Professional Entities

Most states have adopted separate statutes with laws exclusively applicable to licensed professionals. These entities are referred to as professional corporations, professional associations, and professional limited liability companies. Professional organization statutes require that each of the entity's owners be licensed to engage in the same professional practice. Consequently, all shareholders of an urgent care company organized as a professional corporation are required to maintain an active license to practice medicine in the state where the entity is formed. Professional statutes also prohibit the entity from carrying on any activity that is unrelated to the professional practice in which the owners are licensed to perform. As a result, an urgent care business operating as a professional LLC is only entitled to perform professional medical services. Although some statutes allow it, it is uncertain whether an urgent care entity would even be permitted to engage in the rendering of physical therapy (which seems to have become quite common).

Most states do not require that a medical practice be conducted in a professional organization. Because of the operational and ownership limitations imposed on such organizations, it is generally preferable to avoid the professional organization if one's state allows. Not only will doing so provide for a smoother path for expansion (by attracting unlicensed investors), but it will also enable the company to diversify into other lines of business that may not fall within the express statutory definition of the practice of medicine.

Legal Liability

The legal liability of an owner of a professional entity is identical to that previously discussed for the nonprofessional entity. Thus, a member of a professional LLC is subject to the same liability risk as a member of a traditional LLC, and the same goes for shareholders of a professional corporation. It should be noted again, however, that a provider who renders care to patients (in any entity) remains personally liable for his or her own professional negligence. Because this risk is unavoidable, urgent care companies should ensure that adequate insurance is obtained.

Tax Consequences

As is the case with legal liability, professional entities are taxed in the same manner as their nonprofessional counterparts. One potentially divergent entity-structuring consideration, however, exists in those states where the medical practice is required to be operated as a professional corporation. In those states, it is almost always beneficial for the urgent care company to elect to be taxed as an S corporation. Because by virtue of state law the entity will not be entitled to admit nonphysician owners, the entity will not have the opportunity to accept an investment from an entity. Consequently, the S corporation limitation restricting ownership to individuals will have no negative impact on the entity. Furthermore, a portion of an S corporation's income generally escapes payroll taxation if such income is distributed as dividends to the shareholders rather than as salary (as is generally required by an LLC).

Although professional entities may not be preferable because of the applicable ownership restrictions, experienced legal counsel can typically suggest entity-structuring techniques to avoid some of the regulatory hardships. For an additional discussion on a few of these techniques, see Chapter 8 ("Corporate Practice of Medicine and Other Legal Impediments to Nonphysician Ownership").

CONCLUSION

Much of the legal planning associated with urgent care companies is driven by state health-care regulation, legal liability, and tax concerns. In all cases where the choice of entity is not prescribed by applicable state law, the LLC is generally the preferred choice. The governance provisions are flexible, and the owners benefit from the single-level tax regimen applicable to partnerships, all while enjoying the limited liability attributes of a corporation. Furthermore, most states permit an urgent care practice to be conducted through an LLC. In many cases, this is true even in states that previously required that all professional services be rendered through a professional organization.[8]

If the urgent care company (or the management company in states that have adopted the corporate practice of medicine doctrine) chooses to operate as an LLC, the decisions regarding federal tax classification should be made within 75 days of company formation.[9] If the owners anticipate attempting to attract sophisticated investors who will invest through entities, remaining taxed as a partnership (the default status) is likely the preferred choice. If, however, the owners foresee that only individual owners will be involved, it may be prudent to elect to be taxed as an S corporation. Owners should confer with their tax professionals before making any decisions regarding entity and tax classification.

---

8   This is likely true even though the state may have adopted the corporate practice of medicine or a similar doctrine. Owners should consult with counsel to determine regulatory limitations to entity planning.

9   This is the deadline to elect S corporation status without requesting relief for late filing.

Although the preformation entity analysis may initially appear overwhelming, much of the guesswork will be eliminated by consulting competent advisors. Because of the potential financial and legal implications of the decision, the initial choices pertaining to entity selection should not be taken lightly.

KEY POINTS

1. One of the most important decisions in the life cycle of an urgent care business is made before the first patient is treated.
2. Owners of urgent care centers in one state may face a different set of unique challenges from those in another.
3. Corporations and limited liability companies (LLCs), including professional corporations and professional LLCs, are the most common entity choices in the urgent care industry.
4. Owners of corporations are referred to as shareholders or stockholders, whereas owners of LLCs are referred to as members.
5. In general, partnerships do not offer the same liability protection as do LLCs or corporations.
6. Ownership restrictions associated with operating as an S corporation may make this option unattractive to urgent care owners focused on growth.
7. LLCs are either member-managed or manager-managed, and in most cases certain decisions must be approved by at least a majority of the members.
8. Although professional entities may not be preferable because of their restrictions on ownership, experienced health-care and corporate attorneys can typically suggest entity-structuring techniques to avoid some of the regulatory hardships.
9. If the urgent care company chooses to operate as an LLC, decisions regarding federal tax classification should be made within 75 days of company formation.
10. Although in many states choice of entity type is driven by applicable regulations, most urgent care center operators tend to choose LLCs.

CHAPTER 7

Exit Transactions: The Process of Selling an Urgent Care Company

Adam Winger

ALL GOOD INVESTMENTS MUST come to an end. Options for exiting an investment in an urgent care company include transitioning the business to younger generations in the owner's family, selling the company's equity or assets to one or more third parties, or simply ceasing all business operations.

Over the past several years, the exit strategy of choice in the urgent care industry has been the sale to outside investors. This is not surprising in light of the elevated purchase prices that have resulted from the investment interest of private equity investors, hospital systems, and insurance companies.

Although the potential to receive retirement-type money is appealing, the prospect of ending your relationship with a company that has consumed years (and potentially decades) of your life can be both overwhelming and emotional. Further complicating the process of selling your own company in the urgent care context are the many unique regulatory challenges to be overcome to transfer ownership of the business.

This chapter introduces a variety of these challenges. Specifically, it addresses issues relating to transaction structuring, tax, and liability of the seller after the conclusion of the sale. Although the process of selling a business is never without stress, planning for these issues will lead to a smooth transaction that benefits both seller and buyer.

TRANSACTION MECHANICS

Before delving into the various substantive aspects of an urgent care transaction, it may be helpful to provide a bit of context for the discussion. Nearly all urgent care transactions involve the following chronology:

1. Execution of a confidentiality and nondisclosure agreement
2. Completion of preliminary due diligence by the buyer
3. Negotiation and execution of a letter of intent

4. Completion of further diligence by the buyer
5. Negotiation and execution of a purchase agreement and various ancillary agreements
6. Closing of the transaction

Confidentiality and Nondisclosure Agreement

Before an urgent care seller turns over any confidential information concerning the business, it will generally require that the buyer enter into a confidentiality and nondisclosure agreement. These agreements are frequently referred to as CAs or NDAs.

As their titles suggest, these agreements generally establish the ground rules for the buyer's use and disclosure of the seller's confidential information furnished during the course of the parties' relationship. Although the format of these documents varies, most provide for

- A prohibition against disclosure of confidential information
- A definition (which can be somewhat lengthy) of the term *confidential information*
- Limited exceptions to the prohibition against disclosure
- Obligations of the parties if the transaction is not closed
- Legal remedies on a breach of the agreement
- Various miscellaneous provisions including the procedure for amending the agreement

In some situations, it makes sense for the disclosure prohibitions to apply to both the buyer and seller. For example, the seller may require evidence confirming that the buyer is capable of paying the purchase price when the transaction closes. This may involve a comfort letter from the buyer's accountant or provision by the buyer of confidential financial information such as bank statements or bank commitment letter. In these situations, the agreement should provide for mutual disclosure prohibitions.

The following paragraph is an example of a typical provision restricting disclosure of confidential information:

> The party receiving Confidential Information [defined elsewhere in the agreement] shall not: (a) except as otherwise provided herein, disclose, disseminate, communicate, or otherwise publish any Confidential Information received under this Agreement to any third party without the prior written consent of the disclosing party; (b) disclose the fact that Confidential Information has been made available under this Agreement; or (c) use any portion of the Confidential Information for any purpose other than evaluating and implementing the proposed transaction.

Exceptions to the general disclosure prohibition typically include the sharing of information with the receiving party's authorized representatives such as attorneys, accountants, bankers, consultants, and financial advisors, as well as any disclosures required when the receiving party becomes legally compelled to disclose the information.

A final issue frequently addressed in the confidentiality and nondisclosure agreement is the prohibition against either party hiring the employees of the other, typically called a *nonsolicitation* provision. The seller will almost always be required to provide the buyer the right to interview certain of the seller's employees during the buyer's due diligence investigation. If the buyer and the seller operate or plan to operate in competing markets, it is of great importance that the buyer not be entitled to divert or entice away the seller's employees in the event the transaction is not closed. A typical nonsolicitation provision prohibits the buyer (or in some cases both parties) from contacting or attempting to contact active employees and, in some cases, recently terminated employees of the seller within a certain period of time for the purpose of hiring that employee.

Due Diligence

With an executed confidentiality and nondisclosure agreement in place, the parties progress to the due diligence phase. The buyer requests information about the urgent care business from the seller to determine whether to make an offer and the general terms on which the offer will be made. On making the offer and reaching a preliminary agreement under a letter of intent, the buyer will continue with a more detailed review of the diligence information. Although pre- and post-offer diligence is generally conducted in two phases, both are addressed here.

The diligence information requested by experienced buyers is fairly standard, but responding to such requests is time-consuming even for the most seasoned sellers. A diligence request list can range from 2 to 20 pages, and the investigation process may include auditing financial statements and coding practices; reviewing written contracts, organizational documents, and other legal documentation; and interviewing key occupational medicine clients, employees, and medical providers.

It is not uncommon for a practice administrator to spend at least a full workweek responding to preliminary diligence requests and countless hours thereafter responding to follow-up inquiries. In light of these extensive time demands, a seller should ensure that adequate staffing is available to avoid potential disruption to the seller's business. This becomes imperative around flu season, when all resources are needed to successfully operate the business.

To further limit the disruptive effect to the seller's business, the seller and seller's attorney should discuss with the buyer and buyer's attorney how diligence will be conducted. Appointing a single representative from the seller's staff to serve as the diligence point person avoids involving unnecessary personnel and reduces duplication of effort. Another approach involves the furnishing by the seller of a prepared diligence package to each potential buyer. This package will include much of the information that the seller anticipates the buyer will request, such as financial statements and copies or summaries of material contracts. By preparing the diligence package in advance, the seller can strategically determine which information will be provided to the potential buyers. This enables the seller to make the best first impression by presenting favorable information in a clean, organized, and professional manner.

Rather than copying and mailing reams of printed information to the buyer, sellers often use an electronic storage or cloud-based portal, frequently called a *data room*. Among other things, a data room allows the seller both to restrict access to certain information and to monitor who accesses the information and when. Data rooms historically have been hosted by professional technology companies that charge a flat fee or a variable fee based on the amount of information uploaded by the seller and/or the number of users that are afforded access to the information. Fortunately, lower-cost cloud-based options now exist, and parties to a transaction should discuss which options will achieve the desired results. Regardless, the buyer and seller should confirm with their health-care attorney that the uploading, storage, and sharing of information through such an online portal will not violate applicable patient privacy laws.

Using an online diligence platform that enables the seller to track which documents were provided to the buyer (and preferably when the documents were accessed by the buyer) could also reduce post-transaction litigation. For example, assume the seller is successful in negotiating for the inclusion of an *anti-sandbagging* provision. This provision prevents the buyer from suing the seller for a breach of certain provisions (representations and warranties) of the purchase agreement if the buyer knows at the time the transaction is closed that the seller was in breach of such provision.[1] Suppose the buyer requires that seller state (or *represent*) that the financial statements presented to the buyer are "true, complete, and correct." If the buyer is aware that although the accounts receivable are presented as $250,000 on the balance sheet, they are actually only $150,000, an anti-sandbagging provision would prevent the buyer from later suing for the seller's breach of the representation that the accounts receivable were "true, complete, and correct" as presented in the financial statements. A data room provides the seller with a mechanism to prove the extent of the buyer's knowledge. By having not only a record of the specific documents that were made available to the buyer but also the precise time at which those documents were downloaded or reviewed by the buyer, the seller is better able to make use of the protections afforded by the anti-sandbagging provision (and other applicable provisions of law). Continuing with this example, if the seller is able to show that the buyer reviewed an accounts receivable aging analysis as of the closing date and thus the

---

[1] Because of the risk to the buyer, it is generally rare that a seller will be successful in negotiating for the inclusion of an anti-sandbagging provision. Given the current leverage enjoyed by urgent care sellers in the marketplace, however, it is well worth the effort to make the request.

buyer knew that the accounts receivable were overstated, the seller may be able to protect itself from a later suit for breach.

Although responding to information requests can be burdensome and time consuming, the importance of the diligence phase cannot be overstated. The buyer's due diligence gives the buyer the only look into the operations of the seller's business, and it is during that time that the buyer assesses and attempts to quantify the risk perceived in acquiring the business. Such risk involves not only what the buyer can uncover in reviewing the information provided by the seller but also any undisclosed or undetected risk of a lawsuit or other potential financial loss that may arise after the closing of the transaction. The buyer will reach conclusions that are based not only on the information presented but also on the manner in which the seller conducts its business. The seller can significantly reduce the buyer's perceived risk by presenting itself in an organized and competent manner. For instance, if the information furnished is sloppy or incomplete or the seller's response is untimely, the buyer may draw broader conclusions regarding the owner's lack of attention to detail, which may justify a downward valuation adjustment. Although a full analysis of the diligence process is beyond the scope of this chapter, here are a few items generally included in diligence request lists as well as comments on how such items may result in further valuation adjustments.

▶ *Organizational documents*   The buyer will want to review the company's key organizational documents (and any subsequent amendments), such as the certificate or articles filed to form the company, any agreement among the owners (shareholders' agreement or operating agreement), the company's minute book, an organizational chart showing subsidiary or affiliated companies, and a schedule explaining the company's ownership. In general, the buyer's concerns with this information are regarding the seller's authority to sell, any arrangements that may require payment on the closing of the transaction, and the proper organization of the company. Although having all such documents immediately on hand may not be necessary, the seller should be in a position to quickly access and assemble the information.

▶ *Governmental filings*   The buyer will want to confirm, at a minimum, that the seller maintains all appropriate licenses, permits, certificates, registrations, supervision or collaboration agreements and protocols for midlevel providers, Drug Enforcement Administration numbers, and provider numbers. If any such document or number has lapsed or been revoked or suspended for any reason, the buyer will request an explanation. It may be prudent for the seller to maintain a log containing all such documents, permits, and licenses required for the seller to operate its business, their respective renewal or expiration dates, and any other pertinent information concerning the documents.

- *Material contracts* The buyer will request to review all of the seller's material contracts. This will include loan documents, payer agreements, occupational medicine contracts, equipment and real property leases, joint venture agreements, malpractice and general liability insurance contracts, employment agreements, noncompetition agreements, and marketing agreements. In addition to confirming that each agreement is currently in effect (not expired) as of the date of the request, the buyer will be reviewing each agreement to determine (1) whether the agreement requires the consent of, or notice to, the other party (landlord, equipment lessor, etc.) in the event the transaction is closed and (2) how quickly the contract can be terminated if the buyer does not intend to assume it.[2] Any contract resulting in revenue to the company (occupational medicine, on-site clinic, etc.) that has expired will likely result in a downward adjustment to the purchase price if such price was determined by reference to the company's revenue or earnings (i.e., multiple of EBITDA [earnings before interest, tax, depreciation, and amortization]). Furthermore, a contract that either is not in compliance with laws (such as the Stark law [also called the physician self-referral law] or the federal Medicare and Medicaid anti-kickback statute) or requires the consent of a third party that may be difficult to obtain could result in the buyer abandoning the transaction or in a material delay in the transaction's closing.

- *Financial and business information* The buyer will generally request financial information for the previous 3 to 5 years. This may include financial statements (balance sheet, income statement, and statement of cash flows), accounts receivable aging analysis by payer, bad debt and charge-off schedules by payer, profit and loss by service line (urgent care versus occupational medicine), key business metrics (patients per day, charges and collections per patient), evidence of payer mix by center, schedules of assets and liabilities, schedule of 20 largest suppliers, schedule of 20 largest occupational medicine clients, and employee compensation and bonus schedules. Having this type of information either ready or readily accessible will be viewed favorably by a knowledgeable buyer, but an owner's ability to convey the information without review (showing mastery of the business) is potentially more important.

- *Employee matters* The buyer may want to perform a more detailed review of employment agreements, independent contractor agreements, noncompetition agreements, bonus and other incentive plans, 401(k) and other retirement and profit-sharing plans, equity compensation plans, employees and contractors lists, lists of physicians and other providers, staffing schedules, and the seller's employee handbook or policies and procedures

---

2   The considerations and analysis of material contracts are different for buyers of urgent care assets and buyers of equity of the urgent care company.

manual. Employee records should be maintained along with all applicable agreements, and acceptable safeguards should be implemented to prevent theft of employee information. The buyer will be concerned not only with the seller's past business practices and financial obligations relating to payroll but also with whether the employee benefits it intends to offer will be competitive with those currently offered by seller.

- *Litigation* The buyer will want to know about any active or pending litigation, administrative proceedings, or governmental investigations as well as any acts or omissions that the seller believes may lead to litigation or an investigation. Because the potential liability in litigation is largely unpredictable, the seller's valuation could decrease substantially on account of an unresolved legal matter. As a result, it frequently makes sense for all claims to be settled prior to considering the sale of an urgent care business.

Letter of Intent

If on preliminary review of the due diligence information the buyer decides to move forward with the acquisition, it will do so by extending a nonbinding offer in the form of a letter of intent. The letter of intent is often referred to as a term sheet, LOI, offer letter, or a memorandum of understanding.

The letter of intent provides the basic terms and conditions on which a transaction will be effected and generally sets the stage for the more detailed purchase agreement to be proposed by the buyer. The letter of intent will include, among other things, the purchase price, the transaction structure the buyer intends to employ (discussed in the section "Transaction Structure" in this chapter), the plan to transition the business, and certain other obligations of the parties.

Most provisions in the letter of intent will be nonbinding (such as the buyer's obligation to pay the purchase price and the seller's obligation to turn over the business), but because of the time and money the buyer expends during the due diligence phase, the buyer often negotiates for certain terms to be enforceable. For example, buyers frequently require that the seller agree to an exclusivity provision prohibiting the seller from marketing the company while the letter of intent remains in effect. Other enforceable provisions may include an obligation of both parties to negotiate in good faith, a requirement that each party respects the confidential nature of the information shared, a requirement that the buyer be given adequate access to complete its diligence review, and a promise that the seller operate the company in a manner consistent with its past practices. It is appropriate to note, however, that each of these provisions is subject to negotiation, and sellers may find it useful to limit or expand the enforceable provisions under the letter of intent.

Purchase Agreement

On both parties' execution of the letter of intent, the buyer's attorney prepares the initial draft of a purchase agreement. Depending on the structure of the transaction, an urgent care purchase agreement can take the form of either a stock purchase agreement or an asset purchase agreement.

The purchase agreement contains all of the binding provisions on which the transaction will be consummated. A typical urgent care purchase agreement addresses the following concepts:

- The assets or stock to be purchased
- The liabilities, if any, to be assumed by the buyer
- Various *representations and warranties* of the parties
- Additional obligations (or *covenants*) of the parties
- Various conditions relating to the closing of the transaction
- The procedure for closing of the transaction
- Obligations of the parties to indemnify (or make whole) the other party in the event of a breach of certain terms of the agreement

As the party preparing the initial draft of the purchase agreement, the buyer often has the upper hand in the beginning stages of negotiating the transaction. Because the seller is put in a position of responding to the proposed purchase agreement, each sentence of the document must be closely scrutinized to ensure that the terms are consistent with the letter of intent and that they do not inappropriately benefit the buyer.

If, on reviewing the document, the parties disagree on several major business issues, it is generally recommended that the buyer and seller, along with their attorneys, discuss these issues rather than having the seller's attorney propose wholesale revisions to the agreement. Not only do such revisions drive up legal expenses but they also can create tension between the parties if not accompanied with appropriate explanations. After all major deal points are resolved, both parties' attorneys will begin trading drafts of the purchase agreement and negotiating the finer legal points in consultation with their clients until a final agreement is reached and executed.

Ancillary Agreements

Buyers and sellers need to negotiate and execute, in addition to the main purchase agreement, several other documents to close the transaction. Among these documents are the following:

- *Bill of sale* Used by the seller to transfer any tangible personal property purchased by the buyer (generally not executed by the buyer).
- *Assignment and assumption agreement* Executed to transfer any contracts purchased by the seller. As suggested by the document's name, such

contracts will be transferred or *assigned* to the buyer, and the liabilities under those contracts will generally be *assumed* by the buyer.

- *Noncompetition agreement*   If provisions governing the seller's ability to compete with the buyer after the transaction closes are not included in the purchase agreement, they frequently will be detailed in a separate document executed by both parties.

- *Escrow agreement*   If the parties negotiated for the use of an escrow agent, an escrow agreement will be entered into to provide instructions to the agent regarding the disbursement of any escrowed funds. Buyers request that funds be escrowed to ensure that a portion of the purchase price remains available to satisfy obligations of the seller after closing.

- *Management services agreement or lease agreement*   The concepts underlying these documents are discussed in the section "Management Services Agreement or Lease Agreement" in this chapter, but in general, to avoid the financial risk of closing the transaction without appropriate payer contracts being in effect and physician credentialing being complete, buyers and sellers generally agree to certain management or leasing arrangements whereby the seller agrees to manage the center consistent with its past practices for an agreed-on period.

Depending on the complexity of the transaction, the number and sophistication of the ancillary agreements will vary. When the time and energy associated with the ancillary agreements is added to that needed to finalize the confidentiality and nondisclosure agreement, the diligence process, the letter of intent, and the purchase agreement, it is not surprising that closing a sale of an urgent care business transaction can take several months. The process can be disruptive, exhausting, and, during flu season, impossible for physician–owners who continue to treat patients throughout the process. As a result, physicians should consider the impact on their practice before engaging in the process. Although the loss of patients may be insignificant to the seller if the transaction closes, the seller must always consider the long-term risk to the company if the parties walk away from the deal.

TRANSACTION STRUCTURE

Urgent care transactions generally take the form of either an equity acquisition or an asset acquisition.

Equity Acquisitions

Equity acquisitions involve the sale of the equity owned by the urgent care company's seller. Equity represents the seller's ownership in the urgent care company and may take the form of stock, units membership interests, or partnership interests. Transactions involving the sale of equity offer several tax and state law advantages to sellers but are generally not favored by buyers.

Tax Considerations

From a federal income tax perspective, in almost all circumstances the sale of equity results in either capital gain or loss. As of the publication date of this book, transactions involving capital assets are broken down into two distinct categories for federal income tax purposes on the basis of the owner's holding period. An owner's holding period begins on the date the owner acquires the equity and ends on the date of sale. If the owner's holding period is shorter than 12 months, the transaction is subject to the rates applicable to short-term capital transactions. If the holding period is longer than 12 months, the owner is subject to the preferential rate tables applicable to long-term capital transactions.

In general, gains from short-term capital transactions are taxed at the taxpayer's ordinary income tax rate. Consequently, all sales proceeds received from a short-term equity sale are subject to tax just as though the owner earned the income at his or her job.

In January 2013, the American Taxpayer Relief Act of 2012 made permanent (that is, until the next time the legislature changes them) the rates applicable to long-term capital transactions. Beginning in 2013, the maximum long-term capital gains rate applicable to an urgent care equity sale is 20%. This rate applies to all married couples filing joint returns whose adjusted gross income exceeds $450,000. Married couples with adjusted gross income of less than $450,000 are subject to a lower capital gains rate of 15%.

To the extent sales proceeds are received over time, a seller could effectively limit the amount that is subject to the 20% level. If the seller ensures that the proceeds, when added with all of the seller's income from all other sources, do not exceed the applicable annual threshold, the seller's sale proceeds will remain taxed at the 15% level. Other considerations applicable to installment sales are addressed later in this chapter.

Liability Considerations

Aside from the tax benefits, state law also offers post-transaction liability protections to sellers of equity in urgent care transactions. From a state law perspective, an equity purchaser steps into the shoes of the seller. The urgent care entity will stay in existence and the tax identification number will remain unchanged. The effect of this carryover process is that the purchaser, by operation of law, inherits (or assumes) all of the known and unknown liabilities of the seller. Although the transaction document itself may attempt to limit the seller's liability, in general, an equity sale is a best-case scenario for an urgent care seller—he or she gets to walk away without worrying about future legal claims against the company.

The natural corollary to the seller's benefit is the obvious potential burden to the purchaser. On the effective date of the transaction (or the day after), an equity purchaser becomes responsible for any and all existing and future liabilities related to the urgent care company. Perhaps the most significant of these risks relate to malpractice, improper billing practices, the rendering of medically unnecessary services and other regulatory risks, risks associated with unpaid tax obligations, overtime and other employee claims, and the risk of reimbursement or refund to private payers. Of course, appropriate insurance can limit each of these risks, but the potential exposure to the organization can never be fully quantified. As a result of this unlimited hypothetical risk, it is of little surprise that buyers generally require that urgent care transactions be structured as asset acquisitions.

Asset Acquisitions

Tax Considerations

As in an equity transaction, sellers of assets generally are afforded capital gain or loss treatment on the sale of all or substantially all of the assets of an urgent care business. Exceptions to this general rule exist for organizations taxed as C corporations and for sale of certain assets by entities taxed as a partnership for federal income tax purposes.[3]

If the urgent care company operates as a C corporation, the asset sale is taxed both at the corporate 35% level (no preferential capital gain treatment for the sale of the corporation's assets) and again as a dividend when the proceeds are distributed to the shareholder at the 15% or 20% level, depending on the owner's income. If the company operates as a limited liability company or a partnership, generally only the portions of the sales proceeds that are allocated to *hot assets* (that is, accounts receivable and unsold inventory) are subject to unfavorable, ordinary income tax rates. All other proceeds are generally taxed at capital gains rates, and if the owner has held its investment for over 12 months, the maximum capital gains rate of 20% applies.

Liability Considerations

Unlike the case in equity transactions, purchasers in an asset deal are able to pick and choose both the assets they wish to purchase and the liabilities they intend to assume. Typically, the description of the assets purchased in an urgent care transaction will be similar to this: "Purchaser shall purchase all assets used or useful by Seller in connection with Seller's operation of the urgent care business." This broad description results in the purchaser acquiring substantially the same assets it would in an equity purchase, but without the unlimited downside risk associated with the liabilities.

Purchasers generally disclaim all responsibility for liabilities relating to an event that took place prior to the closing of the transaction. For example, the purchase agreement may state that "Purchaser shall have no responsibility to satisfy any claim, loss, or damage if the act or omission giving rise to such claim, loss, or damage occurred prior to the closing date of the transaction." The effect of such a provision is that liability is effectively divided between the parties as of

---

3   Unless a limited liability company (LLC) elects otherwise, it will be taxed as a partnership for federal income tax purposes.

the closing date with the purchaser becoming liable only for those events occurring after the closing.

Because only the assets are purchased (not the entity and its tax identification number), the purchaser's entity will need to enter into new payer contracts (or add the site to its existing contracts), recredential the center's physicians under those contracts, and enter into new supplier agreements and malpractice coverage to operate the urgent care business. Perhaps of most concern to urgent care buyers is the risk that they will be unable to finalize the contracting and credentialing process before taking over the operations of the business. As any urgent care owner knows, the potential financial impact of operating a center without the ability to properly bill payers can be devastating. To mitigate these risks, asset purchasers generally attempt to negotiate one of the following two approaches.

Delayed Sign and Close

The *delayed (or deferred) sign and close* approach is generally considered the more buyer-friendly of the two approaches. Under a transaction providing for a delayed sign and close, the buyer and seller sign the asset purchase agreement, but the closing of the transaction (when the buyer pays the purchase price and the seller turns over title to the assets) does not occur until some later time. The gap between signing and closing is designed to give the purchaser sufficient time to negotiate payer contracts, obtain malpractice coverage, credential providers, and resolve any other issues in anticipation of taking over the operation of the business.

Typical sticking points in the delayed sign and close asset purchase agreement involve the negotiation of the events that permit the buyer to walk away during the period between signing and closing. In legal terms, these events are generally referred to as *conditions to closing* or *conditions precedent to closing*. For example, the asset purchase agreement may state that the buyer has no obligation to close the transaction if the buyer is not able to enter into new payer contracts with all of the third-party payers from which the seller receives payment as of the closing (or signing) date, or if the buyer is not able to recruit and credential a number of providers necessary to operate the center in a manner consistent with the seller's past practices.

Because this approach allocates much of the risk associated with the buyer's ability to take over the business to the seller, the seller will want to confine or limit these conditions. For example, with respect to the buyer's entry into new payer contracts, the seller may want to state that so long as the buyer enters into contracts with payers accounting for 75% of the private-pay revenue, then the buyer will be required to close. Conditions to closing are always a point of heavy negotiation, and a seller should begin contemplating responses to the anticipated requests from the date it first understands how the buyer intends to structure the transaction.

Management Services Agreement or Lease Agreement

The second of the two most common approaches involves the buyer and the seller entering into a management services agreement or what is sometimes referred to as a support services agreement or an office, equipment, and personnel lease agreement. Under these arrangements, the buyer and seller close the transaction before the buyer is able to complete its contracting and credentialing processes. Because at closing the buyer is not in a position to bill payers for the services rendered at the centers, it requires that the seller agree to an arrangement whereby the buyer (now the owner of all the urgent care assets) leases the assets back to the seller and the buyer performs all nonmedical services relating to the business. Under the arrangement, the seller continues to provide medical services and bill payers under its existing payer contracts. This arrangement is described in a management services agreement. In exchange for the buyer's leasing of the assets and the performance of the nonclinical services, the buyer is paid a management fee or rental fee. At the time when the buyer has appropriately credentialed the providers and entered into its payer contracts, the management services agreement terminates and the buyer begins to operate the facility.

Because of the complexity of either approach (or similar alternatives), each party's obligations prior to and after closing should be set forth in great detail in either the purchase agreement or one of the ancillary agreements. Specifically, the duration of the management services agreement, the length of time between signing and closing, and all conditions to closing should be addressed at length prior to execution of documents.

INDEMNIFICATION

In either an asset acquisition or an equity acquisition, the parties will need to address their respective liabilities after the closing of the transaction. In general, the liability of the buyer to the seller after closing is minimal. Aside from the buyer's failure to satisfy obligations of the seller that the buyer expressly agreed to assume in the purchase agreement, there are few instances where the buyer owes the seller any additional money. The seller's exposure, however, can be substantially greater.

The term indemnification refers to an obligation of a party to compensate the other for losses incurred by the other. In the mergers and acquisitions context, the potential for a seller to be obligated to indemnify the buyer for the buyer's losses can add significant risk to the seller. In the most basic of examples, assume an urgent care transaction is closed in which the buyer purchases the assets of the seller. In the transaction, the buyer agrees to pay all liabilities occurring after the closing date but assumes no responsibility for acts or omissions occurring before closing. Within a week after closing the transaction, a malpractice claim is filed against a physician and the seller's entity for negligent care rendered prior to closing. Because the negligent act occurred before the closing date, in all cases the seller will remain responsible for all uninsured damages resulting from the claim because the transaction was structured as an asset sale. Assume, however, that the buyer is named as a plaintiff in the suit under a theory of successor liability (legal theory under which even an asset purchaser can become liable for seller's past acts), and as a result, the buyer spends $50,000 defending itself before being dismissed from the suit. Typically, the seller would be obligated to "indemnify" the buyer for the $50,000 of legal expenses that the buyer incurred in connection with the malpractice suit.

The main source for potential seller indemnification liability arises from breaches of its representations and warranties.

Representations and Warranties

Representations are factual statements made by sellers concerning the urgent care business or the seller's company as of the date the purchase agreement is signed or the transaction is closed. *Warranties* refer to the seller's commitment to stand behind its representations. For example, a buyer's initial draft of the purchase agreement may require that the seller represent that it is in full compliance with all applicable laws, rules, and regulations. If, after the transaction is closed, it becomes clear that the seller was not in fact in full compliance, and the buyer incurs financial loss as a result of such noncompliance, the seller will be obligated to indemnify the buyer for the loss incurred by the buyer. In reviewing the initial draft of the purchase agreement, the seller will want to lessen its potential exposure under the various representations.

For example, the seller's lawyer may revise the representation concerning the seller's legal compliance by adding the language shown here in italics: "*to the seller's knowledge*, it is in *material [delete 'full']* compliance with all applicable laws, rules, regulations *material to the operation of the seller's business*." As revised, the seller's representation is simply that as of the closing (or signing) date, the seller is not aware that it is violating any law that would keep it from operating. This is much more favorable to the seller than a statement that the seller is in full compliance with all laws. Of course, this shifts the risk of noncompliance to the buyer, and buyers predictably resist such a change.

By broadening or softening the representations, the seller reduces the risk that its statement of facts will be found to be untrue. As a result, the risk that it will be required to compensate the buyer as a result of the untrue representation (or "indemnify" the buyer) is significantly reduced.

Other standard representations made by the seller relate to the accuracy of financial information and the nonexistence of any of the following that may affect the urgent care business:

- ▶ Litigation
- ▶ Environmental issues
- ▶ Employee disputes
- ▶ Employee compensation obligations
- ▶ Unpaid taxes
- ▶ Involvement of brokers in the transaction

Survival Period

If the buyer includes a provision in the purchase agreement that the representations and warranties survive closing, the seller will be indefinitely liable (or liable until the end of the applicable statute of limitations) for the factual statements it made in the purchase agreement. To further reduce the seller's post-closing risk, the seller's attorney will negotiate to limit the *survival period* of the seller's representations and warranties.

For example, assume that 4 years after the closing (ignoring any applicable statute of limitations), an employee claims that overtime was improperly calculated by the seller. To avoid any employee disruption, the buyer pays the overtime. Because the purchase agreement includes a representation by the seller that all employee compensation liabilities were satisfied as of the closing date, and also that all representations survive closing, the buyer could seek indemnification for the amount of the overtime in addition to any legal fees it incurs to pursue the indemnity suit.

Although certain representations will generally survive for extended periods, most urgent care representations will survive anywhere from 12 to 24 months. As is the case with all contract terms, however, survival periods are subject to negotiation, and sellers should be intensely focused on limiting this period.

Indemnification Baskets

Sellers can further limit post-closing liability through the use of *baskets*. Indemnification baskets are essentially triggers; they set forth a minimum amount that must be exceeded before any indemnification obligations of the seller arise. For example, the purchase agreement might state that "the buyer may not assert any claim for indemnification unless the aggregate amount of all buyer's losses which, without this provision, would give rise to such a claim for indemnification, exceed $50,000." The purpose of the basket is to prevent the buyer from coming to the seller for minor charges such as a minor miscount in supplies or pharmaceutical inventory and also to shift a portion of the post-closing risk to the seller.

Baskets generally come in two forms: tipping and deductible. Continuing with the same example, a deductible basket would provide that the seller is to be liable for losses only to the extent such losses exceed the $50,000 trigger. The *tipping basket* (sometimes called a *threshold deductible*), on the other hand, would provide that once the $50,000 trigger point is crossed, the buyer can seek indemnification for all damages (including the amount of the $50,000 basket), rather than merely the excess over the $50,000. The tipping basket can be expressed as follows: "Buyer may not assert any claim for indemnification unless the aggregate amount of all Buyer's losses which, without this provision, would give rise to such a claim for indemnification, exceed $50,000, provided, however, that if the aggregate of all such losses exceeds such amount, Seller shall be liable for all such losses."

Another possibility is the use of a partially deductible basket. Under this approach, when the applicable losses exceed the amount of the basket, the seller is responsible for all subsequent losses, but only a portion of the losses that make up the basket must be paid by the seller. Such a provision can be expressed as follows: "Buyer may not assert any claim for indemnification unless the aggregate amount of all Buyer's losses which, without this provision, would give rise to such a claim for indemnification, exceed $50,000, provided, however, that if the aggregate of all such losses exceeds such amount, seller shall be liable for only the amount of such losses that exceeds $25,000."

The basket is an effective mechanism to ensure that the buyer is not harassing the seller for immaterial claims for losses (e.g., the cost of five pencils) and is also a way to shift a portion of the post-closing liability from the seller to the buyer. Perhaps the best way to limit post-closing indemnification risk, however, is to negotiate a cap on all such claims.

Indemnification Cap

Indemnification caps establish a ceiling for the seller's future indemnity liability. Without a cap, a seller could be at risk for more than the seller received in the transaction. Caps are frequently expressed in terms of percentages of the purchase price. For example, the purchase agreement might state that "the maximum aggregate liability of Seller to Buyer for all indemnification claims to which Buyer is entitled to seek indemnification under this Agreement shall be an amount equal to twenty percent (20%) of the Purchase Price."

The buyer may negotiate to carve breaches of certain fundamental representations out of the cap (such as a breach of the representation that the seller's owner had the authority to enter into the transaction), and the seller will desire for all such claims to be counted toward the fulfillment of the cap. In the end, the cap should represent the seller's maximum post-closing liability, and should be considered in conjunction with the scope of the seller's representations, the seller's tax liability as a result of the transaction, and all other potential claims under the purchase agreement.

CONCLUSION

From the confidentiality and nondisclosure agreement to managing the risk of post-closing liability, the process of buying and selling an urgent care practice is anything but simple. Although it is imperative that owners of urgent care companies seek out competent legal and financial representatives to guide them, sellers should understand the process and the various associated risks.

KEY POINTS

1. Nearly all transactions involve the following stages: (1) confidentiality and nondisclosure agreement; (2) preliminary due diligence; (3) letter of intent; (4) further diligence (5) negotiation of purchase agreement and ancillary agreements; and (6) closing the transaction.

2. The confidentiality and nondisclosure agreements establish the ground rules for the buyer's use and disclosure of confidential information disclosed by the seller during the course of the parties' interaction with respect to a potential transaction.

3. The buyer's due diligence provides the buyer with the first full look into the operations of the seller's business, and it is during that time that the buyer determines the offer price for the urgent care company.

4. Although due diligence request lists are fairly standard, responding to such requests can be time consuming for the most experienced of sellers.

5. Before making the decision to market an urgent care company, a seller should ensure that adequate staffing is available to avoid the potential disruption to the seller's business.

6. The letter of intent lays the road map for the transaction, setting forth non-binding provisions concerning purchase price, transaction structure, and other high-level details.

7. The purchase agreement contains the binding provisions on which the transaction will be consummated, and a typical purchase agreement addresses the following concepts: (1) the assets or stock to be purchased; (2) the liabilities, if any, to be assumed by the buyer; (3) the procedure for closing of the transaction; (4) representations and warranties of the parties; (5) additional obligations (covenants) of the parties; (6) various conditions to the closing of the transaction; and (7) obligations of the parties to indemnify (or to make whole) the other party in the event of a breach of certain terms of the agreement.

8. Representations are factual statements the seller makes relating to the seller's business and entity as of the date the purchase agreement is signed and closed. Warranties relate to the seller's agreement to legally stand behind such representations.

9. Two approaches used to manage a buyer's credentialing and contracting risk are the delayed sign and close approach and the management services or lease agreement approach.

10. Post-closing liability to the seller can be limited by such techniques as indemnification baskets, indemnification caps, and limitations to the survival period of representations and warranties.

CHAPTER 8

Corporate Practice of Medicine and Other Legal Impediments to Nonphysician Ownership

Adam Winger

STATE HEALTH-CARE LAWS OFTEN have a dramatic impact on the legal structuring of an urgent care business. This chapter focuses on the legal issues confronted when entities or nonphysician individuals attempt to own an equity interest in an urgent care company. Although the discussion is directed largely toward those in the startup phase, it should also be helpful to those considering either growing their business outside the state in which they currently operate or accepting an investment from one or more nonphysicians.

Several statutory and common law principles limit a layperson's ownership of a company engaged in the business of practicing medicine. Although the principles that have found their ways into state statutes and case law share several fundamental commonalities, each state has devised its own approach to confronting the concerns with unlicensed persons owning interests in medical practices. This fragmented regulatory approach leads to frustration in the urgent care community, especially for those in the startup phase. Having fielded dozens of calls from prospective entrants into the urgent care market, I would like to address this frustration and also provide some insight into the regulatory limitations applicable to ownership of an urgent care business by a nonphysician.

The health-care industry has long been among the most heavily regulated in the United States. From patient privacy laws to the detailed provider licensure and supervision rules, it is clear that our state and federal governments are focused on every aspect of the health-care delivery process. Given the government's intense interest in our medical care, it is of little surprise that the ownership and operation of an urgent care company is also subject to a number of regulatory constraints.

Unfortunately, many of those considering entering the urgent care business are either unaware of or unconcerned with this aspect of the business. In a recent conversation, a prospective client told me, "Owning an urgent care center is really not much different from owning a McDonald's." To this I said, "Although you may be right in some respects, you won't go to jail for owning a McDonald's." The prospective client was exaggerating; I was not.

The nonchalant tone of the McDonald's comment has become somewhat commonplace in my interactions with potential clients, and it continues to disturb me. Anyone entering the urgent care industry should understand that although the industry shares many characteristics of a retail business, the regulations applicable to the medical industry are vast and complex, and the penalties for noncompliance can be devastating. If you are considering involving yourself in the urgent care business, I urge you to gain an understanding of the law before making an investment.

This chapter

- Explains the application and underlying theories of the corporate practice of medicine (CPOM) and similar legal doctrines
- Provides an overview of the common entity and contractual structure used by lay investors in the urgent care setting to comply with the CPOM doctrine
- Gives an overview of potential penalties for noncompliance with the applicable legal provisions

THEORIES UNDERLYING THE CORPORATE PRACTICE OF MEDICINE DOCTRINE

At the forefront of the legal theories restricting a nonphysician's ownership of an urgent care business is the CPOM doctrine. In its most basic form, this doctrine prohibits a corporation from practicing medicine or employing a physician to practice medicine on the corporation's behalf. Although the rationale for this prohibition is explained in a number of ways (several of which are discussed in the following sections), the central concern is that the profit motives of an unlicensed person or entity will somehow interfere with the physician's professional medical judgment. The following questions posed by a Texas judge reflect these and other related concerns that the CPOM doctrine attempts to address by prohibiting the employment of a physician by a business entity:

> To whom does the doctor owe his first duty—the patient or corporation? Who is to preserve the confidential nature of the doctor–patient relationship? What is to prevent or who is to control a private corporation from engaging in mass media advertising in the exaggerated fashion so familiar to every American? Who is to dictate the medical and administrative procedures to be followed? Where do budget considerations end and patient care begin?[1]

---

1 *Garcia v. Texas State Bd. of Medical Examiners,* 384 F. Supp. 434 (W.D.Tex.1974), aff'd, 421 U.S. 995 (1975). See also Texas Attorney General Opinions JM–1042.

In light of these concerns, the CPOM doctrine has been said to serve the following three purposes:

- To protect the physician–patient relationship from interference by unlicensed persons or entities
- To prevent the commercialization of the practice of medicine
- To prevent control of a physician's practice by entities or unlicensed persons[2]

Protecting the Physician–Patient Relationship

One of the central underpinnings of the CPOM doctrine is that a physician's loyalty should not be divided between the patient and the physician's employer. The American Medical Association has stated that "… [t]he relationship between patient and physician is based on trust and gives rise to physicians' ethical obligations to place patients' welfare above their own self-interest *and above obligations to other groups*" [emphasis added]. An employee, on the other hand, is obligated to act in the best interest of the employer.[3] Consequently, a physician's duty to an employer is eternally at odds with the obligation to the patient.[4] As stated by the California attorney general, adding an unlicensed commercial entity between the patient and physician "gives rise to divided loyalties on the part of the professional and would destroy the professional relationship that is based on trust and confidence."[5] At some level, the states that have adopted the CPOM doctrine have determined that the only way to effectively manage the fiduciary conflict between patient and employer is to eliminate the duty owed by the physician to the employer. Those states accomplish this by prohibiting the physician from serving as an employee of a business entity.

Commercialization of the Practice of Medicine

Other objections raised in defense of the CPOM rest in concerns regarding commercialization of the medical industry. The essence of such concerns is that if an unlicensed entity encourages the physician to focus more on advertising, marketing, and profit making, then the quality of the state's health care will diminish. As stated by the American Medical Association, if a business entity is permitted to employ physicians, "…professional standards would be practically destroyed, and professions requiring special training would be commercialized,

---

2   See Fichter A, Owning a piece of the doc: state law restraints on lay ownership of healthcare enterprises, *Journal of Health Law* 2006;39(1):23.
3   American Medical Association, Code of Medical Ethics, Opinion 10.015, stating that the "ethics of any profession is based upon personal or individual responsibility. One who practices a profession is responsible directly to his patient or his client. Hence he cannot properly act in the practice of his vocation as an agent of a corporation or business partnership whose interests in the very nature of the case are commercial in character."
4   See *Carter-Shields v. Alton Health Inst.*, 777 N.E. 2d 948, 956–958.
5   Opinions of the Attorney General of California 08–803 (2008), finding that the employment of a physician "is incongruous in the workings of a professional regulatory licensing scheme which is based on personal qualification, responsibility, and sanction."

to the public detriment." And, stated a bit differently by the South Carolina Supreme Court, "The commercialization of professions would destroy professional standards and the duties of professionals to their clients are incompatible with the commercial interests of business entities."[6]

Corporation Is Not Licensed

It is frequently argued that it is a legal impossibility for a corporation to engage, by itself or through the employment of physicians, in the practice of medicine. The rationale is that a corporation cannot be licensed to practice medicine because only humans are able to satisfy the education, training, and character-screening requirements for obtaining a professional license.[7] Because it is impossible for a corporation to obtain a medical license, it follows that a corporation cannot legally engage in the practice of medicine. Finally, because the acts of the physicians are attributable to the employer, which cannot obtain a medical license, the employment of physicians by business entities is illegal.[8]

STRUCTURING AN URGENT CARE ENTERPRISE

How do the CPOM and related legal doctrines apply to an urgent care business?

Professional Entity Statutes

All 50 states have enacted statutes allowing physicians to practice medicine through professional corporations (PCs), and many have broadened this right to now permit the operation of a professional limited liability company (LLC) or a professional association.[9] Ownership of a professional entity in the medical context is generally limited to licensed physicians.[10] Because the ownership is not "tainted" by unlicensed, profit-seeking persons, exceptions are carved out from the CPOM doctrine permitting employment of a physician by the entity. This exception is compromised, however, when nonphysicians enter the ownership pool.

In addition to the professional entity ownership restrictions and the CPOM doctrine, both of which forbid a layperson from owning an interest in a company that renders medical services, restrictions frequently exist preventing an entity owned by an unlicensed person or entity from sharing in the revenue or profits

---

6   See also *Columbia Physical Therapy, Inc., P.S. v. Benton Franklin Orthopedic Assocs., PLLC*, No. 81734-1 (Wash. 2010), citing *Ezell v. Ritholz*, 198 S.E. 419, 424 (S.C. 1938), stating: "The commercialization of professions would destroy professional standards and that the duties of professionals to their clients are incompatible with the commercial interests of business entities."

7   See 17 *Cumberland Law Review* at 491; see also *Kerner*, 362 Ill. at 454, 200 N.E. 157.

8   See Hall M, Institutional control of physician behavior: legal barriers to healthcare cost containment, *University of Pennsylvania Law Review* 1988;137(431):509–510.

9   See Fichter, at 6.

10 State laws are inconsistent when it comes to whether out-of-state physicians may own an interest in a domestic professional entity, and at least one state (New Jersey) requires that the physician owners all practice in the same or closely related healthcare field. See New Jersey Administrative Code § 13:35-6.16(f)(2), stating, "The professional services offered by each practitioner, whether a partner, member or shareholder, shall be the same or in a closely allied medical or professional healthcare field."

of the medical company. These statutes (called *fee-splitting* statutes) are described in greater detail in the "Fee-Splitting Application" section in this chapter.

Friendly PC Structure

In response to the CPOM ownership restrictions, urgent care businesses frequently use the *friendly PC* structure (also known as the captive PC structure), which involves a two-entity approach. One entity, which I'll call the medical company, is wholly owned by physicians; the other, which I'll call the management company, is owned by one or more unlicensed persons.[11]

Although approaches vary, the medical company is generally organized as a professional entity (usually a PC or a professional LLC), and the management company is an LLC or a corporation. Which entity form is appropriate under the circumstances is driven largely by tax considerations, which are outside the scope of this chapter.

In the friendly PC structure, the medical company and the management company are linked by one or more contracts. Among these contracts is a management services agreement (see the section "Management Services Agreement or Lease Agreement" in Chapter 7, "Exit Transactions: The Process of Selling an Urgent Care Company"). Under the management services agreement, the management company is generally obligated to perform practice-management services for the medical company in exchange for a management fee.

Practice-Management Services

The actual services to be rendered by the management company are described in the agreement, but in general the management company is responsible for handling all of the nonclinical aspects of the medical company's practice. This may include "billing; practice development; negotiating professional services and other contracts; providing nonclinical personnel services; office space and equipment; insurance; accounting and legal services; and similar administrative support."[12] The medical company, on the other hand, is obligated to perform all clinical aspects of the business. This frequently includes rendering of professional medical care to patients, supervision of all health-care providers, ensuring appropriate quality control over clinical operations, hiring and firing of all such providers, operating and supervising laboratory services offered at the center, contracting with public and private payers, and making determinations concerning malpractice insurance.

The division of services in the friendly PC structure is often dictated by state law.[13] For instance, in California, the prohibition of the CPOM doctrine is in-

---

11 Although certain federal and state limitations may apply to a physician's ownership of the management company, the arrangement can generally be structured to allow the physician to participate in both the medical company and the management company.
12 See Fichter, at 10.
13 Both the services and fees set forth in the management services agreement have been the subject of much litigation. Parties should not attempt to negotiate or draft such agreements without the assistance of counsel.

terpreted broadly "to encompass not only direct medical decisions, but 'business' and 'administrative' decisions which have medical implications as well."[14] Specifically, the California medical board has taken the position that it would be impermissible for the management company to perform certain advertising functions for and on behalf of the medical company.[15] Although this interpretation of the CPOM represents a minority view, there are similar restrictions across the country that should be investigated before you draft and negotiate a management services agreement.

Management Service Fee

Perhaps the most difficult aspect of the relationship between the management company and the medical company to address is the determination of the service fee to be paid by the medical company in exchange for management services. State courts and medical boards pay particularly close attention to the structuring and amount of the fee, and an inappropriately constructed fee can violate both the CPOM doctrine and state fee-splitting laws.

Fee-Splitting Application

State fee-splitting laws vary greatly in their language and application, but the most problematic statutes in the urgent care context involve prohibitions against the sharing of professional fees with unlicensed persons or entities. Of particular concern in states that have adopted such statutes are interpretations or specific language that expressly prohibits services fees based on a percentage of the medical company's revenue or profit.

Not only do percentage-based arrangements have the appearance of attempting to leave the unlicensed person or entity in the position of an owner but they also directly tie the compensation of the unlicensed person to the professional services performed by the physician. For these reasons, New York has long maintained a blanket prohibition against paying medical services providers (including entities such as the management company) on the basis of a percentage of either profits or revenue earned by the physician entity.[16]

Rather than investigating the theory and rationale behind fee-splitting laws, it may be useful to analyze the specific provisions of a state statute that directly affects an urgent care management fee. Under Tennessee law

> It is an offense for any licensed physician or surgeon to divide or to agree to divide any fee or compensation of any sort received or charged in the practice of medicine or surgery with any person, without the knowledge

---

14   Materials to the 2011 meeting of the Medical Board of California.
15   Medical Board of California, "Corporate Practice of Medicine," prohibiting "arranging for, advertising, or providing medical services rather than only providing administrative staff and services for a physician's medical practice (non-physician exercising controls over a physician's medical practice, even where physicians own and operate the business)." http://www.mbc.ca.gov/Licensees/Corporate_Practice.aspx.
16   New York State Education Law § 6530 (19).

and consent of the person paying the fee or compensation, or against whom the fee may be charged.[17]

Interpreting the above provision, the Tennessee attorney general found that a physician violated the statute when he paid a management company a fee based on a percentage of that physician's collections.[18] Because this conclusion is foreseeable in any state with this type of statutory provision, any urgent care company operating (or considering operating) in a state that has such a statute should consult a competent health-care attorney before proceeding. Fortunately for Tennessee urgent care providers (or perhaps more accurately, their nonphysician investors), the following section was added to the statute shortly after the attorney general's opinion was released:

> The provisions of this section do not prohibit a physician from compensating any independent contractor that provides goods or services to the physician on the basis of a percentage of the physician's fees generated in the practice of medicine. *The percentage paid must be reasonably related to the value of the goods or services provided*[19] [emphasis added].

The sentence in italics is similar to that found in several other state statutes that permit some degree of fee splitting. Although it is still necessary to understand how the statute has been interpreted in a particular state, in general, so long as the percentage fee reflects the fair market value for the management services rendered, the fee will likely be respected.

Corporate Practice of Medicine Application

States that have adopted the CPOM doctrine will likely object if the amount or structure of the fee suggests that the actual intent of the parties was to shift the profits from the medical company to the management company. The following reflects the logic employed by a Louisiana court (applying South Carolina law) in analyzing a service fee, which is similar to the way other courts have addressed the issue[20]:

- Although the management services agreement claims that the service fee is payment in exchange for services, it is clear that "both parties shared the operating expenses and the practice's profits and losses."

- Because the management company controlled many of the business aspects and shared in the profits and losses of the medical business, it was found that the management company was in fact involved in a partnership with the medical company.

---

17 Tennessee Code Annotated § 63–6–225(a).
18 Tennessee Attorney General, U94–161 (1994).
19 Tennessee Code Annotated § 63–6–225(b).
20 *Kerry White Brown, D.D.S. v. OCA, Inc., et al.*, Civil Action Number 06–2938 (E. Dist. La. 2008).

- Because the parties were found to be in a partnership, (1) the physicians were deemed to be employed by a business entity in violation of the state's CPOM doctrine, and (2) both parties were in violation of the state statute restricting ownership of a PC (or professional LLC) to licensed individuals.

The failure to appropriately structure the management fee can lead to disastrous results in the friendly PC structure. Because the structuring of the management fee involves the analysis of state statutes, applicable case law, relevant attorney general opinions, medical board decisions, and other legal authority, it is highly recommended that those interested in starting an urgent care company consult competent health-care counsel before proceeding.

NONCOMPLIANCE PENALTIES

In nearly all states that restrict ownership of a medical enterprise to licensed professionals, the applicable state medical board, commission, or agency is authorized to sanction health-care providers that violate the state's restrictive ownership laws. Such boards and agencies generally can suspend or revoke the license of the physician involved in the illegal arrangement. Being that the medical license is a physician's most valuable asset, it is surprising how little diligence is sometimes performed before entering into an economic arrangement with unlicensed investors.

The application of the rules and regulations promulgated by the relevant state health-care board is generally limited to the licensed health-care professionals in the state. As a result, the state board generally has no authority to impose penalties or other sanctions against the nonphysician investors.

In addition to the enforcement authority delegated to the applicable medical boards, many state courts refuse to enforce any contract between the physician and the unlicensed individual or entity that is found to violate the CPOM doctrine or other ownership prohibitions. Because many of the unlicensed investors in urgent care startups make substantial financial investments to lease the necessary space, fund the center's build-out, acquire the medical equipment, and provide general startup working capital financing, the risk is severe that a court will deem a contract void and will refuse to require the medical company to repay the management company.

The seminal Texas Court of Appeals case *Flynn Brothers, Inc. v. First Medical Associates* illustrates the point. In *Flynn*, the court set aside the contractual arrangement between a physician and a company that provided staffing and other nonclinical services. The court reasoned that because the relevant contracts attempted to share the profits earned by the physician with an unlicensed entity, the agreements between the two parties were illegal and therefore unenforceable. On reaching its conclusion, the court made the following statement regarding its willingness to compensate one of the parties for its loss in the transaction: "When an attempt is made to bring an action upon an illegal contract, the courts of this state have uniformly held that they will leave the parties where they found them."[21] This approach is common in states that have adopted the CPOM doctrine.

Consequently, if a management company in Texas invests significant capital in the medical company but inappropriately structures its relationship, the court will likely leave the "parties where it found them," potentially disregarding any repayment obligation of the medical company. Because the risk of loss for unlicensed investors is typically substantial, it is advisable to gain a full understanding of how each aspect of one's arrangement will be viewed before investing.

Some state statutes take an even harsher approach to violations of state ownership prohibitions. For example, under New York law, a violation of the CPOM statute is considered a felony carrying a potential jail sentence of 2 to 5 years.[22] This potential sentence applies to both the physician and the nonphysician owner. Similarly, in California, CPOM violations are punishable by 1 to 5 years of imprisonment and/or a fine of $50,000 or double the amount of the fraud, whichever is greater.[23]

Finally, it should also be noted that a private payer that reimburses a medical practice for professional fees could potentially seek to have all such fees returned on a finding that the entity was illegally engaging in the practice of medicine. Because the fees were paid on the basis of medical services rendered to patients, on discovering that the providing company was not authorized to provide such services, the payer could take the position that it is entitled to a refund.

CONCLUSION

State and federal health-care laws often have a dramatic impact on the legal structuring of an urgent care business. Diligence in the planning and execution of urgent care company formation and operation is a must, as is the engagement of a competent health-care attorney experienced in these issues.

KEY POINTS

1. Care must be taken from the start to structure the entity within the state's statutory regulations.

2. Check state health-care laws, which often have a dramatic impact on the legal structuring of an urgent care business.

3. The regulations applicable to the medical industry are vast and complex. The penalties for noncompliance can be devastating.

4. The CPOM doctrine prohibits a corporation from practicing medicine or employing a physician to practice medicine on the corporation's behalf.

---

21 *Flynn Bros., Inc. v. First Medical Associates*, 715 S.W.2d 782, 785 (Tex. App. 1986).
22 See New York State Education Law § 6512.
23 See California Business and Professions Code § 2417.5, as amended by Assembly Bill 2566. See California Penal Code § 550.

5. The CPOM doctrine's central concern is that the profit motives of an unlicensed person or entity will somehow interfere with the physician's professional medical judgment.
6. The CPOM doctrine serves the following three purposes:
    - Protecting the physician–patient relationship from interference by unlicensed persons or entities
    - Preventing the commercialization of the practice of medicine
    - Preventing control of a physician's practice by unlicensed persons or entities
7. The failure to appropriately structure the management fee can lead to disastrous results in the friendly PC structure.
8. Many state courts refuse to enforce any contract between the physician and the unlicensed individual or entity that is found to violate the CPOM doctrine or other ownership prohibitions. In *Flynn*, the court set aside the contractual arrangement between a physician and a company that provided staffing and other nonclinical services. The court reasoned that because the relevant contracts attempted to share the profits earned by the physician with an unlicensed entity, the agreements between the two parties were illegal and therefore unenforceable.
9. A private payer that reimburses a medical practice for professional fees could potentially seek to have all such fees returned if there is a finding that the entity was illegally engaging in the practice of medicine.
10. Do not attempt to structure agreements between an entity and medical provider without the input of a qualified attorney.

CHAPTER 9

Insurance Requirements for the Urgent Care Center

David Wood

Whether you are starting a new urgent care center or currently own one, arranging the various types of business insurance policies can seem challenging and complex. The types of insurance are organized into categories in this chapter so you can focus on the most important policies first and then determine when your budget allows you to purchase other types of insurance. You should consider purchasing all of these, though, as they are all important.

- Must-have insurance policies:
  - Medical-professional liability insurance (i.e., malpractice insurance)
  - Business insurance (property, general liability, auto, umbrella)
  - Workers' compensation
  - Life and disability

- Might-consider policies:
  - Employment practices liability
  - Billing errors and omissions (E&O)
  - Employee benefits
  - Cyber-technology

- Not-sure-at-this-time policies:
  - Directors' and officers' liability
  - Fiduciary liability
  - Crime and fidelity
  - Outbreak expense

Reviewing each type of coverage in detail is beyond the scope of this chapter. This chapter will get you started with the basics of the must-have insurance coverage. But please ask your insurance representative about the others that are listed.

MUST-HAVE INSURANCE POLICIES

Medical-professional Liability Insurance

There are three sources of medical-professional liability insurance:

- *Commercial insurers*   These can be found by using an insurance agent.

- *Local mutual insurance companies*   These are normally the main in-state providers of medical-professional liability insurance.

- *Risk retention groups (RRGs)*   These were created by the federal Liability Risk Retention Act. RRGs must form as liability insurance companies under the laws of their charter state. The benefits of RRGs include the ability of members to
    - Manage their own programs
    - Obtain premium stability
    - Implement risk-management practices
    - Pay dividends for good loss experience
    - Access reinsurance markets
    - Maintain a consistent source of liability coverage
    - Operate on a multistate level

Insurers' Financial Condition

The first evaluation of any of these three insurance sources is their financial stability and strength. The easiest way to determine this is to find out each insurer's A.M. Best rating. A.M. Best rates insurers on their financial strength, stability, and experience. There are several other rating firms, but A.M. Best is one of the largest and most commonly used by the industry and third parties you might contract with that will incorporate insurance requirements in their contracts.

Purchase coverage from insurers that hold an A.M. Best rating of A (excellent) VIII or higher. The letter *A* represents how well they run their company, and the roman numeral represents their financial size. The roman numeral *VIII* means that they have between $100 million and $250 million in policyholder surplus. The roman numeral *XV* is the highest category ($2 billion or more in surplus). Some insurers have an A–, A+, or A++ rating. If an insurer is A– rated (still excellent), make sure that it has a roman numeral rating of X or higher and that the A.M. Best outlook regarding the insurer is "stable." An A+ or A++ (superior) rating means that the insurer is highly regarded because of the way it operates.

Mainstream insurers offering insurance to the health-care industry try to maintain a high A.M. Best rating. Selecting a financially stable insurer and using A.M. Best for financial rating is a good standard to use.

Sometimes an insurer without any rating will talk about how highly its reinsurance is rated. But consider the rating of the insurer that provides the policy, not the rating of the company's reinsurers. Rated reinsurers are great, but the insurer's reinsurance agreement can be terminated, leaving you with a policy provided by an unrated insurer.

An RRG typically asks you to invest in the RRG in addition to paying a premium. Some RRG insurers say that their policy won't cover losses in the event that the RRG goes out of business. Because this claim is often brought up by an RRG, you should consider investigating this claim more thoroughly. To verify that the RRG is not assessable, ask for written confirmation from your lawyer (one with expertise in insurance law in your state) that the nonassessable feature of the RRG means that no third parties can pursue you in the event of the RRG's failure.

Types of Insurance Products

After you complete your financial review of the insurer you want to receive a quote from, you must determine whether the insurer has a product designed for your type of operation. Some insurers try to make their current products fit what an urgent care center needs. This does not always work well.

Several types of coverage are available:

- *Occurrence*   This insurance provides coverage for insured events occurring during the policy period, regardless of the length of time that passes before the insurance company is notified of the claim.

- *Claims-made*   This insurance provides coverage for insured events occurring on or after the specified policy's retroactive date, when the insured events are *reported* during the policy period.

- *Modified claims-made*   This insurance provides coverage when a claim is made, with an included tail or extended reporting endorsement.

- *Extended reporting period (or tail) coverage*   At the expiration of an insured's final claims-made policy, it is necessary to obtain coverage for any as-yet unreported claims that may occur as a result of past medical incidents. This coverage closes the gap between claims-made and occurrence coverage.

- *Prior acts (nose) coverage*   This insurance may be purchased when the insured is changing policy carriers and continuing to practice. This type of coverage extends to events that may have occurred prior to the initial date of the policy.

Occurrence coverage (if structured properly) and modified claims-made coverage are the options for an urgent care center. The issue with occurrence coverage is that it is often rated on a per-provider basis and starts at the top of the cost scale. Per-provider rating is not a financially attractive approach for a policy for an urgent care center. If you consider an occurrence policy, make sure that the insurer has a very high A.M. Best rating, because you are counting on them to be around for a long time after you purchase their policy. Even if all the right qualities are available and there is no tail charge if the group policy is terminated, the cost of an occurrence policy is prohibitive for the budget of an urgent care center.

Modified claims-made coverage is like traditional claims-made coverage in that there is a tail to purchase in the event the group policy comes to an end and no new insurer is assuming the prior acts liability. The difference is that the tail charge is not made when the providers depart during the active life of the policy. The departed providers stay covered as long as the group medical-professional liability policy is still active and in force. In a true claims-made policy there is a tail charge each time a provider leaves. This is generally not sustainable or affordable.

An urgent care center should consider a group policy that covers the entity, the staff members, and the providers under a single policy. Having separate policies for each provider and the entity can be a management challenge and poses a risk for varying levels of coverage and an inability to verify whether each separate policy is actually in force. (A certificate of insurance is only a snapshot of coverage on the day the certificate is issued.) You cannot manage the departed provider's insurance after they leave. If you have a claim in subsequent years, it can be troublesome if the departed provider's insurance has lapsed or changed in a manner that does not provide coverage. Please note that most insurers do not offer the tail if a policy is canceled for nonpayment of premium.

Developing a Premium

The best starting point for developing a premium is for the insurer to rate the policy on the number and type of visits you encounter during the year. A policy that rates on hours or number of providers does not properly reflect your center's true full-time equivalent status or the staffing variability of an urgent care center. Some insurers mix the rating between per provider, hours, and visits, but the best method is per visit.

In a modified claims-made policy, the per-visit rating is lower in the first year and goes up each year over a 4- to 5-year period. This is because of the aggregation of patient encounters you see over this time period and because there are more possible patients that might make a claim in the future. A patient treated in the first year is less likely to make a claim after the fifth year. This is why the rates level out.

The types of services you offer can affect the per-visit rate. The higher the intensity of services, the more the rate will be. Activities like x-ray overread, patient follow-up, use of an electronic health record, written discharge instructions, and diligent hiring protocols can mitigate your cost. Accreditation can also lower your cost.

During the application process, evaluate the applications and determine whether they are applicable to an urgent care center and not an adaptation from another health-care segment. This indicates whether the insurer is trying to understand your operations.

Limit of Liability

Choosing the limit of liability for your medical-professional liability policy can be complex. There are many variables: state requirements, contract requirements, structure, amount, assets, affordability, and availability. The most common limit is $1,000,000 per occurrence and $3,000,000 in the aggregate for any policy year. There are variations of the common limit that are based on state requirements and apply if there are mandatory patient compensation funds or if you have elected to voluntarily participate in a patient compensation fund. You might choose to purchase limits that will allow you to be part of a state tort cap that is triggered if you carry the correct level of limit. Some health plans require specific limits. Lenders sometimes require specific limits. You can choose to have the limits apply per claim or per provider. The costs go up if there is a higher limit and if the limit is applied per provider.

Sometimes providers come together to start an urgent care center and each provider has their own insurance. Sometimes the provider-owners are emergency physicians. It is best to not have the center's policy assume liability for the providers' work prior to the opening of the center, lest the policy be subject to claims unrelated to the center's operation. Often the provider-owners have different backgrounds and work experiences, which makes it hard to weigh the fairness of exposing the multiowner center to assumption of the varying risks for all owners. The driving force behind the prior acts consideration is the cost of the tail of the owner's policy.

This comes up during the hiring process for new providers. Some applicants will want you to assume prior acts coverage for the time they worked for others, because of the high cost of their tail. You should try to avoid doing so. Some owners offer a 3-year vesting period for reimbursement of the provider's tail premium. This is tied to length of time the employee works full time with you and is conditioned on showing up on time and not having other problems while working at your center. The total percentage reimbursed over 3 years is typically 50%.

Credentialing

Core Specialties

Given the unique demands on urgent care providers, one of the greatest challenges for you as the owner of an urgent care center is to maintain a well-balanced staff of qualified providers. Some medical-professional liability insurers are more diligent than others when it comes to reviewing provider applications. This is often based on experience and how invested the insurer is in the urgent care class of business. The three specialties that seem to make it through the underwriting grid are emergency medicine, family practice, and medical pediatrics. Often there are internal medicine providers with prior primary care, emergency medicine, or urgent care experience working for urgent care centers.

Off-Specialty Providers

Evaluating on-the-job training experience for providers who do not have a specialty that is suited for an urgent care center requires due diligence to determine eligibility. The most common core competency areas that are lacking are shown in Table 1.

All types of providers want to work at an urgent care center, including retired surgeons, anesthesiologists, radiologists, ophthalmologists, and pathologists. In each case, these types of off-specialty providers and others listed in Table 1 bring valuable experience and knowledge to the urgent care center setting but may be lacking in some of the urgent care core competencies. You need to consider additional training to support their working at the urgent care center. Some emerging continuing medical education (CME) programs covering urgent care core competencies can assist in training and bringing new providers onboard.

Third-Year Residents

Resident providers sometimes want to work in an urgent care center. Most insurers believe that a third-year resident in emergency medicine, family practice, or medical pediatrics can be considered for a position. Because the resident is not a fully trained provider and insurers assume you have trained providers treating patients, you have to be sure the resident is being trained in the area that supports the urgent care setting and is far enough along that they are closer to completing their training than not. You also want permission from the residency program that the resident is qualified and approved to work for you. You will want to provide extra oversight and access to supervising providers during their shifts.

Providers With Blemished Records

Providers with prior claims or board actions or who are under state supervision for addiction or other related problems are not necessarily uninsurable and impossible to hire. Some people in the insurance industry (not me) think of urgent care centers as halfway houses for providers with issues and believe that providers who are not board certified tend to end up working at an urgent care center. You must apply extra up-front due diligence before hiring such individuals. Strong credentialing and screening can assist in the protection of the brand and reputation of your center and ensure quality patient care.

Table 1. Specialties That Trigger Underwriting Reviews

Provider's Specialty or Experience	Core Competency That May Be Lacking
Internal medicine	Pediatrics
Pediatrics	Adult care
Non-primary-care specialty	Primary care
Career correctional care	General private health care
No direct patient care for ≥3 years	General private health care

Providers From Locum Tenens and Staffing Firms
Some urgent care centers hire providers through locum tenens and staffing firms. You must apply the same credentialing, screening, and hiring processes for these providers as for others. You should have your insurer review each one for insurability. If possible you want to make sure the medical-professional liability insurance from the staffing firm is primary and noncontributory and has the same or higher limits than you insure for. This means that their insurance pays first and your insurance would be excess of their coverage. If possible, have your entity added as an additional insured.

Midlevel Providers
Most of the issues that apply to physicians also apply to midlevel providers.

Credentialing Considerations
Insurers look at the balance between providers with no issues and those with issues. They look at your ratio of providers that are just right for your center to those who have specific deficits of the kinds described in this section. If there are higher-than-average risk factors related to the claims in your region or if your center's risk-avoidance profile is below average, then some insurers may choose not to offer you coverage because of the level of your provider balance. The more you are out of balance toward more problematic providers, the more you increase your exposure to loss and the higher your premiums are likely to be.

Some emerging CME programs can assist the urgent care center by providing training in core competencies of their providers. These help shore up the weaker skill sets and enable the provider to bring back applicable skill sets that can lift the overall quality of your urgent care center. Some traditional sources for CME are not applicable to urgent care center needs for improving care and staff knowledge.

Although you want the staffing process to be as easy as possible, you also want to have an insurance partner that will provide education and perspective to help you avoid hiring providers who will cause you to risk your insurability.

Business Insurance
Business insurance is associated with your lease and insuring the space you occupy. Some center owners also own the building, but most often they do so through a separate entity from the urgent care business. My focus is on the insurance for the center.

The basic elements of this insurance are

- General liability coverage
- Non-owned and hired auto coverage
- Property coverage for your business personal property, computers, and tenant improvements and betterments
- Loss-of-income and extra-expense coverage
- Umbrella coverage

General Liability Coverage

The policies for this coverage generally offer a great value for the cost. Don't skimp on your budget for this type of policy. You certainly have to meet the lease limit requirements of your landlord, but you should try to obtain at least $2,000,000 per claim or occurrence and $4,000,000 in the aggregate for any policy year for your general liability (if available) and at least $1 million in umbrella coverage (higher limits are affordable).

Non-Owned and Hired Auto Coverage

The non-owned and hired auto limit is typically $1 million, and the umbrella will be in excess of this limit. You should always purchase the liability and physical damage coverage when you rent a vehicle even if you have secured these coverages under your business owner's policy. It is better to transfer a claim to the rental car company than to file a claim under your policy. Insurers are becoming concerned about the non-owned vehicle coverage. This is coverage for employees who drive their personal cars on company business. If they have an at-fault accident, the injured party can claim you asked the employee to drive in a rush to their meeting or that you did not take care to protect the public from a poor driver (if the driver has a poor driving record or lacks insurance). More insurers want you to verify that each employee who drives their own car for your business has at least $300,000 of liability coverage, to verify their driving record before they are allowed to drive for your business, and to verify their record each year. Insurers also want you to have a policy that employees have to advise you regarding tickets and other driving infractions (especially driving while intoxicated). The policy should be written such that if they do not advise you and you find out, their employment is automatically terminated.

Property Coverage

The limit for your business personal property and computer coverage should be high enough to insure 100% of replacement value.

The tenant improvements and betterments coverage should be at least $100 a square foot (or more if your cost is higher). As a rule of thumb you should increase your build-out cost by 25% for the tenant improvements and betterments limit. Do not accept responsibility for the roof or for damage caused by leaks or water damage. Certain parts of the country are highly susceptible to hail damage, and you do not want accept damage to the heating, ventilation, and air-conditioning (HVAC) or to equipment exposed to hail loss in these areas. Do not accept responsibility for anything underground. Do not accept responsibility for loss to property or bodily injury outside your premises. This includes not being responsible for the "good repair" of the sidewalk. This can be a particular problem when there are slick surfaces caused by rain, ice, or snow.

Some landlords try to require certain types of insurance endorsements or certificates. You should try to eliminate these clauses and have them accept the endorsements that are used by your insurer and the current standard Association for Cooperative Operations Research and Development certificates. When you review your lease, look out for words like *all*, *any*, and *all risks*, because these words are not supported in your policy. You should try to have the landlord accept the extent of your policy coverage and not have indemnification or clauses that are broader than your policy. Insurance will not mimic the agreement you sign, and most urgent care center owners do not have enough money to act as the deep pocket for a building owner.

Determine the age of the building and when updates were last made to the roof, plumbing, electrical, and HVAC. Many insurers want these items to have been updated in the last 25 years. If you sign a lease for an older space that is not updated, your insurance cost goes up and your options are limited. For certain areas of the country that have significant wind and hail exposure (Florida, Mississippi, Louisiana, and most coastal counties, plus the second county inland from Maine to Texas), you need to be extra certain of the quality of the construction and the wind rating of the property. If you can see the ocean, can see signs that indicate that ocean beaches are nearby, or can smell the ocean air, your insurance costs are going to be higher than normal, and some key coverages might be limited.

Business insurance for these areas is generally limited to what is offered by local agents who live in your area. This is because insurers have limited capacity to offer the coverage and they want to make sure that local agents have access to the capacity. For these types of special insurance areas, you want to be sure you work with the loss-control department of your insurer to develop a plan in the event of a catastrophic loss. Most qualified insurers will have excellent resources for you and your staff to work with and to be ready for a catastrophic loss (like a hurricane). Most policies have a higher deductible and possibly a co-pay for losses by wind or named storms. Be sure that you understand these terms and are ready for the financial impact.

Loss-of-Income and Extra-Expense Coverage

Centers have closed because of loss of utilities caused by storms and because of the public staying inside the centers as a result of storms and crimes in the community. Most policies do not cover your loss of income unless you incur direct damage to your premises or there are specific endorsements to address the unique loss-of-income claim. In some instances there is no coverage available.

Many centers incur a loss because of utility interruption, but the center has not incurred a physical loss to their premises. Coverage for this situation is generally available, but many centers elect not to purchase the coverage because of a perceived higher cost. The increasing risk of major storms means that you cannot assume that your utilities will be back to normal in a reasonable time. Coverage for this type of business interruption (if it is available to you) is important to purchase.

Loss caused by surface water is not covered under the special-form business owner's policy. You need flood coverage. If your location is in a flood zone, then you need to access the National Flood Insurance Program (go to www.fema.gov/national-flood-insurance-program) to obtain coverage.

General Considerations for Business Insurance

New types of claims that are not specifically listed in the business insurance policy can emerge as a result of changes in the world around us, so it is important to review your business coverage periodically and keep it up-to-date.

Owners of urgent care centers are creating many new corporate configurations. There are holding companies, subentities, staffing entities for the urgent care center staff, and development entities for the equipment and leases. You must be sure that all of your entities are listed on your business insurance policies. The same goes for your medical-professional liability policy. Some entities that do not provide medical services might have more limited coverage under the medical-professional liability policy.

You should keep your insurance source informed of your entity changes, especially change of ownership, because most policies do not automatically grant coverage for that type of change.

Workers' Compensation Insurance

Workers' compensation coverage is a required insurance by law. Some states require that you purchase the coverage from the state insurance program. These are called monopolistic states. In nonmonopolistic states you should apply the same insurance company financial requirements as you would apply to other carriers. When purchasing this coverage, make sure you increase the employer liability limits to $1 million and add blanket waiver of subrogation. Be sure the correct entity is insured, the entity that employs the staff. If you lease your staff, you want to be sure that the leasing company affords these coverages to your entity and that your entity is named on their policy. In the event of a claim, you want to be granted separate defense representation. When signing a lease or entering into a contract that addresses workers' compensation coverage, be sure your insurer or the insurer of the leasing firm (if you lease your employees) can comply with the requirements.

This type of coverage can be difficult to deal with because of increasing claims and rising rates. Pay attention to what discounts are being offered and your experience-modification factor. Needlestick injuries appear to be the most frequent claims for urgent care center staff members. You want to seek out your insurer's loss-control and education sources to assist you with lowering the risk for these types of claims. In a small urgent care center, it does not take many claims to create a poor loss ratio, which leads to much higher insurance costs. You also want to reduce claims regarding staff downtime.

Life and Disability Insurance

Life and disability insurance are important for protecting your income and your family's security. They also come into play for bank loan requirements and buy–sell agreements between partners. Your health status and age affect your eligibility and cost. Some insurance sources want you to combine insurance goals with investment goals. The right decision for you is a personal choice, but it's generally best that you separate your insurance protection needs from your investment needs. You can still use life insurance as an investment vehicle, but you should not combine it with policies encumbered by lenders or tied to partner obligations.

Many owners do not think to have a disability buyout policy in the event that a partner becomes disabled. This is an important additional purpose for disability insurance along with protecting your income. Be sure to review the definition of disability, the definition of your occupation, and how your policy coordinates with other disability insurance sources (group policies).

Disability insurers have had a hard time since the start of the 21st century. The health-care industry has had a significant increase in claims. In addition, the investments of some life and disability insurers (not unlike banks) have put them at risk for financial problems. For life and disability insurance, you want to put the financial strength of the insurer over the cost of the policies. It is best to consider mainline insurers with the highest ratings. A.M. Best ratings of A+ or higher are the standard for life and disability insurers.

OTHER TYPES OF INSURANCE

Although all of the types of insurance listed at the beginning of this chapter are important, owners of urgent care centers have shown the most interest in employment practices liability insurance (EPLI) and billing E&O insurance. EPLI protects you from employee lawsuits for items such as wrongful termination and discrimination. Billing E&O protects you from allegations of wrongful billing from government payers or private health insurers. In the current health-care climate, billing issues are getting a lot of scrutiny. Another type of insurance to consider is fiduciary liability and fidelity protection. If you have a 401(k) plan, you should also add this protection.

CONCLUSION

As an owner of an urgent care center, you should consider several factors when evaluating insurance coverage, policy structure, and representation. The quality of the insurer, the underwriting process, how providers are selected, your region, the nuances of your property location, and the types of contracts you enter into all have a bearing on your policies. Having confidence in your insurance source and understanding the basics of your insurance coverage are important. Decisions about the insurance you purchase and the coverage you choose to delay purchasing should come after you have been provided enough detailed information so that you can make an informed decision.

Stay engaged in your insurance purchases and make sure that those who represent you have experience and expertise in your area of health care. As with running any business, you want to hire the best to work for you. Insurance representation is no different. Hold your insurance representation to a high standard, and understand that not all professionals who work in insurance are qualified as experts in arranging insurance for an urgent care center.

KEY POINTS

1. Must-have insurance includes
   - Medical-professional liability insurance
   - Business insurance (property, general liability, auto, umbrella)
   - Workers' compensation
   - Life and disability

2. There are three common sources of insurance: commercial insurers, local mutual insurance companies, and risk retention groups.

3. The insurers you purchase coverage from should hold an A.M. Best rating of A (excellent) VIII or higher.

4. Do not rely on the rating of the reinsurer as a proxy for the strength of the insurance company.

5. There are three types of coverage: occurrence, claims-made, and modified claims-made.

6. Occurrence (if structured properly) and modified claims-made are the two options for an urgent care center. Occurrence coverage is often rated on a per-provider basis and starts at the top of the cost scale.

7. Modified claims-made is like a traditional claims-made policy in that there is a tail to purchase in the event the group policy comes to an end and no new insurer is assuming the prior acts liability. The difference is that the tail charge is not made when the providers depart during the active life of the policy.

8. It is preferable not to have the urgent care center policy assume the prior acts of the providers for their work before starting at the urgent care center.

9. The three specialties that seem to make it through the underwriting grid with the fewest challenges are emergency medicine, family practice, and medical pediatrics.

10. There are new CME programs for urgent care centers that can help with bringing new providers onboard.

CHAPTER 10

Equipment and Supply Vendor Selection

Sybil Yeaman

Successfully choosing equipment and supply vendors helps to control overhead costs, and building partnerships with vendor representatives through communication and collaboration can bring new ideas and resources into your urgent care center.

It can be a daunting challenge to identify, choose, and negotiate cost-effective agreements with equipment and supply vendors. Taking the challenge and making a systematic effort up front to find the right vendors will be rewarded in the end with cost-effective contractual agreements that increase the center's bottom line and will provide quality service that supports center staff and patient care for many years.

SPECIFY VENDOR SERVICES

Being prepared is a key element to success in purchasing products and services. Before beginning the process of identifying vendors, first determine in writing the specific products and define the services needed for your project. For example, if you are building a new center and are focused on radiology, list the build-out, equipment, installation, and supplies your center will require. Then list additional options, such as service agreements or delivery and timelines for installation, to consider for each area.

A specific list for each project (Table 1) acts like a worksheet for cost and service comparisons and a guideline to use while researching and meeting with equipment and supply vendors. Each vendor will have different offerings and service packages, and a worksheet allows you to compare pricing while staying focused on what your center needs.

When you are developing a new urgent care center, consult these tables of commonly purchased equipment and supplies:

- Table 2: Medical equipment and supplies
- Table 3: Exam room supplies
- Table 4: Intravenous (IV) supplies

Table 1. Sample Vendor Worksheet for Start-Up Radiology

Item	Quantity	Price	Service Contract	Timeline
Drawings and build-out	1	$		
X-ray equipment	1	$	Verify included	
Computed radiography unit	1	$	Verify included	
Installation and training	1	$		
Signs, gowns, aprons	Multiple	$		
Estimated cost with computed radiography		$		

Name of Company:

- Table 5: Life support, triage, and respiratory supplies
- Table 6: Wound care supplies
- Table 7: Specialty supplies
- Table 8: Pharmaceutical supplies
- Table 9: Information technology and electronic equipment
- Table 10: Office supplies and lobby furniture

WHERE TO LOOK FOR VENDORS

Vendors you have worked with successfully in the past should be considered primary vendor candidates if their companies provide services in your local area. Having a relationship with vendors you already trust before you need them will save valuable time in the selection and start-up process for center projects. However, it is important to be careful about choosing vendors who are also personal friends, because the friendship may cloud judgment. Place vendor friends on the vendor list being compiled, but make sure friends fulfill the same demands for stability, competitive pricing, and service as any other vendor being considered.

Successful colleagues are a good resource. Inquire which vendors they are using and whether they are happy with the vendors' prices and ongoing support services. Attending meetings and networking at professional urgent care organization conferences, such as the Urgent Care Association of America (www.ucaoa.org), should provide opportunities to confer with colleagues and meet vendors in the exhibit areas. Medical journals, such as the *Journal of Urgent Care Medicine (*http://jucm.com*)*, advertise vendors specializing in equipment and services for urgent care centers.

RESEARCHING VENDOR COMPANIES

Search engines are excellent research tools to help compile and narrow down a list of potential vendors. Use a search engine to look up and evaluate established

Table 2. Medical Equipment and Supplies

- Antimicrobial soap dispenser, Provon
- Antimicrobial soap dispenser refill, Provon
- Apron, full, large (24″ × 42″)
- Apron, half
- Apron holder and glove rack
- Autoclave
- Blood pressure cuff, child
- Blood pressure cuff, small adult
- Blood pressure cuff, thigh
- Calipers
- Casters for halogen light
- C-fold towel dispenser, 15″, chrome
- C-fold towel dispenser, 8″, chrome
- Chemistry analyzer, Abaxis Piccolo xpress
- Clarity Urocheck urine analyzer, plus bottle strips
- Computed radiography unit and view screen
- Defibrillator, Cardiac Science Powerheart AED G3
- Digital scale with height rod
- Electrocardiograph, interpretive, Welch Allyn CP100
- Electrocardiograph, interpretive and spirometer combination, Welch Allyn CP200 (optional)
- Emergency eye wash unit, double stream
- Exam tables
- Foam wedges (positioning aids)
- Fluorescent ultraviolet lamp, handheld
- Footstools
- Glove box holder, Maxi-Dispenz
- Halogen gooseneck exam light
- Hand sanitizer touchless foam dispenser
- Hand sanitizer touchless foam refill, 1200 mL
- Hematology analyzer, QBC STAR
- Integrated diagnostic system
- IV pole (mobile) with 4 legs and 2 hooks
- Lead blockers
- Lead markers, right and left
- Mayo stand
- Medical stools, adjustable, with wheels
- Mobile cart for electrocardiograph
- Mobile stand with basket for vital signs monitor
- Nebulizer
- Ophthalmoscope
- Otoscope
- Oxygen tank, size E, with full-size cart
- Oximetry sensor, PediCheck
- Pillow cases

(continued)

Table 2. Medical Equipment and Supplies (*continued*)

- Pillow, Dacron-filled, 21" × 27"
- Pregnancy signPulse oximeter, Dura-Y multisite sensor
- Suction machine
- Sundry jars, glass, unlabeled, 7" × 4"
- Table mat
- Temporal artery thermometer, Exergen TAT-5000
- Transformer
- Trash can, 8-gallon, white for triage
- Trash cans, 8-gallon, red for triage, exam rooms, and laboratory
- Vaginal specula dispenser, KleenSpec
- Vaginal specula (disposable) and cordless illuminator, KleenSpec
- Vital signs monitor and 2 cuffs, adult and large adult
- Wall cabinet with alarm for automated external defibrillator, Cardiac Science
- Wall enclosure for sharps, half-gallon and 5-quart
- Warning sign, "Caution: x-ray," 7" × 10"
- Warning sign, "Radiation," 7" × 9.5"
- Weights/sandbags
- Wheelchair, 350-lb capacity
- X-ray equipment

medical companies that are well known and financially stable. Delete any companies on your list that have numerous customer complaints or several name changes. Customer complaints may indicate poor service or substandard quality products, whereas multiple name changes may indicate company instability.

Selection criteria should include

- ► Experience providing urgent care products and services
- ► Longevity and financial stability
- ► Good reputation and customer satisfaction
- ► Capacity to deliver on center timelines
- ► Competitive pricing and payment terms

CONSIDER A GROUP PURCHASING ORGANIZATION

Consider joining a group purchasing organization (GPO) to benefit from the organization's high-volume purchasing power. By using a GPO, small to midsized independent urgent care centers can obtain the same cost savings that large urgent care companies and hospital centers benefit from. A GPO is an excellent choice for start-up urgent care centers or centers expanding to a new location. Joining a GPO will provide one-stop shopping and guaranteed discount pricing for site selection, equipment, and medical supply services.

Table 3. Exam Room Supplies

- C-fold towels
- Deodorizer, CitraStatRx
- Cotton balls, medium
- Cotton-tipped applicators, nonsterile, 6"
- Cover gowns, medium and large
- Disinfectant wipes, EZ-Kill, 160 per can
- Distilled water, 1-gallon bottle
- Earloop face masks
- Earloop face masks with eye shields
- Emesis basin, plastic, 16-oz
- Exam gowns, economy, 30"× 42"
- Exam-table paper, smooth, 21" × 225'
- Facial tissues
- Hot and cold gel packs, reusable, 6"× 10"
- Infectious-waste bag, 18-gallon
- Needles, disposable, 25G × ⅝"
- Needles, disposable, 27G ×1¼"
- Needles, disposable, 30G × ½"
- Sharps containers, 5-quart refills for wall mount
- Specimen containers, sterile, 4.5-oz
- Syringe system, Carpuject
- Thermometer, refrigerator/freezer
- Thermometer, refrigerator/freezer, digital (laboratory)
- Toilet seat covers, Scott
- Toilet tissue, 2-ply
- Tongue depressors, nonsterile, adult
- Trash bags, 7-gallon to 10-gallon, brown
- Washbasins, 7-quart

Look for a GPO that specializes in urgent care product lines, like the Urgent Care Integrated Network (www.ucinet.org), or focuses on the needs of outpatient medical facilities. Use your search engine to evaluate the products and services offered before you join. The GPO should provide opportunities to contract with most or all of the services urgent care centers need. Appraise the vendors to see if they are credible national companies, some of which you may already have on your list of potential vendors. With their buying power, the GPO should offer savings of at least 10% on medical supplies and durable medical equipment and 5% or more on vendor services. A GPO should also be able to offer new or improved lines of business for your urgent care center, such as laboratory services and in-house dispensing of prescription drugs.

WHAT COSTS TO EXPECT

Prices will vary with volume, discounts, and service offerings, but pricing should fall within reasonable ranges of what is anticipated. Start-up urgent care centers should expect the approximate basic price ranges shown in Table 11.

Table 4. IV Supplies

- Blood collection needle, 21G × 1¼″, Vacutainer Eclipse
- Blood collection set, 23G × ¾″, Vacutainer Safety-Lok
- Catheter, Foley, latex, 16F, 5-mL
- Catheter, IV, Introcan Safety, 20G × 1″
- Catheter, IV, Introcan Safety, 22G × 1″
- Catheter, IV, Surflo, 16G × 2″
- Dressing, 1.75″ × 1.75″, Tegaderm
- IV administration set, 15 drops/mL, 93″
- IV armboards, disposable, 3″ × 9″
- Leg bag, 1100-mL, large, with straps
- Luer adapter, Venoject
- Needle, disposable, 18G × 1″
- Needle, disposable, 25G ×1″
- Needle holder, Vacutainer
- Normal saline, half and dextrose 5%, 1000 mL
- Normal saline, half, 1000 mL
- Normal saline, 1000 mL
- Normal saline, 50 mL
- Normal saline, 20 mL
- Small-bore extension sets for peripheral IV catheters, 8″, Ultrasite
- Syringe with safety needle, SurGard2, 23G × 1″
- Syringe and needle, 1-mL, 25G × ⅝″
- Syringes, 3-mL
- Syringes, 5-mL
- Syringes, 60-mL
- Tube collectors, 8.5-mL, red top, Vacutainer
- Tourniquet, stretch, latex-free
- Ureteral catheter tray, 16F

WHAT TO EXPECT FROM VENDOR REPRESENTATIVES

Contact the top two or three vendors and speak to their local representatives. Let the vendors know they have been selected as your center's top candidates and will be competing for your center's business. In some rural areas, there may only be one vendor available for a specialized service, such as biomedical waste disposal. Call and make an appointment to meet with the representative even though the company is not competing for business. It is never a waste of time to start a business relationship on a personal level. The meeting may provide an opportunity to discuss additional savings or credits for unadvertised service packages.

As you review your worksheet of project requirements, consider how you are treated on the phone as a possible indicator of how you will be treated as a customer. Assess whether the vendor representative listens and seriously considers your center's needs or you receive a rehearsed sales pitch instead. Eliminate

Table 5. Life Support, Triage, and Respiratory Supplies

Life support
- Defibrillator, Powerheart AED G3, automatic package, 9146 battery
- Disposable resuscitator with mask, adult, Spur
- Disposable resuscitator with mask, pediatric, Spur
- Electrocardiogram paper, CP100/CP200
- Electrocardiogram resting tab electrodes, 2.2 × 2.2 cm
- Oxygen mask, medium-concentration, pediatric
- Oxygen mask with tubing, adult
- Pediatric pads for defibrillator, Powerheart
- Suction canister, 800-mL
- Suction device, open-tip, Yankauer

Triage
- Blood pressure cuff, adult, DuraShock
- Blood pressure cuff, adult large, DuraShock
- Blood pressure cuff, child, DuraShock
- Blood pressure cuff inflation system, one-piece, small adult
- Oral thermometer probe covers, SureTemp

Respiratory
- Mouthpieces for measuring peak expiratory flow, disposable
- Nebulizer mask, adult
- Nebulizer with reserve, MicroMist
- Peak expiratory flowmeter

undesirable vendors that do not listen and cannot meet your center's needs. Make appointments to meet with each of the suitable vendors separately.

Personally meeting with potential vendors is time-consuming but provides an opportunity to assess the company and to determine if the vendor is truly capable of providing the products and services needed. Just as how you were treated on the phone was a possible indicator of how you will be treated as a customer, the appearance and behavior of the vendor representative may also be an indicator of the service you will receive. If the sales representative comes to the appointment late and unprepared, they may not be the right person to provide the level of service your urgent care center deserves. Having an organized spokesperson does not guarantee that the vendor is competent, but it does demonstrate that the representative cares about your perception and the reputation of their company.

Meeting and negotiating rates with vendors requires a mix of communication, negotiation, and persuasion skills. Your center has a budget to stay within, and the vendor will want to negotiate the highest prices possible. During the meeting both parties need to find fair competitive pricing that fits the center's needs and allows the supplier to retain a reasonable profit margin. Although pricing is important to the bottom line, negotiation has to go beyond pricing. Quality products and ongoing service must take precedence in the negotiation process for the vendor contract to be completely successful.

Table 6. Wound Care Supplies

- Alcohol prep pads, nonsterile
- Anesthetic, topical spray-mist, Pain Ease
- Bandages, adhesive flexible, ¾" × 3"
- Bandages, adhesive flexible, 2" × 4"
- Bandages, adhesive flexible, 3" × 3"
- Bandages, elastic tubular, 1", Surgilast
- Cautery replacement tips for #HIT1, fine
- Chlorhexidine gluconate scrub 4%
- Drape, fenestrated, sterile, 18" × 26"
- Finger ring cutter
- Forceps, Carmalt splinter, straight, 4¼"
- Gauze, conforming stretch, nonsterile, 3"
- Gauze, conforming stretch, nonsterile, 4"
- Gauze, iodoform, ¼" × 5 yd
- Gauze, iodoform, ½" × 5 yd
- Gauze, nonsterile, 2" × 2"
- Gauze, nonsterile, 3" × 3"
- Gauze, sterile, 12-ply, 4" × 4"
- Gauze, tubular, ⅝", Surgilast
- Gloves, clear blue nitrile PF, large, Criterion
- Gloves, clear blue nitrile PF, medium, Criterion
- Gloves, clear blue nitrile PF, small, Criterion
- Hemostat, Kelly, curved, 5½"
- Hydrogen peroxide, 16-oz bottle
- Nail splitter, 4"
- Needle holder, 5", Mayo Hegar
- Packing strip, ¼" × 5 yd
- Packing strip, 1" × 5 yd
- Pads, nonadherent, sterile, 2" × 3"
- Pads, nonadherent, sterile, 3" × 4"
- Razor, disposable, twin-blade, Personna
- Scalpels, disposable sterile #11
- Scissors, iris, standard straight, 4½"
- Scrub brush, povidone-iodine, 15 mL
- Skin staple remover, sterile with gauze, disposable
- Sponges, all-gauze, nonsterile, 8-ply, 4"×4"
- Stapler, 5-count, precise, titanium
- Strip wound closure, ¼" × 3"
- Strip wound closure, ⅛" × 3"
- Suture, 3-0 C7 Prolene
- Suture, 4-0 C6 gut
- Suture, 4-0 C6 Prolene
- Suture, 4-0 FS2 Prolene
- Suture, 5-0 C3P
- Suture, 5-0 C6 Prolene
- Suture, 6-0 C22 Prolene
- Tape paper, 1" × 10 yd, Micropore
- Tissue adhesive, topical, Indermil
- Wire-cutting scissors, 4¾"
- Wound irrigator, Igloo

Table 7. Specialty Supplies

Ear, nose, and throat supplies
- Applicator for silver nitrate, 6″
- Cerumen irrigator, portable, Waterpik
- Curettes, infant scoop, blue, 2-mm
- Ear curettes, yellow, 4-mm, CeraSpoon
- Ear irrigation tips, OtoClear
- Forceps, alligator, 4″, Noyes
- Otoscope replacement bulb, 3.5-V MacroView
- Ophthalmoscope replacement bulb, 3.5-V
- Nasal packing, 10 × 1.5 × 2 cm, extra-large, Rhino Rocket
- Specula, disposable, 2.75-mm, KleenSpec
- Specula, disposable, 4.25-mm, KleenSpec
- Speculum, nasal, medium

Orthopedic supplies
- Ankle brace, universal
- Arm sling, deluxe, extra-large
- Arm sling, deluxe, large
- Arm sling, deluxe, medium
- Arm sling, deluxe, small
- Bandages, elastic with Velcro, LF NS, 2″ × 4.5 yd
- Bandages, elastic with Velcro, LF NS, 3″ × 4.5 yd
- Bandages, elastic with Velcro, LF NS, 4″ × 4.5 yd
- Canes, aluminum, adjustable, with tip
- Cervical collar, adjustable, Perfit ACE
- Crutch, complete aluminum, 37″–46″
- Crutch, complete aluminum, 45″–53″
- Knee support, patella, adjustable
- Padding, undercast, regular finish, 2″, Webril
- Padding, undercast, regular finish, 3″, Webril
- Splints, cast, 3″ × 15′, Techform Orthoroll
- Splints, cast, 4″ × 15′, Techform Orthoroll
- Splints, finger, padded, 3″
- Splints, finger, padded, 4″
- Splints, wrist/forearm splint, medium, left
- Splints, wrist/forearm splint, medium, right
- Splints, wrist/thumb, universal, left
- Splints, wrist/thumb, universal, right
- Surgical shoes, men's, small
- Surgical shoes, men's, medium
- Surgical shoes, men's, large
- Surgical shoes, women's, small
- Surgical shoes, women's, medium
- Surgical shoes, women's, large

Ophthalmic supplies
- Eye chart, kindergarten, 22″ ×11″
- Fluorescein and proparacaine ophthalmic solution, 5 mL
- pH indicator strips
- Snellen wall-mount eye chart

(continued)

Table 7. Specialty Supplies (*continued*)

Obstetrics and gynecology supplies
- Forceps, sponge, 7″
- Lubricating jelly, 4-oz tube
- Obstetrical towelettes
- Specula, vaginal, 590 series, small
- Specula, vaginal, 590 series, medium
- Specula, vaginal, 590 series, large

Respiratory supplies
- Mouthpieces for measuring peak expiratory flow, disposable
- Nebulizer mask, adult
- Nebulizer with reserve, MicroMist
- Peak expiratory flowmeter

While meeting with vendors, it is essential to verify that your urgent care center will not be locked into a long-term agreement if the business relationship doesn't work out as planned. The intent is to develop a long-term working relationship, but in a constantly changing medical marketplace a company may change ownership or be unable to fulfill its contractual obligations. When possible, negotiate a mutual termination clause with a 60- or 90-day written notice of termination. If a short-term notice is not an option, be sure the contractual agreement is for only one year and does not renew unless both parties are in agreement.

At the conclusion of each vendor meeting, consider the following questions to narrow down choices so you can select the winning vendor:

▶ Did the representative listen and understand what you need?

▶ Did the representative seem overly anxious to make the sale?

▶ Are you comfortable with the vendor representative?

▶ Does the company appear to be customer service oriented?

▶ Does the company offer convenient support services?

▶ Does the company serve other urgent care centers?

▶ Does the vendor offer competitive pricing?

▶ Is the pricing within your center's budget?

▶ Is the vendor demanding exclusivity?

▶ Does the company provide a reasonable termination clause?

▶ Does the vendor guarantee their products and services?

CHOOSING EQUIPMENT VENDORS

Purchasing equipment is an expensive financial commitment that can be nerve-racking to make but should be compared to purchasing a car to put the

Table 8. Pharmaceutical Supplies

- Acetaminophen suspension, 80-mg, 4-oz bottle
- Acetaminophen tablets, 325-mg
- Albuterol inhalation solution, 3 mL
- Aspirin tablets, 325-mg
- Bacitracin zinc ointment, single-use
- Ceftriaxone sodium injection, single-dose vial, 1 g/Vl
- Clindamycin injection, single-dose vial, 150 mg/mL, 2 mL
- Clonidine HCl tablets, 1-mg
- Diphenhydramine capsules, 25-mg
- Diphenhydramine injection, single-dose vial, 50 mg/mL
- Diphtheria, tetanus, acellular pertussis vaccine, single-dose vial, 0.5 mL, Adacel
- Donnatol (belladonna-phenobarbital) elixir, 16.2-mg, grape flavor, 1 pint
- Ibuprofen suspension, 100-mg, 480-mL bottle
- Ibuprofen tablets, 200-mg
- Imodium (loperamide HCl) caplets, 2-mg
- Insulin, regular, 100 Units/mL
- Ipratropium inhalation solution, 2.5 mL
- Ipratropium-albuterol inhalation solution, 0.5/3 mg, 3 mL
- Kenalog-40 (triamcinolone acetonide) injection, 40 mg/mL, 1-mL vial
- Ketorolac, 30-mg
- Lidocaine 1%, 50-mL single-dose vial
- Lidocaine 2% with epinephrine, 30-mL single-dose vial
- Maalox antacid, 12-oz bottle
- Medicine cups, graduated, 1-oz
- Ondansetron HCl tablets, 4-mg
- Ondansetron injection, single-dose vial, 2 mg/mL, 2 mL
- Pepcid AC antacid tablets, 10-mg over-the-counter
- Phenergan injection, single-dose vial, 25 mg/mL, 1 mL
- Purified protein derivative tuberculin tests, 10-dose
- Prednisolone oral solution, 15 mg/5 mL, 480-mL bottle
- Prednisolone tablets, 20-mg
- Solu-Medrol (methylprednisolone sodium succinate), 40-mg Act-O-Vial, 1 mL
- Solu-Medrol (methylprednisolone sodium succinate), 125-mg Act-O-Vial
- Unasyn (ampicillin-sulbactam), 1.5-g

purchase into perspective. There are a limited number of car manufacturers but a multitude of showrooms of new-model vehicles in many US cities. The make and model of car you choose is usually defined by the price range you can afford. The sports car may be attractive, but the economy car with good mileage is often the best financial fit. The final selection is usually based on customer service and the vehicle service agreement. It is the same with purchasing medical equipment. The equipment you choose is most influenced by the center's budget, then by the delivery and service agreement. For example, when you evaluate the

Table 9. Information Technology and Electronic Equipment

- Alarm system
- Antivirus software
- Cabling
- Copiers with scanners
- Credit card machines
- Desktop computer systems and monitors
- Digital tablets
- Electronic health record and business management system
- Firewall
- Liquid crystal display (LCD) televisions
- Message board
- Microsoft Office Professional software suite
- Overhead paging
- Phone and fax lines
- Phone headsets
- Phone system
- Phones
- Postage machine
- Power strips
- Power supply
- Primary dedicated Internet access circuit
- Printers
- Privacy filters for LCD monitors
- Router
- Routing switch
- Satellite television receiver
- Uninterruptible power supply, backup
- Uninterruptible power supply, rack-mounted
- Wireless access point
- Wireless Internet

purchase of radiology equipment, there are only a few major manufacturers but many dealers. The equipment you choose is most influenced by the price range the urgent care center has budgeted, and most dealers are competitive. The real choice in equipment vendors comes down to finding a customer-service-oriented dealer that offers reasonable cost of installation and delivery and includes service agreements for inspection and ongoing maintenance as part of the purchasing package.

It is important to pick a well-established and financially sound company when purchasing or leasing equipment. In a volatile economy and constantly changing medical marketplace, new companies that offer exceptionally low prices to establish themselves as competitors may fail to penetrate the marketplace and may go out of business. The service agreements of a failed company may be complicated

Table 10. Office Supplies and Lobby Furniture

Office supplies
- Hand soap
- Mop and bucket
- Napkins
- Plastic knives, spoons, and forks
- Plates, disposable
- Plunger
- Stepladder
- Stirring sticks
- Toilet bowl cleaner
- Toilet brush
- Waste receptacles with lids
- "Wet floor" sign

Lobby furniture
- Artwork
- Chairs, armless
- Chairs with arms
- End tables
- Magazine racks
- Table lamps

or cease to exist unless the vendor is bought out by another company that honors the inspection and maintenance agreements. Be sure to include inspections and a service-level agreement as part of the purchase package or verify that they are included within the contract. Incorporating discount rates for inspections and maintenance agreements during equipment purchase is an important part of a cost-effective purchasing strategy. An enticing purchase price or lease will not be cost-effective over time if maintenance services are expensive add-on costs.

Table 11. Sample Estimated Cost Listing

Basic Equipment and Supplies	*Price Range*
Medical equipment	$52,000 to $55,500
Medical supplies	$13,000 to $14,000
Radiology equipment and installation	$48,000 to $51,000
Office and lobby furniture	$17,500 to $19,000
Computer equipment	$28,000 to $29,500
Audiovisual equipment	$6,000 to $6,500
Estimated start-up costs	$164,500 to $175,500

When evaluating service options, be sure that the representative reviews repair and loaner equipment service timelines. Downtime with equipment repair can disrupt the flow of patient care and is costly to the center. Verify that the company will support the urgent care center in a clearly defined and timely manner in the service-level agreement or within the contract.

The radiology equipment vendor will present both computed radiography (CR) and digital radiography (DR) processing units when meeting with you to determine the center's needs. Start-up centers and centers with low volume (fewer than 10 x-rays per day) should purchase a cost-effective CR unit. Centers with high volume or that include a primary-care practice may consider investing in a DR unit. Factor in the up-front costs as well as ongoing costs when discussing options with the equipment vendor. The representative should be able to provide data to evaluate costs on the basis of volume of use. Carefully evaluate health plan restrictions on use before purchasing computed tomography (CT) or ultrasound equipment. Many health plans enforce strict preauthorization guidelines that prohibit patients from receiving CT and ultrasound services in an urgent care setting. Usually health plans try to control costs by encouraging members needing advanced radiology services to use the plans' own cost-effective contracted vendors. Most independent urgent care centers do not invest in CT and ultrasound equipment because of the low volume of use. If CT and ultrasound equipment is not being purchased, the center does not need an expensive picture archiving and communication system (PACS) reading station.

Use your worksheet to review with each sales representative what your center requires, but understand that sales representatives have a sales range and can only go so far on price to meet your center's needs. Be flexible and consider other offers or services that augment the value of the pricing structure. For example, to win your business, the vendor may be able to offer additional service benefits or a bonus plan that is not normally part of the sales package and offsets the price with service. Such discounts are often as good as cash, and everyone benefits. Take notes on costs, service fees, and promises made by the equipment vendor representatives to verify against the contractual agreement.

For smaller equipment purchases like exam tables, gurneys, and wheelchairs, ask the vendor representative if they offer refurbished as well as new equipment. Consider generic as well as brand-name equipment. The cost difference may be significant.

Also, high-volume urgent care centers may consider creative options that save the center money up front, such as consignment for durable medical equipment, which allows the center to stock shelves at no cost until the equipment is dispensed.

CHOOSING MEDICAL SUPPLY VENDORS

Verify that the medical supply vendor is capable of providing most or all of the medical supplies your urgent care center needs. It is not cost-effective for center staff members to use multiple providers for the medical products that the center requires. The vendor should be competitive on pricing, but also verify that the vendor provides extended hours for ordering medical supplies and provides next-day delivery without incurring additional charges, fuel surcharges, or penalties. Look for vendors that are truly service-oriented and offer quality, not just quantity. Having a customer-service-oriented medical supply vendor that provides extended hours and flexibility in delivery is priceless. A service-oriented supply vendor should offer most or all of the following:

- Competitive pricing
- A single source for all medical supplies
- Extended hours for ordering supplies
- Consistent delivery times
- Ability to supply products overnight
- No shipping or mileage fees except for special orders
- Changes in orders without penalty

Discuss costs for disposable versus reusable items. A deterrent for buying disposables is higher cost, but speed and immediate availability are a plus. Reusable items are less expensive because they can be used repeatedly, but the added staff time to process and increased liability for the sterility process should be considered. Often the differences in price are negligible, and the decision can be based on physicians' personal preferences rather than cost.

CHOOSING VENDORS FOR A NEW LINE OF BUSINESS

For a new line of business, follow the same process of researching and interviewing equipment and supply vendors. If you do not have previous experience in the new line of business and are unable to list the equipment and services you need to create a worksheet, list the pros and cons of adding the line of business to the center as talking points when meeting with the vendor representatives. For example, if you are considering drug dispensing, list the pros and cons of automatic machine dispensing versus maintaining a staffed pharmacy, based on return on investment (ROI). Be aware that automatic dispensing machines may have an ROI that is elusive, although the new technology is compelling.

Laboratory services are usually very competitive, and the laboratory company will provide most or all of what your facility needs in supplies. Meetings with the vendors will be about customer service and which company offers convenient pickup and turnaround times, and technology for laboratory results.

CHOOSING OFFICE SUPPLY AND EQUIPMENT VENDORS

Often office supplies are considered secondary or dismissed with a cursory glance when budgeting or considering costs for a project. However, some office supplies like copiers can increase center costs for years if not negotiated carefully. For example, if you are leasing copiers, negotiate reasonable fees for the expected volume of copies at the time of leasing, or the fee invoices will increase with volume and be costly for the duration of the contract. If your center chooses to purchase, then you should negotiate maintenance, repair, and a loaner agreement as part of the incentive package, the same as when negotiating large medical equipment purchases.

There are some options an urgent care center should never consider when choosing office equipment, such as being a beta site for important products that are necessary for the workflow of the center—for example, a new high-tech phone system and software. The money saved being a beta site disappears when center phones are down for days, sometimes weeks, because of software glitches or software incompatibility issues. It is better to go with technology that has a good record of success in other medical centers, even if it's not the newest technology on the market.

FINALIZING CONTRACTUAL AGREEMENTS

Read your contract carefully. Compare the contract with your worksheet notes to verify the prices, services, and terms promised by the sales representative. Confirm that the center is not locked into a long-term contractual agreement or locked into a long-term agreement that only allows termination with an expensive penalty attached. Never assume a contractual agreement is correct. There are often discrepancies between what was offered by the vendor representative in their enthusiasm to win your business and what is actually presented contractually in writing. This does not mean the vendor is deliberately trying to deceive your center. Vendors often use a single boilerplate agreement for all customers, and the sales representative may not have fully communicated every detail of your negotiations. Highlight the questionable portions of the agreement, write down the discrepancies, and then call the vendor representative to get the contract corrected.

If the vendor sales representative promised prices or services that are not available and misled you to win the business, then terminate the relationship quickly to avoid additional loss of time in the process. Contact the second-choice vendor, keeping in mind that the second vendor's offering may be the most cost-effective in the long run after closer evaluation. Meet with the vendor representative a second time and be willing to compromise with credits and other service discounts to get the best long-term agreement that works for your center.

File completed contracts in individual folders and include a list of contacts and a worksheet of terms, especially with equipment leases or purchases. When equipment fails and the patient workflow is interrupted, the list of contacts for support services and the worksheet of maintenance and loaner equipment terms will be invaluable.

VERIFYING VENDOR SERVICES

It is imperative to follow up the effort spent in choosing the right vendors by routinely and systematically verifying that contractual agreements are being fulfilled and that the urgent care center is getting what it is invoiced for. Consider the following guidelines to maintain the integrity of vendor agreements:

- Routinely review invoices against supplies and services received to verify that the center received what was ordered.

- Look for overpricing by comparing invoices to contractual rates and fees to verify that correct charges are being invoiced.

- If applicable, verify that ordering and delivery times are being honored and additional fees or penalties are not occurring.

- Address any issues immediately with your vendor if the quantity, quality, or prices of the products or services received are not accurate.

- Verify that medical equipment is inspected and maintained according to medical guidelines and that documentation of services is provided by the vendor to keep on file within the center.

VENDOR PARTNERSHIPS

The ROI of the time and energy put into developing vendor relationships cannot be calculated because quality service is difficult to price. The returns often pay out in unexpected customer service over a long period. For example, when your vendor is a long-term partner, they will personally expedite repairs or delivery of loaner equipment when a vital piece of equipment fails and patient care is affected, or they will rush a shipment of vaccine for a flu clinic that was not ordered by staff in a timely manner.

Become acquainted with vendors personally by taking the time to maintain a regular flow of communication and by being respectful and open to compromise when issues occur. Be open to suggestions for improvement, and encourage your vendors to bring their expertise and ideas to your attention for discussion and strategizing. Over time, communication and collaboration will build trust and make your vendor a partner. The vendor partnership should provide

- Cost-effective contracts
- Better customer service
- New center resources
- New lines of business

CONCLUSION

The process of choosing equipment and supply vendors can be complex and time-consuming but is well worth the investment. Choosing the right vendors and building vendor partnerships will create greater opportunity for cost-effective contracts and increased quality of service. Partnership collaboration can be financially transforming for the center by bringing new ideas and resources that are mutually beneficial.

KEY POINTS

1. Successfully choosing equipment and supply vendors will control overhead costs and provide consistent quality of service.

2. List all equipment, supplies, and services needed for each center project to create a worksheet before contacting vendors. Tables 2 through 10 provide lists of commonly purchased equipment and supplies.

3. Ask colleagues for vendor recommendations, and consider vendors you already know and trust.

4. Research and narrow down vendors on the basis of
   - Experience
   - Financial stability
   - Customer services
   - Competitive pricing

5. Start-up and independent urgent care centers should consider joining a GPO for better discounts and pricing than they can achieve on their own.

6. Take the time to meet with vendors personally.

7. Read contracts carefully to verify that they include the promised
   - Pricing and fees
   - Service guarantees
   - Reasonable out clause

8. Be willing to find another vendor if a contract does not reflect the agreed-on pricing and services negotiated.

9. Routinely verify your center is receiving the pricing, quality, and services as contractually agreed.

10. Make your vendor a partner through communication and collaboration.

CHAPTER 11

Urgent Care Accreditation

Michael Kulczycki, Laurel Stoimenoff, and John Shufeldt

EVERY URGENT CARE FACILITY operator will eventually confront the question of whether to get the facility accredited. Accreditation is a process that tells the stakeholders in your business (your patients, your community, your liability insurance company, your staff) that your facility adheres to a certain set of quality standards. These standards are meant to improve patient care and reduce the number of mistakes that can often plague hectic and information-heavy environments like urgent care and other health-care facilities.

For urgent care clinics, accreditation is generally not necessary to have a legally compliant operation, and most managed-care organizations don't require accreditation at this time. Nonetheless, being able to show that your facility adheres to certain standards can help with receiving managed-care reimbursements, lowering your liability insurance expenses, and improving your operations.

BACKGROUND

Accreditation of medical facilities in the United States can be traced back to the Joint Commission, which was formed in 1951 as the Joint Commission on Accreditation of Hospitals. The Joint Commission is a nonprofit organization that creates best practices guidelines for hospitals and medical facilities to ensure high-quality patient care. Although the Joint Commission's original focus was on hospitals, in the mid-1970s the organization began to offer accreditation options that targeted other types of facilities.

However, the Joint Commission is not the only body that can provide accreditation. The Accreditation Association for Ambulatory Health Care (AAAHC) was founded in 1979 and has played an instrumental role in developing best practices policies and providing accreditation, but it does not specialize in urgent care centers.

Another organization, the American Academy of Urgent Care Medicine (AAUCM), developed an accreditation system in 2000 to focus on the needs of urgent care clinics. This was largely because the earlier accreditation requirements, such as those from the Joint Commission, were deemed too broad for the needs of urgent care clinics. Most recently, the Urgent Care Association of America (UCAOA) announced that it was planning to establish its own accreditation program that would combine the Joint Commission's practices with the UCAOA's existing Certified Urgent Care Center guidelines.

Together, these four agencies (Joint Commission, AAAHC, AAUCM, and UCAOA) are likely to continue playing a dominant part in the accreditation of urgent care clinics. Although the Joint Commission and AAAHC are older organizations that have built a reputation for accrediting medical institutions, the AAUCM and UCAOA offer an approach that focuses on the operational dynamics of urgent care clinics. This narrower approach will likely provide more educational and operational value to urgent care facility operators.

OVERVIEW

Regardless of which organization you choose to accredit your facility, the process itself is similar across the board. It involves an application for accreditation, an on-site visit, an opportunity to correct any deficiencies, and follow-up visits or follow-up reports thereafter, until the accreditation needs to be renewed.

The specifics of the application process depend on the accrediting body. Typically, you have to fill out an application that gives the accrediting body enough information about your facility to understand the dynamics of your clinic. In the application, you provide the relevant information that details what kind of facility you operate, what services you provide, how many patients you see, and other useful data that will help the accrediting organization understand your operations.

The on-site visit portion of the process follows submission of the application and is designed for a professional surveyor from the accrediting organization to see firsthand how your facility operates. The representative will review a random sampling of client files, will interview selected medical staff, and will gather any additional information needed to assess how well your facility adheres to best practices.

The surveyor files a report of the findings and issues a list of recommendations for improving the overall operations. If the surveyor's opinion includes findings, you will usually have 4 to 8 weeks to make the necessary changes and provide proof that the appropriate guidelines have been met. The accrediting body may then issue a full approval, may deny accreditation, or may issue conditional accreditation that requires certain aspects of the operations to be improved before full accreditation can be issued.

Once your facility has received accreditation, it will remain in effect until a new site visit needs to be conducted for renewal purposes, after an interval that depends on the accrediting organization you choose. The Joint Commission issues accreditation that is valid for approximately 3 years. There may be random site visits during that time (see the section "How Long Does the Joint Commission

Accreditation Last?" in this chapter), but once you receive accreditation, it will remain in effect for 3 years unless there are major issues afterward. The AAAHC and AAUCM also issue accreditations that are valid for 3 years, but the AAUCM sometimes issues conditional accreditations that last for only a year if there are certain findings that must be corrected by the facility. Overall, accreditation bodies understand the burden that the review process puts on facility operators, and they are not likely to issue accreditation that lasts less than 3 years unless there are problems with the facility that jeopardize patient care or staff safety.

JOINT COMMISSION ACCREDITATION

Although other organizations engage in the accreditation of urgent care facilities, the accreditation method administered by the Joint Commission is a good example of how the process works overall. It's a little more cumbersome than the alternatives, but a description of it shows what you can expect in a serious review. The Joint Commission is the oldest of the four major organizations that issue accreditation, and other organizations tend to build on their process. Therefore, the Joint Commission procedures are useful to understand.

Before the Application

Before starting the application process, obtain the Joint Commission's *Comprehensive Accreditation Manual for Ambulatory Care* (*CAMAC*). This manual is usually provided as part of the application process, but obtaining it before filing a formal application gives you a head start and makes the process smoother. Because there are time limits after your application is filed (discussed in the section "Application" in this chapter), having this manual beforehand can improve the chances of being prepared for the accreditation survey.

The *CAMAC* is full of information about best practices for various aspects of running a medical facility. It covers topics such as proper human resources functions, proper prevention and control of infectious diseases, planning for community emergencies, management of medication, and a number of other topics. Not all of the areas covered by this manual may be applicable to your urgent care facility. The Joint Commission accredits many types of medical facilities, and the guidelines in some cases may be too broad for your situation. Nonetheless, this manual can go a long way in helping you ensure that your facility is ready for the accreditation process.

Application

The first formal step in the accreditation process is to complete and submit an application to the Joint Commission. The application will contain information about your facility, the number of staff and physicians, types of services provided, and other pertinent facts. An application deposit fee ($1,700 in 2013) must also accompany your paperwork to get the ball rolling. It is a good idea to submit your application approximately 4 to 6 months before your initial on-site review by a Joint Commission surveyor. The importance of this timeline cannot be overstated.

If your facility cannot accommodate an on-site survey within 6 months, your application becomes invalid, because the information on it is deemed outdated. If this happens, you will have to submit a new application along with another deposit fee. Your original deposit fee will not be refunded.

Preparation

The Joint Commission will assign an account representative to help you move the process forward. This individual will become your main point of contact for scheduling the survey and answering any questions you may have about the process. Keep in mind that the account representative is not the person who will be conducting the actual survey.

The survey process can seem very hectic, but it becomes easier to prepare if you understand the idea behind it. Throughout the entire time, the main thing that the surveyor will be doing is reviewing your systems to ensure that the processes you have in place are congruent with the best practices outlined by the Joint Commission.

As you're preparing for the survey, you want to tackle the biggest item first: patient safety. Ensure that your protocols for admitting patients, running tests, and providing medication are as tight as possible. A big problem for medical facilities is misidentification of patients as they are handed off to different staff members throughout the treatment process. Misidentification can lead to incorrect test results and incorrect medications that can cause the patient significant harm.

Once you've taken care of ensuring that there are adequate patient safety procedures in place, focus on other procedures, such as contingency plan manuals, human resources review, and other important items. You may want to discuss the specifics with your account representative to gain a better understanding of what review items apply to your unique situation. Work on the most important factors first, and then work your way down to the less-relevant items that will have a less-significant effect on the final accreditation decision.

Use these preparation months wisely. Delaying preparation until the end could leave you unprepared for your survey, thus causing you to spend extra time and money.

Initial Survey

Either shortly before or on the day of the survey, you will receive an agenda that outlines everything that the surveyor will need to assess. You will usually have an opening meeting with your surveyor in the morning to go over the survey process and what is expected of you on those days.

The initial survey lasts approximately 2 days, and the surveyor will ask for various information and backup documentation to gain a comprehensive understanding of your internal processes. They will review organizational charts, your management and emergency contingency plans, your list of active patients, and other information that will help them understand how different patients move through your system and how care is provided. The surveyor will also schedule time to talk to some of your staff members and may elect to interview several patients, chosen at random, to cross-reference the information that is provided in the patient files. Furthermore, the surveyor will likely review personnel records to ensure that the relevant staff members and physicians have met all of their licensing requirements and that all personnel who provide care to patients have the necessary training.

Throughout this process, be honest and straightforward with your surveyor. Some operators make the mistake of being combative and trying to withhold information. This can create a difficult relationship for you with a person who will play a big role in the final decision as to whether your organization should be accredited.

After the Survey

Approximately 2 days after the survey is complete, you will receive an accreditation survey findings report. This report will summarize the surveyor's discoveries and any problems that you need to address. You will have approximately 4 to 8 weeks to correct any issues and submit Evidence of Standards Compliance (ESC) and Measures of Success forms that show how you addressed the findings in the initial report.

Approximately 2 weeks after you submit any post-survey documentation, you will receive one of five possible decisions: accredited, provisional accreditation, conditional accreditation, preliminary denial of accreditation, or denial of accreditation.

Accredited is exactly what it sounds like. It means that your organization was in compliance with the relevant standards at the time of the survey. *Provisional accreditation* means that you have not fully addressed all compliance findings within the allotted time period. This decision would usually be issued when negative findings are not too substantial and don't warrant an outright denial. *Conditional accreditation* is issued when there are substantial compliance problems within your organization and further detailed review (including another site visit) will be necessary to make a final decision. *Preliminary denial of accreditation* is issued when there is significant noncompliance with best practices or when your facility operates in a way that poses an immediate threat to patients and staff members. A conditional accreditation can deteriorate into a preliminary denial if it is not taken seriously and initial problems are not resolved. *Denial of accreditation* means that accreditation for your facility has been denied, and you no longer have any recourse to fix the problems and reengage in the process.

How Long Does the Joint Commission Accreditation Last?

Once your organization has received accreditation from the Joint Commission, it will typically last for a period of 3 years. Approximately 6 months prior to the expiration of your accreditation, you will need to reapply with the Joint Commission and go through the survey process again to receive a renewal.

During the 3 years between accreditation cycles, you will have the opportunity to provide updated reports to the Joint Commission and to speak with their staff members about any potential issues you may have, but this is not mandatory. During this time, a small number of accredited institutions are also chosen for surprise on-site visits, approximately 18 to 36 months after the initial survey. These visits really are a surprise because you find out about them the morning of the visit, and they can only be postponed for major reasons such as a catastrophic event or a facility move to a new location on that day. Another thing you may experience are random ESC validation surveys. These are unannounced visits to ensure that any information you provided in your ESC paperwork regarding your steps to fix problems have actually been addressed and implemented. Only about 5% of initial applicants are chosen for these unannounced visits, and they are chosen randomly to ensure the integrity of the overall accreditation process. Keep in mind that random ESC validation visits are different from random surveys. ESC validation visits are strictly to ensure that any corrective changes you specified actually took place. Random surveys, on the other hand, are a repeat of your initial survey and are much more comprehensive in scope.

How Much Does It Cost?

The cost of the accreditation process with the Joint Commission depends on several factors, including the number of patients you treat and the number of facilities you have. The fee is paid over a course of 3 years, with about 60% of the total fee being payable in the first year and the other 40% spread over the next 2 years. If you have just one facility of medium size, you can expect to pay $10,000 to $20,000 over the course of the 3 years. If your facility is larger or you have multiple locations, you can expect to pay significantly more.

ACCREDITATION BY THE AMERICAN ACADEMY OF URGENT CARE MEDICINE

The AAUCM has its own accreditation procedures and focuses more closely on urgent care facilities. This organization has been accrediting facilities since 2000, which is a significantly shorter time than for the Joint Commission, which was established in the 1950s, or the AAAHC, which was established in the late 1970s. However, the goal of the AAUCM was to make the accreditation process more relevant specifically to urgent care facilities. The organization reviewed the standards used by the Joint Commission and the AAAHC and created a program that was more specific to the needs and dynamics of urgent care clinics.

The AAUCM has created a two-pronged process that focuses on (1) assessing the qualifications of medical care practitioners and the quality of medical care delivered and (2) assessing whether the facility operates according to best practices. Some of the major requirements for AAUCM accreditation are listed here:

- ▶ The facility has been providing health care services for a minimum of 6 months before the on-site survey.
- ▶ The medical care provided at the facility is supervised or directed by a physician who is responsible for the medical facility.
- ▶ The facility is in compliance with applicable laws and regulations (federal, state, local).
- ▶ All required state licenses for operating the facility are active.

In contrast to the five possible decisions you can receive from the Joint Commission, the AAUCM issues one of three accreditation decisions: unaccredited, provisionally accredited, and fully accredited. *Full accreditation* covers the facility for 3 years. However, to have more latitude in the decision, the AAUCM can also shorten the duration of an accreditation. For example, accreditation may be awarded for only 1 year if there are issues that the urgent care facility still must address. Another reason for a 1-year accreditation could be that a facility has a medical practitioner whose medical license is on probationary status.

Early Survey Program

The AAUCM also offers an Early Survey Program (ESP), which is a way for facilities that are still in the ramp-up stages to receive accreditation before fully opening their doors to the public. This program has been made available because many health insurance companies require accreditation before issuing reimbursements. Therefore, not having accreditation before patients are treated can create significant cash flow problems. Some of the requirement for the Early Survey Program are as follows:

- ▶ The building in which care will be provided to patients must be finished and ready to support patient care. (It cannot still be under construction or being remodeled.)
- ▶ All of the policies and procedures (as well as any bylaws) must have been approved by the medical director and have been fully instituted.
- ▶ All equipment must have been tested, must have logged documentation, and must be ready for use.
- ▶ The medical and administrative staff must have been hired by the facility, and all licensure and documentation must be on file at the facility. This is necessary because a survey cannot be complete without review of personnel files.
- ▶ A provisional certificate of occupancy or any other applicable licenses must have been obtained from the state where the facility is located.
- ▶ The date the facility will begin practice must have been established.

Costs

The cost of AAUCM accreditation usually amounts to only several thousand dollars, which is notably less than the cost of Joint Commission accreditation. The AAUCM process was partly derived from the Joint Commission process but was refined specifically for the needs of urgent care facilities. Many facilities were hesitant to obtain accreditation before this program was initiated because of the cost and time involved. This program was specifically designed to be less expensive and less time-consuming but to still hold the facility to high standards.

THE ROLE OF THE URGENT CARE ASSOCIATION OF AMERICA IN ACCREDITATION

The UCAOA is a nonprofit organization that was founded in 2004 to help meet the needs of urgent care centers. Initially, the UCAOA did not provide accreditation; instead it devoted its efforts to working with the Joint Commission to refine accreditation standards. The UCAOA partnered up with the Joint Commission to help review the standards for applicability and to develop an urgent care accreditation process that better reflected the realities of running this type of facility. The UCAOA works with the Joint Commission in the following ways:

- ▶ Collaborating through professional and technical advisory committees for ambulatory care
- ▶ Providing the Joint Commission's Standards Interpretation Group with technical assistance regarding urgent care issues
- ▶ Providing input during field reviews of any applicable standards that are in development or revision
- ▶ Developing applicability grids, process guides, manuals, and other relevant resources

Certification by the Urgent Care Association of America

In 2009, the UCAOA initiated an urgent care center certification program that helped facilities better define themselves as urgent care centers. Accreditation is not the same thing as the current UCAOA certification. Accreditation aims to do a thorough examination of safety control protocols and ensure that a clinic operates according to best practices standards. Certification, on the other hand, helps a facility develop an array of services that better fit under the urgent care center definition. Sometimes, clinics inadvertently structure their services in a way that pushes them into a gray area where they may no longer be defined as an urgent care facility. This can become a problem when it comes to delivering care and receiving insurance reimbursements because the overall nature of the facility no longer correlates to how the facility represents itself. The UCAOA certification program is designed to specifically address that problem and help urgent care centers differentiate themselves from other ambulatory health-care facilities.

Accreditation by the Urgent Care Association of America

In late 2013, the UCAOA rolled out its own accreditation program that was meant to address certain needs of urgent care facilities that the Joint Commission program does not. Mainly, the UCAOA accreditation program was designed to be less costly and time-consuming than the Joint Commission program, and to pair accreditation with UCAOA certification. However, this accreditation program does not necessarily compete with the Joint Commission program, mainly because the Joint Commission accreditation is more widely recognized and has a significantly longer history. Instead, UCAOA accreditation is a steppingstone for facilities that cannot yet undertake the expense and time investment of a Joint Commission accreditation. This creates a good opportunity for newer urgent care facilities to obtain accreditation, whereas before, they would forego the process altogether because of the cost and time investment barriers.

The UCAOA accreditation program has another attribute that makes it different. Because of its ongoing partnership with the Joint Commission, the UCAOA allows organizations that are accredited by the Joint Commission to go through a fast-track process to receive UCAOA accreditation, by eliminating the need for another on-site survey.

Overall, the UCAOA accreditation is poised to have a significant effect on the accreditation landscape. By providing urgent care facilities with a less-expensive alternative, the UCAOA could significantly bolster the number of facilities obtaining accreditation. More centers obtaining accreditation would mean more-standardized patient care in urgent care clinics throughout the country. This, in turn, would help continue building a reputation of quality for urgent care facilities as a valuable part of the health-care system, thus leading to better insurance reimbursement rates and a continued place at the table in the ongoing national health-care dialogue.

CONCLUSION

The process of obtaining accreditation can be lengthy, frustrating, and expensive. As you consider the various options available to you, focus on the needs of your facility above everything else.

No matter which accreditation agency you choose, the process will be detail-oriented and will take time on your end. You will be interviewed about your processes and internal control mechanisms by an outsider, which doesn't always feel great and occasionally provokes angst. A good way to approach the situation is to stop looking at it as a chore, or something that you feel you *have to* do. Instead, look at your on-site accreditation visits as an opportunity to learn and improve your practice. The agencies that provide accreditation may not always have the best solutions or solutions that apply to your situation 100%. But remember: They spend a lot of time designing their best practices guidelines and are likely more experienced than you in addressing problems.

After you receive your accreditation, do not just forget about it. Even if you obtained it solely for licensing or insurance reimbursement purposes, you can leverage it further to build better rapport with your patients and other stakeholders. You've worked hard for it. You've probably lost some sleep over it. So you might as well show everyone the effort that you've put into the process. On top of that, it will give your staff an extra something to be proud of and remind them that your facility does not settle for the status quo.

KEY POINTS

1. Accreditation is not mandatory unless mandated by the managed-care organization. Therefore, if your sole reason for pursuing accreditation is to meet perceived licensing or regulatory guidelines, make sure to double check with your state and local governing bodies to ensure that this is indeed required in your situation.

2. Give serious consideration to which accreditation organization has the best program for your facility. The Joint Commission has a thorough process that can be somewhat cumbersome, yet it is more widely recognized than others and may be more beneficial, depending on which insurance companies you bill for reimbursements. On the other hand, the AAUCM and the UCAOA have less-expensive and more-streamlined solutions. Carefully consider the size and the needs of your facility before you make the decision.

3. Take the accreditation process seriously. It is an opportunity to set your clinic apart from local competitors who don't have accreditation and to develop a system for delivering quality care.

4. Do not mislead the surveyor during the accreditation process. Inadvertent mistakes and errors from inexperience can be fixed most of the time. But if you are misleading on your application or during the survey process, you will clearly show that you have a lack of regard for your patients, and will thus seriously jeopardize the success of the endeavor.

5. The accreditation process does not have to be a chore or something that you *have to* do. Instead, consider it a great learning experience that will allow you to polish your operations, improve patient care, and reduce the potential for medical misadventures.

6. If there are any findings during a survey, do everything you can to correct them quickly. Accreditation decisions are not made by organizations but by the people who work there. People like to be taken seriously and feel that their job matters. If you show them how important the accreditation is to you and that you're willing to go above and beyond to address their requests, they'll be more likely to take you seriously and help you along the way.

7. If your facility is not up and running yet, you should give serious consideration to the AAUCM's Early Survey Program. It is specifically designed for urgent care facilities that are nearing their grand opening. This could save you time down the line and speed up receipt of insurance reimbursements.

8. Don't forget that after obtaining accreditation, you may still be subject to random visits in some cases. It's a good idea to always be prepared. It will help you maintain accreditation and, most importantly, provide better care to your patients.

9. Accreditation is not just a process but a mind-set. If you gear your way of thinking toward using best practices, you will have a significant advantage. Communicate this mind-set to your staff, and ensure that the entire organization is proactive about adhering to best practices.

10. Once your facility is accredited, promote this fact to your patients and your community. Be proud of the fact that you went through the process, and show your stakeholders that you're willing to work harder than most and that your facility holds itself to a higher standard.

CHAPTER 12

Pro Forma Financial Statements: Creating Income, Balance Sheet, and Cash-Flow Forecasts

Glenn Dean

Pro forma financial statements are management's representation of the expected future results of company operations. The statements detail the cost structure, staffing requirements, revenue growth, and predicted cash flows, revealing the capital requirements of operating the business. Preparation of an income statement, balance sheet, and cash-flow statement are necessary for new businesses seeking capital investment through a bank loan or issuance of equity or for existing businesses undergoing a change in their capital structure. More importantly, however, the pro forma financial statements become the benchmark against which financial results are measured. Analyzing the variances between actual results and the pro forma statements yields essential information for making timely managerial decisions.

ACCOUNTING METHODS: CASH VERSUS ACCRUAL

Most start-up businesses use cash-basis accounting. It is simple to administer and easy to understand; it is basically a checkbook register. Revenue is recorded when cash is received, and expenses are recognized when cash is paid. Cash-basis accounting is a common method for managing cash in the business when resources are scarce and bank balances are closely monitored; however, it is problematic to rely on the information to make timely operational decisions. There are significant differences between the time revenue is earned and when cash is received. Similarly, payment of invoices typically happens up to 30 days after the expense is incurred. The combination of these timing differences yields reports that are inaccurate and misleading. Relying on cash-basis reporting to make operational decisions means using inaccurate historical trends to forecast future results.

   Accrual accounting records financial transactions as they happen. Income is recorded when it is earned, and expenses are recognized when they are incurred. This matching principle permits a more accurate assessment of profitability and operational performance and yields the information necessary for important managerial decisions based on historical trends and current results. The challenge with accrual accounting using only a profit-and-loss statement (P&L) is managing cash flow. Successful cash management requires integrating balance sheet and cash-flow statements with the accrual-based income statement. The cash-flow statement supersedes cash-basis accounting by providing the framework for accurately tracking the sources and uses of cash to manage bank balances. Accrual accounting is the foundation for creating pro forma financial statements and the basis for effectively tracking and managing the business.

INCOME STATEMENT

The *income statement*, also the *P&L*, is a measurement of company performance over a particular period, typically over a fiscal year represented by month. Revenue minus expenses is *operational net income*, defined as *earnings before interest, taxes, depreciation, and amortization (EBITDA)*. Interest expense, taxes, depreciation and amortization are subtracted from EBITDA to calculate *net income*.

Table 1 is a 4-month pro forma income statement for a typical urgent care start-up. Visits are estimated by day and calculated on a 30-day month. *Net revenue* is determined by multiplying the monthly visits by the estimate for net revenue per visit. *Operating expenses* are calculated using a *key drivers* section in the financial model (see the section "Revenue" in this chapter). In Table 1, start-up costs and clinic development are funded through an equity investment, equipment is purchased, and no long-term debt is incurred. The interest expense lines are presented as options to account for capital lease and debt financing, and income taxes are included for future use in determining tax expense in a corporate structure or when cumulative net income turns positive.

Revenue

Key drivers are the variables in the financial model that use mathematical equations to create the pro forma financial statements. In urgent care, the key drivers for revenue are patient volume and *net revenue per visit (NRPV)*. *Net revenue* is the number of patients seen during the period multiplied by the average NRPV. The complexity in this equation is in how NRPV is calculated. Net revenue is based on contracted rates with commercial and government payers, self-pay rates, and expected bad debt percentages, not gross charges or fee schedules. NRPV is the net realizable revenue or the amount of cash expected to be received for the average patient visit recognized at time of service. Table 2 is an example of the key drivers for revenue, a forecast of visits per day by month, and a forecast of expected average net revenue per visit. The driver is visits per day, but the revenue formula is based on visits per month. For clarity, variables are in the shaded cells.

Creating a key drivers tab in the financial model workbook and linking the formulas in the financial statements to the associated key driver allows the user to conduct an analysis by changing one or more variables to determine the net effect. For example, if NRPV is decreased by $2, what is the cumulative difference in net income for the year? If the decision is made to close the doors at 4 pm on

Table 1. Pro Forma Income Statement

	Preopening	Month 1	Month 2	Month 3	Month 4
Visits					
Visits per day		5	10	13	15
Total visits		150	300	390	450
Revenue					
Net revenue per visit		125.	125	125	125
Net patient revenue		18,750	37,500	48,750	56,250
Other revenue		—	—	—	—
Total revenue		18,750	37,500	48,750	56,250
Operating expenses					
Clinical salaries and wages	—	47,147	47,147	47,147	47,147
Employee benefits	—	8,486	8,486	8,486	8,486
Medical supplies	—	1,050	2,100	2,730	3,150
Medications	—	281	563	731	844
Laboratory fees	—	300	600	780	900
Radiology fees	—	150	300	390	450
Advertising and promotion	35,000	3,375	3,750	3,975	4,125

(continued)

Chapter 12   Glenn Dean   Pro Forma Financial Statements: Creating Income, Balance Sheet, and Cash-Flow Forecasts

Table 1. Pro Forma Income Statement (*continued*)

	Preopening	Month 1	Month 2	Month 3	Month 4
Information technology	—	975	1,350	1,575	1,725
Legal and professional	10,000	188	375	488	563
Purchased services	—	300	600	780	900
Communications	—	94	188	244	281
Medical malpractice insurance	—	225	450	585	675
Other insurance	—	188	375	488	563
Rent and lease expense	—	8,600	8,600	8,600	8,600
Other expenses	10,000	375	750	975	1,125
Billing	—	1,219	2,438	3,169	3,656
SG&A	—	938	1,875	2,438	2,813
Total operating expenses	**55,000**	**73,889**	**79,946**	**83,579**	**86,002**
EBITDA	(55,000)	(55,139)	(42,446)	(34,829)	(29,752)
EBITDA %		−294.1%	−113.2%	−71.4%	−52.9%
Cumulative EBITDA	(55,000)	(110,139)	(152,585)	(187,414)	(217,166)
Capital lease interest expense		—	—	—	—
Line of credit interest expense		—	—	—	—

(*continued*)

160

Table 1. Pro Forma Income Statement (continued)

	Preopening	Month 1	Month 2	Month 3	Month 4
Depreciation		(5,425)	(5,425)	(5,425)	(5,425)
Net income before tax	(55,000)	(60,564)	(47,871)	(40,254)	(35,177)
Taxes					
Net income	(55,000)	(60,564)	(47,871)	(40,254)	(35,177)
Cumulative net income	**(55,000)**	**(115,564)**	**(163,435)**	**(203,689)**	**(238,866)**

EBITDA, earnings before interest, taxes, depreciation, and amortization; SG&A, selling, general, and administrative.

Table 2. Key Drivers

	Month 1	Month 2	Month 3	Month 4	Month 5	Month 6
Visits						
Visits per day	5	10	13	15	18	20
Total visits	150	300	390	450	540	600
Revenue						
Net revenue per visit	$125	$125	$125	$125	$125	$125

Sunday instead of staying open until 8 PM because of light patient traffic, how much will it decrease operating cost over the next month? These questions can be answered by manipulating the appropriate driver in the key drivers tab and monitoring the effect in the financial model.

Expenses

With the exception of clinic staffing, the key drivers for expenses are arranged to match the income statement. Each driver has an associated multiplier in the income statement; some expense categories have additional drivers signifying multiple types of expenses within a category or as catalysts to generate a result. A catalyst is an additional stimulus to forecast an expense category that is driven by revenue—as an example, when the revenue levels are not yet large enough to accurately forecast expenses—as is common in the early stages of growth.

Clinic Staffing

In Table 3, the clinic is open for 80 hours per week and each employee works 40 hours per week. The staffing model includes one front-office person, one back-office person, and one health-care provider for each shift. Radiology technician is

Table 3. Staffing Cost Drivers

Clinic Staffing	Hourly Rate	Month 1	Month 2	Month 3
Front office	18.00	3,120.00	3,120.00	3,120.00
Front office	18.00	3,120.00	3,120.00	3,120.00
Back office	27.00	4,680.00	4,680.00	4,680.00
Back office	27.00	4,680.00	4,680.00	4,680.00
Manager/back office	32.00	5,546.67	5,546.67	5,546.67
Provider—physician	95.00	16,466.67	16,466.67	16,466.67
Provider—physician assistant or nurse practitioner	55.00	9,533.33	9,533.33	9,533.33
Clinical salaries and wages		47,146.67	47,146.67	47,146.67

rarely a full-time position in an urgent care business; it is preferable to train the right person to perform back-office or front-office duties in addition to radiology in order to save resource cost in a start-up business. A full-time clinic manager is employed to supervise operations and perform all necessary nonclinical administrative duties.

Clinical Salaries and Wages

Each full-time resource is assigned an hourly rate, which can be calculated for a salaried employee, and the expense is calculated by multiplying the hourly rate by the number of hours in a typical month (2,080 hours per year ÷ 12 months = 173.33 hours per month). In this model, resources are assumed to be employees. If contractors will be used, create another expense line below the employee-benefits row to track independent contractors separately from employees; the organization will not incur the same employee benefits obligations for these resources.

Table 4 displays the expense drivers for each category of operating expenses.

Table 4. Operating Expense Drivers

Operating Expenses	Key Driver	Additional Driver	Multiplier
Employee benefits	18.0%		% of salaries
Medical supplies	7.00		$/visit
Medications	1.5%		% of revenue
Laboratory fees	2.00		$/visit
Radiology fees	1.00		$/visit
Advertising and promotion	2.0%	3,000	% of revenue + monthly rate
Information technology	2.50	600	$/visit + monthly rate
Legal and professional	1.0%		% of revenue
Purchased services	1.6%		% of revenue
Communications	0.5%		% of revenue
Medical malpractice insurance	1.50		$/visit
Other insurance	1.0%		% of revenue
Rent and lease expense	8,600		Monthly rate
Other expenses	2.0%		% of revenue
Billing	6.5%		% of revenue
Management	5.0%		% of revenue
Total operating expenses			

Employee Benefits
Included in benefits are all employment-related taxes and the employer portion of Social Security, Medicare, unemployment and workers' compensation insurance, as well as the employer-paid portion of other employee benefits, including health and dental insurance, 401(k) match, and so forth. The key driver is a percentage of salary expense.

Medical Supplies
Whether or not medical supplies are inventoried, they are expensed when used. With electronic ordering from medical-supply companies, same-day delivery, and next-day shipping, inventories can be kept at a minimum. For planning purposes, the average cost of medical supplies per visit is the key driver; the expense scales linearly with visit volume. Experience and years of data have shown that average cost is between $6 and $8 per visit, regardless of reimbursements. The key driver is linked to the income statement tab and multiplied by the monthly visits.

Medications
The *medications* category has two main components: (1) injectable and other medications given at the time of a visit and (2) medications inventoried and dispensed to patients. Because there is a revenue component to administering or dispensing medications, the key driver is a percentage of patient revenue. The key driver is multiplied by the monthly revenue to calculate the monthly medications expense.

Laboratory Fees
There are two major components in the *laboratory fees* category, the cost of performing laboratory tests and maintaining laboratory equipment within the clinic, and the unreimbursed expense of delivering specimens to third-party laboratories for analysis. The key driver is an average cost of performing tests for the period that is then multiplied by the number of visits to predict the monthly expense.

Radiology Fees
Radiology overreads by an unrelated third-party radiology group is calculated in this category. By using these services, you transfer some of the risk to the radiology group; this may result in a lower medical malpractice insurance cost for your urgent care center. On average, 8% to 12% of urgent care patients are given x-rays. If each x-ray is subject to an overread, the average cost will be roughly $1 per patient visit. This driver is multiplied by the number of monthly visits to forecast the monthly expense.

Advertising and Promotion
For urgent care start-up businesses, the most important predictor of success is patient volume during the first few months of operation. One important component of generating patient volume is a well-designed and well-implemented

marketing campaign targeted to the population within the trade area, typically a 3- to 5-mile radius around the clinic in areas of average population density.

There are three elements for predicting expense in this category: two key drivers and a preopening marketing spend. The preopening expense is for traditional methods that reach prospective customers, informing them that a new urgent care facility is opening. The two key drivers are marketing expenditures as a percentage of revenue and a flat monthly expense rate for a period. The purpose of marketing expenditures is to drive patient traffic and thus revenue; therefore, the expense becomes a predictor of future revenue. Because of the lag time between marketing spend and patient volume generated, the engine must be primed with additional marketing expenditures to generate momentum in patient growth for a period—1 year, for example. The key driver as a percentage of revenue is multiplied by the monthly revenue in the income statement and added to the flat monthly expense:

[Income Statement! (adv. and promo. exp. cell)] =
[Key drivers! (adv. and promo key driver cell)] * [Income Statement! (net patient revenue cell)] + [Key drivers! (adv. and promo monthly rate cell)]

In the model presented in Table 4, the advertising and promotion income statement cell for month 1 looks like this:

=D11*Key Drivers!$D45+Key Drivers!$E45

At some point—after month 12, for example—the monthly rate portion of the formula is eliminated.

Information Technology

Electronic health record (EHR) systems are transitioning to a software-as-a-service (SaaS) model. They are more cost-effective and efficient, and they require less hardware on-site than installed systems do. They typically include both electronic medical records and practice-management components. The systems are usually cloud based, hosted in an offsite data center, and accessed via a thin client over the Internet. The revenue models are per transaction, with minimal setup fees. In urgent care the cost scales linearly with patient volume. Monthly expense for information technology (IT) has two components representing different mechanisms to forecast future IT expense. The key driver is an EHR charge per patient visit, which typically includes electronic medical records and the practice-management system. The monthly rate component is for connectivity, the infrastructure required to connect the computers and tablets in the clinic to the EHR system via the Internet.

Legal and Professional

Start-up costs in the legal and professional category are predominantly legal costs related to entity formation and creation of agreements and other legal documents. Once the entity is created, the organizational requirements for business legal work diminish considerably. Expenses in this category after opening are primarily accounting costs not captured in the management—or *selling, general, and administrative (SG&A)*—category.

Purchased Services

Purchased services are those obtained from an outside vendor that are not otherwise categorized in the financial statements. The purchases are small and may be repetitive, but they are tracked collectively because they are insignificant to the forecast by themselves. Examples of purchased services are janitorial, laundry, sharps disposal, delivery of drinking water, repairs, maintenance and service contracts, payroll processing, human resources, drug screens, advisory services, audit expenses, and consulting agreements. This category scales with revenue; the key driver is multiplied by monthly revenue to forecast purchased-services expenses.

Communications

Telephone expenses and the voice communication line are the largest expenses in the communications category. They include all telephones in the clinic, cell phone reimbursement, fax line, check-verification and credit card–processing connection, and long-distance service. These expenses scale with patient volume and revenue; the key driver is multiplied by patient revenue for the period to forecast communications expense.

Medical Malpractice Insurance

Malpractice liability insurance has been historically issued to each provider as a separate policy. In an urgent care center, there are many part-time providers, and physician turnover makes it prohibitively expensive to insure when tail insurance is included in the equation. It is becoming common practice in urgent care to offer malpractice insurance to an entire practice instead of to each provider. This covers the tail insurance for a continuing operation (see Chapter 9, "Insurance Requirements for the Urgent Care Center"). The medical liability insurance cost per patient visit can be determined for a forecast patient volume over the duration of the policy, usually 1 year.

The insurance is purchased up front or financed over the year, and it is allocated in the income statement by the patient visit. In an urgent care start-up, the per-patient charge is low because of the lack of history and low number of patients treated. As the practice matures and the patient history grows, the need for tail coverage grows with it. Therefore, the per-patient charge for medical liability insurance grows commensurate with the risk. For the income statement, the medical malpractice insurance driver is multiplied by the patient volume to forecast the expense. For the income statement forecast, it does not matter when the policy is paid. If the payment is made in the first month of the policy, the total amount will be coded to the balance sheet under prepaid expenses and allocated over the next 12 monthly periods (see the section "Prepaid Expenses and Other

Current Assets" in this chapter) but will not change the expense on the income statement.

Other Insurance

Any insurance that is not medical malpractice is forecast in this category. At a minimum, the entity should carry a business owner's policy that covers general liability and property coverage that includes equipment and tenant improvements (TIs). Additional insurance to consider is emergency management coverage, billing errors and omissions, technology and data liability, directors and officers liability, and an umbrella policy. Some kinds of policies are based on revenue numbers; therefore, the forecast is driven by revenue. The key driver is multiplied by monthly revenue to forecast other insurance expense.

Rent and Lease Expense

The simple method of recognizing lease expense for the space is to expense the monthly cost of the lease, pro rata portion of real estate tax and insurance, common area maintenance, or triple-net charges. For example, if you are leasing 3,000 square feet at a cost of $26 per square foot for the first year, and have a triple-net charge of $4.50 per square foot, your monthly lease expense would be $7,625. It is common to have escalators in the lease of 2% to 3% per year over the life of the lease. Using the previous example, if the escalator for the second year is 3%, and the triple-net charge increases $0.33, the monthly lease expense increases to $7,903. This is the quick and easy method of forecasting lease expense, which also forecasts the cash flow for this category; however, it does not comply with generally accepted accounting principles (GAAP) for accrual-based accounting.

Most small businesses are cash-basis taxpayers; therefore, accounting for lease expense using the cash-basis method accurately projects cash flow for the monthly lease payment but does not create matching issues in other categories. Unless your business is required to comply with GAAP, the cash-basis method is preferred to forecast lease expense. GAAP-compliant lease accounting requires recognizing rent beginning at time of possession in a straight-line fashion for the entire period of the lease, including any automatic renewal options. The calculation includes base rent, escalators, common area maintenance increases, and any tenant improvement reimbursements. The difference between cash payments and rent expense in the early part of the lease is accounted for as a deferred rent asset. It is advisable to consult with your accountant if GAAP-compliant lease accounting is required.

Other Expenses

As with purchased services, other expenses are coded separately in the detail but forecast collectively in this category. Examples of other expenses are office supplies; dues and subscriptions; travel expense including airfare, hotel, car rental, parking and transportation, mileage, and meals and entertainment; uniforms; utilities; licenses and fees; and a miscellaneous category. The key driver for these expenses is multiplied by the monthly revenue to forecast other expenses in the income statement. The financial forecast also includes $10,000 of preopening expenses not included in legal expense or advertising and promotion.

Billing

Revenue cycle management companies typically charge a percentage of collections for billing commercial and government payers and sending statements to patients (although there may be an additional postage fee). Payment is typically due for total net collections received the previous month. There is a significant time lag between the patient visit and the time full payment is received. However, if the revenue is booked correctly on the basis of what is expected to be received, the liability to the billing company is incurred though not yet paid. In accrual accounting and adhering to the matching principle, the expense must be recognized at the same time as the revenue, at the time of visit. Therefore, billing expense is forecast as a percentage of revenue for the period.

Management, or Selling, General, and Administrative

The management category, or SG&A category, is a discretionary one based on the structure of the operation. One way of setting up an urgent care company is to separate clinical operations from management operations. The management company can be a separate entity that would be reimbursed for services provided as a percentage of clinic revenue (see Chapter 6, "Business Formation and Entity Structuring"). In this scenario, the management fee uses a key driver as a percentage of revenue. If a management company structure is not used, the expense may be used to estimate the SG&A expense of the operation. It would be typical for owner–operators to leave cash in the business during the start-up phase and receive compensation only when the business is generating cash in excess of what is required for monthly clinic operations. In this structure, an expense would be accrued on the basis of the revenue generated.

Depreciation

Depreciation is calculated when the assets are put into use (Table 5). The useful life of equipment is estimated at 72 months. TIs have a useful life equal to the duration of the lease, in this case 10 years. Total depreciation expense for the period is the basis of each asset divided by its useful life, and added together. *Net property, plant, and equipment (PP&E)* is net of monthly depreciation expense.

BALANCE SHEET

The balance sheet (Table 6) is the statement of financial position as of a specific date, presented in assets, liabilities, and owner's equity. An important metric derived from the balance sheet is *net working capital*, which is defined as current assets minus current liabilities. In essence, it is the organization's ability to generate cash flow to pay long-term obligations and to fund growth of operations. Creating a balance sheet as part of a package of integrated financial statements

Table 5. Depreciation

	Basis	Useful Life	Month 1	Month 2	Month 3	Month 4
Depreciation—FF&E	163,000	60	2,717	2,717	2,717	2,717
Depreciation—TIs	325,000	120	2,708	2,708	2,708	2,708
Cumulative depreciation			5,425	5,425	5,425	5,425
Net property, plant, and equipment	488,000		482,575	477,150	471,725	466,300

FF&E, furniture, fixtures, and equipment; TIs, tenant improvements.

Chapter 12 Glenn Dean Pro Forma Financial Statements: Creating Income, Balance Sheet, and Cash-Flow Forecasts

Table 6. Balance Sheet

	Preopening	Month 1	Month 2	Month 3	Month 4
Assets					
Current assets:					
Cash and cash equivalents	494,000	399,285	341,908	296,367	259,767
Patient accounts receivable	—	14,063	32,813	45,938	54,375
Inventory	18,000	18,000	18,000	18,000	18,000
Prepaid expenses and other current assets	—	—	—	—	—
Total current assets	512,000	431,348	392,721	360,305	332,142
Net property, plant, and equipment	488,000	482,575	477,150	471,725	466,300
Total assets	1,000,000	913,923	869,871	832,030	798,442
Liabilities					
Current liabilities:					
Accounts payable	55,000	5,000	7,600	9,160	10,200
Accrued salaries	—	23,573	23,573	23,573	23,573
Other current liabilities	—	914	2,133	2,986	3,535
Total current liabilities	55,000	29,487	33,306	35,719	37,308

(continued)

Table 6. Balance Sheet (*continued*)

	Preopening	Month 1	Month 2	Month 3	Month 4
Capital lease obligations	—	—	—	—	—
Long-term debt	—	—	—	—	—
Total liabilities	55,000	29,487	33,306	35,719	37,308
Owner's equity					
Membership interest	1,000,000	1,000,000	1,000,000	1,000,000	1,000,000
Clinic acquisitions	—	—	—	—	—
Retained earnings	(55,000)	(115,564)	(163,435)	(203,689)	(238,866)
Total shareholders' equity	945,000	884,436	836,565	796,311	761,134
Total liabilities and owner's equity	1,000,000	913,923	869,871	832,030	798,442

is crucial in reconciling the accounts through linking a statement of cash flows. The balance sheet and cash-flow statements should be created below the income statement on the consolidated financial statement tab; each column is delineated by month and is consistent for each successive financial statement.

Assets

Cash and Cash Equivalents

The category *cash and cash equivalents* refers to the cash available at the end of the month. The cash on the balance sheet is calculated from the cash at the end of the previous period and the cash flow represented on the cash-flow statement. The mathematical equation calculates the cash at the end of the period. This balance consists of cash in the bank and the reconciling items within the monthly bank statements, including deposits in transit, outstanding checks, and credit and debit card payments not yet reflected on the bank statement.

Patient Accounts Receivable

Create a subschedule below the cash-flow statement on the consolidated tab that links to patient revenue and calculates collections and accounts receivable. The first step is to estimate the percentage of revenue collection that happens during the current month and subsequent months. In this example, 25% of net patient revenue is received in the current month. The amount comprises patient responsibility collected at time of visit; co-pays, unmet deductibles, and payments from self-pay patients. Reimbursements from commercial and government payers as well as additional patient payments are received over the next 2 months at 50% and 25% of the net realizable revenue, respectively. Bad debt is included in the net realizable revenue equation; therefore, the calculations are based on 100% of the collectible revenue.

In this subschedule, revenue is linked for month 1 from the net patient revenue for the same month in the income statement. Collections in month 3 are calculated as follows:

$$(48,750 * 0.25) + (37,500 * 0.50) + (18,750 * 0.25)$$

or, in the model:

$$(L118 * \$J115) + (K118 * \$K115) + J118 * \$L115)$$

The dollar sign before the column identifier holds the column constant when copying the formula to the subsequent months. Revenue minus collections is equal to the monthly *accounts receivable (A/R)*. Total A/R is derived by adding the prior month's total A/R to the current month's A/R. The total A/R calculated in this subschedule (Table 7) is linked to the balance sheet in patient accounts receivable.

Table 7. Total Accounts Receivable

	Current Month	2nd Month	3rd Month			
	25%	50%	25%			

	Month 1	Month 2	Month 3	Month 4	Month 5	Month 6
Revenue	18,750	37,500	48,750	56,250	67,500	75,000
Collections	4,688	18,750	35,625	47,813	57,188	66,563
Monthly A/R	14,063	18,750	13,125	8,438	10,313	8,438
Total A/R	14,063	32,813	45,938	54,375	64,688	73,125

A/R, accounts receivable.

Inventory

As mentioned previously, there are two main methods for tracking medical supplies: (1) expensing medical supplies when they are ordered and received and (2) setting up an inventory of medical supplies with the initial purchase. In this model, medical supplies are inventoried. In the forecast, medical supplies are expensed with patient volume and are presumed to be ordered and received when needed; the inventory remains constant because it is replenished on a just-in-time basis. In reality, medical-supply inventories fluctuate and require inventory management. For purposes of financial planning, however, inventory is assumed to remain constant.

Prepaid Expenses and Other Current Assets

A prepaid asset is something paid in advance for use in a future period—for example, insurance that is paid 1 year in advance. The initial entry would pay the invoice out of cash and create a prepaid asset equal to the invoice amount. Each month, one-twelfth of the original amount would be expensed to insurance expense, and the prepaid asset would be reduced accordingly, until the prepaid asset is extinguished in the twelfth month. For cash planning purposes, if any expenses are prepaid, they should be reflected in the balance sheet. This results in a cash outflow in the cash-flow statement, but the expense is properly spread across the year in the income statement. In our example, there are no prepaid assets.

Net Property, Plant, and Equipment

Net PP&E is the current value of long-term assets, estimated by the original cost of the assets net of depreciation expense. In our example, there are two main categories, TIs and equipment. Using the straight-line depreciation schedule detailed in the income statement section, the value at the end of month 1 is as shown in Table 8. The net PP&E in the depreciation schedule is linked to the net PP&E asset account in the current month.

Table 8. Net Property, Plant, and Equipment

Tenant improvements	325,000
Equipment	163,000
Depreciation (month 1)	(4,972)
Net property, plant, and equipment	483,028

Liabilities

Accounts Payable

Create a subschedule for *accounts payable (A/P)* by taking the total operating expenses for the period and subtracting expenses that are paid in the current month or accounted for elsewhere. This will estimate the invoices coded and expensed this month but not paid until future periods. The two most obvious are salary expense (accrued in its own category) and lease expense (paid monthly in advance). Conservatively, apply a percentage to the product (80% to 90%), allowing for paying some invoices in the current month. Link the A/P calculated in the subschedule to the A/P balance sheet account.

Accrued Salaries

For accounting and reporting simplicity, choose a twice-monthly pay cycle. Employees and contractors are paid on the 25th and 10th of the month for periods ending on the 15th and the last day of the month. In this structure, the monthly salary expense incurred during the last half of the month is not paid until the 10th of the following month. Therefore, the *accrued salaries* as of the end of the month are generally equal to one-half of the monthly salary expense unless there are wide fluctuations in salary expense during the month. The accrued salaries on the balance sheet are one-half of the salary expense on the income statement. Link the monthly salary expense to accrued salaries for the month and divide by 2.

Other Current Liabilities

Although it is a general category for all other liabilities, in this model the *other current liabilities* category consists of billing fees expected to be due and payable in a future period for net patient revenue booked and payments not yet collected. The equation is accounts receivable in the current month multiplied by the billing expense on the key drivers tab. Accounts receivable is the amount expected to be collected in the future and subject to billing fees that are based on the money collected by the revenue cycle management company.

Capital Lease Obligations

In the example model, it is assumed that equipment is purchased and not leased. An alternative to conserve cash is to lease equipment under a *capital lease*. Title

Table 9. Amortization Schedule

Month	Beginning Balance	Monthly Payment	Interest Expense	Ending Balance	Depreciation Expense
1	163,000.00	3,640	1,653.32	161,013.32	2,716.67
2	161,013.32	3,640	1,633.17	159,006.48	2,716.67
3	159,006.48	3,640	1,612.81	156,979.29	2,716.67
4	156,979.29	3,640	1,592.25	154,931.54	2,716.67
5	154,931.54	3,640	1,571.48	152,863.02	2,716.67
56	17,659.04	3,640	179.12	14,198.15	2,716.67
57	14,198.15	3,640	144.01	10,702.16	2,716.67
58	10,702.16	3,640	108.55	7,170.72	2,716.67
59	7,170.72	3,640	72.73	3,603.45	2,716.67
60	3,603.45	3,640	36.55	(0.00)	2,716.67
		218,400			

Interest rate: 12.171656%.

to the asset is transferred to the lessor, and it is accounted for in three different accounts. The first step is to create an amortization schedule (Tables 9 and 10) based on the original asset price, the monthly lease payment, and the length of the lease (typically 60 months). The amortization schedule calculates the categories (the months between 6 and 55 are hidden from the display). The interest rate is derived through an iterative process.

Excel calculates interest expense using the proper formula

[RATE(number of periods, monthly payment (negative number), beginning balance)*number of periods]

or, in the model:

[=RATE(A64,−C5,B5)*12]

Table 10. Column Contents

Column	Column Contents
A	One month for each period in the lease, 60 months
B	Beginning balance in the period, starts with original purchase price. Beginning balance in period 2 equals ending balance in the prior period
C	The monthly payment from the leasing company
D	The monthly interest payment – beginning balance × interest rate
E	The ending balance = beginning balance – payment + interest
F	Depreciation expense = original beginning balance ÷ 60 months

Another method is to use an iterative process to derive the interest rate given the other variables in the amortization schedule. Change the rate in cell A4 (12.171656%) until the ending balance at month 60 is zero. Once this is accomplished, the schedule provides all necessary data for input into the model.

Table 11 connects the financial statement accounts used to track the capital lease obligations with the corresponding columns in the amortization schedule. The asset balance, interest expense and depreciation expense are entered into the financial model in the proper periods. Each month, the asset value is decreased by the depreciation expense and the capital lease obligation is decreased by the amount of the payment that exceeds the interest expense; the integrated financial model will account for the decrease in the cash balance.

Long-Term Debt

If the members, directors, or managers of the organization decide to finance part of the operation or to fund working capital with debt, it will be listed in *long-term debt* in the liabilities section of the balance sheet. A form of amortization schedule similar to what has already been described must be created, but without depreciation expense. The interest rate will probably be fixed and known, the periods may vary, and the payment may be deferred for a period of time. The beginning balance, interest expense, and ending balance formulas remain intact, whereas the periods may need to be expanded (or contracted) and the payments may be discretionary. The output of the schedule will yield the information necessary to create a forecast with one exception. The interest expense will be coded to the income statement, and the ending balance will be coded to long-term debt. Without making any payments, the long-term debt balance will grow because of unpaid accrued interest.

Equity

Membership Interest

In this example, *membership interest* is the original capital investment of the owners of the organization. The investment is represented as equity. Alternatively, the working capital can be financed with equity and debt depending on the creditworthiness of the principals. The equity portion would be represented as membership interest in a limited liability company structure (shareholder interest in a corporation), and the debt portion would be booked to long-term debt,

Table 11. Financial Statement Accounts

Financial Statement Account	*Column*
Capital lease asset and obligation in the balance sheet	Beginning balance
Capital lease interest expense in the income statement	Interest expense
Depreciation expense in the income statement for equipment	Depreciation expense

with a representative debt schedule that lists monthly payments and calculates interest expense.

Retained Earnings

Retained earnings are the cumulative net income of the organization. For the current period, add the current net income to the cumulative retained earnings of the prior period.

CASH-FLOW STATEMENT

The *cash-flow statement* is a reconciliation of net income through tracking changes in balance sheet accounts and other noncash items like depreciation. The statement starts with the beginning cash balance and net income for the period; classifies sources and uses of cash in operations, financing activities, and investing activities; and provides information on the liquidity and solvency of the organization by forecasting future cash flows. One caveat: The cash-flow statement (Table 12) indicates cash flows over the monthly period and cash balance at the end of the period but does not forecast cash deficits that may occur during the period.

- ▶ *Net income (loss)* This is linked directly to the bottom line net income in the income statement and serves as the basis for the statement of cash-flow reconciliation.

- ▶ *Depreciation and amortization* This is linked directly from depreciation expense in the income statement. Depreciation and amortization are non-cash items; thus they are added back to net income to reconcile cash.

- ▶ *(Increase)/decrease in patient accounts receivable* This is the prior month's accounts receivable balance minus the current month's balance. An increase in A/R is a use of cash, a decrease is a source of cash.

- ▶ *(Increase)/decrease in inventory* This is calculated using the same formula as for A/R—prior month's balance minus current month's balance. There is no cash effect because medical supplies inventory is forecast to be the same balance month after month.

- ▶ *(Increase)/decrease in prepaid expenses and other assets* Prior month's prepaid expenses minus current month's prepaid expenses balance yields the net effect on cash.

- ▶ *Increase/(decrease) in accounts payable* This is calculated in the opposite manner from the calculation for asset accounts; this is the current month's balance minus the prior month's balance. An increase in A/P is a source of cash, expenses that were not paid. Conversely, a decrease is a use of cash, more expenses paid than incurred in the current month.

- ▶ *Increase/(decrease) in accrued salaries* Current month's balance minus prior month's balance is the net effect on cash.

Chapter 12 Glenn Dean Pro Forma Financial Statements: Creating Income, Balance Sheet, and Cash-Flow Forecasts

Table 12. Cash-Flow Statement

	Preopening	Month 1	Month 2	Month 3	Month 4
Cash flow from operations:					
Net income (loss)	(55,000)	(60,564)	(47,871)	(40,254)	(35,177)
Noncash items included in net income:					
Depreciation and amortization	—	5,425	5,425	5,425	5,425
(Inc.)/Dec. in patients accounts receivable	—	(14,063)	(18,750)	(13,125)	(8,438)
(Inc.)/Dec. in inventory	(18,000)	—	—	—	—
(Inc.)/Dec. in prepaid expenses and other assets	—	—	—	—	—
Inc./(Dec.) in accounts payable	55,000	(50,000)	2,600	1,560	1,040
Inc./(Dec.) in accrued salaries	—	23,573	—	—	—
Inc./(Dec.) in other current liabilities	—	914	1,219	853	548
Cash provided (used) by operations	(18,000)	(94,714)	(57,377)	(45,541)	(36,601)
Cash flow from financing activities:					
Principal payments on capital lease obligations	—	—	—	—	—
Long-term debt proceeds (extinguishment)	—	—	—	—	—
Equity issuance	1,000,000	—	—	—	—
Cash provided (used) by financing	1,000,000	—	—	—	—

(continued)

Table 12. Cash-Flow Statement (continued)

	Preopening	Month 1	Month 2	Month 3	Month 4
Cash flow from investing activities:					
Purchases of fixed assets	(488,000)	—	—	—	—
Payment for clinic acquisitions	—	—	—	—	—
Cash provided (used) by investing	(488,000)	—	—	—	—
Total cash provided (used)	494,000	(94,714)	(57,377)	(45,541)	(36,601)
Beginning cash	—	494,000	399,286	341,909	296,368
Ending cash	494,000	399,286	341,909	296,368	259,767

- *Increase/(decrease) in other current liabilities*   Same formula for liabilities—current month's liabilities minus prior month's liabilities. An increase has a positive effect on cash balances and is a source of cash.
- *Principal payments on capital lease obligations*   Current balance minus prior balance reflects the change in capital lease obligations as a source or use of cash.
- *Long-term debt proceeds (extinguishment)*   This is the change in the principal balance, or perhaps principal and accrued interest balance if not tracked in another account, reflected here as current month minus prior month.
- *Equity issuance*   The original equity issuance is reflected as a source of cash, occurring in the preopening period, with no changes reflected in future periods, current balance minus prior balance.
- *Purchase of fixed assets*   The changes in the purchase of fixed assets, including the TIs and equipment purchases, are tracked by the prior period's balance minus the current period's balance in PP&E and represent a use of cash.
- *Payment for clinic acquisitions*   This is a section that would show the use of cash for an acquisition of an existing clinic, prior balance minus current balance, or a source of cash by selling a clinic.

CONCLUSION

The financial statements should be integrated and contained within one tab in the forecast workbook. They are presented by month and by category, detailing financial results, balances, and cash flows. The subschedules used to calculate accounts receivable, accounts payable, PP&E, and depreciation are computed below the cash-flow statement and ideally contain no variables within the financial statement tab. Associated amortization schedules and lease payment calculations can be presented in a separate tab and linked to the financial statements.

The variables contained in the mathematical formulas in the financial statements are organized in the key drivers tab for review and analysis, making the financial forecast an output of the key drivers of the business. Mathematical and sensitivity analysis can be performed by changing the key variables on the key drivers tab and examining the changes to the financial model to determine the net effect on cash flow and to demonstrate cash requirements of the business for a given set of circumstances.

KEY POINTS

1. Cash-basis financial statements are generally easiest to implement but have significant limitations in the financial information that they provide for making key business decisions in a timely manner.

2. Pro forma financial statements are based on accrual accounting. Accrual-basis financial statements yield timely financial information and most accurately reflect operational performance. Revenue is booked when earned, expenses are realized when incurred, and assets and liabilities are tracked at current book value.

3. Key drivers in the pro forma financial model are the foundation for generating the financial statements. Each variable used in mathematical formulas to forecast the income statement, balance sheet, and cash-flow statement balances is contained in the key drivers tab in the consolidated financial model.

4. Revenue is the amount expected to be collected for each patient at time of visit and in the future based on contracted rates and the cash-pay fee schedule, not on billed charges. Patient responsibility not collected at the time of visit is the primary source of bad debt.

5. Staffing is the largest expense of the business. While the business is growing and patient volumes are increasing, it is advisable to operate with a lean staff to preserve scarce capital resources. Cross-training clinic managers and radiology technicians to perform multiple functions will save expenses in the short term and create staffing flexibility in the future. Use the model to forecast the growth in staff and health-care providers when patient volumes exceed current resource capacity.

6. The key drivers that have the highest impact on the income statement are the number of patient visits and the net revenue per visit. Most expenses are fixed for the short term—staffing, benefits, rent, and marketing. Other expenses scale directly with patient volume—medical supplies, medications, and billing expense. The additional expense incurred for an incremental patient visit is typically less than 25% of the revenue generated. Success for an urgent care business hinges directly on patient volume. The pro forma income statement will predict break-even patient volumes and provide tools for measuring progress toward profitability.

7. The balance sheet is a snapshot in time and tracks current value of assets, liabilities, and owners' equity. The current assets and current liabilities account balances are used to calculate ratios that provide liquidity information and forecast the need for working capital to manage growth. The fixed asset balance is cash paid for TIs and equipment that is amortized over the life of the assets. Long-term liabilities are usually debt to finance development of the business or to lease equipment and cash infusion that is not part of equity contributions.

8. The cash-flow statement is a reconciliation of the balance sheet accounts using net income and depreciation to calculate and categorize the sources and uses of cash. In conjunction with the balance sheet, the cash-flow

statement reveals cash requirements by period, predicted for a given set of circumstances by the key drivers of the business.

9. Accounts receivable is an important account for predicting the cash needs of the business and the overall health of operations. The subaccount that predicts A/R balances and the timing of cash collections is based on net realizable revenue not yet collected and the estimate of how long it will take to collect.

10. The financial model is a living document. It is intended to be a benchmark against which operational performance is measured. Actual performance will be important feedback to the validity of the key drivers and the predictive capabilities of the model. It may be advisable to update the forecast periodically to create a new benchmark using more timely and accurate operational data.

CHAPTER 13

Financial Management: Internal Control, Performance Measurement, and Evaluation

Glenn Dean

INTERNAL CONTROL

The internal control structure defines how the organization's resources are directed, evaluated, and measured. Effective controls regulate normal operations, are consistent with established policies, and are complied with using the corresponding procedures. Controls have many functions but are primarily instituted to ensure reliability of records, to comply with rules and regulations, to secure valuable assets, or for operational efficiency. Measuring the effectiveness of the control framework relies on accurate and timely financial reporting for evaluating results over the period.

An example of the application of controls is deterrence of employee theft. Roughly 75% of small businesses experience some form of employee theft. The best defense for an organization is to implement internal controls, a series of checks and balances used in daily operations. These controls are designed, implemented, and administered in accordance with a set of principles.

Control Principles

1. *Segregation of duties*   Separating duties among employees is arguably the most important concept of internal control for eliminating errors and combating employee fraud. Responsibility for related activities should be assigned to different individuals; recordkeeping must be a separate task from authorization to purchase or from physical custody of assets.

2. *Policies and procedures*   Policies are guidelines formulated by management to achieve the key objectives of the organization. Procedures are specific methods designed from the policies to create tasks and processes that result in desired outcomes.

3. *Control over information processing* Every employee and contractor with access to information processing systems must be authorized and have a unique user name and password. Authorization for data entry, accounting for transactions, appending patient records, or unlocking patient accounts should be limited to those who require specific privileges. All entries that change records must be tracked by log-in user name and date stamp.

4. *Accurate and timely records* The financial statements must represent actual results in a timely manner. This requires adhering to a monthly closing process that records all transactions incurred in the proper period. Once the revenue earned and expenses incurred are accurately reflected and accruals and allocations have been recorded, the period can be closed and results can be analyzed.

5. *Performance measures* Once the books are closed for the period and the financial statements are prepared, the key performance indicators (KPIs) can be calculated and scrutinized. Variances from forecast and month over month and year over year changes in variances and KPIs are evaluated. The material changes are investigated and explained and the reasons are justified to predict the impact on future results in comparison with the current forecast.

6. *Management review* The final principle is evaluating results and the explanation for variances in financial statement categories and KPIs. As a control principle, the management review process can result in proposed changes to specific internal controls, policies, or procedures, or in undertaking a reforecast. A recalibrated forecast may be necessary if material changes to the forecast drivers are required to more closely resemble expected future results, taking into account recent financial trends, the changing competitive landscape, and other outside influences.

Cash

The handling and processing of cash transactions presents the greatest risk to an organization without suitable internal controls. The proper control is to correctly record cash transactions in the patient records, the financial statements, and deposit slips, and to ensure they balance, while partitioning the duties of accounting for transactions from the custody and control of the cash.

The handling and safeguarding of cash requires adherence to specific procedures and segregation of duties (Table 1). If these are not properly followed, the risk of embezzlement increases dramatically at the front desk, where processing patients includes collecting cash during check-in and check-out procedures. To mitigate the risk, install a security camera that records the area where cash is accepted; embezzlement is arguably less likely to occur if the employees believe their activities are being recorded.

Table 1. Cash Controls

Control	Recommended Practices
Input all types of payments into the patient record on receipt.	• Transactions should be captured by an electronic device such as a credit card terminal, check-verification software, or manual tracking with a numbered receipt book for cash received. • Any cash received should be inserted into a slot in the safe. • Employees who handle cash transactions should not have access to the safe.
Accumulate all patient charges at check-out, on the basis of services provided.	• Use contracted rates with the patient's insurance company or a self-pay fee schedule, including any ancillary services and dispensed medication, to calculate total charges for the patient visit. • Any amount due after co-pay has been processed (usually at check-in) and insurance billing is calculated as patient responsibility. • Collect the amount due from the patient before completing the check-out procedure, and record the transaction appropriately.
Issue a receipt to every patient.	• Once payment has been processed and the patient account has been updated, print an electronic receipt from the practice-management system that includes all charges and payments received from the patient.
Control access to records.	• The system should be set up to lock the patient account on discharge. • The front-desk personnel should not have privileges to unlock the patient account.
Close daily.	• At the end of the day, perform the cash receipts closing. • Print a report from the practice-management system that details and totals all cash transactions in the system for the day. • Perform batch processing for the credit card terminal and check-verification system to list and total all transactions for the day.
Reconcile cash account using a resource not involved with transaction processing.	• This may be a back-office responsibility. • It can be delayed until the following day for the clinic manager. • Reconciliation must include cash received and requires access to the safe, which the front-desk resource should not have. • A proper reconciliation balances the cash posted to the practice-management system and the cash receipts from the batch processing and cash in the safe. • If a discrepancy exists, track it down immediately. Ignoring the imbalance violates the internal control and increases the possibility of embezzlement or uncorrected process errors that will multiply.

Petty Cash

In an urgent care center, the petty cash drawer should be used only for providing change for payments made at the time of service in the form of cash. With this sole purpose, reconciling the cash drawer is as simple as ensuring that its balance is consistent at the end of each business day. Historically, petty cash has been used for small purchases that would otherwise require cutting a check—for example, purchasing paper, printer ink, or other items that are necessary for conducting business. Best practices would dictate the use of a company credit or debit card with a $500 limit in lieu of petty cash. This method provides an electronic tracking of purchases, eliminating the need to reconcile the petty cash account and minimizing the risk of using cash for unauthorized purposes.

Billing and Collection

This chapter is not about the billing process—most small organizations will outsource the function—but the topic is briefly addressed here to cover the receipt of payments and related cash controls. With the exception of a well-designed front-desk process, the most important cash control procedure is to get a lockbox. Essentially, a *lockbox* is a banking service that processes accounts receivable (A/R) payments sent directly to the bank. As part of the service offering, the bank will reconcile the payments received with the explanation of benefits (EOB) or electronic remittance advice (ERA) and deposit the cash directly into the organization's account. The EOB and ERA are also received by the billing group for entry into the practice-management system. Patients' statements for unpaid patient responsibility should list the lockbox as the pay-to address.

Occasionally, patients will send checks directly to the clinic. For this reason, opening the mail is a management responsibility. Checks should be received by a manager without responsibility for input into the system, and should be stamped immediately "For Deposit Only" with the account number. Thereafter, the checks can be sent to the billing company or internal resource with billing responsibility for input to the patient account. If you believe this control is unnecessary, see "Who Should Open the Mail?" in this chapter, which describes a technique that I discovered while performing due diligence on an acquisition target.

Payroll and Independent Contractors

More than half of the cost of operating an urgent care clinic is resource cost: salaries, benefits, and hourly rates for independent contractors. The most effective tool for tracking time and attendance is a biometric time clock. Properly managed, it limits the administrative overhead of manual time sheets and overtime tracking, and it greatly reduces fraud by preventing unauthorized use. Many potential employees may view a time clock as Big Brother watching over them, but setting the expectation in the beginning as a condition of employment solves most of those issues. After all, you want honest employees who have access to cash and medical records; those individuals rarely have problems with a time clock.

Who Should Open the Mail?

The mail is opened each morning at the front desk and sorted, and checks are set aside for input. When patients pay cash for services at time of check-in, no entry is made in the practice-management system and no cash receipt is given. During the patient's visit, or after the patient is checked out without delivery of a receipt, the embezzler will post the checks received in the mail to the accounts of patients paying cash that day and put the cash in their pocket. If a patient calls after a few months of receiving statements and complains that they have paid the bill, the embezzler will tell them that the error has been discovered and will be taken care of, and the embezzler will cover their tracks by simply posting a check received in the mail that day to the complaining patient's account. This is only one example of the ingenuity of embezzlers given latitude without the proper cash controls.

Managers are responsible for making the schedule and approving the time sheets. The variance between the schedule and actual time worked should be explained each payroll cycle. For simplicity, I suggest a twice-monthly payroll cycle. Payments are made on the 25th and 10th of the month for work performed through the 15th and end of the month. This cycle simplifies the monthly accounting in comparison with a 2-week payroll cycle. As a system control, insist on direct deposit. The employees will get their money faster, and the risk of forgery and stealing checks is diminished.

Purchasing and Accounts Payable

The design and implementation of internal controls for accounts payable requires segregation of duties and is important to limit errors and eliminate fraud (Table 2).

The Fictitious Vendor Ploy

One ingenious method for embezzling funds through the accounts payable process is to set up a fictitious vendor. In the absence of internal controls, the embezzler approves invoices, has checks cut, stamps an authorizing signature, and deposits the checks into a bank account using the name of the fictitious vendor but having the embezzler as the beneficiary. This method is hard to detect without the proper controls and segregation of duties.

Table 2. Purchasing and Accounts Payable Controls

Control	Recommended Practices
Segregate accounts payable duties.	• Have different people approve purchases, receive orders, approve invoices for payment, enter invoices into accounting records and prepare checks, sign and mail checks, and review and reconcile financial records. • If the business is not equipped for spreading all of the duties among several staff members, then at a minimum, segregate approving invoices for payment from maintaining accounting records and cutting checks.
Authorize purchases.	• Because urgent care operations are typically too small and understaffed to require purchase orders for requisition of supplies, purchases over a particular dollar amount should require authorization from management through creation of a requisition over a certain dollar amount; $100 is a reasonable standard in an urgent care setting. This helps the manager have an understanding of and control over the cost structure. • The requisition should list the items requested, the reason for the request, and the proposed cost. • The manager should approve the request and place the document in a pending file to be matched with a packing slip and incoming invoice.
Verify purchases.	• When a shipment is delivered, the front-desk resource or manager should verify that the items listed on the packing slip are actually received, and then sign the slip verifying accuracy. • The signed packing slip should be attached to the requisition and set aside for matching with the invoice. • When the invoice is received, it should be checked and approved by the person who ordered the supplies or equipment, for the correct quantity and price, including any discounts. • The approved invoice should be attached to the packing slip and requisition (if created) and delivered to accounting for entry into the accounting system.
Pay invoices based on the weekly aging report.	• On a weekly cycle, the accounts payable aging report should be created. It should list the following for each unpaid invoice currently in the system: vendor, invoice date, amount, and due date. • The clinic manager should approve payment for invoices on the aging report on the basis of several factors, including due date and current bank balance. • The accountant should cut the checks and prepare the approved backup (requisition, packing slip, and invoice) to be assembled with the check and delivered to the manager for signature and payment. • Once the payment is made, the backup should be returned to the accountant for filing.

Check Requests and Expense Reports

As for the accounts payable process, check requests must be accompanied by the proper documentation and approvals. Check requests are usually prepayments for goods or services to be delivered in the future, or for items purchased outside of the normal process. For consistency, it is advisable to limit these purchases, but occasionally they are necessary. At a minimum, the request must be accompanied by an original invoice, and the checks should be cut from the accounting system with sequential numbers. Otherwise, internal controls are compromised and additional risk is introduced.

Employee expense reports should be submitted on an official company form, accompanied by original receipts and approved by a manager. It is advisable to require timely submission of expense reports for expensing in the proper period. Otherwise, the undocumented expenses accumulate, and unexpected expenses appear in future periods.

PERFORMANCE MEASUREMENT

Revenue

Recognizing revenue in health care is confusing and challenging and is misunderstood by many urgent care managers and owners. There are numerous components: gross charges, fee schedule, contracted rates, time-of-service payments (co-pays and unmet deductibles), contractual adjustments, time of payment adjustments, write-offs, and bad debt. The two most common methods of recognizing revenue are cash basis (when cash is received) and billed charges; there are significant disadvantages to both methods. It is common for both methods to be used concurrently.

Cash-basis revenue recognition works well for co-pays, unmet deductibles, and cash-pay patients when payment is received at the time of service, but it creates significant timing differences in reporting that potentially lead to poor decisions that are based on erroneous data. One simple question will point out the inadequacies of this method. What is your average net revenue per visit? The net revenue per visit (NRPV) equation (see the subsection "Revenue" in the section "Evaluation" in this chapter for further explanation) is revenue for the period divided by the number of visits. If your collection cycle averages 45 days and you collect 25% of your payments at time of visit, three-quarters of the numerator of the equation is revenue collected for patients seen 2 months earlier. The timing differences created by this method of revenue recognition yield operational reports that are based on inaccurate data, and they distort historical trends. You will not be able to manage your billing company's efficiency, calculate collection percentages, or recognize changes in reimbursement or increasing bad debt percentages. These may result in decreasing net revenue per visit but will likely remain invisible in the cash-basis financials.

Recognizing revenue based on billed charges creates bigger issues. When a claim is filed with an insurance company, the codes from Current Procedural

Terminology (CPT) and *International Statistical Classification of Diseases and Related Health Problems*, 10th revision (ICD-10) are billed from the fee schedule regardless of the contracted rates. Fee schedules are set in a manner to exceed the highest reimbursement rate for any payer, typically more than 25% higher. With reimbursement compression, the difference between the fee schedule and contracted rates continues to grow.

The reimbursement from the insurance company is the contracted rate for the entity and credentialed provider regardless of the billed amount, provided the billed rate exceeds the contracted rate. For example: The fee schedule for the services provided to a particular patient adds up to $160, and the contracted rate is $120. The claim is filed with billed charges of $160 and coded to revenue, creating a receivable of $160 (ignoring any time-of-service payments). When the claim is paid 45 days later, the $120 of cash received offsets 75% of the receivable. Ordinarily, the $40 difference in the receivable is written off by coding the amount to contractual adjustments, a contra account to revenue.

Patient revenue	160.00
Contractual adjustments	(40.00)
Net patient revenue	120.00

There are fundamental problems with this approach. Revenue and A/R are overstated by 33%, not only for the amount billed to the insurance company on behalf of this patient for 45 days but also for all billed charges over the 45-day payment cycle. Furthermore, revenue and A/R are consistently overstated by one-third of the total billed charges for 45 consecutive days on a rolling basis. If monthly revenue is $100,000, and 25% is collected at time of a patient visit, revenue and A/R will be overstated by $37,500 at a minimum. The compounding factor that leads down a destructive path is what happens if the excess A/R is not written off. This is the formula used to calculate A/R using the gross charges method:

End A/R = Beg A/R + Gross charges − Cash received − Adjustments

Ending A/R (End A/R) equals beginning A/R (Beg A/R) plus all gross charges (revenue) minus the cash collected minus contractual adjustments. Adjustments to the gross charges are made only when cash is received from the payers.

Contractual adjustments recognized as revenue and not yet written off are only one source of excess A/R. The more devastating cause is bad debt. The major source of bad debt is uncollected patient responsibility, payments due from patients that are not collected at the time of a visit. Typical bad debt is between 2% and 5% of total revenue, depending on front-desk process and efficiency in collecting patient responsibility at the time of visit—typically co-pays and unmet deductibles. If not properly written off, uncollectible A/R can grow to several hundred thousand dollars in only a few years. On the balance sheet the business appears healthy with a high A/R balance; however, with the majority being uncollectible, the true picture is being masked by an asset that is significantly overvalued.

The proper method to account for revenue is the amount expected to be collected in the future, realized at the time of service. This is called net realizable revenue. Once the coding and billing process has been completed—typically 48 to 72 hours after the patient visit under an appropriate service-level agreement with the billing group—all the information for properly accounting for revenue is available. Calculated revenue is prepared by patient and includes CPT and ICD-10 codes; fee schedule for each code; the contracted rates for each code, if insured; co-pays and unmet deductibles, if uninsured; the cash-pay schedule; and the amount paid by the patient at the time of service.

To perform these calculations manually is an onerous task, but this is the kind of processing that computers do well. A properly formatted practice-management system integrated with the electronic medical record database will calculate net realizable revenue and all related components (with the exception of bad debt estimates), provided that the patients are properly set up and that the contracted rates are loaded into the system by payer and by code. The system will deliver gross revenue based on billed charges per the fee schedule and net revenue using contracted rates with insurance companies and government payers, and the self-pay fee schedule for cash-pay patients. Gross revenue minus net revenue is the calculated contractual adjustment.

The discretionary input to the net realizable revenue equation is an estimate of bad debt. The major source of bad debt is unpaid patient responsibility. In the following example, bad debt is estimated at 5% of net revenue. The accounts represented there are booked into the revenue section of the income statement.

Gross patient revenue	160.00
Contractual adjustments	(40.00)
Bad debt reserve	(6.00)
Net patient revenue	114.00

Accounts Receivable

In accrual accounting, net revenue booked at time of visit is an estimate of the expected cash collection for each patient. As previously stated, A/R is revenue already recognized and cash expected to be received. Clearly, the revenue-recognition methodology is the most important input to the A/R balance.

Patient payments made at the time of service are an input to the billing calculation and A/R entry. The A/R balance for the patient in the preceding example is calculated before the bad debt reserve and is based on net patient revenue minus time-of-service payments. If the co-pay is $50, the A/R balance is calculated as follows:

Net patient revenue	120.00
Patient payment (cash)	(50.00)
Accounts receivable	70.00

Bad debt reserve is typically a fixed percentage of net realizable revenue; in this example, it is 5% of net revenue. The bad debt expense is a contra account to revenue (reduces net revenue), and the bad debt reserve is a contra account to A/R. The process of recognizing bad debt on the financial statements happens after revenue and A/R are booked. The revenue booked for the month is multiplied by the bad debt percentage estimate of 5%. The entry is

Bad debt expense (contra to revenue)	Revenue × Bad debt %
Bad debt reserve (contra to A/R)	Revenue × Bad debt %

Using this process, bad debt expense is a fixed percentage of net revenue but the bad debt reserve on the balance sheet will continue to grow each month. The reserve is reduced when A/R is written off or there is an adjustment to the bad debt percentage based on the history of collections. If the bad debt reserve account did not exist, A/R would be written off directly to revenue. The reserve method of accounting for bad debt presents a more complete picture of net realizable revenue and provides a more accurate basis for calculating key performance metrics.

Properly managing A/R minimizes the time receivables are outstanding by providing timely information for prompt responses to aging accounts and write-off of uncollectible balances. Table 3 is an example of an accounts receivable aging report summary. This is a snapshot that categorizes balances by payer type and aging bucket, allowing the user to further investigate areas of concern. Any balances over 60 days for commercial payers should be investigated; there may be contracting or credentialing issues that can be solved relatively quickly or some other issue that needs your attention. The small $25 balance for United Healthcare over 90 is a candidate for write-off, but it may be worthwhile to track down the reason it exists.

Table 3. Accounts Receivable Aging Report Summary

A/R Aging Report	1–30	31–60	61–90	Over 90
Commercial payers				
Blue Cross Blue Shield	32,500	25,000	15,000	1,500
United Healthcare	14,000	9,000	500	25
Government payers				
Medicare	3,500	2,500	250	6,000
Medicaid	1,500	1,200	1,000	1,200
Patient responsibility				
All patients with balances	7,000	7,500	5,500	27,500
Totals	58,500	45,200	22,250	36,225

A large balance in the "Over 90" column for Medicare means there is an issue with billing or credentialing. There is a time limit for addressing these issues, so immediate action is desirable. Some Medicaid plans are slow payers; large overdue balances are not uncommon but should be addressed.

The biggest concern in this table should be patient responsibility. Large balances in the "1–30" column (and in other self-pay aging buckets) are indications that the front-office procedures should be evaluated. Clearly, patient payments are not being collected at the time of visit. Because most bad debt is unpaid patient responsibility, actual bad debt percentage of total revenue may be much higher than 5%, particularly when the "Over 90" category is not being addressed.

The "Over 90" patient responsibility bucket is most concerning. A large percentage of this balance is uncollectible; thus A/R is overstated unless the reserve account can absorb the write-off. If proper A/R management procedures are followed, the balance would not be able to grow to this level without someone's assessing the policies and procedures that led to the high balances.

Unless there is a reason to the contrary, such as credentialing issues or billing corrections leading to late submissions, all balances in the "Over 90" category should be written off. Following is the journal entry to write off the over 90 patient responsibility bucket:

Bad debt reserve (contra to revenue)	27,500
Accounts receivable	27,500

If proper A/R management procedures are employed, the bad debt reserve should be between 5% and 10% of the A/R balance. If not, consider changing the bad debt percentage formula. If the bad debt reserve turns negative, more bad debt expense should be recognized to bring the reserve in range; the result will be a write-down of revenue in the current period. If the reserve is too large, bad debt expense should be decreased; this will in turn decrease the reserve. The net effect will be an increase in revenue for the period.

Working Capital

A measure of operational efficiency and financial liquidity, working capital is an indication of the company's ability to satisfy short-term obligations and generate free cash flow. Positive working capital predicts the capability to fund continuing operations without the need for raising capital through issuing equity or incurring debt.

The formula is simple:

$$\text{Working capital} = \text{Current assets} - \text{Current liabilities}$$

Current assets:

- *Cash*   Cash on hand and in the bank
- *Accounts receivable*   Net realizable revenue: net billings and unpaid patient responsibility

- *Inventory* Medical supplies, medications, office supplies

Current liabilities:

- *Accrued payroll* Payroll earned but not yet paid
- *Accounts payable* Expenses incurred but not paid
- *Current portion of debt* Principal payments due within 12 months

In urgent care, once the space is leased, tenant improvements are funded, and the equipment is purchased, working capital is an effective measure of the health of the business. For the working capital equation to be accurate, the underlying categories must be properly calculated.

Current Liabilities

Addressing current liabilities first, accrued payroll is the total amount of salaries and benefits owed to the employees and contractors at the end of the period. If the payroll cycle is twice a month, on average one-half of the monthly payroll is accrued payroll liability. Accounts payable is the liability for expenses incurred and not yet paid. This category is typically for vendors on a net 30 payment cycle. Most operating expenses other than salaries, rent, and prepaid expenses (such as insurance) are candidates for this category. The current portion of debt is the principal payments due within the next 12 months.

Current Assets

For current assets, cash is primarily the bank balance, any patient payments held in the safe, and other deposits in transit. Inventory is typically maintained at a consistent level using just in time fulfillment and effectively expensed when used. By far, the most important category in the working capital equation is the A/R balance.

A/R should ideally reflect the cash that will be collected in the future; an accurate working capital calculation depends on this concept. The A/R balance is the revenue booked but not yet collected minus adjustments and bad debt write-offs. Excluding the treatment of past-due accounts using bad debt reserves, A/R balances are a reflection of the revenue-recognition policy.

Variance Analysis

A key element of performance measurement and evaluation is variance analysis. A variance is a quantitative representation of the difference between actual results and the planned or budgeted amount. The first step in the analysis is to calculate the variance by category over the given period—typically 1 month, but this can also be performed quarterly or annually. Variances are designated as favorable or unfavorable. An increase over budget for revenues or assets over a given period is considered favorable; a decrease is unfavorable. Conversely, an increase over budget for expenses or liabilities is deemed unfavorable; a decrease is favorable. Favorable variances are recorded as positive numbers; unfavorable, as negative numbers.

Once the variance is calculated, the important work begins. For each category, investigate the reasons for the variance from budget. The exercise of discovering and reporting the reasons for the discrepancies accomplishes two important objectives. First, it provides insight into the cause and effect of business drivers, and second, it furnishes important feedback on the key mathematical drivers that are the cornerstone of the predictive nature of the forecast. In other words, it tightens the forecast structure. After all, the productivity of variance analysis is directly correlated with the accuracy of the forecast.

Financial Statements and Variances

Tables 4 and 5 are examples of variance calculations for each revenue and expense category in the income statement, and for each asset and liability category in the balance sheet. To calculate variances in revenue, assets, and owner's equity, subtract the budget from the actual results. For expenses and liabilities, subtract the actual results from the budget. Of particular interest, the favorable versus unfavorable calculation in the balance sheet is not a balancing mathematical formula and does not result in total variance in assets equaling total variance in liabilities and owner's equity. The representation of favorable or unfavorable variances is meant to facilitate investigation to determine the underlying causes.

All large variances should be investigated and explained. With numerous interdependencies between categories and accounts, one business driver may be responsible for variances in multiple functional areas. Small variances do not necessarily signify proper forecasting; the categories should not be ignored solely on basis of the lack of variance.

EVALUATION

With few exceptions, the majority of the data used in analyzing the operational performance of the business comes from evaluation of the financial statements. The validity of the analysis and usefulness of the calculations is dependent on the quality, accuracy, and timeliness of the statements and the use of accrual-based accounting procedures.

In this chapter we have covered the importance of the revenue-recognition methodology on the quality of the income statement, net income, A/R, and the working capital equation. Variance analysis compares actual results to a financial forecast as a benchmark to measure financial performance. The power of this process is in the results derived from investigating the variances and reporting on the specific reasons for the disparities in each category.

Additional mathematical analysis of the financial results is performed using key performance indicators (KPIs) designed to provide data that can be compared over periods and measured against industry standards. The KPIs defined in the following subsections quantify the most important drivers of the business.

Table 4. Variance Calculations for Revenue and Expense Categories in the Income Statement

	September Budget	September Actual	September Variance
Visits			
Visits per day	35.00	39.27	4.27
Total visits	1,050.00	1,178.00	128.00
Revenue			
Net revenue per visit	125.00	123.95	(1.05)
Net patient revenue	131,250.00	146,013.10	14,763.10
Other revenue	—		
Total revenue	131,250.00	146,013.10	14,763.10
Operating expenses			
Clinical salaries and wages	47,146.67	52,147.00	(5,000.33)
Employee benefits	8,486.40	8,525.00	(38.60)
Medical supplies	7,350.00	7,475.00	(125.00)
Medications	1,968.75	2,015.00	(46.25)
Laboratory fees	2,100.00	1,725.00	375.00
Radiology fees	1,050.00	1,128.00	(78.00)
Advertising and promotion	5,625.00	6,368.00	(743.00)
Information technology	3,225.00	3,387.00	(162.00)
Legal and professional	1,312.50	822.00	490.50
Purchased services	2,100.00	1,573.00	527.00

(continued)

Table 4. Variance Calculations for Revenue and Expense Categories in the Income Statement (*continued*)

	September Budget	September Actual	September Variance
Communications	656.25	729.00	(72.75)
Medical malpractice insurance	1,575.00	1,612.00	(37.00)
Other insurance	1,312.50	562.50	750.00
Rent and lease expense	8,600.00	8,532.00	68.00
Other expenses	2,625.00	3,981.00	(1,356.00)
Billing	8,531.25	9,490.85	(959.60)
SG&A	5,250.00	5,840.52	(590.52)
Total operating expenses	108,914.32	115,912.88	(6,998.56)
EBITDA	22,335.68	30,100.22	(7,764.54)
EBITDA%	17.0%	20.61%	-52.59%
Cumulative EBITDA	(214,678)	(184,578)	(192,343)
Capital lease interest expense	—	—	
Line of credit interest expense	—	—	
Depreciation	(5,425.00)	(5,498.00)	73.00
Net income before tax	16,910.68	24,602.22	7,691.54
Taxes			
Net income	16,910.68	24,602.22	7,691.54

EBITDA, earnings before interest, tax, depreciation, and amortization; SG&A, selling, general, and administrative.

Table 5. Variance Calculations for Asset and Liability Categories in the Balance Sheet

	September Budget	September Actual	September Variance
Assets			
Current assets:			
Cash and cash equivalents	215,677.75	231,410.95	15,733.20
Patient accounts receivable	115,312.50	142,322.33	27,009.83
Inventory	18,000.00	18,000.00	—
Prepaid expenses and other current assets	—	—	—
Total current assets	348,990.25	391,733.28	42,743.03
Net property, plant, and equipment	455,450.00	441,883.33	(13,566.67)
Total assets	**804,440.25**	**833,616.61**	
Liabilities			
Current liabilities:			
Accounts payable	20,600.00	20,918.33	(318.33)
Accrued salaries	23,573.33	26,073.50	(2,500.17)
Other current liabilities	7,495.31	9,250.95	(1,755.64)
Total current liabilities	51,668.65	56,242.78	(4,574.14)
Capital lease obligations	—	—	—
Long-term debt	—	—	—
Total liabilities	**51,668.65**	**56,242.78**	**(4,574.14)**
Owners' equity			
Membership interest	1,000,000.00	1,000,000.00	—
Clinic acquisitions	—	—	—
Retained earnings	(247,228.40)	(222,626.18)	24,602.22
Total shareholders' equity	752,771.60	777,373.82	24,602.22
Total liabilities and owners' equity	**804,440.25**	**833,616.61**	

Revenue

$$\text{Net revenue per visit (NPRV)} = \frac{\text{Net patient revenue over a period}}{\text{Number of patient visits in the period}}$$

NRPV should be tracked by payer to distinguish the level of reimbursement from insurance companies, government programs, and self-pay patients.

$$\text{Net collections percentage} = \frac{\text{Patient payments over a period}}{\text{Billed charges} - \text{adjustments}}$$

This formula calculates collection efficiency on the basis of billed charges, an indication of the effectiveness of the billing group. If billed charges and adjustments are properly coded, the formula is an approximation of bad debt percentage.

$$\text{Contractual adjustments percentage} = \frac{\text{Gross charges}}{\text{Net payments}}$$

Tracking the percentage of contractual adjustments by payer indicates the relative level of reimbursement within the same category (commercial, government, self-pay) when compared with other payers, provided the same fee schedule is used. Calculating the percentage in the aggregate and evaluating the percentage over time may indicate a change in the payer mix or the billing efficiency and process.

Accounts Receivable

$$\text{Days receivables outstanding (DRO)} = \frac{\text{Accounts receivable}}{\text{Average daily charges}}$$

$$\text{Average daily charges} = \frac{\text{Net patient revenue over a period}}{\text{Number of days in the period}}$$

Days receivables outstanding (DRO) is a calculated efficiency measure of the entire billing and collections process from patient payments at the time of visit through the billing cycle to collecting overdue accounts. It is a relative performance measure in comparison to the urgent care industry and prior periods for the organization. Industry averages are 35 to 45 days for operations that collect patient responsibility at time of visit and have and efficient billing and collections cycle.

Aging by Payer

As presented in the section "Accounts Receivables" in this chapter, aging by payer (Figure 1) illuminates inefficiencies in the billing and collections process that warrant further investigation. Ideally this report should itemize all payers—at a minimum, insurance companies, government plans, and self-pay patients.

A/R Aging Report	1–30	31–60	61–90	Over 90

Figure 1. Aging accounts receivable by payer to highlight additional information.

Separating the payer types provides valuable information that directs further investigation.

Evaluating the performance of the organization is a continuing process using the financial statements as the foundation for calculating variances and key performance indicators. The power of this process is in comparing the results to the forecast, prior periods, and industry averages through investigating and explaining the reasons for the differences in results and changes in direction of trends.

CONCLUSION

Internal controls ensure that the business operates as designed by managing and giving employees incentive to abide by policies and follow procedures designed to achieve desired outcomes. The financial results for the period are dependent on adherence to operational procedures and the proper accounting of net realizable revenue and the associated expenses incurred during the period. The financial forecast and accompanying schedules are the benchmark against which performance of the business is measured. The forecast must be detailed, must scale with key drivers of the business, and must be identical in structure to the actual financial statements. Evaluation of financial results is dependent on accurate accounting and preparation of the actual statements. The variances and key performance indicators are only useful if the primary data used to calculate them are accurate. The power of this process is in the analysis of results and investigation of unexpected variances and trends to illuminate cause and effect.

KEY POINTS

1. The reliability of accounting and financial records, as well as compliance with regulations and security of assets, is dependent on strong internal controls.

2. Segregation of duties is an important control to limit fraud and human error; this is accomplished through a series of checks and balances that require multiple resources to be engaged in each transaction cycle.

3. Internal controls are created by detailed policies that are the source for operational procedures. The policies are guidelines formulated by management to achieve key objectives of the organization. Procedures are specific methods designed from the policies to create tasks and processes that result in desired outcomes.

4. The accrual-based revenue-recognition methodology is essential for recognizing net realizable revenue at the time of service by using contracted rates for billed services and collecting patient responsibility at time of visit.

This is the only method that records revenue in the income statement when earned and reliably estimates A/R.

5. A/R is the amount of cash expected to be collected in the future for net patient revenue already realized. The A/R balance is reduced by an estimate of bad debt, calculated as a percentage of total revenue for the period.

6. Effectively managing the A/R aging buckets increases the cash collected and thus the revenue recognized for a given patient volume. Detailed reports on A/R aging provide insight into inefficiencies and direct the investigation to discover the causes. DRO is an important metric to monitor; any material fluctuation is an indication of a breakdown in the process.

7. Working capital is an estimate of operating liquidity, the ability of the organization to satisfy current liabilities and generate free cash flow to fund growth. The equation is dependent on accurate revenue and A/R balances.

8. Financial statements are the foundation for the mathematical calculations and subsequent analysis and investigation. They must be timely and accurate. The income statement shows revenue realized when earned (time of visit) and expenses recognized when incurred, regardless of when they are paid. The balance sheet and integrated cash-flow statement reveal current asset and liability values and sources and uses of cash.

9. Variance analysis is the process of investigating differences between actual and forecast operational results. For the variances to be meaningful, the forecast must be a benchmark using key drivers that predict revenue and expense categories from volume multipliers such as visit volume, NRPV, or staffing levels. The process of investigating and explaining variances from expected results produces valuable information for making managerial decisions.

10. Key performance indicators are results from mathematical formulas that reveal operational results over a particular period. The indicators are compared with forecast, and with industry averages, and are used to develop trends over multiple periods. The discrepancy between actual and expected results, or a trend that is diverging from the expected path, is an indication to management that the underlying results should be further investigated to discover the underlying causes.

CHAPTER 14

Physician Leadership

DeVry C. Anderson

IN EVERY URGENT CARE setting, certain physicians have responsibilities beyond clinical patient care. These physicians are responsible for supervising and managing other physicians and staff members within the group and are considered the *physician leaders* of the organization. The abilities and competencies needed to be an effective physician leader in this setting combine general leadership skills and those particularly required to address the challenges unique to urgent care. Great physician leaders help good urgent care groups become great ones; they are catalysts for success and are responsible for developing future physician leaders. The goals of great physician leaders in the urgent care sector are to model, mentor, monitor, motivate, and multiply not only other physicians but everyone else in their working environment.

Quality physician leadership, however, is not always easy to come by. Leadership skills are often lacking, or at least underdeveloped, in the urgent care setting and in the culture of medicine as a whole. The challenge of producing good physician leaders has deep roots; the criteria for physicians' advancement into leadership positions often focus on academic and clinical accomplishments rather than the competencies needed to lead organizations. Furthermore, medical training can interfere with a physician's developing leadership skills. Physician training is long and typically takes place in a strictly hierarchal culture. This indoctrination tends to suppress the type of team goal-oriented freethinking that is so critical to organizational leadership.

Physicians outside of the urgent care setting are extensively evaluated on individual performance rather than group or team performance. This may reinforce the idea that individual performance and achievement are more important to clinical and business success than team performance. Physicians are also prone to experience the *extrapolated leadership* phenomenon in which they extend the clinical authority that is conferred to them through patient care to settings in which it does not apply; they are prone to assume they have authority in areas in which they have no actual experience, competence, or training. Physicians are typically trained to think in terms of deficits, specifically as they apply to differential diagnostics; that is, "What's missing, what's wrong, and what shouldn't be here?"

This deficit-based thinking is useful in clinical medicine, because it encourages physicians to identify problems. Physician leaders, however, must look beyond solving individual problems. They must also seek to manage multiple systems within the urgent care setting to better accomplish the organization's goals.

Understanding some of the obstacles that physicians face as leaders is helpful when selecting, preparing, and evaluating them in the urgent care setting. Urgent care organizations have multiple employees with individual specialties. Leadership in this environment often relies less on the individual prowess of the leader and more on the leader's ability to empower others to use their own talents and skills to advance the team toward an established goal. Although many aspects of physician training promote competition and independence, physician leaders have to promote collaboration, which is critical for effective teamwork. Physician leaders must harness these collaborative relationships to effect positive organizational change.

Urgent care today faces a number of challenges. Responding to these challenges quickly and effectively calls for great physician leadership at multiple levels. The future growth and success of urgent care will depend not only on how well we identify and train physicians in the art of leadership but also on our ability to develop a culture of strong corporate leadership. In selecting, developing, and promoting physician leaders in the individualized urgent care setting, there are two major areas that should be addressed: selecting and hiring the right physician leader and managing the leadership culture.

SELECTING AND HIRING THE RIGHT PHYSICIAN LEADER

Selecting and hiring a physician leader or health-care provider at any level of your organization requires that you establish job criteria, interview candidates, and hire the health-care provider. Each of these steps is important in establishing firm leadership for the organization.

Establishing Job Criteria

Organizational leaders must agree on the job description and expectations of any health-care provider or physician leadership position before the selection process can progress. The selected and agreed-on core behavioral competencies are specific predictors for physician success in the urgent care setting. Job criteria should be specific and reflect the vision and strategy unique to the organization. It is important during this process to ensure that any potential new hire has a clear understanding of the job responsibilities as they relate to technical industry knowledge, health-care knowledge, and problem-solving skills.

Technical Industry Knowledge

Urgent care is slightly different in scope and practice from emergency medicine, family medicine, pediatric medicine, occupational medicine, and other health-care disciplines that engage patients at the primary-care level. So it is important for both pure clinicians and prospective physician leaders to demonstrate understanding of urgent care medicine in the interview setting. Physicians should have a fundamental understanding of the business operations and legal issues as well as public and health-care policies surrounding the organization and the general practice of urgent care medicine. In addition the physician should have an understanding of the financial environment, which includes insurance billing, reimbursement patterns, and regulations, as well as case rate and contracting norms for their respective regions. Physicians in this setting must demonstrate familiarity with the current information technology systems that their organizations use and should stay abreast of evolving changes within that organization as well as within the industry because they will be viewed as subject-matter experts by other health-care professionals and staff members.

The goals of service delivery in urgent care are multiple and potentially competing, a situation that makes delivery of health care challenging. The ever-present tension between expense, clinical care, and patient quality can generate quagmires. The physician leader serves as a connector among the domains of competent clinical care, business profitability, and a compassionate patient–client interface.

Health-Care Knowledge

To lead, the physician-leader must display a general understanding of the practice of medicine as it pertains to urgent care. Specifically, the physician should have some experience with primary-care emergencies and their management as well as screening-level laboratory and radiographic evaluation practices. Physician leaders are also often called on to function as laboratory directors or quality-assurance reviewers for subordinate physicians and staff members, and should have some familiarity with these practices as well. The selected leader's track record and collaborative style should inspire confidence from subordinates, colleagues, and superiors.

Problem Solving

Leaders are problem solvers, and they can be either decisive or contemplative, depending on the situation. One key component to problem solving in the urgent care sector is adaptability. The dynamic nature of urgent care calls for physician leaders and health-care providers who can shift gears quickly in response to emerging priorities. An urgent care physician should demonstrate personal flexibility and be comfortable handling some level of risk and uncertainty. It takes personal courage to both identify and act on situations that involve risk. Urgent care providers should be skilled at making sound and defensible decisions in a timely fashion, especially in such times of uncertainty. In addition, problem solving in any medical arena requires some degree of honesty and authenticity. The ideal leader in the urgent care setting should be known for integrity and for fulfilling stated promises. The selected provider should demonstrate the tact, finesse, and boldness of character to say what needs to be said to whom it needs to be said and when it needs to be said. Physician leaders in the urgent care setting will deal with many different organizational systems and therefore should have a mind-set for identifying patterns and relationships that may be responsible for observed events. Lastly, a sound urgent care physician leader should have solid business acumen, bringing a business perspective to the urgent care system and a demonstrated understanding of the financial implications of clinical practice patterns.

Interviewing Candidates

Once the organization has agreed on the physician's job criteria, it will need to create an interview team. Unlike staff physicians and pure clinicians, the physician leader in the urgent care setting will be expected to interact regularly with other nonphysician department leaders. Therefore, there should be some members of the interview team who are not clinicians. Members of the team should include the chief medical officer or medical director, selected health-care providers, and pertinent department leaders, such as operational officers or regional managers. Physicians selected to participate in the interview process should be those who have been identified as high-performing contributors to the urgent care group and who model the standards of the organization in attitude and behavior as well as clinical competence. Here are some general guidelines for conducting a successful physician interview:

- *Start on time*   High-performing candidates arrive early. Remember that the physician you are evaluating for a leadership position is also evaluating you and your organization.

- *Listen and be attentive*   Silence your smartphone and hold your calls. The candidate should get the impression that the interview is important to you. Remember that problem solving is part of the skill set you are evaluating, so allow the candidate to talk through responses without prompting.

- *Be prepared*   Have at hand the candidate's application or curriculum vitae, the job description, some prepared questions to ask, and note-taking provisions. Ask about any information related to the candidate's professional background, and request any additional information on past experience that may be relevant but not included in the curriculum vitae.

- *Introduce yourself*   Attempt to establish rapport with the candidate. Talk about your role within the organization and how long you have worked there. Make an effort to smile and make eye contact, and avoid closed or disinterested body language like crossing your arms or turning away from the candidate.

- *Take specific notes*   Your notes should summarize the key points made by the candidate, as well as points you want to confirm. Your notes should also identify specific words and examples used by the candidate as opposed to your general impressions, so you can better recall what was actually said at a later time.

- ▸ *Ask questions about past job performance* Consider that past actions are strong predictors of future performance. Use interview questions that explore how the applicant performed in real situations in the past so that you can predict how similar future situations within your organization will be handled.

- ▸ *Ask open-ended questions* Use key phrases such as "Can you tell me about a time when…?" and "Can you tell me exactly how you dealt with…?"

- ▸ *In every question, probe for three critical elements* Ask about a specific situation, the action taken by the candidate in that situation, and the result of the action.

- ▸ *Do not ask inappropriate or unnecessarily personal questions* Remember that any question that is not related to the performance of the job itself may be inappropriate or even illegal.

- ▸ *Ask the candidate, "What questions do you have for me?"* Many successful candidates will have taken time to learn about the organization and will likely have questions.

- ▸ *Close the interview graciously* Thank the physician for taking the time to meet with you. This is an important part of the process. You want to leave a good impression whether or not the candidate is hired. Remember that the candidate will talk about your organization to colleagues and acquaintances. Be sure to outline the steps that will happen next and when to expect to hear back from you regarding a decision.

Hiring the Health-Care Provider

Discuss compensation and contracting after a candidate has been selected for hire. Take time to consider regional compensation norms for similar leadership positions before deciding on a salary or hourly wage. Physician leaders are a valued part of the organization, and loyalty is important. The value of the physician to your organization should be reflected at all stages of your selection process, including contracting. Be sure to highlight and explain any benefits or incentives included in your offer so that the candidate can give them the appropriate consideration. Remember that quality people are difficult to find, so it is important to get and keep the right people on board.

MANAGEMENT OF THE LEADERSHIP CULTURE

Leadership might be defined as organizing a group of people to achieve a common goal. Quality physician leadership involves the ability of an individual or individuals to rally and unify teams and entire organizations around a single platform. *Management* is, in essence, the efficient and effective use of available resources to accomplish desired goals and objectives. Management consists of planning, organizing, staffing, leading or directing, and controlling a group of one or more people, entities, or efforts for the purpose of accomplishing these goals, and involves building effective teams, understanding the individual competencies required for success in key positions, and recognizing and leveraging each team member's strengths.

Management can also be defined as influencing the human actions employed to produce useful outcomes from a system. In this construct, an effective physician leader must be able to first manage his or her individual actions as a prerequisite to managing the actions of others to accomplish objectives within the organization. A culture of personal responsibility and empowerment starts at the top and is often inspired and demonstrated more than it is spoken or taught. Physician leadership and management in the urgent care setting is composed of four phases: setting organizational goals, establishing organizational responsibility, communicating effectively, and evaluating providers.

Setting Organizational Goals

Selecting the right physician for your organization is a process. The first step occurs before the physician is ever interviewed or hired. It is unlikely that an organization will identify, select, train, or produce a physician capable of leading if the organization has not first clearly established its goals. The process of defining appropriate leadership expectations and the standards for physician leadership success starts with creating such goals. It is unfair to expect a physician leader to meet your performance expectations without your first being specific about what those expectations are. It is difficult to be specific about what you are asking someone to do if you yourself do not have a clear picture of the desired action or outcome. Conversely, if clear expectations are projected, modeled, and reinforced, then a culture of leadership-influenced behavior begins to form within an urgent care corporation. Unfortunately, many providers are interviewed and hired without ever being presented with a clear corporate vision or with specific performance objectives that they will be expected to meet. Organizational goal setting is critical to physician leadership. It can be further subdivided into four categories: vision, strategy, tactics, and performance measures.

Vision

Vision can be defined as the overarching aspiration of the organization. It is the desired end point that the business wants to achieve. Typically this vision is expressed in the form of a vision statement, a mission statement, or core values that are disseminated to every member of the corporation. The vision originates with the organization leader (chief executive officer or board) and is the goal toward which the physician leader should be guiding the company.

Strategy

Strategy consists of a broad set of organizational plans for achieving the organization's goals. If we think of *goals* as "what we want to do," then we can think of strategy as "how we plan to do it." Although vision and mission statements are beneficial, they are not a substitute for strategic plans outlining specific employee actions for achieving the ultimate goal. Physicians and all organizational staff need to be able to relate their daily functional performance expectations to the overall organizational strategy and goals.

Organizations may have similar objectives but employ different strategies to reach them. The specific qualities needed for the physician to perform effectively within those respective organizations may also differ based on the identified objectives and strategies for accomplishing them. The vision of a particular urgent care organization originates from its leader or leadership team, but setting strategy should always be a collaborative affair. Leaders across the organization should be involved in strategic planning, and physician leaders are a critical part of that planning team.

Tactics

A *tactic* is a conceptual action or method employed to implement a specific strategy. The physician leader is responsible not only for modeling tactical behaviors that support strategic goal accomplishment but also for mentoring, monitoring, and motivating other employees to do the same.

Provider Performance Measures

Performance measures are objective, measurable, realistic, and clearly stated outcomes that can be tracked and evaluated to determine whether the provider's actions are meeting expectations. It is important to measure the performance of the provider in an objective way and to provide feedback to help shape the provider's actions.

Establishing Organizational Responsibility

The word *responsibility* in this setting implies the exercise of authority and accountability. The *organizational hierarchy* (Figure 1) is the line of authority and responsibility along which orders or directives are passed within an organization or between different organizations. An effective organizational hierarchy helps fuel clear and direct communication, decreases confusion, and ultimately aids senior physician leaders in guiding and controlling their organizational staff as they attempt to accomplish objectives.

The typical urgent care model groups organizational personnel into three distinct categories: health-care providers, operational leadership, and clinical staff (Figure 2). Health-care providers consist of physicians, nurse practitioners, physician assistants, radiologists, and other health-care professionals. Clinical staff may include medical assistants, radiology technicians, laboratory technicians, and front-desk staff. The size of an operational staff varies according to the size

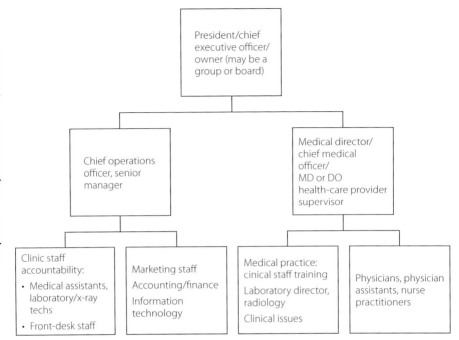

Figure 1. Generalized urgent care organization chart.

of the organization, but often includes marketing and information technology personnel, clinic managers, and finance and operations officers. Although it is helpful to categorize personnel in this way, it is also important to note that many of these defined roles overlap in the everyday function of an urgent care clinic. Most notably, the physician leader functioning in the role of medical director or chief medical officer will often interact with and function within all three areas of urgent care personnel. To maintain a definable line of both responsibility and authority for everyday functions, it is important to establish an organizational hierarchy.

Even though everyone in the organization can and should interact on a cordial basis to share ideas and discuss issues, this cross-talk and intercommunication should not be confused with the directives. Information can and should flow up, down, and across all levels of an urgent care organization; however, directives should only be transmitted down the organizational hierarchy. In general, organizational personnel are expected to give directives only to those below them and receive orders only from those above them. The goal of an organizational hierarchy is to allow the leader to exercise control over the organization. *Control* is the ability of an individual to regulate actions and influence outcomes within an organization. The leader who is able to exercise control can strategically utilize the tactical actions of the personnel in the corporation to achieve

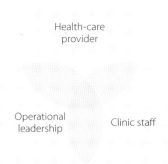

Figure 2. Typical personnel grouping in an urgent care operation.

the corporate objectives. To achieve control, however, the leader must employ effective communication.

Communicating Effectively

Communication is the exchange or transfer of thoughts, messages, or information by speech, signals, writing, and behavior. It is the way influence is conferred from leaders to organizational staff members. Communication is used by leaders not only to create and relay a compelling and inspired vision or sense of core purpose but also to provide logical reasons for choices and to fully articulate ideas. Clear communication allows physician leaders to effectively delegate authority to subordinates and to extend their influence beyond their personal actions.

Evaluating Providers

The goal of a provider evaluation is not only to measure provider performance but also to influence provider behavior. We seek to evaluate our physicians and physician leaders either to change their current behavior or to reinforce the current behavior in an effort to move the organization toward some defined measure of success. Tracking and measuring the effects of the practice habits of providers includes everything from ensuring that practice standards are maintained to determining whether the provider's behavior is influencing the return of patients, the clinic environment and attitudes, the speed of patient encounters, or provider billing. Providers are where the rubber meets the road in urgent care, and they play a large part in determining the experience patients have with the organization. It is difficult to manage things that are not measured; hence, managing providers requires some form of measurable data. Those data are usually obtained via performance tools and metrics, provider self-evaluation, and personal mentoring relationships.

Performance Tools and Metrics

Physician leaders are responsible for moving the organization toward stated goals. Typical health-care provider organizational goals such as efficiency, competency, productivity, and professionalism are difficult to measure without quantifiable metrics in each area and the use of performance measurement tools for objectivity. To measure the provider's actions in relation to the organization's goals, the goals must be broken down into more-specific strategic performance objectives. Performance objectives can be further translated into measurable actions that often correlate with organizational core values. The process of measuring these actions and the indicators used to quantify the actions are referred to as *metrics*. It is these specific performance metrics that are used as a basis for health-care provider evaluation. A *performance measurement tool* is a written or computer-generated instrument that can be used to objectively assess performance metrics. In general, a performance measurement tool addresses metrics that assess quality, quantity, timeliness, and cost-effectiveness as they relate to specific provider actions and performance.

Provider Self-Evaluation

Effective leaders exhibit a high degree of self-reflection. Providers' self-assessment of their own performance in reference to their stated personal goals, practice goals, and perceived barriers and needs is a requisite trait of an effective leader. The ability of physician leaders to self-manage has been referred to in business circles as *emotional intelligence* and is composed of five essential components: self-awareness, self-regulation, self-motivation, empathy, and social skill.

- ▶ *Self-awareness* is the ability to recognize and understand your moods and emotions as well as their effects on others. Great leaders understand that there is a moment between a stimulus and personal response or action. Knowing what provokes you and recognizing the moment when you can regulate your actions makes you better able to control negative emotions and focus on the task at hand. This form of self-management allows a leader to see situations clearly. Self-awareness means having a thorough understanding of one's emotional strengths and weaknesses.

- ▶ *Self-regulation* is the action of verbal and physical self-management. It is the ability to control or redirect disruptive impulses and moods, the propensity to suspend judgment and to think before acting, while taking responsibility for personal performance. It is not only recognizing the moment for self-regulation but is the actual action of regulating. It is also in part the propensity for learning, openness to change, and the demonstrated commitment to ongoing personal development.

- ▶ *Self-motivation* is a passion for work that stems from reasons beyond money or status. Its hallmark is the inclination to pursue goals with energy and persistence. Self-motivated leaders are passionate about their work and will often exceed expectations without prompting or overt incentives.

- *Empathy* is the ability to related to another person's experiences and emotions. Empathetic leaders are experts at reading body language and truly want to hear what people have to say. They are good listeners and respond appropriately to the concerns expressed by other people. Empathy is a key to retaining talented individuals at all levels of an urgent care organization.
- *Social skill* can be defined as proficiency in managing relationships and building networks. It is an ability to find common ground and build rapport with other people or other groups of people. Physicians with sound social skills understand that anything important to the urgent care organization is not accomplished alone. Common tools employed by leaders with social skill include persuasion, conflict management, influence, and cooperative team building.

Mentorship

Mentors are useful regardless of where you are in your career. Mentorship is an interpersonal and developmental interaction in which a more experienced or more knowledgeable person helps to guide and shape a less experienced or less knowledgeable person. It involves an ongoing relationship of learning, dialogue, and professional challenge. Mentoring is a conduit for the informal transmission of knowledge and support in the form of informal personal communication over a sustained period of time between a person who is perceived to have greater relevant knowledge, wisdom, or experience (the mentor) and a person who is perceived to have less of these (the mentee). To develop and sustain a culture of trust, it is important that the physician leader be both a mentor and a mentee.

Key leaders are developed by their early management and administrative leadership experiences in the form of service as medical directors or program directors. Mentors play a key role in guiding junior physician leaders toward and through these formative experiences. Likewise, by becoming a mentor to others, physician leaders are afforded the opportunity to reflect on lessons learned and to reinforce the culture of leadership that is so important to organizational growth. Firsthand experiences and early mistakes and recovery often fuel the passion that drives good physician leaders to become great ones. Mentorship allows for learning to take place apart from formal evaluation and corporate critique and can serve as a farm system for internal leadership development. In his December 2001 article, reprinted in 2011 in *Harvard Business Review*, John P. Kotter states that "successful corporations don't wait for leaders to come along. They actively seek out people with leadership potential and expose them to career experiences designed to develop that potential."[1] This is the essence of mentorship and the heart of sustained leadership.

---

1   Kotter JP. What leaders really do. *Harvard Business Review*. December 1, 2001. Available from: http://hbr.org/2001/12/what-leaders-really-do/ar/1. Accessed February 8, 2014.

COMMON PITFALLS

Physician leadership is critical to the corporate growth of urgent care. When you select leaders to move your organization forward, be aware of some personal characteristics that have proven to be ill-suited to leadership roles in the dynamic and multifaceted systems inherent to urgent care medicine. When identified in physician leaders, certain problematic traits should be remediated, eliminated, or avoided when possible.

- *Leaders who are risk adverse.* Leaders by definition are called on to make decisions when it counts and cannot allow fear to become a prime motivator.

- *Leaders with a limited self-awareness.* The inability to self-manage and to be honest about personal strengths and weaknesses is a liability in the field of urgent care medicine.

- *Leaders with the inability to manage change.* Urgent care is a relatively new health-care specialty and is still in evolution. Everything from the laws that govern the way urgent care is practiced to the technology that determines how information is transferred and evaluated is constantly changing. A leader who is not adept at managing change will soon be left behind.

- *Leaders who are impatient and inflexible.* Physician leadership is about engaging and managing people. Leaders must be able to cooperate and collaborate when needed without compromising values and outcomes. Such skill requires patience and flexibility.

- *Leaders who are individualistic and self-centered.* Organizational leadership in the corporate urgent care setting depends on multidisciplinary collaboration.

- *Leaders who value the tactical over the strategic.* Leaders who focus solely on day-to-day operational activities at the expense of seeing, understanding, and adjusting to the bigger picture are like oxen wearing blinders. They are great for pulling the wagon but not very effective at leading or steering it toward the goal.

- *Leaders who have unclear role expectations.* If a physician leader is not clear about what is routinely expected, it is unlikely that successful results will be predictably reproduced.

- *Leaders who are poor communicators.* Leadership is influence, and influence is accomplished via effective communication. To regulate actions and influence outcomes within an organization, the authoritative exchange of thoughts, messages, and information via speech, writing, and behavior must occur with some degree of clarity. This is communication, and it is the essence of physician leadership.

CONCLUSION

Leadership is a cultivated art. It is a process of constant improvement and the progress of a group toward stated goals via personal communication and social influence. Selecting and hiring the right physician leader is a critical part of this process. Physician leaders help to both establish and propagate the mechanisms by which the people within an urgent care center are organized and engaged in providing fast, efficient, quality health care while maintaining profitability. Management of the leadership culture is equally critical to the art of leadership. Cultures change and evolve because of circumstances, events, and individuals who influence those cultures. Managing the culture of leadership involves empowering individuals to create processes, circumstances, and events that offer the proper stimulus to move an urgent care organization toward its stated goals.

KEY POINTS

1. Organizational leaders must agree on the job description and expectations of every health-care provider in their organization; those job criteria should be specific, reflecting the vision and strategy unique to the organization.

2. Physicians in the urgent care setting should have a fundamental understanding of the financial, operational, legal, and information technology issues surrounding the general practice of urgent care medicine.

3. Urgent care physicians should have enough experience with primary-care emergencies and their management to inspire confidence in their leadership from those working around them.

4. Leaders are problem solvers, and an urgent care physician leader should be comfortable shifting gears quickly and responding to emerging priorities with integrity.

5. Urgent care physician leaders should be interviewed by an selected interview team, with the interview focusing on competencies specific to the job, before the decision to hire is made.

6. Physician leadership in the urgent care setting is best considered in four phases: setting organizational goals, establishing organizational responsibility, communicating effectively, and evaluating providers.

7. Organizational goal setting is critical to physician leadership and is divided into four distinct categories: vision, strategy, tactics, and provider performance measures.

8. Effective communication is critical for leaders to influence personnel actions within a corporation.

9. Managing providers requires some form of measurable data. That data is usually obtained via performance measurement tools and metrics, provider self-evaluation, and personal mentoring relationships.

10. Mentors are useful regardless of where you are in your career. Leaders who are mentored and who mentor others throughout their careers are better leaders than those who go it alone.

CHAPTER 15

Human Resources Overview: Key Labor and Employment Issues

Laura Schiesl

This chapter outlines some key labor and employment issues that are relevant to the urgent care employer. The intent is to set forth some of the best employment practices that are instrumental in the urgent care marketplace and to suggest policies and procedures accordingly. No matter how big or small the urgent care company, having employee policies in place provides structure to the working relationship between the organization and its employees. Once the proper policies are in place, employee expectations are clearer, confusion about proper workplace conduct is decreased, and the company has more of a foundation to defend against disputes that may arise from the employment relationship. The policy suggestions and other best practices recommendations below in no way encompass the entire universe of employment practices that an urgent care employer should implement; however, these are necessary proactive steps to afford the employer and employee some of the important and required protections.

FAMILY AND MEDICAL LEAVE ACT

The Family and Medical Leave Act (FMLA) generally requires providing qualified employees up to 12 weeks of unpaid leave per year for the birth of a child; adoption of a child or placement of a foster child; care of a spouse, parent, or child with a serious health condition; or recovery from an employee's own serious health condition. Employers with *50 or more* employees are covered by the FMLA. In addition to FMLA protections, employees may also qualify for additional state protections. For example, qualified employees in California are also covered by the California Family Rights Act and the California Pregnancy Discrimination Act.

Employees are covered if they have worked at least 12 months for the employer, even if not consecutive, have worked at least 1,250 hours during the 12 months immediately preceding the commencement of the leave, and are employed at a worksite where 50 or more employees are employed by the employer within 75 miles of that worksite.

The employee must provide the employer at least 30 days' notice before taking a foreseeable leave. When the leave is unforeseeable—for a medical emergency, for example—the employee must provide the notice "as soon as practicable," which is ordinarily within 1 or 2 days of learning of the need for leave. The employee need not provide detailed notice or specifically mention that they have a medical condition for which they need time off.

To determine whether your urgent care center or organization is covered and, if it is, what type of benefits are required, it is best to consult with an attorney. It is also prudent to investigate any family and medical leave requirements governed by other state or local laws. Once these determinations are made, the best approach is to formalize the family leave policy and include the policy in your employee handbook.

AMERICANS WITH DISABILITIES ACT

The Americans with Disabilities Act (ADA) prohibits employers that have at least 15 employees from discriminating against a qualified individual with a disability because of such disability. The ADA covers employees who have a physical or mental impairment that substantially limits one or more of the major life activities of the individual, have a record of such an impairment, or are regarded as having such an impairment.

The ADA also requires that employers make reasonable accommodations for disability-caused limitations, if those accommodations will enable the individual to successfully perform the essential functions of their job and do not pose an undue hardship for the employer. Reasonable accommodations may include, among other things, permitting the use of accrued paid leave or additional unpaid leave for necessary treatment, flexible work or part-time schedules, reassignments to vacant positions, and similar accommodations.

The employee requesting an accommodation need not use the specific words *reasonable accommodation*. The request, however, must be specific enough that two things are clear to the employer: The individual has a disability that is causing a work-related limitation, and the individual believes an accommodation is needed in order to do the job.

It is also important to investigate what other disability protections are afforded employees under state law. For example, in California, the California Fair Employment and Housing Act prohibits employers from discriminating against employees and applicants on the basis of physical and mental disabilities. It also prohibits an employer from failing to provide reasonable accommodations to the known physical or mental disability of an applicant or employee, unless the employer can demonstrate that the accommodation would cause undue hardship to the operation of the business. The California Fair Employment and Housing Act covers employers with five or more employees and offers job applicants and employees significantly greater protections than the ADA does. Employers should consult with an attorney to determine whether the employee requesting an accommodation has a covered disability according to either state or federal requirements, and then, if necessary, implement a reasonable accommodation for the employee or another suitable solution.

FAIR LABOR STANDARDS ACT

More than 130 million workers in more than 7 million workplaces are protected or *covered* by the Fair Labor Standards Act (FLSA), which is enforced by the Wage and Hour Division of the US Department of Labor. For the FLSA to apply, there must be an employment relationship between the *employer* and the *employee*.

There are two types of FLSA coverage: enterprise coverage and individual coverage. If an enterprise is covered, all employees of the enterprise are entitled to FLSA protections. Even if the enterprise is not covered, individual employees may be covered and entitled to FLSA protections.

Enterprise FLSA coverage applies to enterprises with at least two employees and at least $500,000 a year in business. It also applies to all hospitals, businesses providing medical or nursing care for residents, schools, preschools, and government agencies (federal, state, and local).

Individual FLSA coverage applies to all workers who are engaged in interstate commerce or the production of goods for commerce, in a closely related process or occupation directly essential to such production, or in domestic service. Engaging in "interstate commerce" may include making telephone calls to other states, typing letters to send to other states, processing credit card transactions, or traveling to other states.

Almost every employee in the United States is covered by the FLSA. However, employees working for small, independently owned retail or service businesses may not be covered, assuming that they do not meet the requirements for enterprise or individual coverage.

With the increase in number of FLSA claims, it is crucial to craft policies governing work schedules and employee breaks. Employers should address the specific schedules that employees are expected to work, including the employer's right to modify those schedules, and the parameters governing employee breaks.

Under the FLSA, employers must pay employees for all time "suffered or permitted" to work, including the following: travel time, working through meal breaks, checking email or voice mail away from the office, donning and doffing uniforms or safety equipment, attending pre-shift and post-shift meetings, and standby time. Covered, nonexempt, or hourly employees must receive one and one-half times the regular rate of pay for all hours worked over 40 in a workweek. In light of the increased vigilance of the Department of Labor's enforcement of the FLSA, employers must pay particular attention to their policies regarding employees' start and stop times and mealtime and rest time policies. It is important to confirm what your state law requires and to verify that your policies satisfy those standards. Employers are not required to grant rest times under the FLSA, but some state laws, including California—as directed by a recent California Supreme Court decision, *Brinker Restaurant Corporation v. Superior Ct.*—require that employers provide (but are not obligated to ensure) for rest and meal breaks. An employer's failure to properly account for break times may subject it to investigation by the Department of Labor, which may result in significant back wages owed to employees, as well as penalties and fines.

The best approach is to set forth in the employee handbook the employer's rules governing breaks and meal periods, including how employees log their time in and out, the number and timing of permissible breaks, and length of breaks. Additionally, the handbook should clarify the eligibility requirements for overtime for nonexempt employees and provide a short explanation for exempt versus nonexempt employees. For example, for nonexempt employees who work overtime, payment and calculation of overtime hours must comply with the FLSA, but exempt employees typically are not compensated for working overtime.

An attorney familiar with local wage and hour laws should be consulted to ensure compliance with pay requirements for rest and meal periods.

TITLE VII: NONDISCRIMINATION POLICY

Title VII of the Civil Rights Act applies to employers with 15 or more employees. Not all employers are liable under Title VII. Under Title VII, an *employer* is defined as "a person engaged in an industry affecting commerce who has fifteen or more employees for each working day in each of twenty or more calendar weeks in the current or preceding calendar year, and any agent of such person…." Employers should implement a clear policy prohibiting discrimination in the workplace. Here is a sample nondiscrimination provision.

> In order to provide equal employment and advancement opportunities to all individuals, employment decisions at [employer name] will be based on merit, qualifications, and abilities. [Employer name] does not discriminate in employment opportunities or practices because of race, color, religion, sex, national origin, age, or disability.
>
> [Employer name] will make reasonable accommodations for qualified individuals with known disabilities, unless doing so would result in an undue hardship. This policy governs all aspects of employment, including selection, job assignment, compensation, discipline, termination, and access to benefits and training.
>
> Employees with questions or concerns about discrimination in the workplace are encouraged to bring these issues to the attention of their supervisor. Employees can raise concerns and make reports without fear of reprisal. Anyone found to be engaging in unlawful discrimination will be subject to disciplinary action, including termination of employment.

TITLE VII: SEXUAL HARASSMENT

Employers that do not meet the eligibility requirements of Title VII would not be subject to charges of sexual harassment under federal law.

Most states also have their own laws against sexual harassment that may differ slightly from federal law. Some states, for example, subject all employers to sexual harassment liability. Other states provide protection against sexual harassment for workers who provide services pursuant to a contract, such as independent contractors (ICs) or employees of a temporary services agency.

Two recent Supreme Court decisions are discussed briefly here, and although they may be described as victories for employers, it remains crucial for employers to maintain proactive and preventative sexual harassment policies in the workplace.

Recent Supreme Court Decision: Definition of Supervisor for Purposes of Title VII Harassment Claims

The Supreme Court of the United States has stated that employers are liable for sexually harassing behavior by their supervisors because supervisors have the ability to participate in such misconduct by the authority that the employers delegate to them.

In two 1998 decisions—*Burlington Indus. v. Ellerth*, 524 US 742 and *Faragher v. City of Boca Raton*, 524 US 775—the court held that in cases involving workplace harassment, employers are directly responsible for harassment by a supervisor; if harassment is committed by a coworker, employers are responsible only if they fail to control working conditions.

Because the Court did not define *supervisor*, a split over the definition has developed in the federal courts since those two decisions. One group of courts has held that a supervisor is someone who directs and oversees an employee's daily work, and other courts have held that a supervisor is only someone who has the authority, on behalf of the employer, to hire, fire, demote, transfer, or discipline the employee.

In a June 24, 2013, Supreme Court opinion, *Vance v. Ball State University*, the issue came before the Supreme Court again: Who is a supervisor under Title VII, for whose actions an employer may be held vicariously liable? In a closely divided majority, the court defined *supervisor* very narrowly: A person who merely has the authority to direct and oversee the complainant's daily activities is not a supervisor for Title VII's vicarious liability provisions. The court's decision means that when employees bring claims involving those who direct and oversee an employee's daily work but who do not have decision-making authority, employer liability depends on whether the employer failed to control working conditions.

Recent Supreme Court Decision: Causation Analysis in Retaliation Claims for Purposes of Title VII Harassment Claims

In the second decision, *University of Texas Southwestern Medical Center v. Nassar* (June 24, 2013), the Supreme Court addressed how employees may prove retaliation on the basis of protected activity under the discrimination statutes.

Under the anti-retaliation provisions of these laws, it is unlawful for employers to fire, demote, harass, or otherwise take adverse actions against employees because they have complained about discrimination. Retaliation charges submitted to the Equal Employment Opportunity Commission have risen a great deal, from around 18,000 in 1997 to nearly 38,000 in 2012.

In a sharply divided five-to-four ruling, the court held that employees must show that "but for" the employer's improper motive—that is, the *retaliation*—the employer would not have taken an adverse action against the employee. The lower courts had been divided over whether the "but for" standard was the correct one, or whether employees could prove retaliation under a more relaxed standard that would require proof only that the improper motive was a motivating factor for the employer's decision.

Suggested Provisions for Sexual Harassment Policy

Although those two decisions may be described as pro-employer, it remains essential for employers to maintain clear and proactive policies on harassment in the workplace. The following are recommendations for some essential components that employers should include in their harassment policy. This is not an exhaustive sample of what should be included in a sexual harassment policy, and it is necessary to consult an attorney to develop a sexual harassment policy well suited for the specific employer and workplace. A comprehensive policy on sexual harrassment should do at least the following things:

- Have a clearly defined purpose
- Have a clear definition of harassment
- Provide for reporting and investigating harassing conduct

Cleary Defined Purpose

[Employer name] is committed to providing a workplace free of unlawful harassment. This includes sexual harassment (which includes harassment on the basis of sex, gender identity, pregnancy, childbirth, or related medical conditions), as well as harassment on the basis of such factors as race, color, creed, religion, national origin, citizenship, ancestry, age, physical disability, mental disability, medical condition, marital status, sexual orientation, domestic partner status, family care or medical leave status, veteran status, or any other basis protected by federal, state, or local laws.

[Employer name] strongly disapproves of and will not tolerate harassment of employees by managers, supervisors, or coworkers. Similarly, [employer name] will not tolerate harassment by its employees of nonemployees with whom [employer name] employees have a business, service, or professional relationship. [Employer name] also will attempt to protect employees from harassment by nonemployees in the workplace.

Clear Definition of Harassment

Harassment includes verbal, physical, and visual conduct that creates an intimidating, offensive, or hostile working environment or that interferes with an employee's work performance. Such conduct constitutes harassment when (1) submission to the conduct is made either an explicit or implicit condition of employment; (2) submission or rejection of the conduct is used as the basis for an employment decision; or (3) the harassment interferes with an employee's work performance or creates an intimidating, hostile, or offensive work environment.

Harassing conduct can take many forms and may include but is not limited to the following (when based on an employee's protected status, as noted earlier): slurs, jokes, statements, gestures, assault, impeding or blocking another's movement or otherwise physically interfering with normal work, pictures, drawings, cartoons, violating someone's "personal space," foul or obscene language, leering, stalking, staring, unwanted or offensive letters or poems, and offensive email or voice mail messages.

Sexually harassing conduct in particular may include all of these prohibited actions, as well as other unwelcome conduct, such as requests for sexual favors, conversation containing sexual comments, and other unwelcome sexual advances. Sexually harassing conduct can be by a person of either the same or opposite sex.

Provision for Reporting and Investigating Harassing Conduct

[Employer name] understands that victims of harassment are often embarrassed and reluctant to report acts of harassment for fear of being blamed, because of concern about being retaliated against, or because it is difficult to discuss sexual matters openly with others. However, no employee should have to endure harassing conduct, and [employer name] therefore encourages employees to promptly report any incidents of harassment so that corrective action may be taken.

Any incidents of harassment, including work-related harassment by any [employer name] personnel or any other person, should be reported immediately to [employer name]'s human resources or personnel manager, who is responsible for investigating harassment complaints. An employee is not required to complain to the personnel manager if that person is the individual who is harassing the employee, but may instead report the harassment to his or her immediate supervisor or any other member of management. Supervisors and managers who receive complaints or who observe harassing conduct should immediately inform the personnel manager or other appropriate [employer name] official so that an investigation may be initiated.

Every reported complaint of harassment will be investigated thoroughly and promptly. Typically, the investigation will include the following steps: an interview of the employee who lodged the harassment complaint to obtain complete details regarding the alleged harassment, interviews of anyone who is alleged to have committed the acts of harassment to respond to the claims, and interview of any employees who may have witnessed or who may have knowledge of the alleged harassment. The personnel manager, or other official responsible for the investigation, will notify the employee who lodged the harassment complaint of the results of the investigation. The investigation will be handled as *confidentially as practicable* in a manner consistent with a full, fair, and proper investigation.

The practice of keeping investigations confidential has come under scrutiny by the National Labor Relations Board (NLRB). In *Banner Health System dba Banner Estrella Medical Center and James Navarro*, 358 NLRB No. 93 (July 31, 2012), the NLRB found that Banner's "generalized concern with protecting the integrity of its investigations is insufficient to outweigh employees'... rights." The NLRB went on to hold that Banner committed an unfair labor practice because the hospital used, in all investigations, a form that reminded interviewers to inform employees that they could not discuss the investigation with anyone else.

This does not mean that employers can never keep investigations confidential; instead, employers are barred from automatically applying the same standards of confidentiality to every investigation. In the *Banner* case, the NLRB indicated that employers must make an individualized determination about the need for confidentiality in each investigation. This focus on the individualized determination analysis makes clear that confidentiality may be necessary in some investigations and not as important in others.

In light of the *Banner* decision, employers should review their investigation policies and revise, as needed, any provisions that require confidentiality in every case.

Provision for Corrective Action

[Employer name] will not tolerate retaliation against any employee for making a good faith complaint of harassment or for cooperating in an investigation. If harassment or retaliation is established, [employer name] will take corrective action. Corrective action may include, for example, training, referral to counseling, or disciplinary action ranging from a verbal or written warning to termination of employment, depending on the circumstances.

Not only is it important to implement a comprehensive and clear sexual harassment policy that provides employees with the necessary information and tools but it is also in the interests of the employer to prevent the costly outcome of litigation involving these types of claims. A successful Title VII plaintiff employee may recover monetary relief such as compensatory and punitive damages, back wages, front pay, damages for pain and suffering, attorneys' fees, and other costs and interest. A successful plaintiff employee may also obtain equitable relief such as reinstatement. The employer should consult with its attorney to develop a sexual harassment policy that is well suited for the individual company.

DEFENSE OF MARRIAGE ACT

On June 26, 2013, the Supreme Court ruled that Section 3 of the Defense of Marriage Act (DOMA) is unconstitutional. Specifically, Section 3 provided that same-sex marriages were not recognized for all purposes of federal law and related regulations. This included the Employee Retirement Income Security Act of 1974 (ERISA) and federal income tax law.

Because of the Supreme Court's ruling, if an employee and a same-sex domestic partner are married under state law, the employer will be required to recognize the same-sex partner as the employee's spouse for purposes of ERISA, as well as for related tax purposes. Employers should identify potential DOMA issues in their workplace and plan accordingly.

IMMIGRATION ISSUES

Each state has specific immigration requirements. Depending on those requirements, the employer should include policies stating the company's commitment to compliance with those statutes and regulations. Also important, the employer should check if the state or states they do business in mandate the use of E-Verify, which is an Internet-based system that compares information from an employee's federal I-9 form against data maintained by the US Department of Homeland Security and US Social Security Administration records. This immigration law compliance policy should detail the employee's responsibilities and be clearly articulated to the employees in a written provision in the employee handbook.

SOCIAL MEDIA AND TECHNOLOGY IN THE WORKPLACE

Technological advances in today's workplace have made it necessary for employers to address employees' use of computers, the Internet, and social networking sites. As a result, every employer should work with legal counsel to craft policies regarding computer, cell phone, Internet, email, and social media use.

Social networking policies have recently come under scrutiny by the NLRB, which has issued guidance about these emerging issues and what constitutes a lawful social media policy. Many employers respond by saying that NLRB guidance doesn't apply to them because their company is not unionized. However, the National Labor Relations Act, which is administered by the NLRB, applies to most employers even if the company, like most private US companies, does not have union workers.

Under the National Labor Relations Act, "Employees shall have the right to self-organization, to form, join, or assist labor organizations, to bargain collectively through representatives of their own choosing, and *to engage in other concerted activities for the purpose of collective bargaining or other mutual aid or protection…*" [emphasis added]. Concerted activity, commonly referred to as Section 7 activity, is when two or more employees take action for their mutual aid or protection regarding terms and conditions of employment. Simply put, if the employee is engaged in concerted activity, the employer cannot discipline an employee for the conduct.

The NLRB wants employers to understand that social media policies should not be overly broad, and that social media policies that are too sweeping in scope may have an impact on employee rights. Specifically, the NLRB is concerned about the right of employees under federal labor law to discuss wages, hours, or other working conditions with each other. The board has concluded that employee discussions of these issues on Facebook and other social networking sites may be protected under federal labor law.

The best approach for employers is to reduce legal accountability by anticipating issues, carefully drafting effective policies, and then enforcing the policies uniformly. If the social media interaction has any of the following conditions, contact counsel before disciplining the employee:

- The post is about workplace conditions and terms of employment.

- Coworkers are responding to the posting.

- The post is a comment or response about something that happened to a group at work.

These are all potential issues that could involve Section 7 (protected concerted activity).

A social media policy should set limits suitable to the organization's needs and expectations. To help employers avoid legal, regulatory, and employee relations pitfalls associated with social networking policies, the NLRB has offered guidance by posting a sample social media policy at http://mynlrb.nlrb.gov/link/document.aspx/09031d4580a375cd (third report issued May 30, 2012, "Social Media Policy Updated: May 4, 2012").

The report examined seven employer policies governing the use of social media by employees. The NLRB General Counsel found that certain provisions were unlawful when they interfered with the rights of employees under the National Labor Relations Act, such as the right to discuss wages and working conditions with coworkers.

When the NLRB recommendations are used as a foundation, these are some acceptable policies that companies can implement:

- They can prohibit employees from posting statements on social media sites that violate the company's nondiscrimination and anti-harassment policies.

- They can bar employees from making untrue statements about the company.

- They can limit employees' use of their personal social media accounts while at work.

- They can communicate to employees that what they say about the company may have an impact on the company.
- They can require employees to respect the confidentiality of the company and fellow employees.

As explained later in this section, employers should be wary of doing any of the following:

- Asking employees for the passwords to their personal social media accounts
- Obtaining unauthorized access to employees' social media accounts
- Prohibiting employees from discussing wages, hours, or working conditions through their social networks

Employers also must proceed with great caution when requesting a user name or password to a social media or email account from an applicant or employee. Legislation restricting employers from asking for this information has been introduced or is pending in at least 28 states.

In April 2012, Maryland passed the first law in the nation to prohibit employers from asking for social media user names and passwords as a condition of employment when both houses of the General Assembly approved two social media privacy protection bills, Senate Bill 433 and House Bill 964. In August 2012, Illinois became the second state to prevent employers from requesting social network account information from current employees and job applicants when Governor Pat Quinn signed House Bill 3782.

In September 2012, California Governor Jerry Brown signed Assembly Bill 1844 (AB 1844) to increase privacy protections for social media users in the state by prohibiting employers from demanding user names, passwords, and information related to social media accounts from employees and job applicants. At that point, California joined Maryland and Illinois in prohibiting employers from requiring job applicants and employees to disclose social media information.

AB 1844 became effective January 1, 2013, and is now codified in California Labor Code section 980. Social media is defined as electronic content, including but not limited to videos, photographs, blogs, podcasts, text messages, email, online accounts, and website profiles. California also bans employers from firing or disciplining employees who refuse to divulge social media information.

At the federal level, HR 5050, the Social Networking Online Protection Act (SNOPA), would prohibit employers from requiring or requesting that employees provide a user name, password, or other means for accessing a personal account on any social networking website. This bill was reintroduced as HR 537 on February 6, 2013, and SNOPA is currently pending in committee.

Company policies should also make clear that the policy is not intended to restrict any employee rights under federal or state labor laws. Finally, the employer should expressly reserve the right to monitor employees' use of the company's computer systems and address privacy expectations in the workplace. The employer should consult with counsel to ensure that its computer, Internet, and social media policies are delicately worded to comply with the NLRB recent mandates and also protect the legitimate business interests of the employer.

INDEPENDENT CONTRACTORS

Workers are either employees or ICs. In classifying a worker in one of those two categories, several factors come into play, including federal and state laws such as tax laws, liability considerations, workers' compensation, and wage and hour compliance, among others. Use of ICs has increased dramatically, in large part because of the economic advantages of using ICs, whose earnings are reported to the Internal Revenue Service (IRS) on a Form 1099 instead of on a Form W-2. Employers are not required to withhold taxes, make Social Security or Medicare contributions, or pay unemployment or workers' compensation premiums for ICs. Similarly, employee benefit plans, including group health insurance and 401(k) retirement plans, cover only employees, not ICs. These economic inducements have led many businesses to unwittingly classify many workers as ICs even though they may fall within the definition of employees under the tax and labor laws. Undoubtedly, some businesses knowingly misclassify employees as ICs, but many pay insufficient attention to this subject or have mistaken conceptions of the laws in this area.

With the implementation of the Affordable Care Act, however, coupled with the increased activity by the Department of Labor in investigating misclassification claims, employers should pay particular attention to their contractual arrangements with ICs in an effort to eliminate the possibility of creating an employer–employee relationship.

The IRS provides guidance as to common law rules that establish the type of business relationship (employee versus IC). The common law rules fall under the following three general categories:

- *Behavioral*   Does the company control or have the right to control what the worker does and how the worker does their job?

- *Financial*   Are the business aspects of the worker's job controlled by the payer?

- *Type of relationship*   Are there written contracts or employee-type benefits?

Courts will look to a variety of factors, depending on jurisdiction, including the following:

- The extent of control that, by the agreement, the employer may exercise over the details of the work

- Whether the one employed is engaged in a distinct occupation or business
- The kind of occupation, with reference to whether, in the locality, the work is usually done under the direction of the employer or by a specialist without supervision
- The skill required in the particular occupation
- Whether the employer or the worker supplies the instrumentalities, tools, and the place of work for the person doing the work
- The length of time for which the person is employed
- The method of payment, whether by the time or the job
- Whether the work is a part of the regular business of the employer
- Whether the parties believe they are creating an employee–employer relationship
- Whether the principal is or is not in business

It is important to note that although you may attempt to address all of these considerations in an employment agreement, the conduct of the business and worker will be determinative, and the courts and the IRS examine all of these considerations in conjunction and look to the totality of the circumstances.

In the short run, classifying workers as ICs is typically less costly than classifying them as employees. However, in seeking to avoid payroll taxes, overtime pay, employee benefits, and other obligations, employers risk significant liability if, for example, a misclassified contractor later claims to be an employee entitled to overtime.

Risks include liability for many years of unpaid federal, state, and local income tax withholdings and Social Security and Medicare contributions, unpaid workers' compensation and unemployment insurance premiums, and even unpaid work-related expenses and overtime compensation. Any one of these types of liabilities (plus interest and penalties for noncompliance) can be potentially devastating for businesses that make substantial use of ICs.

Additionally, certain states are implementing even more severe penalties. In California, if the employer is found liable for "willful misclassification" of employees as ICs, the employer can be subject to penalties up to $25,000 per violation. Government agencies, such as the Wage and Hour Division of the Department of Labor, are increasingly vigilant in identifying employers that misclassify employees as ICs, resulting in potential penalties for many businesses. In addition, some agencies have announced new information-sharing agreements, raising concerns among some businesses that properly reclassifying a worker with one government agency will catch the attention of another agency, such as the IRS. The risk of incurring liability for unpaid wages, payroll taxes, penalties, and interest, combined with other employment-related costs, makes many businesses with evolving workforces even more reluctant to reclassify ICs as employees.

For each potential worker, the employer should analyze the business need and make a realistic decision as to how much control the business wants to maintain over the worker. If the control is substantial, the business may have a difficult time carrying the burden of proving an IC relationship. If, however, the business is able to establish a true IC relationship, the employer should work with counsel to draft a solid and enforceable IC agreement.

CONCLUSION

Delineating employment policies and procedures will serve as a framework for the employer–employee relationship and promote a positive employment relationship. It is imperative for the employer to have a solid grasp of what federal and state requirements are applicable to the company and to implement policies accordingly.

Material contained in this chapter is for general instruction and is not intended to constitute legal advice. Laws and local practices vary by jurisdiction and are subject to frequent modification. The sample provisions contained here are for illustration only and should not be used without prior advice from a qualified attorney. For an urgent care employer to have fully compliant employment practices, it is vital to consult an attorney for employment counseling that is specifically tailored to the individual urgent care center.

KEY POINTS

1. Employee policies provide structure to the working relationship between the organization and its employees.

2. Investigate your organization's requirements under the FMLA, formalize the family leave policy, and include the policy in your employee handbook.

3. The ADA covers employees who have a physical or mental impairment that substantially limits one or more of their major life activities.

4. Under the FLSA, employers must pay employees for all time "suffered or permitted" to work, including the following: travel time, working through meal breaks, checking email or voice mail away from the office, donning and doffing uniforms or safety equipment, attending pre-shift and post-shift meetings, and standby time. Covered, nonexempt employees must receive one and one-half times the regular rate of pay for all hours worked over 40 in a workweek.

5. The best approach is for employers to set forth in their employee handbook the employer's rules governing breaks and meal periods, including how employees log their time in and out, the number and timing of permissible breaks, and length of breaks.

6. The Supreme Court of the United States has stated that employers are liable for sexually harassing behavior by their supervisors because supervisors have the ability to participate in such misconduct by the authority that the employers delegate to them.

7. Under the anti-retaliation provisions of these laws, it is unlawful for employers to fire, demote, harass, or otherwise take adverse actions against employees because they have complained about discrimination.

8. The NLRB determined that it is an unfair labor practice for the employer to use, in all investigations, a form that reminds interviewers to inform employees that they cannot discuss the investigation with anyone else.

9. Because of the Supreme Court's ruling, if an employee and a same-sex domestic partner are married under state law, the employer is required to recognize the same-sex partner as the employee's spouse for purposes of ERISA, as well as for related tax purposes.

10. If SNOPA becomes law, it will prohibit employers from requiring or requesting that employees provide a username, password, or other means for accessing a personal account on any social networking website. This bill was reintroduced as HR 537 on February 6, 2013, and SNOPA was pending in committee at the time this chapter was written.

CHAPTER 16

Urgent Care Duties, Staffing Mix, and Ratios

John Shufeldt

How you staff your urgent care center is an integral component of the smooth and efficient day-to-day operation. Finding the right balance between the number of staff members necessary for an optimal patient experience and prudent financial stewardship is one of the key metrics in successful urgent care management.

The kind of staff members you employ is as important as the number of staff you employ and may weigh into your staffing metrics. For example, is a registered nurse (RN) in the back office as efficient as 1.5 medical assistants (MAs)? Is a physician 1.2 times as efficient as a physician extender (PE)? Do your managed-care plan contracts require a physician, or does the managed-care organization pay at 85% of the physician rate if a PE is used? Does your front-office manager fill in for lunches and breaks for your front-office staff? Do you open the doors on day 1 with a full complement of staff members, or do you scale up the number and capabilities of your staff members as the patient volume grows? Does your staffing formula follow the ebbs and flows of a typical day, and does it account for the historical busy days of the weeks and times of the year?

Although staffing an urgent care facility seems on the surface to be straightforward, it is a complex undertaking, particularly if you are trying to be as fiscally conservative as possible in your pro forma financial plan. It is easy to throw more staff members at prolonged patient waiting times; however, most operators do not have the luxury of staffing up every time patient volume transiently increases. Historically, most hospital-run operations have staffed their urgent care centers richly. In comparison, provider-owned centers, because of their economic model, are forced to staff with a minimal team that grows and fluctuates with patient volume.

STAFF COMPOSITION

How an owner or manager elects to staff the urgent care center has a material effect on patient flow and cost. This cost is magnified when overtime wages are added to the mix. Arguably, the more efficient the staff, the less overtime a center pays. Also, a more efficient staff generally costs more per hour than a less highly trained or educated staff. Balancing these tendencies is the key to finding the most appropriate ratio of staff to providers and staffing mix to patients.

Most centers divide the work into some variation of the following functions:

- Front office
  - Reception
  - Billing
  - Triage
- Back office
  - Medical assistance
  - Radiology
  - Patient scheduling, follow-up, referral
  - Pharmacy (i.e., dispensing medications or transmitting prescriptions)
  - Laboratory work
- Clinic management
- Medical provider (physician, physician assistant [PA], nurse practitioner [NP])

The number of people performing those functions can vary. In smaller operations or in centers with a lower patient volume, most of these functions are shared among the core staff members. The core staff members in every center are

- The front-office person
- The back-office person
- The medical provider

OVERVIEW OF FUNCTIONS AND DUTIES

Front Office

The front office is the gateway to the center. Utmost care should be used when hiring team members for that function. The quality, efficiency, and customer-service skills of the front-office team can make or break your office. The first and often most lasting impression that patients and visitors have of your center is driven by their perception on walking in.

Reception and Billing

The role of the front-office person is to manage the look and feel of the reception area, warmly greet the patients, enter and verify the data, collect co-pays and deductibles, manage patient queuing, discharge patients, and welcome them to return should they have further issues. The front-office leader should also monitor any negative interactions with staff members or providers and assess the general satisfaction of patients when they leave. Dissatisfied patients should be quickly identified and their concerns should be addressed before they leave the center in order to mitigate negative patient outcomes and reviews.

Individuals hired into this role generally have at least a high school education and previous experience. This role is one of the most challenging in the clinic, and the individuals hired to fulfill the role need to be both highly experienced and trained. Many dollars are lost and many opportunities for service recovery and for rectifying potential medical misadventures are missed at the front desk.

The following is a sample job description for the front-office role. The individual in this role

- Warmly greets all people entering clinic
- Demonstrates exceptional customer service in a highly stressful environment
- Performs visual screening and asks patients about their health status to ensure that the patients are not experiencing a medical emergency
- Performs patient registration, scheduling, insurance verification, charge posting, over-the-counter collections, electronic practice-management inputs, and general administrative functions
- Performs all duties corresponding to the appropriate skills-competency checklist
- Maintains established policies and procedures; the center's objectives; its quality-assurance program; and safety, environmental, and infection-control standards as described in the clinic operations manual
- Obtains data from patients and inputs information in the required format in the appropriate practice-management or billing system
- Manages the flow of patients, including placing patients into rooms as needed
- Processes patients financially for discharge, including preparing charges, collecting co-pays and deductibles, obtaining all necessary signatures, and issuing receipts for funds collected
- Completes all necessary forms for registration in the patient-care process and to ensure reimbursement from payers
- Prepares daily deposit, reconciliation, and daily statistical information
- Prepares customer comment cards or electronic surveys for patients
- Maintains a safe, comfortable, and therapeutic environment for patients and families in accordance with facility standards
- Keeps patients and families informed of waiting times
- Ensures an adequate stock of supplies and proper functioning of equipment

- Cleans and prepares front-office area at the end of the shift to ensure preparedness for receipt of patients
- Fields phone calls, using customer-service skills
- Ensures that the patients' waiting area and restrooms are clean and reflect a positive image of the clinic
- Treats patients and coworkers in a manner consistent with the urgent care center's mission statement, vision, values, and performance standards

Triage

Many urgent care centers assign a person to perform triage on arriving patients. This person typically checks vital signs and collects data and may be tasked with obtaining urine, drawing blood, and performing simple tests like a streptococcal screen or influenza test. If the clinic uses symptom-driven care paths, this person may initiate laboratory tests and radiology procedures. For example, if a patient reports a sprained ankle on presentation, the triage person may initiate an ankle x-ray if this is called for in the center's guidelines.

One crucial aspect of this role is to identify the "sick" patient. This is based on parameters for vital signs, the patient's reported symptoms, visual cues that the person "looks sick," and gestalt. It is imperative that if a patient presents in extremis, the provider is notified immediately. The providers must be coached so that they don't chastise the triage person for crying wolf. When identifying the sick patient, it is better to be overly cautious than not cautious enough. Nothing is harder to defend than the suffering or death of a patient who was waiting to be seen by a provider. The literature is replete with reports of patients dying of an acute myocardial infarction, sepsis, or epiglottitis while sitting in the waiting room of a clinic or emergency department.

Individuals hired into this role generally have training as an emergency medical technician, paramedic, licensed practical nurse (LPN) or licensed vocational nurse (LVN), RN, or MA, as well as on-the-job training. Customer-service skills, patient-assessment skills, and technical skills are a must.

The person in the triage role

- Demonstrates exceptional customer service in a highly stressful environment
- Greets patients arriving in the clinic lobby in accordance with clinic policies
- Performs triage assessment, including a patient interview and a brief physical assessment relevant to the chief reported ailment and the signs and symptoms of illness or injury within 15 minutes of a patient's presentation
- Determines the priority of patient rooming on the basis of triage assessment and available resources

- Performs indicated diagnostic screening, such as pulse oximetry, blood glucose testing, or electrocardiogram, as indicated in the center's guidelines or as directed by the provider, and tasks other back-office personnel with completing more-complex procedures as outlined in the center's guidelines
- Collects specimens as indicated in the center's guidelines or as directed by the provider, such as urine, blood, streptococcal screen, and other point-of-care testing
- Administers supplemental oxygen as indicated in the center's guidelines or as directed by the provider
- Places patients at ease and seeks ways to serve patients and make them more comfortable
- Administers first aid to control bleeding and splint injuries as indicated in the center's guidelines or as directed by the provider
- Administers analgesics to patients as indicated in the center's guidelines or as directed by the provider
- Assists in the treatment of patients in cardiopulmonary arrest, including performance of assisted ventilation, performance of compression, application of an automated external defibrillator, use of suction, and retrieval of indicated medications and supplies from the crash cart for the provider's use
- Communicates observations and medical care of patients to other staff members
- Documents observations and medical care of patients using approved forms or tools
- Monitors and reassesses patients in the lobby, administering additional care as indicated or directed by guidelines or as directed by the provider
- Attends to those patients in the reception area and those who are roomed prior to seeing the provider, ensuring that no one is left unattended longer than 15 minutes
- Assists in lifting and carrying patients out of their private vehicle and into a wheelchair
- Assists in transferring patients from a wheelchair to an examination table
- Cleans, stocks, and maintains the triage room or area to ensure preparedness for patient assessment and care

► Ensures that there is adequate stock of supplies and that equipment is properly functioning

Clinical Back Office

While the front office manages greeting and discharge, the back-office team handles the medical care and flow of the patients through the urgent care center. A high-functioning team and thoughtful process can move a large number of patients efficiently through a well-designed center. The movement of patients through the center and the time required for each phase of care determines the door-to-door time. An additional 3 minutes per patient of staff time, in a center visited by 60 patients per day, adds up to 180 minutes—or 3 hours—per day of staff time.

Thus, performing care concurrently (multiple phases happening at the same time) as opposed to sequentially (finishing one step before starting the next one) is imperative to clinic efficiency and controlling staffing cost. For example, triaging the patient while verifying insurance information and initiating tests while waiting for the provider to see the patient saves hundreds of dollars per day in staffing costs, because one team member is not waiting for another to finish their job before they can start. The downside is that you will occasionally start treating a patient who does not have a verifiable payer source. Generally, every patient who presents should at minimum have a screening exam. Even though most urgent care centers do not have to comply with the Emergency Medical Treatment and Active Labor Act, seeing the patient and ensuring that they do not have an emergency medical condition is the right thing to do.

Medical Assistance

Arguably, the better trained the staff, the less time it will take to effectively treat patients and the less the clinic will have to pay in overtime and benefits because fewer staff members and less overtime are necessary.

The training among the variety of potential back-office teammates varies considerably. But some things are required of all of them: an ability to multitask, a specific technical skill set, and an ability to provide extraordinary customer service.

The back-office role is typically fulfilled by an MA, LPN, or LVN, and this person

► Demonstrates exceptional customer service in a highly stressful environment

► Performs all clinical-care duties corresponding to the appropriate skills-competency checklists

► Maintains established policies and procedures; the center's objectives; its quality-assurance program; and safety, environmental and infection-control standards as described in the clinic operations manual

- Ensures that the clinic meets regulatory and accreditation standards; completes and reports the results of monitoring activities and audits
- Follows the guidelines and requirements of laboratory and clinical accreditation policies
- Inventories and orders as necessary to ensure that an adequate level of supplies and equipment are present in the facility
- Trains new and existing back-office employees in clinical procedures
- Completes laboratory training checklists, proficiency checklists, and laboratory 6-month initial and annual reviews of compliance with the Clinical Laboratory Improvement Amendments through COLA (formerly the Commission on Office Laboratory Accreditation)
- Attends education programs and staff meetings as required
- Dispenses prescriptions and medications per policy
- Performs patient-care duties within the scope of practice and clinic policy as needed
- Treats patients and coworkers in a manner consistent with the urgent care center's mission statement, vision, values, and performance standards

Radiology

In many urgent care centers and depending on state statutes, the back-office MA, LPN, or LVN can be cross-trained to obtain plain radiographs. Conversely, practical and licensed radiology technicians can be cross-trained to perform basic back-office skills. As volume ramps up, clinics often separate these roles so that the most highly trained individuals are performing the appropriate tasks.

It is imperative that images are taken correctly, that the right patient is matched to the correct film, that errors in technique are identified and corrected, and that the appropriate information is given to the overread radiologist to allow them to correctly identify the issue for which the film was taken.

Depending on the state and license requirements, individuals performing radiology tests must enroll in and complete specific classes on anatomy, radiation physics and safety, positioning, and equipment troubleshooting.

The following is a sample job description for the radiology technician role:

- Performs radiology duties within the scope of practice as stated in clinic policies and procedures, as well as the state-appropriate radiation rules and regulations
- Performs the essential functions, including back-office clinical duties, as defined by the appropriate skills-competency checklists

- Complies with established policies and procedures; the center's objectives; its quality-assurance program; and safety, environmental, and infection-control standards as described in the clinic operations manual
- Observes and communicates changes in the patient's condition to the provider on duty
- Assists provider with exams, procedures, and other processes related to direct patient care under direct supervision
- Participates in the completion of the daily tasks, as well as any assigned duties and tasks necessary to maintain compliance with federal and state regulations
- Participates in education programs and attends meetings as required
- Follows and complies with guidelines
- Dispenses prescriptions and medications per policy
- Follows guidelines and requirements of laboratory and clinical accreditation policies
- Treats patients and coworkers in a manner consistent with the urgent care center's mission statement, vision, values, and performance standards
- Performs other related duties as assigned or described by the company policy

Medical Providers

The medical providers are essential to the urgent care center. No care can take place, and generally speaking, no payment can be obtained for services unless those services are ordered by and performed by an appropriately licensed and trained medical provider.

Competent, efficient providers will drive the patient experience and add to the bottom line. Conversely, burned-out, inefficient, or negative providers will quickly ruin the clinic's culture and drive off staff members. Take extreme care during the hiring process for providers. Even when you are desperate, the "can they fog the mirror" test has no utility in hiring.

Physicians

Much has been written about the best possible background for an urgent care physician. Should the physician have emergency medicine board certification, or is family medicine or a combined medical-pediatrics residency the best? It may not matter. The bottom line is that the provider must be able to efficiently treat a variety of patients using well-developed diagnostic skills and gut instincts, have solid technical skills, monitor the care that other members are providing, multitask, and give great customer service, all while being attuned to the presence of the subtly but truly ill patient among the thousands of walking well. The provider who can manage all of those tasks will make a great urgent care physician no matter their background or training.

The following is a sample job description for the physician role:

- Demonstrates exceptional customer service in a highly stressful environment
- Maintains established policies and procedures; the center's objectives; its quality-assurance program; and safety, environmental, and infection-control standards as described in the clinic operations manual
- Provides input into the performance evaluations of the front-office and back-office staff to the clinic manager
- Supervises PEs as required by state regulation
- Interacts with the clinic manager regularly and keeps the clinic manager and medical director informed of concerns and potential liability situations
- Renders medical care to all patients who present to the urgent care center during all assigned shifts; if unable to do so, makes arrangements to have that shift covered and notifies the medical director
- Arrives at the urgent care center on the scheduled day at the start of the shift and leaves after the clinic closes and the last patient has left the premises, or in a split-shift scenario, appropriately hands off the patient to the next provider
- Obtains an adequate medical history and performs an appropriate physical exam for the presenting problem
- Orders pertinent laboratory and radiographic studies as needed on the basis of the initial evaluation
- Makes appropriate therapeutic decisions in conjunction with the patient on the basis of the information gathered
- Administers appropriate medication or treatment
- Completes and signs the superbill and discharge instructions
- Reviews and signs diagnostic reports and follows up on patient care as indicated
- Agrees to participate in periodic staff meetings
- Maintains a safe, comfortable, and therapeutic environment for patients and families in accordance with urgent care standards; abides by universal precautions and promotes the use of the precautions

- Ensures accurate maintenance of patients' medical records and treats these records as protected health information (PHI)
- Participates in the development of education programs for the urgent care staff
- Maintains professional growth and development through continuing medical education (CME) and complies with all state CME statutes
- Participates in the orientation and training of newly hired personnel
- Participates in the orientation and training of students

Physician Extender (Physician Assistant or Nurse Practitioner)

Many clinics in the United States elect to use a PE-only model. Others use a combination of physicians and PEs. No matter the model, PEs are an integral part of the team because of the valuable role they play and the perspective they bring to patient care.

As is true for physician background and training, much has been written about which background—PA or NP—is best suited for the urgent care environment. The same question applies here: If they can do the job in an exceptional manner, what difference does it make? Providers from both backgrounds work exceptionally well in the urgent care setting.

The following is a sample job description for the PE role:

- Demonstrates exceptional customer service in a highly stressful environment
- Maintains established policies and procedures; the center's objectives; its quality-assurance program; and safety, environmental, and infection-control standards as described in the clinic operations manual
- Provides input into the performance evaluations of the front-office and back-office staff to the clinic manager
- Interacts with physician supervisors as required by state regulations, case complexity, and patient's request
- Interacts with the clinic manager regularly; keeps the clinic manager and medical director informed of concerns and potential liability situations
- Renders medical care to all patients who present to the urgent care center during all assigned shifts; if unable to do so, makes arrangements to have that shift covered and notifies the medical director
- Arrives at the urgent care clinic on the scheduled day at the start of shift and leaves after the clinic closes and the last patient has left the premises, or in a spit-shift scenario, hands off the patients to the next provider

- ▶ Obtains an adequate medical history and performs an appropriate physical exam for the presenting problem
- ▶ Orders pertinent laboratory and radiographic studies as needed on the basis of the initial evaluation
- ▶ Makes appropriate therapeutic decisions in conjunction with the patient on the basis of the information gathered
- ▶ Administers appropriate medication or treatment
- ▶ Completes and signs the superbill and discharge instructions
- ▶ Reviews and signs diagnostic reports and follows up on patient care as indicated
- ▶ Agrees to participate in periodic staff meetings
- ▶ Maintains a safe, comfortable, and therapeutic environment for patients and families in accordance with urgent care standards; abides by universal precautions and promotes the use of the precautions
- ▶ Ensures accurate maintenance of patients' medical records and treats these records as PHI
- ▶ Participates in the development of education programs for the urgent care staff
- ▶ Maintains professional growth and development through CME and complies with all state CME statutes
- ▶ Participates in the orientation and training of newly hired personnel
- ▶ Participates in the orientation and training of students

Clinic Management

The clinic manager sets the tone and culture for the entire center and is an integral component of the urgent care team. Many clinics promote managers from within, typically moving a successful front-office or back-office person into a clinic manager position. Although this often works well, occasionally gaps in knowledge become evident. The promoted front-office person does not have an understanding of patient care and the related functions, or the promoted back-office person is focused only on the clinical aspect of care and does not have an appreciation for the front-office tasks. Finding that rare individual who understands both the front and back offices, demonstrates superior customer-service skills, and can manage the medical providers is difficult. Once you find someone with the complete package of needed skills, treat that person incredibly well.

Individuals hired into this role typically come down one of two pathways, clinical or administrative, and acquire knowledge in deficient areas either through on-the-job training or formal education.

The following is a sample job description for the clinic manager:

- Demonstrates exceptional customer service in a highly stressful environment
- Maintains established policies and procedures; the center's objectives; its quality-assurance program; and safety, environmental, and infection-control standards as described in the clinic operations manual
- Ensures that staff members and providers maintain standards as outlined in the urgent care center's mission statement, vision and values statements, and performance standards
- Ensures that adequate staffing is present through the scheduling of receptionists, MAs, practical radiology technicians, radiology technicians, occupational medicine coordinators, and any additional staff members needed
- Ensures that the clinic meets regulatory and internal standards, including guidelines of the US Department of Health Services and COLA; fulfills dispensing and corporate compliance programs; and participates in regulatory and insurance audits and inspections
- Manages programs as necessary to ensure that an adequate level of supplies and equipment are present in the facility; makes suggestions for additions to and replacement of equipment
- Evaluates staff performance on a regular basis; provides oral and written disciplinary or corrective action as needed
- Provides input to the medical director regarding the performance of all providers working at the clinic
- Conducts preliminary, entrance, and exit interviews of staff members; participates in other interview processes as requested
- Interacts with the medical director regularly to ensure appropriate operational and clinical service delivery
- Addresses client concerns promptly, using customer-service skills; makes recommendations for or implements resolution as necessary
- Participates in the development of education programs and attends meetings as required; attends education programs as needed
- Maintains professional growth and development through seminars, workshops, and professional affiliations to keep abreast of the latest trends
- Ensures accurate maintenance of patients' medical records and treats those records as PIII

- Obtains statistical data about the facility and compiles information into the required format
- As applicable, maintains skills in back-office and front-office departments so as to provide backup for these positions
- Participates in interviewing, hiring, orientation, and training of personnel
- Ensures appropriate clinic expense and revenue management, including input in the annual budget process and monthly review of profit and loss statements
- Manages financial reporting and profit and loss control
- Treats patients and coworkers in a manner consistent with the urgent care center's mission statement, vision, values, and performance standards

OTHER ROLES AND STAFF

Depending on the scope of practice a clinic wants to achieve, a number of other team members may be necessary. Dedicated laboratory personnel, dispensing or pharmacy technicians, patient-referral coordinators, and customer-service representatives may be used effectively, depending on their financial and service return on investment. Alternatively, front-office and back-office team members can also perform these roles.

STAFFING RATIOS

There is no magic formula for staffing ratios, because so much depends on case complexity; patient volume and timing; provider and staff-member efficiency; and the functionality of the clinic, practice-management, and medical record platforms. Some providers see four patients per hour, day after day, have short waiting times, provide great care, and give exceptional customer service. Others struggle to see just one patient per hour and still manage to have long waiting times and poor customer-service scores.

A three-person team (front office, back office, and provider) should be able to efficiently treat 30 patients per day. The challenges of the three-person model are when many patients present at once and when staff breaks are necessary. When the 30-patient-per-day level is consistently exceeded, a front office–back office float is cross-trained to pitch in where necessary. Alternatively, and depending on the number of tests ordered, a radiology technician is used in the back office and a part-time front-office person is used during peak times. A more expensive approach is to hire a clinic manager who steps in to help when staff members are busy or need breaks.

CONCLUSION

Staffing is a complex, dynamic undertaking driven by a lot of variables. Most owners or managers, because of financial constraints, tend to err on the side of lean staffing. This is prudent, provided the center does not lose patient volume and its reputation for great service as a result. No matter how you staff the center, the care delivered depends on the individuals involved, and you should devote careful attention to selecting new team members.

KEY POINTS

1. Model your decisions, remembering to include an appropriate amount of allotted overtime hours.
2. Understand that the leaner the center is staffed, the more likely the center will be paying overtime.
3. Hiring the best people mitigates many of the staffing ratio challenges.
4. Lean staffing models during the patient ramp-up period is desirable, provided the center has the opportunity to increase its staffing model as necessary to accommodate patient volume.
5. Defined job descriptions and skills checklists are crucial because the center will benefit from better-defined roles and accountability.
6. Treat all team members with respect and courtesy to demonstrate your expectation of how they should treat other team members and the patients.
7. Do rapid-cycle testing on staffing ratios to determine the best mix for your center.
8. The ratio or staffing mix does not have to be the same on every day of the week.

CHAPTER 17

Physician Extenders in the Urgent Care Center

John Shufeldt and Adam Winger

THE UTILIZATION OF PHYSICIAN assistants (PAs) and nurse practitioners (NPs) in clinical settings across the United States has grown tremendously since the first decade of the 21st century, and urgent care companies are among the biggest beneficiaries of such growth. This group of professionals treats tens of thousands of patients every day in centers across the country, and it is no surprise that their involvement has become integral to the success of the urgent care industry.

Not only do physician extenders (PEs) increase patients' overall access to health care but they also do so at a lower cost than care by physicians alone. Unfortunately, in many states, payers use the decreased payroll expenses associated with midlevel providers to justify reduced reimbursement rates for patients treated exclusively by a PA or NP. As a result, many urgent care companies use midlevel providers as much as possible but, to obtain the higher reimbursement levels, require that the physician treat each patient.

Most analysts agree that under the Affordable Care Act, at least 30 million more Americans will be eligible for health insurance than ever before. This additional patient population will only exacerbate the existing problems associated with our country's physician shortage, and the use of midlevel providers seems to be a significant part of a credible solution.

There are more than 85,000 trained and certified PAs in the United States and more than 155,000 practicing NPs. PAs can prescribe certain medications in all 50 states, but they can work only under the supervision of a licensed physician. In 12 states plus the District of Columbia, NPs can work independently, but they may need a formal collaborating agreement with a medical doctor. In either case, the midlevel provider may perform (and the physician may delegate) only those tasks coming within the individual's authorized *scope of services*. In general, the state board of medicine will govern the activities of the PA and the board of nursing will regulate those of the NP.

Before engaging with or employing a PE, review your state supervision statutes and notify your medical malpractice carrier to ensure that you are covered for claims of negligent supervision. Generally speaking, when a midlevel provider is sued, the physician and the urgent care company itself will also be named for a claim of negligent supervision or negligent hiring. Physicians ought to remember the legal truism that "although you can delegate responsibility, you cannot, under the law, delegate liability."

The good news is that PAs and NPs are less likely to be sued than are their physician counterparts. These data come from a 2009 study by the Federation of State Medical Boards, which looked at claims data from 1991 through 2007. During that period there was, on average, one payment for every 2.7 physicians, compared with one for every 32.5 certified PAs and one for every 65.8 NPs.[1] However, in a review of closed claims by the Physician Insurers Association of America, the average indemnity payment, unadjusted to present value, was $174,871 for PE suits that also named a physician. This amount was greater than the amount when only a physician was named. The take-home message is that when the plaintiff can attach the physician to the claim, the award is increased.

CAUSES OF ACTION WITH PHYSICIAN EXTENDERS

Generally, in order to successfully file a lawsuit, the plaintiff must show that the patient and physician had established a prior physician–patient relationship. However, many states have expanded the nature of this relationship in order to capture the negligent acts of on-call and attending physicians while supervising medical students, residents, and midlevel providers. This makes sense. If a physician is on the phone, giving orders and opining about the treatment to be rendered, they share some of the responsibility even if they have not actually laid hands on the patient.

Vicarious Liability

Under a *vicarious liability* cause of action, the physician is responsible for the negligent acts of employees or contractors under his or her control. This doctrine is referred to as *respondeat superior* ("let the master answer"). The bright-line test is whether or not the employer directs and controls the actions and performance of the employee. The Maryland appellate court in 1957 established the following criteria for determining whether a master–servant relationship exists:

- ▶ Did the employer select and hire the employee?
- ▶ Does the employer pay the employee's wages?
- ▶ Does the employer have the power to terminate the employee?
- ▶ Does the employer control the employee's conduct?
- ▶ Is the work of the employee part of the regular business of the employer?

---

1   Hooker R, Nicholson J, Tuan L. Does the employment of physician assistants and nurse practitioners increase liability? *Journal of Medical Licensure and Discipline.* 2009;9:6–16. Available from: http://www.paexperts.com/Nicholson%20-%20Hooker%20Article.pdf. Accessed September 14, 2013.

The issue is one of control. If the employee is performing tasks in furtherance of the employer's business and at the employer's direction, than the employer is deemed to *own* the liability for the employee's bad actions.

Negligent Supervision
Liability on the part of the physician can also be imputed under a *negligent supervision* cause of action. Even if the PE is not found to be negligent, the supervising physician can retain liability for negligently supervising the PA or NP. If the company does not have policies and procedures in place regarding the PE's scope of practice or the medications which the PE may prescribe, or if policies and procedures are in place but are not followed, the physician-supervisor will almost always remain liable. Additionally, if the physician is not following prescribed state statute–mandated supervisory duties, they can be sanctioned by the state medical board, which may involve a suspension or revocation of the physician's medical license.

Negligent Hiring
A company and supervising physician can be named if it is determined that the PE was performing services outside their scope of practice or if the PE did not have the requisite skills or training necessary for their assigned duties or roles. The same holds true for all employees. It is imperative that the employer exercise the appropriate level of diligence regarding background checks, training, and verification of prior employment, and that the supervising physician assign only those tasks that the PE is competent to perform.

MITIGATING YOUR RISK
Before hiring a PE, you should ensure that the candidate has the appropriate level of training and certification necessary to perform the required duties. If an employer fails to exercise reasonable care in the hiring process, a cause of action for negligent hiring may ensue. At a minimum, the following nine areas should be addressed before employing a PE:

- ▶ Review requirements set forth in relevant state statutes and board regulations concerning utilization of PEs.
- ▶ Confirm that the individual holds the requisite licenses and that all are current and in good standing.
- ▶ Determine what duties and authority may and may not be delegated to a PE by a supervising physician.
- ▶ Review education, training, and experience of the PE.
- ▶ Determine the appropriate setting in which the PE may competently work.
- ▶ Confirm skills and knowledge during a mandatory proctoring process.

- Understand the collaborative nature and limitations of interactions between PEs and physicians, including limitations on PEs' ability to prescribe controlled substances.
- Delineate the scope of practice and methods of communication; consider creating certain protocols listing the medications that the PE may prescribe and the actions to be taken in given situations (for example, contact the physician immediately when a patient presents with chest pain).
- Have both the physician and the PE sign documents outlining the nature of their relationship.

Many PEs are reluctant to call the supervising physician when they have questions or concerns. Therefore, establishing specific and well-delineated medical protocols removes this barrier and can help minimize risk.

PEs should always present themselves using the title *physician assistant* or *nurse practitioner*. Name tags should also clearly delineate the title and role of the medical provider, and under no circumstances should patients be led to believe that they have been seen by a physician when they were actually seen by a PE.

ANALYSIS OF RELEVANT STATE STATUTES REGARDING SUPERVISION OF NURSE PRACTITIONERS AND PHYSICIAN ASSISTANTS

Nurse Practitioner Supervision

In 12 states plus the District of Columbia, NPs do not require physician supervision.

- Alaska
- Arizona
- District of Columbia
- Hawaii
- Idaho
- Iowa
- Montana
- New Hampshire
- New Mexico
- Oregon

- Rhode Island
- Washington
- Wyoming

In Maine, once a nurse practitioner has 2 years of practice, they no longer need supervision. In Colorado and Maryland, the NP needs to attain an attestation from their supervising physician. In Utah, if the NP is prescribing controlled substances, they need to have an agreement in place with their supervising physician. The remainder of the states' requirements are on a continuum from constant supervision (Oklahoma) to meeting semiannually (Ohio). Please consult your state statutes or our website, at www.urgentcaretextbooks.com, for further clarification.

Physician Assistant Supervision

All states require PAs to have physician supervision, and the details of the requirements vary by state. Some states require that 100% of the PA's charts are reviewed and cosigned for the first 3 years, whereas other states have no requirements for cosigning. Most states require that a supervisory agreement is consummated between the PA and physician; however, the constant physical presence of a physician is not required under any state's statute. Please consult your state statutes or our website, at www.urgentcaretextbooks.com, for further clarification.

CONCLUSION

Physicians and PEs must check their state statutes and the applicable rules and regulations of any governing body regarding supervision and collaboration requirements. Lawsuits involving PEs will likely increase as the scope of practice for PEs expands and as more and more patients receive primary, urgent, and emergency care from highly trained PAs and NPs.

KEY POINTS

1. Before hiring, ensure that you are knowledgeable about reporting and supervising requirements.
2. Document compliance with state-mandated supervision statutes.
3. Post notices or signs in the waiting room regarding the level of providers on site.
4. Understand the three causes of action: *respondeat superior*; *negligent supervision*; *negligent hiring*.
5. Draft clear guidelines for the appropriate use of PEs.
6. Check training, prior experience, and work history on all PEs.

7. Ensure that the supervising physician is meeting state-mandated supervising duties.
8. Have clear titles (*physician assistant*, *nurse practitioner*) on name badges, and use titles while making introductions to patients. Do not let patients believe they are being seen by a physician when a PE is the treating provider.

CHAPTER 18

Provider Compensation

John Shufeldt

MANY FACTORS PLAY A role in the success of your urgent care clinic. Choosing the right location, developing a complementary array of services, and having competent administrative staff help determine the profitability of your facility and your return on investment (ROI). However, a big chunk of the final outcome rests squarely on the professionalism and competence of the providers you hire to take care of your patients. Their daily interactions with patients, their ability to effectively deliver exceptional care, and their willingness to help you build a proactive, compassionate culture among support staff members will all make a big difference in your facility's reputation, patient volume, and revenue.

Your ability to attract good providers will depend on, among other things, the compensation structure within your facility. If you want top-quality providers, your compensation methodology has to make sense, has to be competitive, and has to encourage the desired behavior. This is why the development of an appropriate pay structure for your clinic is essential for attracting and retaining quality physicians who will help your clinic grow and will cultivate a positive image within the community.

When it comes to designing a pay structure, you have many choices. Clinics can compensate their providers via fixed hourly pay rates or performance structures, can create hybrid models that incorporate various hourly and performance features, and can even add bonus components. As you go through the process of designing the right pay structure for your clinic, or redesigning an existing one, you will need to carefully weigh the pros and cons of the various options available to you because each will have different ramifications. For example, some structures give providers more earning stability but less earning potential, thereby possibly discouraging proactive and efficient behavior. Other structures can create more incentives for providers but at the same time could inadvertently encourage negative behavior that may lower quality of care by promoting a *turn and burn* mentality.

As you consider the various approaches, keep in mind that the option (or mix of options) you choose will be unique to your specific needs. This is an area of practice-management that you can design to give you more negotiating room when you hire providers. It is an opportunity to build your team in a way that maximizes the long-term potential of your facility and stability of your staff.

OVERVIEW

There are two general types of compensation structures within medical facilities: straight hourly, which pays a fixed rate for every hour of work, and performance-based structures, which aim to more closely tie provider compensation to volume of work.

Straight hourly structures are quite simple to understand and administer because the provider receives only a set rate of pay for each hour of work; there are no profit-sharing elements and no other variables to calculate. The hourly structure simplifies payroll and allows for easier and more accurate projections of payroll expenses for internal budgets and cash-flow estimates.

However, the hourly structure has its downside, mainly because it doesn't provide any upside potential for the medical professional and therefore offers no incentive to deliver exceptional care or service to patients or to increase patient retention. Of course, every provider realizes that if they don't perform well, they may lose their job. But even high-caliber employees are rarely motivated by losing their job, especially when they know that if they leave the practice, the facility operator will be forced to deal with many logistical headaches. Therefore, straight hourly compensation is best suited for hiring providers who are just starting out, don't have an established patient base, and value the stability of a regular paycheck. Providers with more experience will be less likely to accept a straight hourly pay position unless either the hourly rate is very competitive or there are other significant perks, like schedule flexibility.

Performance-based (or volume-based) compensation is different in that it largely aims to tie provider pay to volume of work completed by that provider (with the exception of quality metrics, which are not based on volume). It looks at different metrics and uses compensation formulas to derive actual pay on the basis of the volume of specific metrics the provider achieved. This type of structure can be much more complex and can vary significantly between clinics, mainly because performance can be measured in many different ways. Some clinics will pay their providers on the basis of the total number of patients or office visits, some will pay on the basis of revenue generated by the provider, and others may use relative value units (RVUs) to measure the total work contributed by the individual.

Many clinics use performance-based structures with varying degrees of success. Some make the provider's entire compensation dependent on performance measures, thus placing a strong emphasis on measurable results to the clinic.

RELATIVE VALUE UNITS

RVUs have gained wider utilization in performance pay structures since 2008. If you've billed Medicare or Medicaid before, you're likely familiar with RVUs, but it's nonetheless helpful to have a refresher on the topic if you are going to implement it as part of a performance-based structure within your facility.

RVUs have their origin in the studies commissioned by the US Health Care Financing Administration in the late 1980s. The goal of the study was to develop a more standardized Medicare reimbursement system that would create a closer correlation between the amount of resources used by a provider to deliver care and the payment the provider received for their services. Various medical procedures were analyzed for difficulty, time to complete, and the necessary skill level, among other considerations. Essentially, the study aimed to ascertain all the resources that were needed to complete a medical procedure, and then to quantify those resources into one number for that procedure: the total RVU. The more resources used in a procedure, the more RVUs it was assigned, and the higher the total RVU value.

The total RVU value is further broken down into components: the work RVU, the practice expense RVU, and the liability insurance RVU. The work RVU focuses on the time it should take a physician to perform a procedure, the stress associated with it, and the level of skill necessary. The practice expense RVU looks at the average amount of resources a practice needs to devote to a certain procedure. This helps account for overhead associated with the procedure, including the time of nonphysician staff. The liability insurance RVU takes into account the cost of the malpractice insurance premiums allocated to the procedure.

Although the formula details for each procedure can get a bit tricky, the core idea was quite simple: to quantify medical procedures into consistent and uniform measuring units. Think of it as comparing apples to apples. For example, hip-replacement surgery in New York will not cost the same dollar amount as the same procedure in Ohio, but the amount of *resources* used, and hence RVUs, should be the same.

When incorporating RVU measures into the compensation structure, you should focus on the work RVU. This component can help you better gauge the contribution of your provider to the clinic, especially if you have more than one physician on premises. Let's say you have two providers in your office, one a family physician who sees patients only for common symptoms, and the other an orthopedist who is regularly involved in the repair of bone fractures. The two could be working exactly the same hours, but because of the types of patients she sees, the orthopedist cannot accommodate as many patients as the family practitioner. Therefore, if both providers were paid strictly on the basis of the number of patients, the orthopedist would always have an inherent disadvantage and would earn less simply because her procedures take longer. This could therefore be unfair because her amount of work, if measured in RVUs, could be the same as, if not more than, that of the family practitioner, yet she would be paid less.

The approach of breaking down procedures into RVUs strives to measure the volume of work and effort but not necessarily the revenues generated by the provider. Of course, the connection between RVUs and revenue is implicit—the more difficult and time-consuming procedures usually generate more revenue. However, this connection between RVU and revenue is indirect within the confines of your pay structure. In effect, this measures how much of the *workload* the provider has handled. Different patients will come in with different complaints, and some problems will be more complicated and time-consuming to resolve. When you use RVUs in your compensation structure, you're no longer just asking, "How many patients did this physician see?" or "How much in billing did that physician generate?" but instead can ask the more meaningful question, "How much of the overall clinic workload did this provider handle?"

Because RVUs allow for a more direct comparison of effort between physicians (by focusing on resources used) they can be a valuable tool within your performance compensation structure. Keep in mind that RVUs are only a measurement tool, not the full solution. The way that you tie RVUs to actual pay and the extent to which you use them within your practice may vary significantly-fromthe ways others do so.

HYBRID STRUCTURES

Some clinics create hybrid pay structures in which a provider's compensation is partly based on hourly rates and partly based on performance measures. For example, your structure might pay a provider a straight hourly rate but also include an incentive component by paying a set dollar amount to the provider for each RVU (or other metric, like number of patients seen) in *addition* to their hourly earnings. The provider receives some stability in the form of a regular, albeit smaller, hourly paycheck but also has the motivation to contribute as much as possible to the clinic in order to receive more incentive pay.

Another way to build a hybrid model is to pay straight hourly but to also add a bonus component when the clinic meets or exceeds certain goals, like the number of patients or profitability. Note that a bonus is different from earning additional compensations on RVUs, described earlier. In the previous example, the provider earns a predetermined amount for *each* additional value unit they contribute. With a bonus structure, the provider is incentivized less directly, by being encouraged to help the clinic meet its overall goals, and usually receives a predetermined dollar amount if those goals are met.

PERFORMANCE-BASED STRUCTURES AS A MANAGEMENT TOOL

It is likely that your clinic will use performance measures in one way or another to determine compensation. A big reason for this is that by tying compensation to performance, you are incentivizing your providers to be more proactive, in the hopes that their drive will contribute to the success of your facility. However, the effectiveness of performance structures ultimately depends on how well the providers' interests are aligned with yours.

Think of it this way: Performance-based compensation encourages providers to make more money by changing their behavior to maximize their reward.

But whether this behavior actually provides benefit to your clinic largely depends on the metrics you decide to use to measure performance. For example, if you pay providers strictly on the basis of the number of patients they see, then they could end up providing substandard care by rushing patients out or making mistakes in the medical record. Or they could end up asking the patients to come in repeatedly for rechecks, thus driving your clinic to becoming a patient mill, with very low quality of care and possible patient safety events.

Therefore, if your compensation structure has a performance component, do consider whether the behavior it encourages is the behavior you want. Ask yourself about your vision for your facility and what you would like it to become in the next several years. Then figure out which metrics are important for your staff to meet in order to get your clinic to the place you want. Note that your goals should not just include revenue levels. Your revenue is important, but there are numerous other metrics that define your business. Do you want your clinic to have the highest quality of care in the city? Then work a quality-of-care score into the compensation formula. Is patient satisfaction important to you? Then work that into the compensation formula as well. These don't have to be huge components of the overall formula, but if your providers understand that these metrics play into their final earnings, they are more likely to adjust their behavior accordingly. Carefully selected compensation metrics can play a big role in cultivating the attitudes you would like your providers to have, so that you can build the right type of culture within your facility. Consider an example in which the base hourly salary is $80 and there is a bonus of up to 25% of base salary ($20 per hour in addition), broken down as follows:

Patient satisfaction:	30%
Quality indicators:	25%
>3.5 patients per hour:	15%
Door-to-provider time:	10%
Door-to-door time:	10%
Clinic profitability:	10%
	100%

In that model, if a provider meets all of their goals, their hourly rate for the month measured is $100 per hour, because they earned 100% of their bonus, which is based on an additional 20% of their base salary.

COMPENSATION STRUCTURE CONSISTENCY

Once your compensation structure is ironed out, try to keep it as consistent as possible. Of course, centers do change their compensation practices from time to time, but you don't want to have a straight hourly structure one year, a straight RVU structure the next, and then switch again the year after that.

There are several reasons why you want to limit major changes from occurring often. The main reason is because people like consistency. The providers working in your clinic have their own goals and dreams in life, and having a relatively predictable way to estimate their earnings helps bring stability to their personal plans. They know what they have to do, how many hours they have to work, or how many patients they have to see or RVUs they have to generate, and they structure their time accordingly and develop certain expectations. When pay structures change too much too quickly, it can be very frustrating for providers because they may now need to focus on a completely different set of goals and change their practice patterns and thought processes.

MAKING YOUR COMPENSATION STRUCTURE COMPETITIVE

When you hire a provider, you have to offer a compensation structure that is competitive so that you can attract the best talent. You want the best quality providers in your clinic so that your facility offers exceptional care and builds a strong reputation within your community. If the compensation is not competitive, you'll attract providers with a lower level of skill and possibly an attitude that will rub patients the wrong way. Hiring and firing providers can consume a lot of your time and resources, so it behooves you to build a competitive compensation structure, or at least a comparable one to your immediate competitors.

An important step in developing the provider compensation structure includes surveying predominant pay structures in your local geographic market. The providers you hire will likely look for positions within your geographic vicinity and will have likely applied to other clinics in their job search. Consequently, having a good idea of what other clinics offer can increase your chances of hiring top-quality staff by adjusting your own structure accordingly. It's essential to realize that you're not just looking at pay structures and copying the one with the most prevalent usage in your area but rather taking a look at what others are doing to make your own structure more competitive.

Once you're ready to start staffing your clinic with quality providers, keep in mind that you have wiggle room beyond just the pay figures when it comes to negotiating the positions. Ask the candidate about what's important to them. Maybe they need scheduling flexibility to take care of their children, or perhaps they'd like to devote more time to certain types of procedures. The final amount of their pay is only part of the equation, and if your compensation rates are not the most competitive, you can sometimes make the offer more appealing by addressing other needs the prospective provider may have.

THE BIRD'S-EYE VIEW

Figuring out the right compensation structure for your clinic may be frustrating at first. One helpful step is to realize that a good compensation structure is all about measuring a physician's contribution to the clinic. Sound measurements help you ensure that the provider is paid fairly and that your clinic receives its fair share as well. The real challenge is to build your structure around metrics that directly correlate to your desired results. After all, when you incentivize someone, you are asking them to produce more volume of one thing or another, with the idea that more volume will equal a bigger benefit to your facility.

For example, when you're paying a provider a straight hourly rate, you're really paying for volume—the volume of hours worked. Why are you doing this? Because ideally, the number of hours worked should directly correlate to the benefit that the provider brought to the clinic. The more hours they work, the bigger the theoretical benefit to the clinic, and hence the more they should get paid. The only problem is that the volume for which you are paying (volume of hours) is probably not very closely correlated to the overall benefit your clinic received.

Performance-based structures have the same goal of paying the provider for volume except that they measure volume differently in the hopes of more closely correlating work and pay. Instead of measuring volume in hours, their focus is shifted toward results. They'll consider the volume of patient visits or total revenue generated by the provider. These approaches are just an attempt to more closely correlate provider compensation with benefit to the clinic, but they still have limitations. RVU measures further try to bridge the gap between provider work and benefits to the facility, although not always accurately, and with their own set of potential issues.

The goal for all of these methodologies is the same: to find a way to measure the benefits to the clinic and pay each provider fairly for their work. Keep this in mind as you think about the various strategies available to you. This will help keep the provider happy while ensuring that your clinic is not inadvertently paying too much for too little. If you focus your thought process on bridging the gap between measuring provider effort and measuring the benefit to your clinic, you will be much more likely to develop a structure that is a good fit for the unique attributes of your facility.

CONCLUSION

The compensation structure for your facility will play an integral part in your clinic's ultimate success. Everything from your ROI to quality of care will be affected by how you design your structure and by which metrics, if any, you choose to include in the compensation formula. Your final structure will be affected by your local competitors because you cannot attract quality providers if your overall package isn't up to community standards. However, this does not mean that your structure has to be the same as everyone else's—your clinic is unique, and you can choose performance metrics that best reflect your clinic's operations.

As you consider various structure alternatives, make sure to run financial forecasts based on these alternatives. You have to understand how the different pay structures will affect your finances and your cash flow. This is an important step because it can have significant long-term implications for your ROI.

As you design and then implement your structure, don't forget to plan time and energy to make minor adjustments. The process will be stressful and sometimes downright confusing. You could even design a structure only to find out that it doesn't work the way you intended in real life and that you will need to change it again. But eventually, you'll get to a solution that will be a good fit, even if it takes some time.

KEY POINTS

1. The complexity of the compensation plan and the number of metrics used will directly affect how difficult it is to implement. Complicated plans can take a lot of time to administer and may be prone to errors. Such errors are especially dangerous when they happen to be in your favor, as that can breed distrust in providers.

2. Incentives should align the providers' interests with yours. Your clinic will only thrive if everyone is working toward its success. Choose the metrics for performance-based structures carefully.

3. Include quality measures in the pay structure. Compensating providers strictly on volume can have a negative impact on the quality of care and can lead to malpractice lawsuits. Communicate the importance of quality and service by making patient satisfaction part of the pay formula.

4. A provider cannot be paid on the basis of any radiology or laboratory tests ordered. Do not include these in your compensation structure under any circumstances.

5. Make sure you are competitive by surveying pay structures in other facilities within your area. This is a vital step in acquiring good talent and showing candidates that you are in touch with the overall market.

6. Invest some time in developing your structure carefully the first time. Changing it once your facility is up and running, and once your providers have been hired, could create unnecessary tension and potential headaches if providers choose to quit. Doing a thorough job ahead of time reduces chances of future problems.

7. Although the use of RVUs in pay structures has become more common, this measure has its own limitations. As technological advances significantly simplify some procedures, official RVU figures have not necessarily been updated to take these developments into account. Therefore, the number of RVUs generated by the provider's work may be somewhat inflated because the RVU figures for those procedures may not accurately reflect the difficulty of the work.

8. Don't confuse bonuses with per-RVU payments. Bonuses reward the provider when the clinic meets its goals as a whole, whereas per-RVU

structures pay a specific dollar amount for each RVU generated by the provider.

9. For per-RVU performance structures, you could also consider a laddered approach, in which the per-RVU dollar amount increases at each threshold level. This can further incentivize providers to meet minimum thresholds and gives them a larger potential paycheck, and it also limits your downside if baseline goals are not met.

10. Include the compensation in your financial forecasts. Create different scenarios based on various structure options you are considering to see how they will affect your financials. Your providers will be one of the biggest expenses in operating the facility, and you need to clearly understand how different pay structures will affect not only the center's profitability but also any temporary cash-flow shortfalls that could arise.

CHAPTER 19

Hiring and Managing Medical Providers

John Shufeldt

Without the right medical provider, an urgent care clinic can struggle and even fail. This chapter discusses challenges in hiring and managing medical providers.

THE PHYSICIAN SHORTAGE

In 1997, the federal government placed a cap on Medicare funding of hospital residency training programs. Since the cap was put in place, the number of physicians trained in the United States has grown only marginally, whereas population size and population aging have increased significantly, driving up demand for physician services. This has also fueled the demand for midlevel providers.

The Association of American Medical Colleges (AAMC) believes that by 2025, the United States will face a shortfall of nearly 160,000 physicians, of which more than 50,000 are in primary-care specialties. According to the AAMC, the Affordable Care Act will increase the shortage by 31,000 physicians. The American Academy of Family Physicians projects a global deficit of 149,000 physicians by 2020, and the US Health Resources and Services Administration projects a shortage of 65,000 primary-care physicians by the same year.

Moreover, a study published in *JAMA* by Staiger et al showed a 5.7% decrease in hours worked by nonresident physicians in patient care. Given a workforce of approximately 630,000 in 2007,[1] this is equivalent to a loss of approximately 36,000 physicians from the workforce.[2] The authors of the study postulate that declining physician reimbursement in real dollars and decreased job satisfaction are directly correlated to declining work hours.

The way physicians practice also affects physician supply. The private-practice model is rapidly being replaced by hospital and large medical group employment. Many younger physicians prefer the set hours and controllable lifestyle typical in large-practice employee settings to the longer hours characteristically associated

---

1   *Physician Characteristics and Distribution in the US*. Chicago, IL: American Medical Association; 2009.
2   Staiger DO, Auerbach DI, Buerhaus PI. Trends in the work hours of physicians in the United States. *JAMA*. 2010;303:747–53.

with private, small group, or lone-physician practices. In addition, the influx of female physicians into the workforce also has had an inhibiting effect on overall physician full-time equivalents.[3]

Finally, a white paper published by Merritt Hawkins & Associates on behalf of the Physicians Foundation disclosed that only about 25% of the physicians surveyed plan to continue with their current mode of practice. Close to 75% plan to take steps likely to reduce the number of patients they see or to remove themselves completely from patient care.[4]

These data reveal that the need for urgent care centers, staffed by both physicians and midlevel providers, will be an important component of the continuum of care in the near future—even more than it is today.

HIRING QUALITY PROVIDERS

The good news is that because of this supply–demand imbalance, in the near future medical providers will be able to demand a premium for their services. It is evident that physician practice patterns are not the same as they were at the start of the 21st century and will be even more different as time passes.[5] Providers today, particularly those wanting to practice in an urgent care or primary-care walk-in clinic, are often looking for a work–life balance that providers of the past may not have viewed as important.

Given this trend, a leader tasked with staffing and managing an urgent care center has to be creative to ensure that the center's hours are properly covered. Staffing the center may require hiring a variety of physicians and midlevel practitioners and scheduling them on the basis of their disparate practice preferences. For a variety of reasons, the practice of staffing, in one week, one provider for four 12-hour shifts and another provider for three 12-hour shifts and then flip-flopping them the next week is probably coming to an end. This is not necessarily a bad thing, inasmuch as studies have shown that an individual's effectiveness starts to deteriorate significantly after 8 to 10 hours of patient care.

How, then, does one find and hire the medical staff to meet both the needs of the practice and the needs of the providers? In an ideal world, the urgent care center would be staffed by full-time, employed medical providers who have some sort of equity stake in the smooth operation and financial viability of the center. For smaller-scale operations, this may in fact be the way providers are engaged. However, this becomes less realistic and less feasible with larger-scale operations.

The key is to hire or contract with providers who act *as if* they are owners. This is a two-way street. For medical providers to act as owners, they should be

---

3   Fowler D. A revealing 2011 survey on locum tenens physicians. *Journal of Urgent Care Medicine*. Available from: http://jucm.com/web/?id=20. Accessed February 4, 2014.

4   Physicians Foundation. Health reform and the decline of physician private practice: A white paper examining the effects of the Patient Protection and Affordable Care Act on physician practices in the United States. Available from: http://www.physiciansfoundation.org/uploads/default/Health_Reform_and_the_Decline_of_Physician_Private_Practice.pdf. Accessed July 28, 2013.

5   Fowler D. A revealing 2011 survey on locum tenens physicians.

treated as owners. This treatment may involve engaging them in a collaborative discussion about how best to operate the center, rewarding or incentivizing them for the desired metrics or as part of their compensation, or giving stock options or phantom stock[6] in the center.

It is the rare person who has the ability to consistently perform as if they own the business. Thus, center managers must use a variety of creative staffing tools to ensure that the center always has a provider on-site during hours of operation. There are a variety of ways to accomplish this goal, including the use of locum tenens, search firms, part-time providers, residents, and direct recruitment.

LOCUM TENENS

Locum tenens (a Latin phrase roughly meaning "to take the place of") is a growing style of practice in which physicians fill temporary duties that can range from 1 day to 1 year, filling in when permanent physicians are difficult to recruit or are otherwise absent.[7] Historically, physicians worked locum tenens as a professional courtesy, filling in for colleagues or peers who were temporarily absent because of illness or vacation.

In the 1970s, locum tenens staffing began to be organized on a larger scale through staffing companies supplying providers, mostly in rural areas. At that time, locum tenens physicians were still something of a novelty.[8]

Health-care facilities use locum tenens physicians for a variety of reasons. This reflects an evolution in the locum tenens market that is linked to the physician shortage. Today national provider shortages have prompted hospitals, medical groups, and others to use temporary physicians to maintain services because permanent physicians are increasingly difficult to find.

Many physicians today are working fewer hours and are interested in a controllable lifestyle featuring regular vacations. Fifty-three percent of those surveyed indicated they use locum tenens physicians to fill in for vacationing physicians, a trend that may accelerate as a growing number of physicians move toward the employment model (with its set vacations and hours), and away from private or small group practice.

Generally speaking, locum providers are more costly than using the clinic's providers. In addition to high cost, there are other challenges. Because they are coming into the hospital or practice cold, locum tenens physicians may be unfamiliar with the equipment and prevailing practice patterns. They therefore must learn to be adaptable and open-minded, quickly absorbing the practice culture and working within it—a historically difficult task for many physicians.

---

6   Phantom stock is a form of compensation in which a company promises (in lieu of actual stock) to pay cash at some future date, in an amount equal to the market value of a number of shares of its stock. Like other forms of stock-based compensation plans, phantom stock encourages employee retention through alignment of interests.
7   Fowler D. A revealing 2011 survey on locum tenens physicians.
8   Fowler D. A revealing 2011 survey on locum tenens physicians.

Here are some statistics about locum utilization from "A Revealing 2011 Survey on Locum Tenens Physicians," by Daryl Fowler, on the *Journal of Urgent Care Medicine* website:

- 63% of respondents reported using locums to fill in for provider shortages until a permanent provider is found.
- 53% reported using locums to fill in for vacationing providers.
- Only 4% responded that they use locums to increase coverage during peak times.
- 73% said that they use locums to prevent disruptions in patient care during times that providers are not available. This may be particularly helpful for urgent care centers during hard-to-fill shifts or peak patient flow times.
- Most respondents cited cost as the major drawback to using locums. Per diem rates run between $850 and $1250.
- Most respondents (72%) rated the quality of locums as either excellent or good. It has been my experience that locum tenens companies rigorously screen applicants; this prevents some of the challenges of the past regarding the quality of locum providers.
- The respondents were almost evenly split regarding the productivity (patients and charges) of locums; however, these data may be skewed by the shifts or hours staffed by the locums.
- The majority of those surveyed (72%) work with more than one staffing company when seeking locum tenens physicians. Staffing companies work on a contingency basis, with payments due only when the physician is in place seeing patients and generating revenue.
- The majority of respondents believed that locums have a positive return on investment.

Today an effective staff plan may embrace the strategic use of locum tenens physicians and all the various other types of providers and contractual arrangements that address our increasingly diverse medical workforce.

As Alan Ayers pointed out in his excellent review in the *Journal of Urgent Care Medicine*,[9] along with the positive aspects of locum tenens come some challenges:

- There may be a turn and burn mentality toward patients, meaning that no effort is made on collaborative care or follow-through. Or there may be the converse, a one-pace-fits-all approach, where no matter the patient volume, the locum provider goes at one speed only.

---

9   Ayers A. Making the most of locum tenens in your urgent care. *Journal of Urgent Care Medicine* 2012;7:21–4. Available from: http://jucm.com/magazine/issues/2012/1212/files/23.html. Accessed February 4, 2014.

- There may be an extreme aversion to risk. In this scenario, all patients except those with the most benign and straightforward conditions are sent to the emergency department, or every patient gets every test because locums are practicing defensive medicine.
- There can be a failure to take any ownership regarding the quality of the documentation or diligence in evaluation and management coding, which often manifests in undercoding, missed procedures, and ancillary codes.
- There may be referrals to out-of-network specialists or inappropriate referrals for conditions that don't warrant specialty care.
- There can be extended wait times if the locums are not appropriately incentivized or indoctrinated into the culture or trained in the use of the electronic health record.

Staffing a center using locums as the primary providers is a recipe for financial ruin. Unless you are fortunate enough to find providers who are as engaged and dedicated as your full-time, employed providers, for the same price and without crippling travel and lodging expenses, you will have difficulty maintaining a viable practice given today's declining managed-care rates.

The key to success using locums is to find a partner–vendor who understands your needs and who performs thorough background checks and primary-source verification. Moreover, finding a vendor who has flexible payment and bonus methodologies is preferable to being restricted to the per diem payment structure.

SEARCH FIRMS

If you are planning for growth or know you will be experiencing a provider shortage, it is imperative to start the hiring process early. One way is to engage a search firm to assist in the hiring process. As with locum tenens companies, there are some upsides and downsides to using provider search firms.

Most search firms are engaged by the practice or center needing a provider. Search firms contract in one of two ways: retained agreement or contingency agreement.

Retained Agreements

Under the retained method, the search firms are paid a percentage of the service fee to begin the search. Using this model, the search firm often demands an exclusive commitment from the group or institution so as not to find itself expending resources to find a provider who is not ultimately engaged.

Under such a retained exclusive search, all candidates are contacted and screened by the search firm. In this scenario, the physician does not make the decision to use a search firm but rather receives the recruitment services, initial interview, and primary-source verification as engaged by the institution or practice at no cost to the provider.

The monthly retainer ranges from $4,000 to $6,000 or in some cases is a percentage of the total search fee. The balance of the search service fee is paid on contracting with a provider. Depending on the recruitment company and the services rendered, the total search fee ranges from $20,000 to $30,000 per provider.

Contingency Agreements

Under a contingency arrangement, the total fee is paid to the recruitment company on completion of the recruitment process, and the firm carries the entire cost of the search until the candidate is hired. The total fee amount is similar to the retained arrangement. Under a contingency recruitment agreement, few (if any) performance guarantees are provided by the search firm. Essentially, it is a full-risk expense contract for the search firm in the event a successful candidate is not hired.

If you have a great practice with a positive work culture in a fairly reasonable location and compensate in a reasonably competitive methodology, you should not need to engage a search firm unless there are extenuating circumstances.

GOING IT ON YOUR OWN

You can engage and hire providers without using search firms or locum tenens groups. The best way is through word of mouth from the providers currently working in your center. Having an organization with a positive culture that values the employees and patients and is open, caring, and reasonable is the best thing you can do to help your hiring process. Your providers are your best recruiters and should be actively engaged and rewarded by their efforts to build the practice.

Here are other tips and suggestions:

- ► Have a fair and balanced contract. Know the market and what your competitors offer. Onerous and restrictive covenants, termination clauses, and employee-paid tail provisions are deal breakers for all but the most desperate providers.

- ► Encourage your providers to have the contract reviewed. This gives you free legal advice on what the market will bear.

- ► Have a frank discussion before hiring the provider. Go over expectations, productivity requirements, communication expectations, and the ethical and compassionate treatment of patients and staff members.

- ► Check background, education, and references. In health care most providers are separated by only a few degrees. You pretty much always know someone who trained or worked with a prospective employee. Find references and contacts not listed on the curriculum vitae and ask them for honest feedback.

- ► Conduct a behavioral interview. You will learn a lot about a prospective employee by how they spend their free time, their altruistic engagements and projects, the books they read, and how they have faced adversity. Note that there are some questions that the prospective employer cannot ask during an interview.[10]

When you have exhausted the word-of-mouth search for providers, look at the following sites, which were provided by a veteran provider-recruiter.[11]

RESOURCES TO FIND PROVIDERS

Physician Job Boards

- www.practicelink.com
- www.physiciandepot.com
- www.practicematch.com
- www.locumtenens.com
- www.healthecareers.com
- www.mdsearch.com
- www.careermd.com
- www.mommd.com
- www.physicianemployment.org
- www.physemp.com
- www.doctorshangout.com
- www.doximity.com
- www.physiciancareerjobs.com
- www.physiciancrossroads.com
- www.mdcareercenter.com
- www.usadocjobs.com
- www.physicianjobboard.com
- www.primarycareopenings.com
- www.edphysician.com
- www.nejmcareercenter.org
- www.do-online.org

---

10 Prospective employers cannot ask about race, color, sex, religion, origin or birthplace, age, disability, or marital status, because basing a hiring decision on a candidate's answers regarding any of those issues is discriminatory.
11 Maisch L. Email communication. July 30, 2013.

- www.aafp.org
- www.ucaoa.org (for urgent care physicians)
- State MD and DO association sites

Midlevel Job Boards

- www.healthecareers.com
- www.paworld.net
- www.npworld.us
- www.paboard.com
- www.healthjobsnationwide.com
- www.npjobs.com
- www.pajobsite.com
- www.pa-exchange.com
- www.aapa.org

POST-HIRING CHALLENGES

Hopefully all the providers you hire turn out to be the competent, caring providers you knew they were when you hired them. However, if you are like everyone else who has hired and managed medical professionals, you will get the wool pulled over your eyes once in a while. Now that you have hired them, how do you manage your disruptive medical providers?

DEALING WITH THE DISRUPTIVE PROVIDER

There is no universally accepted definition of a disruptive physician. In 2000, the American Medical Association (AMA) defined a disruptive physician as a physician whose behavior "interferes with patient care or could reasonably be expected to interfere with the process of delivering quality care."[12] Note that this definition focuses on the overt behavior of the physician and the impact of this behavior on patients and the health system in which the physician works. Given the simplicity, clarity, and breadth of this definition, identifying physicians who meet these criteria should be relatively easy.[13]

Among the categories of behavior that could result in disruptiveness are psychosis, clinical depression, drug or alcohol abuse or addiction, personality

---

12. American Medical Association. Opinion E-9.045—Physicians with disruptive behavior. Available from: www.ama-assn.org/ama/pub/physician-resources/medical-ethics/code-medical-ethics/opinion9045.page. Accessed June 9, 2011.
13. Goodstein LD, Shufeldt J. Dealing with the disruptive provider. *Journal of Urgent Care Medicine*. 2011;5:17–23. Available from: http://jucm.com/magazine/issues/2011/0811/files/19.html. Accessed February 4, 2014.

disorders, excessive stress and burnout, and behavioral changes due to aging. Within these categories, examples of disruptive behavior include disrespectful and profane language; angry outbursts; threats; inappropriate criticism of care given by other professionals; sexual harassment; drunkenness; throwing objects; failure to observe patient–physician boundaries; failure to respond to calls while on duty; failure to show up punctually for work; unauthorized absences during the workday (e.g., long lunches, habitually leaving early); and unkempt, disheveled, or otherwise unprofessional appearance.

By displaying inappropriate emotions and uncooperative behavior in the workplace, disruptive physicians jeopardize the provision of quality health care. The Joint Commission mandates that each health-care delivery system must "have a code of conduct that defines acceptable, disruptive, and inappropriate behavior." In addition, each system must "create and implement a process for managing disruptive and inappropriate behaviors."[14] At the end of this section of the chapter, there is a list of tips for actions to take when a physician is disruptive.

Large-scale, sound, research-based data on the incidence of disruptive physicians do not exist. On the basis of their survey of the literature, Leape and Fromson conclude that 3% to 5% of all physicians evince problematic disruptive behavior.[15] In another literature review, Williams arrives at a significantly higher estimate: 6% to 12% of physicians are "dyscompetent"—that is, not performing at an acceptable standard for providing patient care.[16]

These estimates do not suggest an epidemic of unruly behavior, so it is easy to conclude that the problem of disruptive physicians is a tempest in a teapot. Not so. According to the US Bureau of Labor Statistics, physicians and surgeons held approximately 661,400 jobs in 2008 (the latest year for which statistics are available).[7] If only 3% of those physicians are disruptive, that means 19,842 physicians in the United States are behaving poorly.

Estimates of the number of disruptive physicians do not take into account the ripple effects of their unruly behavior, which adversely affect a far wider circle of people than the physicians in question.[17]

A 2011 survey of a regional group of hospital emergency departments found that more than half the respondents (57%) had observed disruptive behavior in physicians.[18] One-third of the respondents felt that disruptive behavior could be linked to the occurrence of adverse events, 34.5% to medical errors, 24.7% to compromises in patient safety, 35.8% to poor quality, and 12.3% to patient mortal-

---

14 Leadership committed to safety. The Joint Commission. *Sentinel Event Alert*. Issue 43, August 27, 2009. Available from: www.jointcommission.org/sentinel_event_alert_issue_43_leadership_committed_to_safety. Accessed June 9, 2011.
15 Leape LL, Fromson JA. Problem doctors: is there a system-level solution? *Ann Intern Med*. 2006:144:107–15.
16 Williams BW. The prevalence and special educational requirements of dyscompetent physicians. *J Contin Educ Health Prof*. 2006;26:173–91.
17 Goodstein LD, Shufeldt J. Dealing with the disruptive provider.
18 Rosenstein AH, Naylor B. Incidence and impact of physician and nurse disruptive behaviors in the emergency department. *J Emerg Med*. 2011;3:287–92.

ity. Disruptive behaviors "have a significant impact on team dynamics, communication efficiency, information flow, and task accountability," the investigators conclude, "all of which can adversely impact patient care."

Although studies of disruptive physicians have primarily been conducted in hospital settings, problem physicians pose significant risks to any health-care organization—including urgent care clinics—in patient safety, quality of care, staff morale, and community confidence and support, not to mention the potential for lawsuits brought by patients or even members of a clinic's staff. Failure to deal promptly and effectively with an unruly physician undermines staff confidence in the center's leadership and sends a tacit message: "No one here seems to care about how we treat patients, so why should I?" Once allowed to take root, such permissiveness can quickly permeate and undermine a clinic's culture.

Problem physicians severely reduce the job satisfaction of nursing and ancillary staff members, further lowering morale and increasing staff turnover.[19] Williams and Williams found that a disruptive team member not only leads to decreased morale of other team members but also reduces their commitment to the profession and to the workplace.[20] This is something that no health-care facility in a competitive market environment can afford.

Here are actions to take when a provider is exhibiting disruptive tendencies:

- *Don't ignore*   This behavior, if unaddressed, tends to get worse. During the intervening time, you will lose other providers, staff members, and patients. Moreover, your risk of a patient-safety issue increases dramatically.

- *Document the behavior in clear, unambiguous terms.*

- *Counsel the provider and have a witness present*   Discuss the behavior, not the root cause.

- *Document the outcome of the discussion and the actions that will be taken if the behavior or similar behavior occurs again.*

- *Use a two- or three-strike rule*   This behavior does not usually improve. It may wax and wane, but it seems to rarely go away.

- *Learn from your mistake*   How did you miss the patterns or signs during your recruitment or interview?

CONCLUSION

Hiring and managing medical providers will occupy a large portion of the managers' and medical directors' time. There are a number of actions you can take to help you meet your hiring goals. Foremost among them is to have a collaborative and open work environment.

---

19 Rosenstein AH, O'Daniel M. A survey of the impact of disruptive behavior and communication defects on patient safety. *Jt Comm J Qual Patient Saf*. 2008;34:464–71.
20 Williams BW, Williams MV. The disruptive physician: conceptual organization. *Journal of Medical Licensure and Discipline*. 2008;94:12–20.

KEY POINTS

1. There is a looming shortage of medical providers. Plan ahead—form and document a provider engagement game plan.

2. Review your current provider employment agreement. Review termination, noncompete, and medical liability language; and work with your attorney to look for alternative language that still suits your needs.

3. Perform diligence on the locum firms. Look at their screening processes, their track records, and their current talent pools.

4. Work with your locum company on creative ways to compensate providers that align incentives with the practice.

5. Perform due diligence on your search firm, and review the fine print. Understand their guarantees and the time frame within which to request a new hire.

6. Check references beyond those provided by the applicant. No one purposely chooses references who will not give them glowing recommendations.

7. Perform behavioral interviews. You can learn a lot about a person by asking questions not directly related to the practice of medicine.

8. Ensure that you have a great culture and work environment. Your current providers are your best (or worst) advocates.

9. Deal firmly and fairly with disruptive physicians.

10. When dealing with a disruptive provider, do not ignore the problem and hope it will go away. Address the issue immediately. At some point, irreparable damage will be done by the disruptive provider.

CHAPTER 20

Strategic Talent Management: Talent Makes All the Difference

Marty Martin

STELLAR CLINICAL OUTCOMES, STUNNING patient experiences, superb employment experiences, and smart design of clinical and business processes depend on talent. It's that simple. Hence urgent care leaders and managers are responsible, and will be held accountable by the market, for strategically managing the talent they offer at their centers.

Since a group of McKinsey consultants[1] coined the phrase "the War for Talent" in 1997, talent management has received noteworthy attention among academics and practitioners. *Strategic talent management*, also referred to as *human resources management*, is the systematic identification of key positions that contribute to the competitive advantage of your urgent care center. Strategic talent management depends on the ability of your urgent care center to attract and retain high-performing employees—employees who are dedicated to your vision, mission, and strategic goals and who are invested in the success of every member of the team as well as to the overall well-being of your patients. The evidence is clear: Strategic talent management is a source of competitive advantage.[2]

Figure 1 shows the six major functions of strategic talent management, all of which revolve around the core elements of every organization: its mission and strategy.

These functions are described in the sections that follow, along with three evidence-based best practices for each—a total of 18 best practices for you to consider implementing in order to strategically manage your talent.

The success—or failure—of your urgent care center depends on the individuals you engage. Chief executive officers of major companies across the globe choose to spend over 20% of their time on talent management.[3] If you are not

---

1 Axelrod B, Handfield-Jones H, Michaels E. A new game plan for C players. *Harvard Business Review.* 2002;80;80–8.
2 Becker BE, Huselid MA. Strategic human resource management: where do we go from here? *Journal of Management.* 2006;32:898–925.
3 Economist Intelligence Unit. The CEO's role in talent management: how top executives from ten countries are nurturing the leaders of tomorrow. London: *The Economist*; 2006. Available from: http://graphics.eiu.com/files/ad_pdfs/eiu_DDI_talent_Management_WP.pdf. Accessed February 21, 2014.

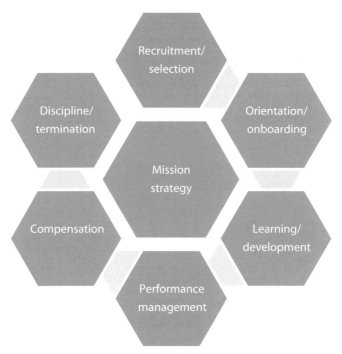

Figure 1. The six major functions of strategic talent management.

doing so, then you're either congratulating yourself on a job well done…or asking yourself this question: Who is *really* responsible for driving the success of my urgent care center?

The War for Talent is critical in the health-care industry because of these challenges confronting its leaders:

- The projected shortage of 91,500 physicians by 2020, including 45,400 primary care physicians[4]

- The growing demand for primary care services as a result of the 32 million patients who receive coverage or better coverage because of the Affordable Care Act and the projected 80 million baby boomers who will be retiring by 2035[5]

- The redesign of clinical services that is increasingly moving away from higher-cost hospitals to lower-cost ambulatory centers—and even to patients' homes.

---

4 Kirch DG, Henderson MK, Dill MJ. Physician workforce projections in an era of health care reform. *Annu Rev Med*. 2012;63:435–45.

5 Schwartz MD. Health care reform and the primary care workforce bottleneck. *J Gen Intern Med*. 2012;27:1–4.

- ▶ The alarming impact of 12-hour shifts for health-care employees, particularly nurses, where an empirical association has been found between such lengthy shifts and increased levels of burnout, job dissatisfaction, and intention to quit the job altogether[6]

Signals like these demand that urgent care leaders and managers initiate change to adapt and thrive.

Strategic talent management means understanding that competition exists for the talent we want. It means understanding that the level of talent makes all the difference in determining the level of our outcomes in

- ▶ Clinical quality
- ▶ Patient satisfaction
- ▶ Employee and physician engagement
- ▶ Resource management
- ▶ Creativity and innovation

It is the talent inside a particular urgent care center that enables it to rise to whatever challenges come its way. It is also the level of talent that enables that center to achieve stellar results for its three key groups—patients, employees, and the community.

The future of urgent care rests on the increasingly competitive race for patients and workers. Beyond the quality of your leadership and the talent of your staff members, the implementation of evidence-based human resources practices also plays an important role. But such practices alone do not suffice in meeting the challenges we face in the health-care delivery system and the urgent care industry. Creativity, innovation, and risk-taking must be embraced to spark disruptive innovations in human resources practices within urgent care in much the same way that urgent care itself has been regarded as a disruptive innovation.[7]

EVIDENCE-BASED HUMAN RESOURCES PRACTICES

The theme here is that urgent care companies will soon adopt evidence-based human resources practices in much the same way they are adopting evidence-based medicine and nursing practices. Most organizations do not implement such evidence-based practices, even though they have been scientifically proven to be associated with higher employee productivity and better financial performance.[8] That is why it is so important to emphasize that strategic talent management is not about doing that which is common but about differentiating your human

---

6   Stimpfel AW, Sloane DM, Aiken LH. The longer the shifts for hospital nurses, the higher the levels of burnout and patient dissatisfaction. *Health Affairs*. 2012;31:2501–9.
7   Hansen E, Bozic KJ. The impact of disruptive innovations in orthopaedics. *Clin Orthop Relat Res*. 2009;467:2512–20.
8   Pfeffer J, Sutton RI. *The Knowing-Doing Gap: How Smart Companies Turn Knowledge Into Action*. Boston, MA: Harvard Business School Press; 2000.

resources practices to attract, retain, and engage your workforce to deliver safe, high-quality, delightfully satisfying care every single day, every single hour, and every single minute.

Recruitment and Selection

You will know that your recruitment and selection function is successful when the right employees are hired at the right time in the right way by the right individuals. Sound easy? Perhaps; perhaps not. Certainly there is a job for nearly every urgent care professional. But not necessarily in *your* urgent care facility. Why? To hire and keep the right talent, base your recruiting and selection on the following formula:

$$\text{Employee effectiveness} = \text{Will} + \text{Skill} + \text{Fit}$$

The effectiveness of a new hire depends on their willingness to do what is required—and then to do a bit more without being asked. Effectiveness also hinges on the hire's underlying knowledge, skills, and abilities brought to the job. New hires must be able to demonstrate not only that they know how to learn but also that they embrace learning—in effect, that they are intellectually curious. The effectiveness of new hires relies on their being in alignment with your center's mission and strategy and in productive harmony with all members of your urgent care team. There is more to effective recruitment and selection than searching for a new hire who is licensed and breathing.

How do you attract and select a new candidate who has it all: possesses the will, has the skill, and fits? First, a *seducing signal* must be sent out into the labor market, using diverse channels ranging from job boards to trade journal advertisements, that you are seeking an urgent care professional, regardless of current position, to provide top-drawer patient care and, equally as important, one who is looking to benefit from an employment experience second to none.

Remember, health-care professionals work for the patient as well as for themselves and their family members. When designing a recruitment campaign, it helps to view it as what might be called *rings of recruitment* (Figure 2).

Each ring represents a branded message, created and then disseminated through various channels, such as paper or online application forms, websites, job announcements in trade journals, and advertisements posted on job boards like CareerBuilder or Monster. Unique messages that correspond to each ring (branded message) are necessary because individuals are attracted to work for all these reasons—and more. Each ring you address makes it more likely that you will attract candidates. If you focus too much on one ring at the expense of the other three, your chances of attracting top talent decreases. Although it is true at least in part that recruitment is a numbers game, attracting and retaining top talent with more than credentials and a pulse requires far more attention.

Once you've attracted some top-drawer talent in response to your search campaign, your second step is to select the best from the group. These evidence-based selection guidelines will help you predict which candidate is likely to perform

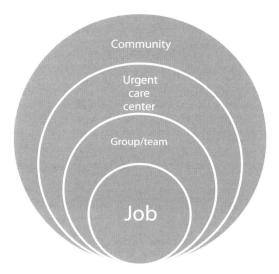

Figure 2. Your seducing signal consists of branded messages focusing separately on the job, the team, your urgent care center, and your community.

with excellence and which candidate is likely to sit around and suck up oxygen and money.

- *Use structured rather than unstructured interviews*   The goal of the selection interview is to predict performance and fit; it is not to decide whether you like the individual. It has been proven that assessing a candidate's fit with the center and its staff improves retention in the long run.[9]

- *Be up front with the candidates*   Share the good, the bad, and the ugly about the urgent care center, the team, and the job. This is known as a *realistic job preview*. Researchers have found an association between realistic job previews and retention numbers, so if you're embarrassed about your center or your staff, don't hide the dirty laundry. Clean it up.

- *Design a job so that it is meaningful*   To want to stay in a job, the person who holds it must be able to derive meaning from its tasks, obtain feedback from those tasks, and recognize how the tasks fit into the bigger picture of the urgent care center. The way jobs are designed can be directly linked to higher performance.

Two words of caution before you proceed on this path: One, obey the law. Two, take selection seriously.

---

9   Kristof-Brown AL, Zimmerman RD, Johnson EC. Consequences of individuals' fit at work: a meta-analysis of person–job, person–organization, person–group, and person–supervisor fit. *Personnel Psychology* 2005;58:281–342.

Obeying the Law

There are a number of legal dos and don'ts when it comes managing your talent. Though it is beyond the scope of this chapter to detail all the relevant federal and state laws pertaining to workplace discrimination, disability, occupational safety and health, and labor unions, note that when interviewing candidates for a job, your focus should be on predicting their performance if they are selected rather than on asking questions that may be illegal—and that provide little valid information about what you really need to know: whether this candidate will perform.

Illegal questions include those about marital status, parental status, religion, national origin, race or ethnicity, and disability status. However, asking illegal questions is just the tip of the iceberg. If you do decide to hire this candidate, you will have entered into a relationship based on certain prescribed legal considerations.

From a strategic talent management perspective, you need to know when specific federal statutes apply to your facility. For example, Title I of the Americans with Disabilities Act kicks in when your center has 15 or more employees. This 15-employee threshold also applies to Title VII, the Civil Rights Act of 1964, but the Age Discrimination in Employment Act of 1967, protecting workers over the age of 40, has a threshold of 20 employees.

The health-care industry is different from some others in that it gives rise to the complication of whether to treat physicians and other medical providers as employees or independent contractors. Designating providers as independent contractors allows the center to escape liability, because the 15- or 20-employee threshold is not met. When providers are designated as employees and legal thresholds are achieved, the center opens itself up to liability. The only way to answer the question as to whether to qualify a provider as an employee or independent contractor is to study a totality of factors, including how much autonomy the provider has, how the provider is regarded with respect to compensation and benefits, how the provider is supervised, and to what degree the provider is restricted from working in other urgent care or health-care settings.

The first general recommendation in this regard is to classify providers and other workers appropriately in part on the basis of what some consultants call the Internal Revenue Service 20-point test (see Internal Revenue Service publication 15-A, available from http://www.irs.gov/pub/irs-pdf/p15a.pdf) and advice from legal counsel. The second general recommendation is to develop, communicate, and train every worker in your center about policies originating from federal and state laws like the Civil Rights Act and the Equal Pay Act (of 1963). But this is only the beginning. In addition to disseminating policies and educating and training staff members, you must also offer complaint handling and investigative and disciplinary processes essential for addressing any allegations or incidents that arise. It is also best to ensure that a complainant can bypass the chain of command if the complaint is lodged against the person's direct supervisor or the owner of the center.

The Financial Impact of Recruitment and Selection

The cost of recruiting, selecting, and training new hires is often more than their first year's salary. For instance, if a newly hired nurse is paid $45,000, then you can assume that you have spent more than $45,000 to recruit, hire, and train that nurse. If this is true, then you can also assume that if the average nurse in your urgent care center has worked there for 4 years, your center has already expended nearly a quarter of a million dollars per full-time nursing position during that time. In most organizations, managers cannot spend $225,000 on anything without going through an extensive approval or capital budgeting process. Yet most managers hire talent without questioning the burden of such high costs—and do it with very little oversight. From this perspective, it is essential that recruitment and selection be taken more seriously.

Orientation and Onboarding

Orientation and onboarding are successful when the new hire is regarded as fully prepared to work as productively as possible and has gotten to that point as soon as was *reasonable* to expect. After all, it is both unreasonable and unfair to expect that new hires will hit the ground running relative to the details of their new job; all of the unique policies, procedures, and processes particular to your specific urgent care center; and all the hidden dos and don'ts that make up its culture (usually expressed by "that's just the way we do things around here"). A robust orientation and onboarding process addresses a number of essential elements, ones that cannot be addressed in a half- or even full-day session by a human resources person or by sending the hire to a website packed with huge amounts of interactive content. Following these three evidence-based guidelines will enhance your center's orientation and onboarding process as well as the eventual productivity of your new hires:

- *Orient new hires* to the job, the urgent care center, and the staff by engaging as many fellow new employees as possible in the process.[10]

- *Give the new hire positive, performance-based feedback* as early as possible to ease the transition into the urgent care center.[11]

- *Offer signals to new hires about how specific tasks and each job contribute* to the center's overall mission and strategy.

The process of orienting and onboarding should not be undermined by approaching it as just a way to get the hire the necessary information to perform and a way to introduce all the key players. The real goal is to increase the chances that your new hire will contribute and add value as quickly as possible by feeling

---

10 Allen DG. Do organizational socialization tactics influence newcomer embeddedness and turnover? *Journal of Management*. 2006;32:237–56.
11 Kammeyer-Mueller JD, Wanberg CR. Unwrapping the organizational entry process: disentangling multiple antecedents and their pathways to adjustment. *J Appl Psychol*. 2003;88:779–94.

connected to the tasks, the job, the team, and the center. You should view this process as one that is ongoing and generally lasts about 6 months, rather than as a single event, a binder, a manual, or a thumb drive.

Learning and Development

You cannot ignore the need to ensure that every member of your urgent care team stays up-to-date with changing laws, rules, and regulations as well as advances in technology, communication, and urgent care medicine. Learning and development is continuous, because change is continuous, and the evidence-based practices that will keep your team on the cutting edge are simple and direct.

- Provide job-specific training.[12]
- Offer opportunities to update skills in order to increase retention.[13]
- Allow employees to change the nature of their job, in toto or in part, as a way to increase engagement and performance. This is known as *job crafting*.[14]

Furthermore, learning and development consists of more than an in-service training program on new technology, a new policy, or a new guideline. Though in-service programs have their place, so do designing and delivering education (targeting awareness and knowledge), training (targeting skill building), and coaching (targeting performance).

If you are a larger or better-off urgent care center, consider offering tuition reimbursement for credit or noncredit courses that are aligned with achieving the center's strategic goals. In addition, offer classes both on-site and off-site that range from stress management to personal financial management; enhancing your employees' overall development sends a clear signal that you value your employees as individuals.

Performance Management

Performance management is more than a performance appraisal or evaluation. Although these are valid tools for documenting performance and making decisions related to compensation, promotion, demotion, and even termination, they generally occur on a single day and typically for a single hour—out of the approximately 2000 hours the full-time employee works each year. You cannot afford *not* to manage performance for all those other hours. Figure 3 illustrates the five key steps in managing performance. These stages are not meant to serve as stand-alone tools but as part of a combined program.

---

12 Home PW, Griffeth RW. *Employee Turnover*. Cincinnati, OH: South-Western College Publishing; 1995.
13 Home PW, Griffeth RW. *Employee Turnover*.
14 Wrzesniewski A, Dutton JE. Crafting a job: revisioning employees as active crafters of their work. *Academy of Management Review*. 2001;26:179–201.

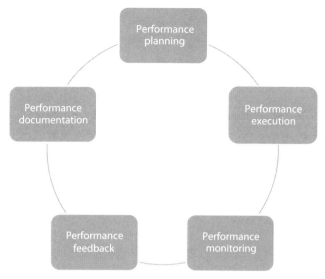

Figure 3. Five key steps in managing performance.

Performance Planning
Establishing and communicating behavioral and performance expectations is the essence of performance planning. These expectations can be set at the individual employee level or at the group or team level. Regardless of the level, it is critical that expectations be aligned with the strategic goals of the urgent care center.

Performance Execution
Once performance expectations (some or all of which may have been embedded in the center's job description for a position) have been communicated, it remains to be seen whether the employee or the team will perform in or out of alignment with these expectations. Employee performance can then be described as meeting, exceeding, or failing to meet expectations.

Performance Monitoring
To determine an employee's or team's level of performance, you need a way to observe or capture it in the form of an evaluation. Think in terms of catching the employee doing something right rather than catching the employee screwing up. Monitoring gives you, the urgent care leader, data you can use when providing feedback and coaching.

Performance Feedback
After performance-related information has been collected, it must be validated. Once it is validated, the individual employee or team receives feedback. At a

minimum, performance should meet expectations; ideally, it should exceed expectations. Develop a coaching style in which feedback is delivered in a collaborative and nonjudgmental manner and is accompanied by active listening and leveraging the strengths of the individual employee or team.

Performance Documentation

Finally, all expectations, monitoring, and feedback must be documented. This documentation is used for internal purposes like making decisions about compensation and promotions and for external purposes such as responding to discrimination complaints and unemployment claims. Remember, the magic of performance does not occur by focusing only on one of these five steps *but on all five together*. Once the process is in place, consider adopting the following evidence-based performance management practices.

- *Set clear, behavior-based performance goals at both individual and team levels*   Goal setting is more effective for improving performance than employee participation in decision making, especially when the goals are challenging ones.[15]

- *Train managers on how to develop good working relationships with those who report directly to them.*[16]

- *Support managers in coaching employees to achieve the goals of the urgent care center as well as the goals of their fellow workers*   Managers are fundamental in generating employee commitment to the goals of the organization.[17]

Compensation and Benefits

People's actual behavior suggests that pay is much more important to them than they imply in surveys. In view of such information, we know that our urgent care staff members experience compensation and benefits relative to their perceptions of fairness and justice, their conclusions about being able to live comfortably, and their confidence in current income security and future retirement security.

When employees perceive they are not being compensated fairly for their time and work, complaints are not uncommon. You might hear it directly, as in "I'm not being paid enough." But often such feelings also reveal themselves in an employee's performance. Either way, it is important to dig deeper, especially if the complaint is lodged directly or highlighted in an employee satisfaction survey or exit interview, because perceived unfairness covers too much territory for only

---

15   Locke EA, Latham GP. *A Theory of Goal Setting and Performance*. Englewood Cliffs, NJ: Prentice Hall; 1990.
16   Aquino K, Griffeth RW, Allen DG, Hom PW. An integration of justice constructs into the turnover process: test of a referent cognitions model. *Academy of Management Journal*. 1997;40:1208–27.
17   Barber L, Hayday S, Bevan S. From people to profits, IES Report 355. 1999. Available from: http://www.employment-studies.co.uk/pubs/summary.php?id=355. Accessed October 19, 2013.

the cursory glance. Fairness—or lack thereof—is usually experienced in one (or all) of these three ways:

▶ *Staff members believe that there is lack of equity between the amount of energy expended on the job and the total compensation package*   In other words, "As hard as I work, I'm not paid enough." Unfairness can also be experienced as the lack of equity between the employee who is doing the complaining and another employee's wage. In other words, "I work harder than she does, so either I should get paid more or she should get paid less." Finally, the perception of unfairness can be based on what the employee believes wages to be at other centers. In other words, "Our pay stinks. Look at what everyone else makes at the other centers and hospitals."

▶ *Staff members feel that the bar for high performance is unreachable*   Feeling that expectations are unreasonable only results in feeling that it's not worth expending the energy to do better because the payoff seems impossible to achieve. In other words, "Why bother?"

▶ *Staff members feel confused about what is expected or how expectations are measured*   Not understanding one's job description or the center's rules and regulations or performance measurements, not fitting into the culture, and not having received enough training are all fodder for confusion around expectations. Such a state of disorientation generally results in an overall diminishing focus on the task at hand—the job.

It's easy to see how perceptions of fairness and unfairness have an impact on focus, how focus, or lack thereof, has an impact on performance, and how performance has an impact on outcomes. Outcomes drive success or failure. That is why if you want to succeed by providing safe, high-quality, satisfying care to your customers, you cannot afford to have your urgent care staff members distracted or anxious about their compensation and benefits package. Distractions increase errors and decrease employee satisfaction, which ultimately undermines patient satisfaction as well.

Some urgent care centers are implementing variable, incentive-based pay-for-performance (P4P) compensation programs. These compensation programs generally align the interests of the employee with the organization. But the evidence is mixed as to the effectiveness of P4P programs in health care. What we do know is that

▶ Incentives are more effective than disincentives, in which there are winners or losers[18]

▶ Larger incentives yield greater participation[19]

---

18   Van Herck P, De Smedt D, Annemans L, et al. Systematic review: effects, design choices and context of pay-for-performance in health care. *BMC Health Services Research*. 2010;10:247–59.
19   de Brantes FS, D'Andrea BG. Physicians respond to pay-for-performance incentives: larger incentives yield greater participation. *Am J Manag Care*. 2009;15:305–10.

- Incentives appear to be more effective initially with lower than higher performers[20]

The key to making this decision is to determine the target of the incentive: Is it for an individual, a group or team, or an organization? Evidence has shown that P4Ps targeting individuals and groups can be extremely effective.[21]

Discipline and Termination

Of all the tasks that managers do in any organization, including urgent care organizations, the one they hate doing the most comes under the heading of discipline and termination. After all, who likes to be responsible for being the heavy—the bad guy?

- Given the already stressful nature of disciplining and terminating employees, the primary challenge confronting many urgent care managers becomes how to compose one's own emotions and avoid being impulsive in the desire to punish the employee in some way. The goal of employee discipline is to encourage, or perhaps direct, the employee to perform in a different manner based on the expectations set forth by the urgent care center and as communicated by you (the manager or chief executive officer), the team leader, and even fellow workers. Furthermore, from everything we now know, it is apparent that a punitive approach to employee discipline does not work. In fact, researchers[22,23] have found that the only result of punishment is fear and anger, not the shift in behavior or performance we're looking for. Employees perceive managers to be more effective if they use a coaching-oriented management style.

The other interesting aspect of disciplining employees is that it benefits not only other employees but also the patients you serve. Health-care employees who experience bullying at work are more likely to quit. Can you afford to have your employees quit because of bullying and leave your patients in the lurch? Bullying and abuse of subordinates by managers is counterproductive, and such managers should be terminated.

CONCLUSION

Your job as an urgent care leader and manager is to provide safe, high-quality, satisfying care as the rule, not the exception, knowing that the advantages are revealed financially, clinically, and operationally. One way to achieve such results

---

20 Lindenauer PK, Remus D, Roman S, et al. Public reporting and pay for performance in hospital quality improvement. *N Engl J Med.* 2007;356:486–96.
21 Van Herck P et al. Systematic review.
22 Redeker JR. Employee Discipline: Policies and Procedures. Washington DC: Bureau of National Affairs; 1994.
23 Grote D. *Discipline Without Punishment: The Proven Strategy for Turning Problem Employees Into Superior Performers.* 2nd ed. New York: AMACON; 2006.

is to purposefully design a strategic talent management system with the aim of increasing work engagement among all your employees. Do not confuse work engagement with job satisfaction, however. Whereas job satisfaction is passive, work engagement is an ongoing and active process.

KEY POINTS

1. Strategic talent management consists of six interlocking human resources management functions:
   - Recruitment and selection
   - Orientation and onboarding
   - Learning and development
   - Performance management
   - Compensation and benefits
   - Discipline and termination

2. Evidence-based human resources practices should be used by urgent care leaders.

3. Distractions on the part of your urgent care workforce undermine your attempts at providing safe, error-free, high-quality, and satisfying urgent care.

4. Employee performance is driven by a combination of will plus skill plus fit.

5. Higher performers are waiting for urgent care leaders to address chronic low performers.

6. Retention is as important as recruitment.

7. Compensation is more than paying more money and offering greater benefits; it also includes the psychological experience of employees.

8. The perception of unfairness among workers can be corrosive if not addressed by urgent care leaders.

9. Discipline is important because what you permit, you promote.

10. The result of strategic talent management is high workforce engagement, which results in higher-quality care.

CHAPTER 21

Employment Contracts and Compensation

Adam Winger

RECRUITING AND RETAINING TOP clinical talent is a crucial step in establishing a competitive presence in the urgent care marketplace. To do so, an urgent care employer must offer an appropriate package of benefits and incentives while balancing the company's overall performance objectives. This chapter addresses issues associated with the employment relationship between an urgent care company and its medical providers.

EMPLOYEE VERSUS INDEPENDENT CONTRACTOR

A threshold question in any discussion involving employment agreements is whether the individual rendering the services is actually an employee of the urgent care company. This determination is meaningful for both legal liability and tax purposes.

Legal Liability

Inappropriately classifying an independent contractor as an employee may result in the urgent care employer unnecessarily assuming all liability for the provider's actions. In general, employers are liable for the negligent acts of their employees but not for those of an independent contractor. Although it is common for independent contractors to be added as insured parties to an urgent care company's malpractice policies, there is no requirement that the company do so. Whether a provider is an employee or independent contractor for legal liability purposes is a matter of state law. Most states, however, analyze the issue by considering factors similar to those used by the Internal Revenue Service (IRS), which are discussed in the following section.

Tax Consequences

If a provider is classified as an employee for tax purposes, the urgent care employer must withhold income and payroll taxes (Social Security tax and Medicare tax from the provider's compensation), and pay Federal Unemployment Tax on it. The taxes must be remitted to the IRS, and substantial penalties exist for the employer's failure to do so. As is the case under state law, a worker who is not appropriately classified as an employee is deemed to be an independent contractor for tax purposes. If the employer incorrectly classifies an employee as an independent contractor or the employer fails to withhold and remit payments, the IRS holds the employer liable for the entire amount that should have been withheld and imposes penalties and interest.

Although applicable treasury regulations plainly state that physicians who "offer their services to the public are independent contractors and not employees,"[1] in making its classification determination, the IRS continues to focus on whether "the person for whom services are performed *has the right to control and direct the individual* who performs the services."[2] For over 25 years, the IRS has employed a 20-factor test to analyze whether the extent of a service recipient's control rises to the level of an employer.[3] Although a full discussion of each of the 20 factors is beyond the scope of this chapter, here are a few of the pertinent factors to consider in making worker classification decisions in the urgent care context:

- The degree of instructions given to the worker by the urgent care company
- Whether the urgent care company pays for continuing medical education and other training for the worker
- Whether the urgent care company is entitled to dictate the time, date, and location that the services are rendered
- The extent to which the worker is entitled to share in the profit or loss in the business
- Whether the company furnishes supplies, equipment, or other materials to be used in the worker's performance of their duties
- Whether the worker makes their services available to more than one company while working for the urgent care company

The IRS recommends that before the start date for each new worker, a process be followed to reach a reasonable and informed conclusion regarding the worker's classification. Perhaps the simplest and most prudent approach might be to adopt a policy in which each of the 20 factors set forth by the IRS is considered. Although doing so may add to the already extensive list of administrative burdens associated with bringing on new workers, the risk of misclassification can be costly. Add to this cost the promise of further IRS audits because of the US Supreme Court's upholding of the Patient Protection and Affordable Care

---

1 Treasury Regulation § 31.3121(d)–1(c)(2). Interestingly, in Private Letter Ruling 9149001, the Internal Revenue Service found, in response to an argument that the corporate practice of medicine doctrine eliminated the potential for the physician to be deemed an employee for state law purposes, that "the laws that may govern a state in defining the relationship between a physician and a corporation *do not control how that same relationship is treated under federal law*" (emphasis added).
2 Treasury Regulation § 31.3306(i)–1(b) (emphasis added).
3 Revenue Ruling 87–41.

Act (commonly called the Affordable Care Act). Because certain employers are now obligated to either pay a fine or offer health insurance to all employees, the differentiation of independent contractor from employee will now carry added significance.

Because of the significant state and federal tax law implications, you should obtain the guidance of a competent professional in developing a prudent employee classification compliance plan.

EMPLOYMENT AGREEMENTS

Assuming that the urgent care company reaches the conclusion that the worker is in fact an employee, the next step is to determine whether a written employment agreement is necessary. In general, if the urgent care employer believes the worker could potentially dispute the terms of the individual's arrangement, it will almost always benefit the employer to insist on a written agreement. For example, because compensation arrangements involving formula-driven incentives are typical sources for dispute, each such arrangement should be put in writing.

Provisions of an Employment Agreement

Once you have concluded that a written agreement is warranted, you will need to consider the terms of such an agreement. The following paragraphs discuss and provide examples of some of the more frequent issues and concepts addressed in a medical provider's employment agreement.

Employee Duties

One of the first concepts typically addressed is the various obligations (or "duties") the employee will be required to perform while the agreement remains effective. The degree of specificity used to describe these duties is largely a matter of style and preference. Certain employers choose to list the obligations in great detail in the body of the agreement, although others take a more casual approach, including a simple bulleted list in an exhibit or schedule attached to the agreement. In reality, not much more needs to be said other than (1) the employee will render medical services to patients at one or more of the employer's urgent care centers, and (2) the employee will perform all other duties and services as may be assigned, from time to time, by the employer. For those who take a more detailed approach, the following additional duties may be included:

- Creating and maintaining appropriate patient charts and records for services rendered
- Making proficient use of the employer's electronic medical records system
- Preparing, submitting, and attending to, in a timely manner, all reports, claims, and correspondence necessary or appropriate to the successful operation of the employer's business

- Working with the employer's other employees in a cooperative, constructive manner, consistent with the employer's stated policies and procedures
- Complying with the employer's clinical protocols, policies, and procedures designed to promote consistent and efficient treatment of patients and reduce patient wait times
- Complying with the employer's quality-assurance and quality-improvement programs
- Supervising and training nurse practitioners, physician assistants, nurses, and other clinical personnel for the employer
- Submitting to periodic, random drug testing in accordance with the employer's written policies and procedures

The duties section of an employment agreement frequently addresses the time that the employee is expected to devote to the business. In the urgent care context, this may take the form of either a number of shifts or a minimum number of hours expected to be worked in a given period. For full-time providers, the provision may state that the provider "shall devote all of Employee's working time, energies, and skills to the furtherance of Employer's business."[4]

Provider Qualifications and Requirements

The employment agreement should require that the provider confirm (or "represent") that they are appropriately licensed in the relevant state to perform the services for which they are hired. Furthermore, because unlicensed providers are generally not entitled to bill public or private payers, the employee should be required to notify the employer immediately on any change to the employee's licensure status.

Billing and Collecting for Services Rendered

The employment agreement should also assign the employer the right to bill all payers in the employer's name and under the employer's provider numbers, for all services rendered by the employee.[5] Without this assignment, the medical provider would remain entitled to collect for the professional services performed.[6] A typical assignment provision might be drafted as follows:

---

4   Frequently allowances are made for a reasonable amount of charitable service.
5   Glasgow LE. Physician employment agreements and related issues. Annual Health Law Conference, April 1997.
6   Note that Medicare specifically provides for the payment of fees to an employer on assignment of such fees:
    Medicare may pay an enrolled physician supplier's employer if the physician is required, as a condition of employment, to turn over to the employer the fees for their services. This right to reassign claims and rights to receive payments also extends to independent contractors, subject to satisfaction of certain additional requirements stated in the regulations. See "Reassignment of Medicare Claims by Employed Physicians." 42 Code of Federal Regulations § 424.80; Form CMS–855R.

The Physician hereby assigns to the Employer any current and future right the Physician might have from time to time to bill and receive payment from any individual patient or other third-party payer, including, without limitation, any managed care payer and the Medicare and Medicaid programs for professional services rendered by the Physician under this Agreement.

In addition, the section addressing billing should also give the employer the exclusive right to establish the amount and timing of the fees to be charged for the services rendered by the provider.[7]

Patient Medical Records

Provider employment agreements should also address which party owns, and, after termination, will own, the patient records and the rights of each party to access such records. Typically, provisions addressing records state that all records produced by the employee are and will remain the property of the employer, and that the employee is required to turn over any records in the provider's possession at the time their employment is terminated.

On termination of the employment relationship, a provider's rights to access patient records are generally provided for under state law. Often, however, the agreement will give the terminated provider access for a specific duration. An example of such a provision is as follows:

All right, title, and interest in and to the records, case histories, charts, documents, and all personal or professional files pertaining to the patients of the Employer are hereby assigned to the Employer, and shall remain the property of the Employer following the termination of this Agreement; provided, however, that for the longer of thirty (30) days or the period provided for under applicable law, following the termination of the Employee's employment with the Employer, at the Employee's sole cost and expense, the Employee may reproduce any records of such patients to whom the Physician has rendered professional services during the Employee's employment with the Employer, at times agreeable to the Employer, subject to applicable state and federal confidentiality and privacy requirements.

Provider Compensation

The structure, amount, and form of the compensation in an individual employment agreement is largely driven by local market factors and the ability of the provider to negotiate the arrangement. At a minimum, however, every provider compensation package will involve cash payments, equity, or both.

Cash Compensation

A provider's cash-based compensation generally includes a fixed component, a variable component, or both. Employers using a purely fixed approach (such as base salary or hourly pay) may find it difficult to retain top talent because of

---

7   Dasco ST. Physician employment agreements. Annual Health Law Conference, April 2009.

the absence of any meaningful connection between performance and pay. Those tying compensation too closely to variable components, however, risk losing seasoned talent because of a lack of income security. They also risk encouraging their providers to engage in unethical billing and coding practices and risk encouraging a reduction in the overall quality of care rendered at the urgent care center.

Recognizing the difficulty in managing the compensation balance, the American Medical Association has offered the following list of objectives in the construction of an effective provider compensation arrangement:

- Provide compensation that is consistent with recognized benchmarks for the physician's experience and specialty.
- Offer a sufficient base salary to promote income security.
- Establish incentives that promote physician productivity and efficiency.
- Base the arrangement on objective criteria that are easily understood by all.
- Promote a sharing of risk between the physician and the organization.
- Provide a mechanism for performance measurement and feedback to the physician.
- Distribute bonus or incentive compensation on a periodic basis.
- Promote a long-term commitment between the physician and the organization.
- Promote the physician's involvement in the overall direction of the organization.[8]

FIXED COMPONENT: SALARY

The provisions setting forth the fixed component of the employee's compensation generally describe the amount, timing, and frequency (monthly, biweekly, and so on) of the payments to be made. Here is an example of such a provision:

> The Employee shall receive an annual salary in the amount of Two Hundred Thousand and No/100 Dollars ($200,000.00), payable in equal installments, on the first and 15th day of each month, subject to state and federal income tax withholding, employment taxes, and such other deductions that may be required by law or that may be otherwise agreed by the Employer and the Employee.

Although many urgent care employers will find it difficult to retain top talent without some variable component, some employees may prefer a fixed arrangement. For instance, providers nearing retirement may find a larger base

---

8 Dasco S, Owens P. Physician employment agreements. Houston: Health Law Conference, April 15, 2009. Citing American Medical Association, Physician Employment, Compensation, Contract Benefits and Incentives, 2004. Available from: http://www.ama-assn.org/ama1/pub/upload/mm/34/compensation_benefit.pdf. Accessed March 26, 2012.

salary much more attractive than a package designed to compensate production through incentive formulas. Employers should be aware of the varying requests and needs of potential employees and should maintain a fair amount of flexibility to accommodate such providers.

VARIABLE COMPONENT: BONUS COMPENSATION

Variable components of compensation plans are generally thought to more effectively align the interests of the employee with those of the employer. Although variable approaches used by urgent care organizations vary, the most effective models all tend to incorporate some element of transparency. For example, an incentive plan that provides for bonuses determined at the sole discretion of management is unlikely to drive production, because the providers are unable to link their actions with increased compensation. Bonus compensation that is transparent in its tie of performance metrics to compensation, however, will appropriately incentivize and motivate the provider. Examples of such approaches are presented later in this chapter.

In addition to being transparent, the variable component must be easily understood and administrable. Perhaps the most straightforward productivity formula is one based on the number of patients the employee treats in a given period. For example, this provision may state that the employee is to receive $10.00 for each patient the employee treats after treating 25 patients in any shift. In this example, the employer may take comfort in knowing that it will reach or almost reach financial break-even before paying bonus compensation. Even this simple approach, however, can lead to complexities. For instance, should patients who are only given flu shots count toward the 25-patient threshold? Also, should there be an adjustment if one of the employee's shifts is longer than others? Finally, if the provider is a physician responsible for supervising a midlevel provider, does that physician receive credit for all patients that they supervise, even if no treatment is rendered?

Other productivity-driven approaches may focus on the financial results of the employee's efforts. For example, an employee may be compensated on the basis of a percentage of the charges or collections attributable to the employee's services. A variation of the percentage-based approach is to compensate the provider on the basis of a tiered formula. For example, the provider may receive 2% of the first $150,000 of collections, 3% of collections between $150,001 and $350,000, and 4% of all collections in excess of $350,000.

A third approach is the use of relative value units (RVUs). RVUs are generally calculated on the basis of the resources used to provide a given service. In the Medicare context, the following three components are incorporated in determining the RVUs attributable to a given billing code: the physician's work to perform the service, the expenses of the urgent care practice attributable to the rendering of such service, and the professional liability insurance that must be carried to provide the service. Historically, RVUs have been used predominantly by hospital systems and multipractice specialty groups because of the calculation complexities. As urgent care electronic medical records systems have become more sophisticated, however, the use of RVUs appears to have become more common. A full description of RVUs is outside the scope of this chapter, but interested urgent care center operatrors should consult their electronic records suppliers to determine whether this approach is administratively feasible.

Equity Compensation

In addition to cash compensation, urgent care companies provide incentives in the form of equity in the employer. Urgent care equity compensation generally takes the form of either stock or options. In either case, such equity is usually issued with restrictions limiting both the provider's ability to transfer the equity as well as the right to participate in the financial results and voting of the employer for a stated period. Certain of these restrictions will be removed (will *lapse*) either on the employee's or the employer's reaching a stated performance milestone (such as a specified number of shifts having been worked or the employer's reaching a financial objective) or on the employee's continued employment with the employer through a certain date. When the restrictions lapse, the equity will be deemed to have been vested. At that time, the employee typically will be entitled to participate in the employer's organization in the same manner as all other owners.

Some restrictions, however, may never lapse. For example, assume an employment agreement grants 1000 shares of stock that are to vest ratably over a 5-year period, and that when the employee is vested, they will share in all financial aspects of the company. If, however, the provider's employment with the company terminates for any reason, the provider must sell all vested stock to the company at its then-existing fair market value and all nonvested stock shall be forfeited without compensation. In this example, even though 200 shares will be vested after the first year, the provider will be obligated to sell those shares to the employer on the termination of the employment arrangement. Because the condition governing the sale back to the employer (or the employer's *redemption option*) will never lapse, the provider will naturally want to limit the company's ability to terminate their employment. The employer, on the other hand, will want to ensure that it has sufficient authority to end the relationship. A common middle ground for these competing interests is that the company's redemption option arises only if the employee is terminated *for cause*. What constitutes sufficient cause is subject to negotiation, but a few typical provisions are covered in the following section.

Termination

The provisions of the employment agreement applicable to its expiration or termination are frequently among the most important to both parties.[9] Both the employer and the provider should consider not only the specific events that may lead to the termination of the employment relationship but also the various rights and obligations of the parties when the agreement is terminated.

---

9   Dasco S, Owens P. Physician employment agreements.

Employment agreements typically provide both commencement and termination dates. When an employment agreement terminates automatically on a certain date (or *by its terms*), it is said to *expire*. Some provider agreements will include what is referred to as an *evergreen* provision, which provides for the automatic renewal of the agreement if either party fails to provide notice to the other that it intends for the agreement not to renew. When the agreement renews, the original terms and conditions will normally remain effective for the stated renewal period.

In addition to the provisions addressing expiration, the agreement will also enumerate several events that will lead to the ability of the employer, the provider, or either party to terminate the relationship. Although both parties are generally given the opportunity to terminate the relationship for any reason ("without cause"), the party electing to terminate is normally required to provide advance notice to the other. The notice required to be given by the employee is generally longer than that required by the employer, and urgent care employers operating in rural areas should negotiate hard to extend this period to ensure that they have sufficient time to recruit a substitute provider. Here is an example of mutual termination right subject to advance written notice:

> The Employer may terminate this Agreement without cause upon at least thirty (30) days' prior written notice to the Employee. The Employee may terminate this Agreement without cause upon at least ninety (90) days' prior written notice to the Employer.

The employment agreement can usually be terminated immediately by the employer for cause, and, if the employee was awarded restricted equity, termination for cause will almost always trigger a buyback of any vested portion of such equity, with any unvested portion simply being forfeited. The following is a list of events that might trigger the employer's immediate right to terminate for cause:

- ▶ The provider's material breach of any covenant or negative covenant contained in the agreement

- ▶ The provider's failure, refusal, or inability to perform duties under the agreement to the reasonable satisfaction of the employer

- ▶ The revocation, restriction, or suspension of the provider's registration with the US Drug Enforcement Agency

- ▶ The provider's engaging in conduct that the employer determines, at its sole discretion, constitutes professional malpractice; is in any way unprofessional or unethical; or is detrimental to the reputation, character, and standing of the employer or the health, safety, or welfare of any patient

- ▶ The suspension, limitation, revocation, or cancellation of the provider's license to practice medicine in the state in which the center is located or any other state, or the institution of disciplinary proceedings against the provider by any governmental agency having jurisdiction over the provider's professional license or conduct

▶ The provider's being or becoming uninsurable from time to time at a cost deemed to be reasonable under the employer's professional liability insurance policies in effect

▶ The provider's engaging in any act constituting a gross neglect of duty or professional standards, dishonesty, theft, fraud, or embezzlement with respect to the employer, any patient, or any third-party payer

▶ Rejection or suspension for any reason of the provider's application for participation or continued participation in any governmental or nongovernmental payer program

HEALTH-CARE REGULATORY LIMITATIONS

State and federal laws and regulations applicable to health-care providers govern the relationship between the urgent care employer and the provider. As a result, it is not uncommon to see several statutory references in the employment agreement relating to compliance obligations of both parties.

Failure to comply with the laws and regulations applicable to provider employment agreements can result in potential civil and criminal penalties. Although several state and federal statutes may apply, included below are some of the more common legal limitations implicated in the drafting and implementation of provider employment agreements.

Physician Self-Referral: Stark Law

Perhaps the most notable of these regulatory limitations is the Stark law. Under Stark, a physician is not permitted to refer patients for "designated health services" covered under Medicare or Medicaid to an entity in which the physician (or an immediate family member of the physician) has a "financial relationship," unless an exception is met.[10] A financial relationship, for Stark purposes, exists if the physician obtains either a direct benefit through compensation or an indirect benefit through an ownership interest.[11] *Designated health services* in the urgent care context generally involve clinical laboratory services, physical therapy services, occupational therapy services, x-ray and other imaging services, durable medical equipment and supplies, and outpatient prescription drugs. To summarize, if the physician's compensation arrangement results in the physician's receiving increased compensation as the result of their referral of designated health services that are payable by a governmental entity, the arrangement violates the Stark law.

The Stark law is a *strict liability* statute. Consequently, the government is not obligated to show that a physician intended to violate the statute. In fact, Stark

---

10 42 United States Code § 1395nn.
11 42 United States Code § 1395nn(h)(5).

penalties can be imposed even if the physician is completely unaware that the arrangement is in violation of the Stark law. Penalties for physicians who violate the Stark law include fines and the potential exclusion from participation in all federal health-care programs.

Anti-Kickback Statute

Unlike the Stark law, which has only civil implications, the federal Anti-Kickback Statute is a criminal statute. The Anti-Kickback Statute prohibits the exchange (or offer to exchange) of anything of value in an effort to induce or reward the referral of business that is reimbursable by a federal health-care program.[12] Although exceptions (or *safe harbors*) to the statute exist, protecting most physician employment arrangements, the introduction of multispecialty urgent care practices could result in violations. In general, if a physician is paid fair market value for his or her professional medical services, a violation of the Anti-Kickback Statute is close to impossible. If, however, an urgent care physician is paid an amount in excess of fair market value, and such excess is attributable to the parties' effort to reward the physician for making higher-yielding referrals that are reimbursed by a governmental entity, a violation may exist.

Conviction for a violation under the Anti-Kickback Statute may result in a fine of up to $50,000 for each violation and imprisonment for up to 5 years.[13] Even more damaging for the physician, a conviction may result in their immediate exclusion from participation in all federal health-care programs.[14]

A fortunate distinction from the Stark law is that the Anti-Kickback Statute is an intent-based statute requiring that the party "knowingly and willfully" engage in the prohibited conduct.[15] Although courts have differed in their interpretation of the terms *knowingly* and *willfully*, the government must prove that the physician intended to violate the law.[16]

Corporate Practice of Medicine Doctrine

Finally, the corporate practice of medicine doctrine, which affects so many decisions regarding corporate structure in the urgent care industry, can also be implicated in the employment context. At its core, the doctrine is little more than a prohibition against a layperson's influence over the professional medical judgment of a licensed provider. To avoid such inappropriate interference, each

---

12 See 42 United States Code § 1320a–7b; Anti-Kickback Statute, American Health Lawyers Association. Available from: http://www.healthlawyers.org/hlresources/Health%20Law%20Wiki/Anti-Kickback%20Statute.aspx. Accessed May 8, 2013.
13 See 42 United States Code § 1320a–7a(a)(7); 42 United States Code § 1320a–7b(b).
14 See 42 United States Code § 1320a–7(a).
15 See 42 United States Code § 1320a–7b(a); *Hanlester Network v. Shalala*, 51 F.3d 1390, 1400 (9th Circuit Court of Appeals, 1995).
16 In 2010, the Patient Protection and Affordable Care Act added a provision clarifying that actual knowledge that one's conduct violates the Anti-Kickback Statute or the specific intent to commit a violation of the Anti-Kickback Statute is not necessary for conviction under the statute. It remains true, however, that an intent to violate the law must be shown. See *Patient Protection and Affordable Care Act,* Pub. L. No. 111–148 (2010); Anti-Kickback Statute, American Health Lawyers Association.

agreement to which a licensed health-care provider is a party should include language evidencing the lack of authority the employer has on the clinical aspects of the employee's duties. Furthermore, it is also sensible to include a provision that guarantees that the profit motives of the corporate entity will not conflict with the independent medical judgment of the health-care provider. Here is a sample provision addressing these concepts:

> The Physician shall make any and all decisions relating to the practice of medicine and the care and treatment of patients. Notwithstanding anything in this Agreement to the contrary, the Physician shall perform all services with respect to the diagnosis and treatment of patients in such manner as the Physician, in the independent exercise of the Physician's medical judgment, deems to be in the best interests of the patients. The parties specifically agree and acknowledge that the Physician shall have final authority over all medical decisions made in the course of the Physician's rendering care and treatment to patients at the Centers.

Although the negotiated terms of an employment agreement such as compensation will be the primary focus at the commencement of the employment relationship, both the urgent care employer and the provider should hire competent counsel to ensure that all applicable laws and regulations are appropriately respected. Finally, the parties should consider which negative covenants or restrictive provisions are appropriate to protect the business interest of the employer after the termination of the relationship.

Noncompetes and Other Negative Covenants

As urgent care market saturation continues across the United States, negative covenants in employment agreements become increasingly relevant and important. Negative covenants are essentially promises not to do something, and in the urgent care employment context these provisions generally come in the following three forms: nondisclosure, nonsolicitation, and noncompetition. Although brief descriptions of the initial two follow, the primary focus of this section is on noncompetition provisions.

Nondisclosure Provisions

A *nondisclosure provision* prohibiting the inappropriate disclosure of protected, confidential information of the employer will generally go hand in hand with a paragraph addressing confidentiality. In addition to regulatory obligations involving patient privacy, providers will often be obligated to refrain from disclosing any company trade secrets, business plans, contractual rights, or other information that the urgent care employer has defined as confidential. Although confidentiality and nondisclosure provisions will generally benefit all urgent care employers, an employer that has disclosed future business plans to a key employee should strongly consider the use of such a provision.

Nonsolicitation Provisions

Nonsolicitation provisions generally prohibit the employee from hiring or attempting to hire other employees of the urgent care employer during and for a period after the termination of the employment relationship. Frequently, indirect solicitations such as through a website advertisement or a third-party recruiter are carved out from the restrictive provision. Urgent care employers that are unable to enforce noncompetition because of jurisdictional restraints may find that nonsolicitation provisions offer a somewhat useful alternative by prohibiting the poaching of productive employees.

Noncompetition Provisions

Noncompetition provisions prevent the provider from engaging in competitive activities with the urgent care employer both during and after the termination of the employment relationship. Provisions limiting a provider's ability to compete in the marketplace have been disfavored as a matter of public policy for decades. Not only does enforcement of such a provision restrict the physician's ability to earn a living, but it also reduces the community's access to competent health care. As a result of these policy considerations, many states have adopted blanket prohibitions against agreements and clauses prohibiting physician competition. In states that enforce such provisions, judicial precedent generally reflects a heightened degree of scrutiny and will restrict the applicability of the provision only to the extent the judge finds necessary to protect the legitimate business interests of the urgent care employer.[17] If a court finds that the provision is excessive in its attempt to protect the employer, it will either render the entire provision void or will rewrite the provision to the extent necessary to enforce it. In determining whether the restrictive language is limited to that necessary to protect the employer's business interests, courts generally focus on the provision's geographic scope, the duration of the restriction, and the scope of the activities restricted.[18]

With respect to geographic focus, in general, a noncompete provision must not extend beyond the area from which the urgent care company's patients are drawn. Although credible arguments may be made to extend this region, anything extending beyond the existing patient catchment area would likely be deemed not necessary to protect the employer's legitimate business interests.

When considering the durational aspect of a noncompetition provision, employers should be mindful that the restriction is only legally enforceable for the time period in which it protects the employer's valid business interest. Consequently, to enforce the provision, an urgent care employer may need to prove that the length of the provision was no longer than necessary to hire and train a replacement physician and to enable the urgent care company to demonstrate

---

17 Schaff MF et al., Representing physicians: potential perils and pitfalls: life cycle of a physician practice. American Health Lawyers Association, 2012.
18 As a result of the unpredictability in determining what a court will deem reasonably necessary to protect the employer's legitimate business interests under the circumstances, many state legislatures have removed the judicial risk by enacting specific statutes that define the parameters of an enforceable noncompete provision.

its effectiveness to its patient base without the terminated provider. Without demonstrating these two elements, it may be difficult to prove that the employer's business would be negatively affected.

Finally, with respect to the nature of the activities restricted, only the services that are competitive to those offered at the urgent care center will be subject to the noncompetition provision. Consequently, a physician who leaves an urgent care company to return to their practice as a surgeon would likely not be subject to a restriction against the provider found in the urgent care employment agreement.

CONCLUSION

An effective employment arrangement can serve as the mechanism to both attract and retain top talent. Recording the arrangement in a written employment agreement not only protects the legal rights and interests of the urgent care employer but also avoids potential disputes with the provider. Although provider employment agreements tend to favor the employer, urgent care companies will find that a balanced, well-constructed agreement is a great tool in staying competitive.

KEY POINTS

1. The improper classification of employees as independent contractors carries both legal liability and tax risks.
2. In general, the degree of control the urgent care company exercises over a provider will determine whether or not the provider is or is not an employee.
3. If the urgent care employer believes the worker could potentially dispute the terms of the individual's arrangement, it will almost always benefit the employer to insist on a written agreement.
4. The employment agreement should require that the provider confirm (represent) certain issues such as that they are appropriately licensed in the relevant state to perform the services for which they are hired.
5. Provider employment agreements should address which party owns the patient records and the rights of each party to access such records after the termination of the employment agreement.
6. A provider's cash-based compensation generally includes a fixed component, a variable component, or both.
7. Variable components of compensation plans are generally thought to more effectively align the interests of the employee with those of the employer.
8. Equity compensation is usually issued with restrictions limiting both the provider's ability to transfer the equity as well as their right to participate in the financial results and voting of the employer for a stated period.

9. Although the negotiated terms of an employment agreement such as compensation will be the primary focus at the commencement of the employment relationship, both the urgent care employer and the provider should hire competent counsel to ensure that all applicable laws and regulations are appropriately respected.
10. Negative covenants are essentially promises not to do something, and in the urgent care employment context these provisions generally come in the following three forms: nondisclosure, nonsolicitation, and noncompetition. Although noncompetition provisions are generally disfavored in American courts, if drafted in a manner that protects the legitimate business interest of the employer, they will likely be enforceable.

CHAPTER 22

Health Plan Contracting

Sybil Yeaman

NEW CHALLENGES IN THE health-care industry are driving sweeping changes in the models of how medical care is provided. Government pressure to provide medical care to the uninsured, an aging population, and health plans aggressively seeking cost containment all profoundly affect urgent care contract negotiations and their reimbursement. Understanding contracting and developing a successful negotiation process are more critical now than ever before.

Successful negotiation of contracts requires urgent care owners to understand their costs for providing medical care, their medical marketplace, the provider relationship with the health plan, the population and competition in their geographic area, and contract language. The time taken up front to prepare for contracting with health plans will provide leverage to negotiate more advantageous provider agreements and more favorable reimbursement.

PREPARATION FOR CONTRACTING

Understand Utilization and Costs to Provide Medical Care
Gaining a clear understanding of utilization and knowing the average cost per patient for doing business are the first steps in preparation for contract negotiations. If your center has not already established an effective utilization review process by payer and procedure, as well as an understanding of the costs to provide care, then start now.

Understanding utilization and the costs to provide medical care helps you determine if health plan fee schedules or higher-risk reimbursement rates cover the true costs of doing business or if they are unacceptable. This gives you leverage when renegotiating established contracts. For example, presenting a health plan's utilization data at renegotiation time will help demonstrate the need to renegotiate and provide leverage for higher reimbursement rates.

Knowing the cost of doing business is especially important as new reimbursement and health-delivery systems are being created that attempt to transfer greater financial risk for health-care services to health-care providers.

Gather Information About the Health Plan, Payment Methods, and Reputation

Reviewing a health plan's website will often provide knowledge of the payer membership and covered population volume. Using search engines will help reveal a plan's public image, types of coverage, and reputation with members and providers in the marketplace. This simple step may reveal useful information before negotiations and help to create leverage for your center in the negotiation process. For example, if the health plan is targeting a new market or is attempting to sell a new product line, the health plan may provide more favorable reimbursement terms to health-care providers who help them compete in the marketplace or establish a new plan network. Being willing to support the new plan also gives your center additional value from the plan's perspective in the marketplace.

Compare the health plan fee schedules to Medicare and to other well-established payers to determine if the fee schedules are consistent with other plan payment rates. Determine if the volume of membership in the plan will potentially increase center volume. The larger the plan and the greater the percentage of enrollees, the more important negotiating a contract will become and the more important it is to protect the center's revenue stream.

Most health plans list their providers online. Locate the other urgent care centers in your geographic area and, if possible, contact several providers to discuss their experience with the payer. It is useful to obtain firsthand knowledge of the financial and operational history of the plan to determine whether the plan is provider-friendly, keeps its contractual obligations, and reimburses claims in a timely manner. Some physicians may be willing to share their reimbursement information, which would be helpful in developing a negotiation strategy. However, it's important to remember that independent physicians are not allowed to collectively determine what rates or contracts to sign; if they do so, they are in violation of antitrust laws. Therefore, gathering information must be done in compliance with state and federal guidelines.

Be Familiar With the Various Payment Models

Urgent care centers carry the financial risk and responsibility for providing high-quality medical care and diagnostic testing before being paid. As the economy has shifted, there has been increasing governmental pressure to create new medical delivery and payment models to provide health care to the uninsured and to an aging population. Health plans are moving away from fee-for-service reimbursement and creating new risk-based payment models that shift greater risk to providers for their enrollees.

Health plans strive to manage medical care in order to manage the cost. Transferring the risk of managing care to health-care providers means urgent care centers will not only need to know what it costs to provide care but will also need to understand the risk involved with the various payment models they may be offered.

The most common managed-care products for urgent care centers are

- *Preferred provider organizations (PPOs)*   Medical care is managed through contracted providers who agree to follow guidelines for prior authorization and referral. Payment to providers is based on a fee schedule, often a percentage of the Medicare fee schedule, in return for access to health plan enrollees. Patients are responsible for deductibles and co-pays, which vary according to the plan they have enrolled in. *Note:* Smaller PPOs will often contract with (piggyback on) larger established networks, and providers are responsible to provide care to the affiliate PPOs at the same reduced contracted rates as the contracted PPO health plan.

- *Health maintenance organizations (HMOs)*   Medical care is managed through a strictly controlled network of providers, prior authorizations, and predetermined medical services. Payment to providers is often through capitation (a flat rate fee paid per member per month) or a reduced fee schedule that may include bundled services for specific medical treatments. Urgent care centers are not usually included in capitation unless they have opted to contract for higher risk through a physician network or in return for a high volume of enrollees. Instead of capitation, the HMO may use a *withhold* of a percentage of the center's reimbursement, to be paid if the costs of medical care are managed within the HMO's estimated costs. *Note:* Capitation shifts significant financial risk to health-care providers, and an experienced professional should be contacted to evaluate and assist in negotiating any capitation plan or any plan contracting case rates.

- *Point of service (POS) plans*   Medical care is managed through a contracted network of providers, and prior authorization may be required for specialty services. However, the plan member may have an *open-access POS plan* that also allows them to obtain medical services outside the provider network in return for the member paying a higher percentage of the fees for their services. Payment is made on a reduced fee schedule in return for access to health plan enrollees. *Note:* A *risk pool*, or a withhold, of a percentage of reimbursement may be used to give contracted providers incentive to control medical costs. Surplus funds are distributed to providers at the end of the contracted accounting periods, but often utilization exceeds estimated funding, so providers should understand that they risk the loss of any withheld reimbursement.

Establish Center Objectives and Determine Leverage in the Marketplace

The better health plans have objectives and understand their leverage in each medical marketplace. Before negotiation, it is important to consider objectives and evaluate what leverage your center may or may not have in its geographic area. Even in a saturated urgent care market, you may be able to create value if your center objectives line up with those of the health plan. For example,

- The center is seeking to increase patient volume. Is the health plan seeking to increase percentage of market share or marketing a new product line?
- The center is looking to increase visibility in its geographic area. Is the health plan looking to increase name and logo recognition in the marketplace?
- The center is looking to develop relationships within the medical community. Is the health plan looking to develop better relationships with providers and medical organizations?
- The center is striving to compete with urgent care centers already contracted. Is the health plan contracted with an urgent care network that allows additional centers in return for shared risk in cost control, quality management, and outcomes analytics?
- The center is striving to support public health and awareness. Is the health plan seeking providers and organizations to assist in running preventive care programs, providing newsletter articles, and fulfilling health-care initiatives?

CONTRACT REVIEW AND ESTABLISHING ACTION POINTS

Careful review and evaluation of current and new managed-care terms and provisions in contracts will help protect the urgent care center from financial risk and will provide a stronger foundation for contract negotiations. Providers should never sign a contractual agreement with a health plan without calculating their center's cost of medical care against the fee schedule and assessing the contractual obligations.

Provider agreements are developed by the health plans, so they are slanted in favor of the plans' best legal and financial interests even if they are provider-friendly. Because the law requires that boilerplate agreements not be used and health plans must negotiate in good faith with health-care providers, many provisions can be amended in the negotiation process to be mutually beneficial.

Recitals and definitions at the beginning of the contract don't just provide basic explanation for mutual understanding by all parties. They also are carefully drafted to clarify the terms that will be most significant to the fundamental provisions that will follow in the agreement. Understanding the significance of these terms and how they can affect your center is imperative. Understanding how to negotiate mutually beneficial contractual terms for advantageous agreements is priceless.

Affiliates

Affiliate usually refers to any subsidiary of a company. In the health plan contract, the term may also be defined as any related entity. This means the center is contracting with the health plan as well as any subcontracted entities it owns or manages. If the center negotiates a reduced fee schedule in return for access to a large volume of health plan enrollees in the center's geographic area, this reduced fee schedule will apply to all other entities the health plan is related to. The center will be obligated to provide care to members of multiple other entities, such as small PPOs and employer groups that contract to use the health plan's medical network. The upside is additional volume, but the downside is that the same patients would normally pay higher fees. This change in reimbursement can usually be absorbed by the center in return for additional volume. Often affiliate member cards clearly indicate the affiliate, and the actual health plan network is noted in a less obvious place. Administration costs for center claims rise when there is confusion about what company or health plan to bill, and the center is then at risk for untimely claims filing.

Action points:

- ▶ Negotiate more favorable rates because the inclusion of multiple smaller entities affects the center financially. These smaller entities would normally have to reimburse at higher fee schedules but will now obtain reduced fees that the center will have to absorb.
- ▶ Verify that the health plan name will be clearly printed on all affiliate membership cards, along with specific billing instructions for each affiliate, by requesting to see a sample copy of an affiliate member's card.
- ▶ Negotiate a stipulation that both parties have to agree with prior written consent before additional affiliates are added.

Arbitration

When an appeal regarding a breach of agreement or other grievance occurs during the contractual period, having an arbitration clause is beneficial. Most appeals and alleged breaches of agreement occur over claims reimbursement issues and utilization management issues. The larger the health plan, the greater number of lawyers the plan may have contracted or have on staff. However, urgent care centers do not have the same financial capabilities, and litigation is both arduous and expensive, so resolving issues through an arbitration process before they go to litigation is faster, less expensive, and mutually beneficial for both parties.

Action points:

- ▶ Review the agreement and verify that it states that providers have the right of appeal.
- ▶ Verify that there is a clause requiring an arbitration process to resolve grievances before litigation.

- Negotiate a stipulation that each party is responsible for its own legal fees in arbitration and litigation, so that the center is never required to pay the legal fees of the health plan.
- Verify that the contract contains a reasonable timetable for the arbitration process.
- Verify that a neutral arbitrator will be proposed that has a medical specialist with experience in emergency medicine.

Capitation and Carve-Outs

Reimbursement based on a per-member, per-month fee is not a common payment model for most independent urgent care centers, although pressures and changes in the health-care industry may change how HMOs and accountable care organizations contract with urgent care centers in the future. When an urgent care provider network or large group of urgent care centers can cover a geographic area, HMOs will seek to carve out urgent care to a specific network or group of providers in order to share the financial risk with the network for managing the care and costs.

Action points:

- Seek an experienced professional to evaluate and assist in negotiating capitation or carve-outs that share risk. Capitation shifts financial risk for medical care from the health plan to health-care providers.
- Consider joining a network to participate in capitation contracts and secure patient volume.

Clean Claims and Claims Provisions

Health plans are responsible for paying claims only as stipulated in their contractual agreements. Therefore, claims submission, claims processing, timely payment, adjustments, and claims appeal processes must be clearly defined to avoid denials and disputes. Some health plans severely limit the claims submission period, which allows for automatic claims denials for all claims outside the time period. A general guideline is to seek claims submission and payment periods that are opposites, allowing more time for claims submission and less time for prompt payment of claims.

Action points:

- Verify that the contract clearly indicates what items render a clean claim and that no burdensome coding or billing requirements are imposed.
- Verify that fee schedules are clearly defined, readily available, and reasonable.
- Negotiate a reasonable claims submission period of at least 90 or 120 days. Some health plan contracts stipulate only 30 days.

- ▶ Verify that the health plan pays or denies claims within 30 days of submission.

- ▶ Negotiate payment of interest on any claims not paid or denied within 30 days. Be cognizant of the state laws, and use them to negotiate interest payments if they do not appear in the contract.

- ▶ Negotiate a reasonable appeals process time of 90 days or less, so claims issues are resolved in a timely manner.

- ▶ Verify that the health plan is responsible for coordination of benefits when its members have coverage under more than one health plan.

- ▶ Negotiate a claim-adjustment period of 12 months for payment and denials.

- ▶ Negotiate that the plan must notify the provider of any offsets (recoupment) at least 45 days in advance and provide an opportunity for the provider to make direct payment. *Note:* This will avoid the administrative complexity and confusion of offsetting reimbursement in accounts receivable and accounting.

Covered Services

Health-care providers and health-care plans may differ on their definitions of what covered services actually include. An urgent care center considers any medically necessary services and supplies rendered to plan members as covered services. The health plan may have additional limitations and exclusions on what are considered covered services, to limit its medical costs. Some provisions in contracts work for primary-care providers or specialists but should not be applied to urgent care. A common provision, such as limiting covered services to the services under the member's benefits, is unreasonable in an urgent care setting.

Action points:

- ▶ Negotiate covered services to include all medically necessary services that the providers and center are licensed to provide.

- ▶ Verify that the health plan does not have the right to change the definition of covered services or amend the language.

Credentialing

The gathering of information on health-care providers and the verification of professional qualifications are standardized by the Joint Commission, but each managed-care organization has its own process. Health-care providers should be aware that the credentialing process can be lengthy, often taking 4 to 6 months. Once they have completed the credentialing process, approved providers should anticipate a wait of 30 to 45 days for activation in the health-care system.

Action points:

▶ Initiate credentialing as soon as possible.

▶ Follow up on credentialing progress and status monthly.

Eligibility and Verification

Verification of member eligibility is the joint responsibility of the health plan and the health-care providers. Beyond the traditional insurance identification card or verification over the phone, new technologies such as electronic eligibility are cost-effective for the health plan and efficient for providers. Immediate online access to current member information helps providers verify insurance coverage and accurately determine members' payment responsibilities.

Action points:

▶ Verify that the health plan provides phone and website access for immediate verification of membership coverage, deductibles, and co-pays.

▶ Negotiate a stipulation that the health plan cannot deny claims for ineligible members if the center verified eligibility at the time of service.

Evergreen and Renewal Provisions

An evergreen provision stipulates that a contract will renew automatically and allows the center to continue to see health plan members without interruption. It also protects the center financially by guaranteeing the volume of the members available in its geographic area. However, automatic renewal also means that the center does not have the opportunity to renegotiate the contract and fee schedule.

Action points:

▶ Review and verify provisions for contract renegotiations before renewal.

▶ Negotiate an additional provision for renegotiation of the contract 90 to 120 days before the contract renewal date, allowing the center to renegotiate unfavorable terms or rates without losing the contract. *Note:* It is the center's responsibility to seek renegotiation within the contracted time frame.

Indemnification and Mutual Liability

Indemnification or hold-harmless clauses are very important in contracting, because they determine liability. Health-care providers need to be aware that health plan contracts may pass additional indirect liability through to them. One-sided indemnification can be very detrimental if the health plan and its affiliates are protected from potential risks and liabilities and the health-care providers are contractually responsible for acts outside their control. All indemnification and hold-harmless clauses should be mutual, so that each party has indemnification from the acts of the other party. Each party should be responsible for its own legal fees.

Action points:

▸ Review indemnification provisions to verify mutual indemnification.

▸ Negotiate a mutual indemnification clause to be added if the contractual indemnification only protects the health plan and its affiliates.

▸ Verify that each party is responsible for its own legal fees.

Medically Necessity

Health-care providers are responsible for providing the services that they determine are medically necessary at the time of service. Health plans control costs by paying for services that are medically necessary and denying services that are not medically necessary. Ever since payments were first connected to medical necessity, conflicts over the definition of medical necessity and who makes the determination of what is medically necessary have become an ongoing issue of contention between health plans and health-care providers. Although health-care providers have traditionally determined medical necessity on the basis of their professional discretion, government programs (Centers for Medicare & Medicaid Services) and state laws also define what is medically necessary. Physicians, health plans, and government all have a risk in the determination of what is medically necessary, but the burden of proof has fallen on the shoulders of health-care providers. To verify medical necessity, physicians have to follow increasingly complex coding guidelines, fulfill detailed documentation requirements, and undergo the scrutiny of data analysis, as well as peer and utilization management reviews.

Action points:

▸ Verify that the contractual definition of *medically necessary* is based on generally accepted medical practices and treatments, given the nature of the diagnosis and severity of symptoms at the time of service.

▸ Verify that the contract clearly indicates the health-care provider has the right to appeal and the right to go to arbitration for any decisions on medical necessity (see the section "Arbitration" in this chapter).

▸ Negotiate the right to appeal services that the health plan has determined are not medically necessary.

▸ Negotiate a stipulation that recoupment of funds will not occur automatically and will not occur until reconsideration is completed.

▸ Negotiate an option to avoid offsets by making direct payment.

New Plans and Product Lines

Health plans seek to bind their health-care providers both to current products and to future products, which may have new reimbursement models that may or may not be favorable for the center. Although automatic participation in a new plan is an opportunity to increase volume, it may also adversely affect the center's bottom line.

Action points:

▸ Verify that the health plan gives 90 days' notice of proposed new plan implementation, to allow time to review the plan and reimbursement structure.

▸ Negotiate the first right of refusal for all new health plan products, to allow the center to opt out of participating.

Policies, Procedures, and Obligations

Health plan contracts contain clauses that bind health-care providers to comply with all of the plan's policies and procedures (P&Ps). These detailed and obligatory items are not always included in the actual contract but are provided separately or on request if not included in the contracting packet. Often health-care providers do not read the P&Ps or give them only a cursory review until an issue of compliance occurs. This is a common and exceedingly detrimental mistake, because the P&Ps contain all the details of the contractual relationship that are not in the contract itself. Once the contract is signed, the P&Ps are enforceable, and the health-care provider may need to wait until renegotiation to negotiate changes unless there is a legal or mutual liability issue that the parties must address for compliance with state and federal guidelines. Before negotiating or renegotiating a contract, always carefully review all of the P&Ps. Some health plans may post their P&Ps online for the convenience of their participating providers.

Action points:

▸ Verify that each of the P&Ps is acceptable and reasonable.

▸ Negotiate the removal of any clauses binding health-care providers to all updates or changes to the P&Ps at the health plan's discretion without prior written notification of changes.

▸ Negotiate the right to terminate without penalty for unacceptable new P&Ps, with a mutually reasonable exit strategy.

▸ Verify that the P&Ps are consistent with the provisions in the provider agreement.

Professional Liability Coverage

Professional liability coverage varies by state, and a health plan contract may demand higher coverage limits than are standard.

Action point:

▸ Review and verify that the requirements are equivalent to the coverage.

Termination Without Cause

Every contract should have a termination-without-cause provision that gives the urgent care center a reasonable exit strategy. In a rapidly changing health-care industry of rising costs and lower reimbursements, it's important for health-care providers to have the right to terminate a relationship with any health plan that becomes financially unfavorable. The health plan is required to maintain the stability and availability of its provider network for its members, so it may not have a termination-without-cause provision.

Action points:

- Verify that terms and termination provisions include termination without cause.
- Negotiate a termination-without-cause provision that is mutually reasonable (90 to 120 days) for both parties.
- Consider a compromise of termination without cause after 1 year, if you are signing a long-term contract or have an evergreen renewal provision.

Unilateral Modifications

Many health plan contracts contain clauses that unilaterally bind health-care providers to comply with all current and new provisions and policies. These may include a requirement to provide services for new affiliates; automatic participation in new product lines and reimbursement models; and accepting modified terms and termination provisions, a revised list of covered services, and adjusted fee schedules.

Action points:

- Negotiate the removal of any clauses unilaterally binding health-care providers to changes in any contractual provisions and P&Ps without prior written notification.
- Negotiate the right to refuse unacceptable new provisions and P&Ps.
- Negotiate the right to terminate without penalty for unacceptable new P&Ps, with a mutually reasonable exit strategy.

NEGOTIATION

The negotiation process is the point where the cost of providing medical care meets the health plan's needs to provide coverage to its members. Urgent care center contracting priorities are a balance between the need to meet the bottom line and securing patient volume. Health plan priorities are based on cost containment, fulfillment, and growing market share. Both parties must work together for success, but the health plan is in the stronger negotiation position.

Health plans' strength comes from their market share. The more enrollees a health plan has in a center's geographic area, the greater is its power to demand its standard contract terms. Often urgent care centers are unable to negotiate from a position of strength unless they are the only urgent care centers in their geographic area or they join an integrated network that can offer high-quality management and data analytics and can carry a portion of risk in return for higher reimbursement and better terms. There is always a center that doesn't understand its costs and so accepts low rates or is willing to take a reduced fee schedule to compete for patients in hopes of making up the difference in volume. This center drives its own reimbursement down along with the compensation for all urgent care centers in the area, because the health plan will use the new reduced fee schedule as its standard.

Although most urgent care centers do not have a position of strength, it does not mean that they do not have the ability to negotiate more favorable terms in their agreements. By law, plan contracts cannot be boilerplate agreements that do not allow modification, and they must be negotiated in good faith. Thus health-care providers have the right to negotiate modifications to the plan's standard contract but must prioritize their objectives in advance to determine what terms should be argued to make the contract more favorable and which terms can be accepted.

An urgent care center that offers more than its location to the health plan will meet with greater success at the negotiation table, especially at contract renegotiation time. For example:

- Being available to write articles for the plan's newsletter or sponsoring a local health fair helps the plan increase visibility and members' participation in understanding and managing their own care.

- Participating in prevention programs and public awareness programs creates value, with plans seeking cost containment through preventive care.

- Providing utilization management and outcomes analytics helps health plans fulfill health-care initiatives and government contract requirements.

Providing more than urgent care not only creates leverage in negotiations but also helps develop a partnership beyond the contractual relationship. In future contract negotiations, keeping your business will be more important to the health plan, because your center brings more value to the table than just another urgent care location.

CONTRACT FOLLOW-UP

Contract obligations and requirements should be reviewed with all health-care providers and staff members to ensure that all who work at the center, from those in the reception area to those in claims billing, are aware of their responsibilities in fulfilling contractual requirements. Guidelines and policy changes should be made readily available for reference as needed.

Expiration and renewal dates should be checked monthly and carefully monitored to give plenty of notice of the renegotiation period and expiration date. This will give the center time to review member utilization and average cost of care and to remind its health-care providers not to sign any health plan paperwork until it is reviewed by administration and a new agreement is negotiated.

Monitoring claims processing and denials, verifying appropriate fee schedule reimbursement, monitoring volume of claims in appeals, and monitoring timeliness of payment should be done monthly as part of the center's revenue cycle management process. Utilization review should be done on a quarterly basis, and the results should be compared with member utilization results for other health plan contracts. Only consistent review and monitoring will protect the center from the financial loss of underpaid or denied claims and save the center from the administrative accounting complexity of offsets for overpaid claims. Centers with an electronic health records system should automatically get notification of fees being overpaid or underpaid if the fee schedule has been built into the system.

CONCLUSION

Understanding the contracting and negotiation process is critical to the financial stability of urgent care centers because pressures for cost containment drive changes in how medical services are provided and reimbursed. Complacency or a wait-and-see attitude in the face of these sweeping changes is self-destructive, and it is a myth that independent urgent care centers cannot effectively negotiate more favorable terms with health plans. Simple changes in terms of liability or arbitration can protect the center. Any increase in reimbursement when fee schedules are consistently being reduced is a victory and is beneficial financially.

KEY POINTS

1. Health plans are required by law to negotiate in good faith with health-care providers and not impose boilerplate agreements.
2. Health-care providers should always attempt to negotiate or renegotiate their contracts for more favorable terms and fee schedules.
3. Learn the language and common terms used in health-care contracting for a clear understanding of the liabilities and obligations in your contract.
4. Carefully review all contracts, especially the P&Ps.
5. Successful negotiation requires urgent care centers to understand their utilization and average cost per patient to provide medical care.
6. Gather information about each health plan: its payment models, contracting and credentialing timelines, and reputation.
7. Start credentialing as soon as possible. The credentialing process often takes 4 to 6 months for completion.
8. Compare health plan fee schedules with Medicare and other health plan fee schedules.

9. Establish action points to negotiate with the health plans and prioritize which provisions are the most important to amend.
10. Create leverage in the marketplace by providing more than urgent care services.
11. Create long-term relationships with health plans to create mutual value.

CHAPTER 23

Choosing the Electronic Health Record

John Shufeldt

Only a small number of physicians in the United States fully use an electronic health record (EHR), even though EHRs have been widely available for years. Common barriers to adoption have included excessive setup and maintenance costs, disruption to physician productivity, legal concerns, and insufficient demonstrable financial or clinical benefits. However, thanks to technological progress, as well as incentives offered by the Health Information Technology for Economic and Clinical Health (HITECH) Act, consumer demand is finally overcoming resistance and spurring adoption.

The General Accounting Office estimated that over $200 billion could be saved annually in the United States with more widespread adoption of EHR systems by physicians. In addition, the General Accounting Office estimates that nearly 100,000 lives could be saved annually. Couple those predictions with EHR vendors' promised positive return on investment (ROI) and productivity improvements, and what's not to love? Apparently, given some of the challenges in EHR adoption, quite a bit.

For example; a 2013 study from the University of Michigan School of Public Health found that practices that implement an EHR without a well-thought-out plan and dedicated focus on enhancing revenue and cutting costs are likely to lose more than $43,000 over 5 years. In other words, 73% of those surveyed failed to see an ROI.[1] Notably, a 2012 user satisfaction survey of the American Academy of Family Physicians showed that only 38% of respondents were highly satisfied with their EHR systems.[2]

This chapter offers a road map to successful EHR selection, adoption, and implementation. It reviews today's EHR competitive landscape, including both

---

1   Adler-Milstein J, Green CE, Bates DW. A survey analysis suggests that electronic health records will yield revenue gains for some practices and losses for many. *Health Affairs*. March 2013. Available from: http://content.healthaffairs.org/content/32/3/562.long. Accessed February 22, 2014.
2   Edsall RL, Adler KG. The 2012 EHR user satisfaction survey: responses from 3,088 family physicians. American Academy of Family Physicians. *Fam Pract Manag*. 2012;19:23–30. Available from: http://www.aafp.org/fpm/2012/1100/p23.html. Accessed February 22, 2014.

opportunities promulgated by the HITECH Act and the hazards of adopting the wrong solution. It then suggests ways to plan for and select an EHR partner that provides your practice with clinical insight and operational efficiency while ensuring accurate documentation and compliant coding.

The process of vetting and implementing an EHR system is challenging for any medical group. But the right EHR solution can help your practice generate more revenue, improve efficiencies, and provide access to better metrics, allowing you to focus on patient care.

TAXONOMY

Before going further, it is important to note the difference between *electronic medical records (EMRs)* and *EHRs*, because multiple terms with overlapping definitions have been used to define electronic patient care records. Both terms, *EHR* and *EMR*, have gained widespread use, with some health informatics users assigning the term *EHR* to a global concept (think: personal health records) and *EMR* to a discrete *localized* record.

Others prefer to define an EMR as the physician interface, and once you add a patient portal to your EMR, you get an EHR. This builds on the idea that once the patient is submitting information, it's no longer a medical record but at that point becomes a health record. For most users, however, the terms *EHR* and *EMR* are used interchangeably. For the purposes of this chapter, *EHR* denotes the patient's medical record and the system employed to capture the information and formulate a billable encounter.

BACKGROUND

In 2004 President George W. Bush called health information technology a national priority. Despite this announcement, few steps were taken toward nationwide EHR implementation until 2009, when the American Recovery and Reinvestment Act earmarked as much as $36 billion for the expansion of health information technology in the United States. This was one of the most notable steps toward widespread EHR implementation, and it ultimately led to the HITECH Act. The HITECH Act was signed more than a year before President Barack Obama signed the Patient Protection and Affordable Care Act into law and is not part of the Affordable Care Act.

The HITECH Act is a $19.2 billion provision within the American Recovery and Reinvestment Act that was designed to encourage the widespread adoption of EHRs as a pathway for lowering costs and improving the quality of health care in the United States. According to the provisions, physicians would be eligible for up to $44,000 in reimbursements from Medicare and $65,000 from Medicaid for "meaningful use" of a "certified" EHR starting in 2011. Requirements for meaningful use include such things as e-prescribing, electronic exchange of patient health information, and reporting on clinical data.

The main provisions of the HITECH Act are as follows:[3]

- Use health information technology (IT) to support and foster quality measures.
- Develop standards for enrolling and checking the eligibility of individuals before or at the point of service.
- Use health IT to test new or more effective health-care delivery models.
- Facilitate the use of health IT in long-term-care settings through financial incentives.
- Provide for risk assessment for Medicare beneficiaries using health IT.
- Encourage health-care providers and health plans to use health IT to improve outcomes.
- Provide assistance in training medical students in health IT.

BENEFITS OF AN ELECTRONIC HEALTH RECORD

What are some of the benefits of EHRs? The right EHR can deliver

- *Stronger practice profitability*   With more accurate clinical documentation, a practice can bill at appropriate and compliant service levels. Implemented correctly, an EHR can also create workflow efficiencies that contain or reduce the costs of delivering care.
- *Better patient care*   Improved access to patient information and clinical data means reduced medical errors, better patient safety, and stronger support for clinical decision making, as well as the ability to measure performance among health-care providers more accurately.
- *Process integrity*   An EHR can help ensure that things are done the same way each time and are based on best-practice workflows and clinical quality.
- *Health-care provider and staff member satisfaction*   A successfully implemented EHR can provide more time for direct patient care and reduce administrative burdens.
- *Practice growth*   Access to clinical and financial data can provide direction for growth by giving the practice greater control over, and visibility into, practice operations.

---

3   Healthcare Information and Management Systems Society. Health IT provisions included in healthcare reform legislation. March 24, 2010. Available from: http://www.himss.org/files/HIMSSorg/content/files/3_23_HealthITProvisionsIncludedHealthcareReformLegislation.pdf. Accessed February 22, 2014.

GETTING STARTED

As you begin to consider various EHR solutions and how they fit into your overall operational strategy, keep the bigger picture in mind. For a practice to undertake the requisite EHR adoption challenges, the system should do the following at a minimum:

- ► It should allow for an incremental adoption within the office.
- ► The incremental adoption should cause minimal disruption to office workflow and practice patterns.
- ► Adoption of the EHR must either improve efficiency or reduce cost. Improving patient safety is a given.
- ► The system must have interoperability and conform to national standards.

Selecting and implementing an EHR solution requires effort and dedication. The ultimate success of your EHR implementation is disproportionately dependent on the time and effort you invest in the beginning stages of the process. Selecting the right EHR solution for the needs of your clinic, selecting the right vendor, and thoughtfully transitioning your staff's workflow to the new system all will play an integral role in generating ROI and workflow efficiencies from this undertaking.

Here is a general overview of the steps for successfully choosing and implementing the right solution for your clinic:

1. Establish that your practice is ready. This may be 3 months before opening or years after opening.
2. Select internal champions who can help you gain buy-in before implementation. Without staff buy-in, your EHR implementation is doomed to failure.
3. Establish a budget and a timeline.
4. Manage (and promote) the change.
5. Redesign workflow in anticipation of going electronic.
6. Choose the right vendor partner (not a product).
7. Think about the future. Where is health care moving, and which partner has the bandwidth to take you there? (Network-based trumps software-based.)
8. Ensure that your partner is equipped to adapt to, and even lead, changing reimbursement patterns.
9. Spend the majority of your efforts on the practice-management solution. It should be scalable, shareable, and well established.

10. Finally, look for a vendor partner whose exit strategy is not selling its business. The vendor partner's windfall will become your nightmare when you are forced to adapt to the new owner's ideas or systems.

WHICH SOLUTION IS RIGHT FOR YOUR PRACTICE?

With over 400 EHR vendors in the marketplace, each advertising a variety of must-have options and price points, the selection process can initially seem daunting. However, a lot of the frustration can be eliminated by approaching the process in steps. The first and most important step is to write down your functional needs. What are the top 15 to 20 things you need your EHR to do for you? What specific changes would you like to see in your practice's workflow after the solution is implemented?

To differentiate one product from another to see if it will meet your needs, you need an understanding of common EHR features and functionalities. A useful list of nomenclature can be found in the analysis reported by Mark Anderson, chief executive officer of AC Group, Inc., in his 2008 white paper, "EHR Pricing—What Can You Afford?" He classifies different EHRs by functional level.[4] His taxonomy was very useful to me during our internal EHR review. Table 1 summarizes some of the general features of EHR solutions and can be a useful tool for you in the beginning stages of the research process.

Once you have a clear understanding of what you would like the EHR solution to do for you, start evaluating the various products based on their ability to meet your functional needs. Whatever you do, don't simply pick a solution that the majority of urgent care centers or primary care offices are advertised as using, because a randomly picked solution is unlikely to address the specific needs of your practice. The cost to switch an EHR is very high, so simply determining how many centers use a particular system means little when the pain, friction, contractual obligation, and cost associated with switching are so high. This is why it is so important to choose wisely the first time.

SELECTING THE RIGHT VENDOR

Once you have identified your functional requirements, make a list of the vendors who have the EHR solution that addresses your needs. At this point, your focus should be on identifying the vendor that will not only give you the solution you need from a functionality perspective but will also become a real partner in your effort to transition seamlessly and will take an interest in helping you build efficiencies. Given this objective, you will first need to pare down your original list of vendors to eliminate those that do not fit this profile. Many of these vendors can be eliminated on the basis of their length of time in business, the number of practices using their system, their financial strength, and their prominence in the industry.

---

4   Anderson M. EHR pricing—what can you afford? Montgomery, TX: AC Group, Inc. January 22, 2008. Available from: http://www.emrupdate.com/media/p/78580/download.aspx.

Table 1. Common Features of EHR Solutions

	Level 1	Level 2	Level 3	Level 4	Level 5
Scans documents into a file or a series of subfolders by patient name or number	•	•	•	•	•
Records patient-related clinical information via voice dictation, typing, and handwriting either by following a template design or by using a blank e-form by clinical category	•	•	•	•	•
Allows recording of E&M codes, but the E&M code is not suggested on the basis of the data entered		•	•	•	•
Can print patient prescriptions, but there is no knowledge base for drug alerts and formulary compliance	•	•	•	•	•
Can capture a patient's family, social, and medical history using a defined format		•	•	•	•
Provides baseline tracking of orders and health-maintenance alerts		•	•	•	•
Provides laboratory ordering and results plus two-way orders and results reporting with specific laboratories		•	•	•	•
Checks for medical necessity, checks health-care plans for ABN requirements, and prints ABN if required		•	•	•	•
Provides a view of laboratory results in a flow sheet over time and can graph labs results over time		•	•	•	•
Provides baseline eRx charting of prior medications ordered by the health-care provider, the ability to order new medications, and the ability to print prescriptions in the office; does not provide drug alerts		•	•	•	•
Provides baseline alerts and clinical support based on the EHR vendor's clinical databases			•	•	•
Baseline charting with practice-specific clinical alerts			•	•	•

(continued)

Table 1. Common Features of EHR Solutions (continued)

	Level 1	Level 2	Level 3	Level 4	Level 5
Provides simple documentation that follows templates that can be modified by the practice and by the individual provider				•	•
Provides a baseline orders and results reporting capability			•	•	•
Provides a patient summary page, making it possible to review prior visit reasons, active medications, active laboratory results, next appointments, etc.			•	•	•
Provides advanced eRx documentation, drug alerts that are updated by the EHR vendor (no national standard alerts), and the ability to electronically send prescriptions to specific pharmacies				•	•
Includes the medication history of the patient ordered by the service provider *and* other health-care providers outside the clinic			•	•	•
Provides advanced clinical orders capability that is based on national guidelines and that follows guidelines for confirming medical necessity			•	•	•
Tracks all orders and indicates when an order result is past due; provides alerts and CDS plus advanced features that are based on user-specific customizable guidelines			•	•	•
Provides advanced E&M and coding guidelines designed to ensure that the actual charges match the clinical charting			•	•	•
Includes advanced templates that can be customized by either the vendor or the practice on the basis of specific practice requirements				•	•
Follows national documentation guidelines like CCD, SNOMED, and CCHIT; software provides an advanced patient summary page plus strong health-maintenance alerts, prior vital signs, patient messages, chronic diseases, and other patient-specific information					•

(continued)

Table 1. Common Features of EHR Solutions (continued)

	Level 1	Level 2	Level 3	Level 4	Level 5
Provides advanced, practice-customized, two-way laboratory interfaces with companies like LabCorp and Quest, along with order guidelines based on practice preference lists and the patient's condition; automatically posts results in the patient's chart and sends a note or message to the provider or nurse that is based on practice-alerts guidelines					•
Tracks all ordered tests and alerts the practice if test results are not back within a specific time					•
Provides advanced eRx capability with nationally updated drug alerts based on multiple parameters, insurance-specific formulary compliance as outlined by companies like RxHub, preauthorization alerts, and personalized eRx preference lists by provider; can transmit eRx via Surescripts to the patient's preferred pharmacy					•
Provides advanced orders and results that are based on practice guidelines and national best practices, according to the patient's condition				•	•
Provides health-maintenance alerts that are based on patient conditions and identifies orders on the basis of national guidelines				•	•
Provides advanced alerts and CDS that are based on nationally recognized sources that are updated on a routine basis, including drug alerts, clinical best practices, health-maintenance alerts, and disease-management guidelines				•	•
Provides advanced charge capture for both nurses and physicians that follows the 1997 E&M coding requirements				•	•
Tracks the number of points per E&M coding category and provides the provider with a one-page summary of the appropriate E&M code				•	•
Enables advanced documentation, with nationally recognized templates based on best practices and clinical guidelines that are customizable to physicians' practicing patterns					•

(continued)

Table 1. Common Features of EHR Solutions (continued)

	Level 1	Level 2	Level 3	Level 4	Level 5
Provides hyperlinks to outside clinical knowledge databases; links problems to orders; provides the ability to view summary information regarding the patient's conditions on one customizable screen					•
Provides documentation that follows national guidelines like CCD, SNOMED, and CCHIT					•
Allows the patient to enter data via a kiosk or via online web-based personal health record; provides a patient summary page plus the ability to customize the page on the basis of the physician's and practice's unique needs; provides laboratory orders that are based on best practices and national guidelines					•
Receives laboratory orders electronically; can post the data automatically in a flow sheet and graph data results over time; can visually compare laboratory results to eRx; can combine results from different laboratories using the same format					•
Provides advanced, nationally recognized, practice-customized eRx with the ability to create customized preference lists that are based on the clinical findings for the patient; allows the patient to request eRx refills via a secure website; can track when a patient does *not* pick up their medication from the pharmacy					•
Provides advanced, practice-customized clinical orders and results reporting that are based on national best practices and nationally accepted standards					•
Bases orders on the patient's condition, personal preference lists, and advance features; provides advanced, nationally recognized, practice-customized alerts and CDS that can meet all current and future guidelines via simplified advanced reporting or building of a new alert template					•

(continued)

Table 1. Common Features of EHR Solutions (continued)

	Level 1	Level 2	Level 3	Level 4	Level 5
Provides advanced, nationally recognized, practice-customized E&M coding tied to the patient's specific health-care plan for maximizing charge capture via preauthorization alerts and guidelines					•
Provides advice on charge capture that is based on best practices and practice guidelines and reports variances from guidelines; provides advanced, nationally recognized, practice-customized clinical reference content with clear labeling of the levels of evidence for facts and assertions and grades for recommendations made, and these levels and grades are clearly and transparently based on the quality of the underlying evidence using reproducible processes					•

ABN, advance beneficiary notice; CCD, continuity of care document; CCHIT, Certification Commission for Healthcare Information Technology; CDS, clinical decision support; E&M, evaluation and management; EHR, electronic health record; eRx, electronic prescription; SNOMED, Systematized Nomenclature of Medicine.

You can find a lot of useful information about vendors by reviewing unbiased industry reports and corporate financial statements. In this business, size and longevity matter, so take the time to do your homework. The vendor's ability to continuously invest significant dollar amounts into implementation, infrastructure, and research is critical. For example, if your EHR vendor becomes insolvent or experiences significant funding issues, it will directly affect your EHR and ultimately your center's ability to survive.

Consider the following facets of the vendor's financial and operational viability[5]:

- *Spot marketing hype over substance*   Marketing is expensive, but smaller niche players attempt to compete with the large players by spending heavily on marketing campaigns and vendor events. This may mean less spending on new software releases.

- *Review stock analysts' assessments, if available*   If a publicly traded company has poor results, that will affect its stock price and its ability to scale to meet demands.

- *Ask yourself if the vendor has a balance sheet strong enough to support the ever-changing needs and demands of its client partners*   Technology changes rapidly. If a vendor cannot effectively upgrade and improve its EHR solution, it will become less competitive, which will in turn lead to fewer sales. The vendor's decreasing revenue will then directly affect its cash flow and ultimately its ability to provide you with effective customer support and the upgrades you will need to stay current.

- *Compare year-over-year sales and check whether the company met promised releases dates and implementation time frames*   Delays are often an early indication of financial or operational issues. Also, evaluate the vendor's revenue recognition strategy. Some vendors will recognize sales and support revenue long before actually receiving the funds. Or conversely, they will charge the practice for support service before the software is implemented.

- *Watch out for special deals*   Many practices have fallen for the side letter or special deal in which the vendor allows them an early out. Although compelling on the surface, this should cause your alarm bells to go off. These offers almost always mean that the product is not ready and that the vendor's finances are shaky. If the vendor files for bankruptcy after taking your money, you are probably out of luck.

---

5   Anderson M. Financial questions for vendors. Montgomery, TX: AC Group, Inc. January 22, 2008. Available from: http://www.acgroup.org/images/2008_ACG_White_Paper_-_Vendor_Financial_Questions.pdf. Accessed February 22, 2014.

▶ *What is the vendor's exit strategy?* If the company is not publicly traded, consider how and when the owners want to exit. Chances are that any strategic acquirer will force a change in the system architecture, release frequency, or support.

IS THE VENDOR CERTIFIED BY THE CERTIFICATION COMMISSION FOR HEALTHCARE INFORMATION TECHNOLOGY?

To help ensure the adoption of common standards, three leading industry associations in health-care information management and technology have launched the Certification Commission for Healthcare Information Technology (CCHIT). CCHIT has undertaken the task of outlining the important functional components of an EHR, how it should interface with other electronic systems, and how it should protect and store patient information. The CCHIT criteria consist of a list of functional product capabilities against which all EHRs are measured. It is also the only federally recognized certification body for EHRs and is therefore important to any medical practice seeking to participate in payment incentive programs from the Centers for Medicare & Medicaid Services. CCHIT-certified EHRs also qualify for a special exemption from the Stark and anti-kickback laws, so that local hospitals or health systems can subsidize a physician's EHR purchase.

CCHIT certification is based on approximately 300 measures of EHR functionality, interoperability, and security. An EHR product must pass all CCHIT-required capabilities. Certification is an all-or-nothing test; there is no partial or feature-by-feature certification.

The CCHIT certification changes each year. That a vendor is certified in the current year does not mean that the same product will meet the upcoming year's certification. Therefore, if you are considering CCHIT certification as part of your selection criteria, you should inquire whether the EHR vendor is currently certified, and if it is not, then determine when the company plans to obtain the subsequent year's certification. If the vendor cannot give you a sufficient answer, you might want to look elsewhere. *Note:* If a hospital or other entity is considering subsidizing the cost of EHRs for its community physicians, the Stark law requires that the EHR product have been certified within the last 12 calendar months. To find which vendors are CCHIT certified, go to https://www.cchit.org/find-onc.

As CCHIT certification continues to gain acceptance, most EHR buyers are using CCHIT certification as a bright-line standard with which to filter EHR products during their selection process. At present many managed-care organizations, accountable care organizations, and health-care information exchanges are also mandating CCHIT certification in order to participate. Considering CCHIT certification in your selection process can be a powerful tool to help you make your decision.

CLIENT SERVER OR APPLICATION SERVICE PROVIDER MODEL?

When buying EHR software, which is better—cloud or application service provider (ASP) or client–server? There is no right or wrong answer, because the solution you choose depends on what's important to your practice.

Using a client–server model is similar to buying software at the store and installing it on your computer. In this kind of model, the software is installed on a server located in your office, and the workstations access the software directly on the server. With this kind of setup, once you purchase the software, there are usually no ongoing fees except for upgrades or support when you need it. The client–server model also gives a practice control over its data. But with this control comes the responsibility of safeguarding that data, because the center is open to the risk of theft, fire, hard drive failure, and data corruption.

The ASP model, on the other hand, is based on remotely hosted software that is accessed through a web browser. This is similar to the model used in online banking, and you can access all of your information at any time, from any place with Internet access. The server is secure and compliant with the Health Insurance Portability and Accountability Act, and it is not located in your office. All technical aspects of the server are managed by a professional IT company, and you pay a monthly access fee (or per-occurrence fee) for the company's services. One of the other benefits of the ASP model is that almost all computing is done in the cloud or on the remote server, thereby reducing the minimum computer hardware requirements of the clients (workstations).

Unlike a client–server model, this remotely hosted system requires a regular rental or service fee. Therefore, the cost of a cloud or ASP-based system is relatively low in the beginning, because you don't pay for the software up front. However, because the regular fees never stop, the cost over the long term adds up and can be greater than with a client–server system.

One disadvantage in cloud or ASP models is the loss of significant customizability. Because the host server is being accessed by many users, the EHR provider has to consider the needs of all users and cannot always customize the system to your needs. Accountability issues are also a consideration for ASPs. If the company experiences financial or operational problems, service degradation is felt more acutely by its clients, and such things as vendor bankruptcy could have a more drastic impact on your practice as a whole. If you choose an ASP-based solution, check the stability of the EHR software vendor periodically and ask for a backup copy of your data regularly.

ARRANGE A PRODUCT DEMONSTRATION

Once you have determined your functional requirements, selected your internal champions, and narrowed down the field of prospective vendors, it is time to arrange a product demonstration. Typically, these are done virtually and are conducted by a salesperson who usually has a good, albeit basic, understanding of the system's attributes.

You will likely be shown a standard, scripted encounter designed to walk you through a typical patient scenario. You can be sure that this scenario will have been previewed many times and will be bug-free by the time of your demonstration. A good way around this is to give the presenter your own encounters to see if the system can stand up to the vagaries of day-to-day practice. Try a few different organ system–based interactions: worst headache of the patient's life, being sent to an emergency department, a young girl with a urinary tract infection and without a legal guardian present, a patient paying with a health savings account card who requires a laboratory send-out and an imaging referral, and so forth.

VISIT SITES USING THE ELECTRONIC HEALTH RECORD

One way to obtain more truthful feedback about the usability and limitations of the software you are considering is to visit other sites that already use it. The reason this is useful is not just because you are getting the opinion of someone who uses the product every day but also because you are not talking to a trained salesperson. Because, for one reason or another, not everyone will be completely truthful with you about their opinion, make sure to ask many different types of questions—not just generalities about their level of satisfaction. How long did their implementation take? What was their biggest problem during implementation? What are their biggest issues with the EHR software right now? Where did they see the biggest improvement in their workflow? Did they achieve their ROI?

Be aware that some current clients may not be completely transparent about their software vendor because they may know that the only way for the EHR vendor to survive is to sell their way out of their financial difficulties, or the clients may be contractually bound to not disparage their EHR provider. That said, other clients may complain far more than is warranted, so approach this aspect of the vetting process with some skepticism. Nonetheless, talking to someone who is already using the software you are considering can be a great source of information, and it is absolutely essential during the selection process.

HOW MUCH WILL IT COST?

Software costs can vary significantly. In addition, many practices fail to accurately anticipate the hidden costs of the EHR, such as ongoing maintenance, upgrade fees, or additional IT support and staff members, all of which will drag down the potential ROI.

When AC Group analyzed the cost of support and maintenance, they found that the average vendor charges between 15% and 20% of the list price of the software. However, when they compared the actual annual support fees to the price, they found that it was between 18% and 35%. This disparity often occurs because vendors offer discounts on the price of the software but no discounts on the support fees. Therefore, you may be expecting to pay 15% to 20% of the purchase price, but in reality, the support fees will be based on the *list* price. If the software price is based on a per-user or per-license methodology, then in a five-license practice, the difference between what was promised and what the practice is actually paying becomes significant.

Consider vendors who simply charge a percentage of collected charges as their fee to use their EHR. Arguably, this aligns incentives, inasmuch as it is easier to document. In addition, the more efficient your health-care providers become, the more patients they can treat, with less downtime spent completing the medical record, and both your center and the EHR vendor will be better off financially. If the vendor offers a percentage-of-collection financial model that includes practice management and no charge for adding more health-care providers or workstations and no extra hidden charges, then you may have found the cleanest and easiest way to implement an EHR and practice-management solution for your center.

When it comes to making the final decisions about which EHR solution is right for you, make sure to include price negotiation as part of the process. Whether it's reducing the up-front costs or negotiating support costs, any concessions you can obtain will directly help you increase the chances of meeting the promised ROI. Remember that the EHR market is fragmented, with over 400 vendors competing against each other. This means that you have significant leverage when it comes to negotiating pricing or having extra services built into the package free of charge. However, be wary of vendors that offer discounts up front, before you ask for one. On the one hand, it could be because the salesperson is near the end of a sales period and wants to meet their quota, but on the other hand it could mean that the company is struggling and is desperate for clients.

COSTS OF IMPLEMENTATION

When it comes specifically to implementation, there is a broad range of costs[6] associated with the purchase and deployment of a system, including the following:

- ▶ *Software licenses,* which are typically sold on a per-provider or a per-workstation basis. This can be particularly challenging in an urgent care environment, where staff turnover is commonplace.

- ▶ *Hardware,* consisting of both individual personal computers for office and exam rooms, as well as central database servers, network hardware, and modems. One argument for cloud-based computing and storage is that the additional purchase of network hardware and servers becomes unnecessary.

---

6   Anderson M. EHR pricing—what can you afford?

- *Training and implementation,* which involve pre-installation planning as well as on-site training of individual users. This cost is often hidden during the sales process; the practice can spend a significant amount of money on training and implementation, which are typically billed at an hourly rate.
- *Software support,* represented as an annual contract typically sold as a percentage of the total sale, providing both help desk functions (technical support) and software updates. Support of these can also be significant.
- *Third-party software* for external knowledge bases and clinical decision support. Fees associated with additional software vendors such as Epocrates, UpToDate, and ExitCare can also add up.

A study conducted by AC Group, based on a sampling of 142 contracts, determined that the software is usually about 36% of the cost of the entire 3-year project. Infrastructure cost runs about 30%, and support costs run about 34%. Therefore, when considering overall costs, health-care providers should multiply the software costs by 3 to estimate the total cost over a 3-year period.

To calculate the total cost of ownership, review these three separate areas:

1. Software cost
   a. Actual vendor software
   b. Necessary interfaces
   c. Third-party or additional software
2. Infrastructure
   a. Hardware—servers and connections
   b. Networks
   c. Communications
   d. Security and associated insurance for breaches
   e. Workstations
   f. Printers and scanners
3. Support
   a. Workflow and process review and revision
   b. Installation
   c. Configuration
   d. Audit and post-audit reviews

e. Support (ongoing)

f. Upgrades

INDIRECT COSTS OF ELECTRONIC HEALTH RECORD IMPLEMENTATION

In addition to the direct, out-of-pocket costs to implement your solution, EHR deployment can also carry indirect costs that will affect your long-term ROI on the project. Some of the more prominent ones include reduced productivity, duplication of processes because of incomplete implementation of an EHR, and decreased access to important patient information.

Reduced productivity is often a by-product of adopting an incorrect patient–provider encounter procedure by basing it strictly on the EHR vendor's suggestions, without taking into account the specifics of your practice. Most EHR software focuses primarily on the provider exam—that is, on creating an electronic interface for the physician to document everything during the patient encounter. These EHRs encourage physicians to adopt the full electronic encounter immediately, which fundamentally changes the physician's encounter workflow (and not always for the better). In addition, the number of clicks to get through the medical record matters. The more clicks required to get through an EHR, the longer the encounter takes and the less productive the provider is—and the more chances there are for errors in the medical record.

Incomplete adoption of the EHR can also drag down the ROI. If new workflow processes are not developed to optimize use of the EHR, the practice duplicates work (using both paper and electronic systems interchangeably), thus failing to optimize the EHR and failing to provide a full ROI. Such reduplication can often be attributed to the fact that many EHR vendors currently seem to be narrowly focused on updating the data entry component of the provider exam with overstructured, noncustomizable elements that don't meet the broader needs of the practice. Or conversely, the EHR vendor has a completely customizable solution that requires hundreds of hours of configuration before the go-live date. This means that the practice may not have access to all the features it needs, or could be stuck in buffering mode, waiting for the solution to finally be customized.

One of the biggest issues that can become a big problem over the long term is the *potential decreased access to important patient information* when the EHR solution is not correctly optimized for the practice. For practices that do not successfully implement their EHR, patient safety can suffer because of diversion of resources and reduced access to critical information, which often occurs in multiple areas within the medical record. Even with EHR software–driven prompts, staying on top of laboratory work, orders, and results requires a significant amount of staff time. Without a closed-loop order-and-results-management system, the cost of managing and tracking documents can be prohibitive. Proper implementation and a carefully thought-out deployment are essential for avoiding these issues.

MEDICOLEGAL PITFALLS

It must be noted that although EHRs have opportunities to improve outcomes and reduce costs, they also come with liability. One area of concern is inappropriate access to a patient's medical record. These privacy issues are compounded for EHRs relative to paper, because the exposure may be in many physical locations simultaneously. Ensure that your EHR requires appropriate practice and network credentialing before anyone can open the patient's medical record. The following areas should also be addressed when selecting an EHR vendor or using an EHR:

- The ability for health-care providers to turn off patient alerts
- Failure to identify laboratory issues that may affect drug dosing—for example, flagging a high serum creatinine level when dosing gentamicin
- A lack of correspondence between the patient's medical history and the patient's physical exam—for example, 2 years previously, the patient had an eye enucleated, but the physical exam states: PERRLA (pupils equal, round, reactive to light, and accommodation).
- Time synchronization problems—for example, the time stamps on the chart may be out of sequence with the care that was delivered
- Delays in documenting the care of a patient, so that it appears that patient care was delayed for those 4 hours
- Cutting and pasting from one document to another or within the same document that leads to inappropriate and inaccurate documentation
- The use of macros, in which entire systems or exams are preloaded into the software, which can lead to inappropriate upcoding as well as inaccurate and inappropriate documentation
- Shared passwords—if the documentation is typed under your password, it is difficult to prove that you do not own what is on the chart
- The fact that *all* alterations are captured—every time that the chart is accessed, changed, or viewed, this is documented in the EHR's metadata, and this can be used in a medical malpractice claim

CONCLUSION

When selected carefully, a good EHR solution can add significant value to your practice. It can reduce costs, improve patient care, and create efficiencies that are not possible to achieve with a paper file system. However, implementing a solution does not guarantee positive results. For your investment in EHR software to provide an ROI, you must make a significant effort up front to select a solution that best fits the needs of your office. If this is not done, or if corners are cut during the initial phases, the solution can drag down productivity and become an expensive mistake.

A big part of this initial process also lies in the selection of the right vendor. The solution must address the needs of your office but also should be provided by a vendor that can adequately meet the ongoing demands of improving the software and providing sufficient customer support. Having a good vendor is absolutely vital to the success of the implementation, because the usefulness of EHR software is heavily dependent on the vendor doing its part in preserving the integrity of your database and electronic workflow.

Overall, the implementation process requires a careful approach that will further develop your practice's infrastructure in the long term. The solution should address real issues that are specific to your practice and should enhance your overall operations and client care. The key is to approach this process from the perspective of what you actually need, rather than focusing on what all the various EHR providers offer. When you are focused on your practice's needs, you will be much more likely to have a positive experience and ROI, even if there are issues along the way.

To further assist you in your research, here is a list of additional resources where you can find comprehensive third-party reports on this topic:

- ► AC Group, Inc.: www.acgroup.org
- ► HIMSS Electronic Health Record Association: www.himssehra.org
- ► Certification Commission for Healthcare Information Technology: www.cchit.org
- ► KLAS: www.klasresearch.com
- ► Forrester Research: www.forrester.com

KEY POINTS

1. Ask staff members (back-office technicians, front-office workers, and billing and coding specialists) to participate in the decision. Health-care providers are not the only users of the EHR and account for only a fraction of the time spent in the medical record.

2. Spend time investigating before going through a demonstration so that you know what to ask. Remember, demonstrations are set up to impress you and get you to buy. The demonstration will be flawless; the product won't.

3. Make sure you go on urgent care reference site visits without the representative of the company. Talk to staff members, the administrator, and health-care providers.

4. Part of the conversion or installation should be to improve workflow. Many practices have not invested the time to optimize processes, forms, procedures, or workflows. Determine where technology can make you more efficient and exploit these opportunities. Even saving 30 seconds per patient adds up over the course of the day.

5. Ensure that the system has a large selection of scripted or built-in macros. Don't rely exclusively on voice recognition to complete your charts. Although systems like Dragon generally work well, they are not flawless.

6. Skimping on training will set you back for weeks, if not months. Make sure that all of your staff members are well versed in the system, including its flaws and idiosyncrasies, and understand the workarounds. Budget for and schedule time outside of office hours for everyone to train. On go-live day, you will be much more productive and efficient if you spend the appropriate training time prospectively.

7. Conversions are stressful. They take months. Don't underestimate the human factors involved in making a conversion or instituting an EHR. Even in the best circumstances and with the best preparation, conversions provoke angst.

8. Continue to take the pulse of users during and after the process. I used a particular EHR system for years, and eventually, a relatively new user showed me things that made me much more efficient. Never underestimate the power of one-on-one training in the trenches.

9. Although standards are important, most EHRs allow the user to get to the same end point in a variety of different ways. Thus, don't choose a one-size-fits-all EHR. Get the data you need but allow users to have some customization.

10. This takes time and is not easy. You will want to give up. Don't. Your team will get there, you will overcome the challenges, and ultimately the EHR will help you better care for your patients and improve your outcomes.

CHAPTER 24

Revenue Cycle Management and Partnership

Sybil Yeaman

Understanding the revenue cycle, controlling its increasing complexity, and choosing the right revenue cycle management partner are critical for the financial stability of every urgent care center. Although the right location and viable health-care contracts are vital for success, systematic clinical and financial oversight of the revenue process and disciplined revenue cycle management ensure continuous cash flow for operating the center.

An urgent care center is a very complex and constantly changing combination of health-care information, medical documentation, and billing and claims services. A clearly defined and efficient workflow of patient information and documentation will make the reimbursement difference between a successful business and a center on the edge of insolvency.

THE REVENUE CYCLE

The revenue cycle (Figure 1) begins when a patient enters the urgent care center for medical care and ends when all medical services and diagnostics tests are paid for. The urgent care center bears complete financial responsibility up front for all medical services that patients receive during their physical exam and treatment. This financial commitment for equipment, staff, supplies, and diagnostic testing is expensive. The financial risk is high, and the responsibility to meet regulatory requirements is intense. Controlling the revenue cycle, from patient registration to payment, is critical for the financial stability and growth of the center. How you manage your patient information, operations workflow, and billing will determine your level of success in managing your center's revenue cycle process.

CONTROLLING THE REVENUE CYCLE PROCESS

Successful management of the revenue cycle process for your urgent care center and for your revenue cycle management partner, if you outsource the management function, requires development of a detailed operational process and protocols to be strictly followed in the following areas:

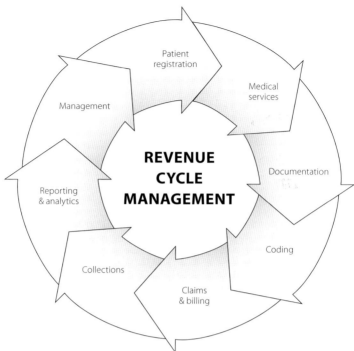

Figure 1. The revenue cycle.

- Patient registration
- Medical services and documentation
- Coding, billing, and collections
- Revenue analytics and management

Patient Registration

Patient registration is a key component of controlling the revenue cycle process. As health-care plans and government-funded programs become increasingly complex, urgent care centers must be able to handle that complexity and the additional responsibility of gathering pertinent patient health plan information before providing medical care. Failure to gather the correct data and payments in the registration area undermines the entire revenue cycle system.

Successful management of the registration area is driven by data and staff experience, which necessitates the development of a standardized process. Guaranteeing success at the beginning of the revenue cycle requires the following:

- A predefined process and a clear set of guidelines for the reception staff to follow (Figure 2)
- Training and ongoing guidance in adhering to uniform procedures to guarantee health-care information, data, and payment collection

Registration Goal

It is the goal of the (Company Name) Registration Team to ensure all patients/guarantors receive the highest quality of service while assisting them in verifying insurance coverage prior to receiving medical services in a caring and professional manner and efficiently processing urgent care patients/guarantors for medical services.

Registration Policy

It is the policy of the (Company Name) Registration Team to verify insurance coverage, and collect co-pays, noncovered services, and deductibles for all patients/guarantors prior to receiving medical services.

Insurance Verification Procedures

All patient/guarantors must fill out registration forms and provide copies of insurance coverage. The Registration Team will scan both sides of the insurance card and will verify insurance coverage, co-pays, covered services, and deductibles for every visit by utilizing electronic eligibility verification and/or online insurance websites.

(Note: If electronic eligibility verification is in place, the following sample website list may be unnecessary.)

The most common websites are as follows:

Insurance Company	Web Address	Username	Password
ABC Health Plan.........	http://webaddress	Center ID #	Sample
EFG Health Plan.........	http://webaddress	Center ID #	Sample
JKL Health Plan.........	http://webaddress	Center ID #	Sample
PQR Health Plan.........	http://webaddress	Center ID #	Sample
XYZ Health Plan.........	http://webaddress	Center ID #	Sample

Phone Verification

If the health plan does not have an online website available for eligibility verification or the website is down, the Registration Team will contact the health plan directly by phone to verify coverage, co-pays, and deductibles by calling the provider phone number listed on the patient's insurance card.

Provider Information for Phone Verification

Physician Providers	NPI Number
Number One, MD......	0000000000
Number Two, MD.......	0000000000
Number Three, DO.....	0000000000

CPNP Providers	NPI Number
Number One CPNP.....	0000000000
Number Two CPNP.....	0000000000

Incorrect Insurance Coverage Resolution

When the insurance coverage does not correspond with the health plan information or coverage has been terminated, the (Company Name) Registration Team member will inform the patient/guarantor all services will be provided on a cash payment basis and obtain signed documentation of the patient/guarantor's agreement to payment terms.

Documentation of Insurance Information

The Registration Team member will enter the insurance verification information into the _____ system, followed by their initials. If the insurance verification information is not documented and initialed, the verification process will not be considered done.

Figure 2. Sample guidelines for registration staff.

- Standard health-care forms, such as advance beneficiary notices, available for noncovered services, readily available at the registration desk
- Technology such as software for real-time electronic eligibility verification (to guarantee accurate insurance data collection) and multiple computers with online access (to verify patient benefits, co-pays, and deductibles)

To establish control at the beginning of the revenue cycle, the registration staff should be given training in a predefined process to follow when gathering patient data. With each health plan having different requirements and guidelines for their members and different health-care product lines, staff members can easily become confused. Clear guidelines (Figure 2) and mandatory eligibility verification guarantee that the urgent care center is following the health plan requirements for each patient. This is particularly important for the collection of co-pays and deductibles. When co-pays are not collected or deductibles are not applied, they fall into the end of the revenue cycle, resulting in the delay or loss of payment to the center.

Use of technology such as electronic eligibility verification will help the registration staff verify insurance cards and patient payment responsibility information more efficiently by using the health plan membership databases instead of health plan websites. Patients without health plan eligibility become cash-pay patients. The collection of cash payments allows the center to receive payment up front and saves the expense of going through the collection process because of denied and unpaid claims.

When patient volume is high, usually after school or during the hours when most primary-care practices are closed, the registration staff is under increased pressure to process patients into the center as quickly as possible. This often translates into attempts to save time by skipping entry of key elements of information required by health plans for claims processing. Thus, using software that requires entry of data into critical information fields before registration can be completed is highly recommended because entering all necessary data into the computer system before the patient is treated is vital to the success of the revenue cycle management process.

Medical Documentation

Medical documentation that is accurate and complete in the patient medical record will provide supporting documentation for claims submission. A well-documented medical record will meet core compliance and quality-assurance measures. The record should also support appropriate payment if a claim for medical services or supporting diagnostic tests are denied. Each year physicians and medical providers are required to produce more and more complex clinical documentation and coding to support the medical care they provide. Comprehensive and accurate documentation will help the center avoid delayed payments, and more importantly avoid refunds, audits, and penalties by payers.

The following are considered key components of all evaluation and management (E&M) services and therefore are required in the medical record to support E&M codes:

- Patient medical history
- Physical exam
- Complexity of diagnosis and treatment plan

So that the maximum appropriate charge can be captured in the revenue cycle, the following should also be clearly documented:

- Coordination of care
- Time spent counseling patient and family members

Having a software system that requires essential patient medical information fields to be completed before the medical record can be closed will protect the center from E&M coding denials because of inadequate supporting documentation. Using technology to close the loop on orders for laboratory and x-ray services will ensure that diagnostic test results and charges are not lost between medical documentation and the claims processes of the revenue cycle.

Billing and Claims

Billing and claims processing have increased in complexity as more regulations, health plans, and new pay-for-quality programs have been put in place. With hundreds of government and health plan coverage nuances, standardization of internal urgent care center processes and more advanced technology are necessary to keep up with changing billing and claims complexities.

Your center's billing and claims process should be clean and consistent if established revenue cycle management protocols have consistently been followed for patient registration and medical documentation. The percentage of clean claims paid on first pass through the claims submission process can be used as a basic test for success. Successful billing and claims reflect a successful revenue cycle process. If more than 90% of all electronic and paper claims are processed on the first-pass scrubbing (i.e., the validation process) and submission, your revenue cycle management is working. It is important to continue to review and strive to improve the performance of all aspects of the revenue cycle to drive the percentage of clean claims submissions higher and the costs of denials and collections lower.

If a test of your first-pass clean claims submission fails, remember that the revenue cycle is complex and that changing staff routines and workflow takes time and consistent effort. Look closely at unpaid claims to determine why they were rejected by the payer. Unpaid claims may be a simple data entry issue in registration, a medical staff compliance issue, claims system errors, or health plan claims-processing issues. Pay special attention to denials because of lack of medical necessity. These may indicate that the diagnosis codes are not being linked to the correct procedure codes. Denials because of lack of timely filing indicate a deeper problem between medical documentation, completion of data entry charges, and billing delays.

Revenue Cycle Analytics

Revenue cycle analytics is management that is based on performance measurements, starting with the entry of data when patients enter the center for an appointment and ending in accounts receivable when services are paid for. Performance measurements and analytics must include management oversight of incorrect health plan payment issues, such as lost claims and errors in allowed amounts during claims processing. This requires consistent and systematic analysis of denials, claims in the appeals process, and requests for medical documentation.

When evaluating denials and unpaid claims, identify where the issues are occurring: in the registration area, in medical documentation in the clinical areas, or in the billing and claims process. Take immediate action to communicate expected changes with staff members, and make sure that they understand where and why breakdowns are occurring in their standardized workflow in the revenue cycle. The expected changes should be carefully designed and implemented without creating upheaval for the staff or making drastic changes in the workflow.

Beyond tracking the percentage of first-pass clean claims and denials, the percentage of accounts receivable beyond 90 days overdue is an indicator of unresolved issues such as uncollected deductibles or a high volume of claims in appeal because of coding errors, such as diagnosis codes not being linked to the correct Current Procedural Terminology (CPT) codes, or data entry errors. Once unpaid claims are overdue by more than 120 days, collection rates decrease rapidly while the time and cost to obtain reimbursement increase drastically. Make corrections until the revenue cycle management process is working and your center is generating consistent revenue to run daily operations and fund future growth.

CHOOSING A REVENUE CYCLE MANAGEMENT PARTNER

Choosing the right revenue cycle management partner for billing, claims, collections, and reporting management services will help your urgent care center keep up with the increasing complexity of documentation requirements, coding changes, and reimbursement structures. The right partner can reduce operating costs by eliminating the need for billing personnel and staff benefits, the purchase and maintenance of computers and specialized software for claims processing, and the time spent juggling the changing health plan billing and coding requirements.

The right partner will allow the urgent care physicians and staff members to focus on patient medical care and diagnostic services rather than on billing. With the focus on medical care, the center should increase patient volume and the bottom line while expediting claims processing to ensure continuous cash flow. The wrong partner, with inadequate performance, will grow your overdue accounts receivable with denied claims that become increasingly more difficult and expensive to collect. There are three steps to guide a center in finding, choosing, and maintaining the right partnership:

- List services and research options
- Meet with the potential partners
- Verify contract and services

The first step in choosing a revenue cycle management partner is to take the time to list and research the services your urgent care center needs from a partner, which may include

- Credentialing
- Health plan contract review and negotiation
- Electronic claims submission
- Collection services
- Compliance audits
- Financial reports and analytics

Once you have identified needed services, start searching for compatible revenue cycle management companies. Consider both local and national companies. Be sure to ask successful colleagues who they work with and look up the recommended companies online. Be careful about choosing vendors who are also personal friends because friendship can cloud judgment. Make sure that friends fulfill the same demands for price and services as any other revenue management company being considered. Use a search engine to check reputation and customer satisfaction. Dissatisfied customers often complain about poor service or high fees in online venues, and multiple complaints should be heeded.

To narrow down the options, contact only companies that offer

- Extensive experience with urgent care billing
- Financial stability and well-established services
- Comprehensive technology and support services
- Customer satisfaction and good reputation
- Compliance and quality-assurance programs
- Competitive pricing rates at 4% to 6% of collections
- Reasonable hourly fees for credentialing and contracting services

Create a list of potential partnership companies and criteria to track and compare price and services (Figure 3). Cost is not the only factor to consider when choosing a revenue cycle management partner. Consider the level of service, resources, and best fit for your center's culture.

Consider using an electronic health record (EHR) service as a revenue cycle management partner that offers a seamless management process from registrations through documentation and claims processing. If your center is currently using an EHR system or planning to switch to electronic records, evaluate whether the system has robust back-office and analytic services. Using an EHR billing solution allows your urgent care center to eliminate the time and cost of double data entry from the charge sheet into the computer system for claims submission. The right EHR system as a management partner should be able to provide a seamless revenue cycle process, from electronic eligibility verification to clinical and financial analytics, by providing

- ▶ Electronic eligibility verification
- ▶ Data entry controls to guarantee key patient information
- ▶ Alerts for missing medical records information
- ▶ Computer-assisted charge sheet and coding
- ▶ Electronic claims scrubbing and submission
- ▶ Payment reconciliation
- ▶ Extensive reporting capabilities
- ▶ Backup and disaster-recovery measures
- ▶ Industry knowledge and analytics
- ▶ Cloud technology without software update expense

The second step in choosing a partner is to personally meet with a company representative to discuss your center's management needs. Meeting face-to-face will provide an opportunity to evaluate whether the representative is competent and service oriented. Trust your instincts in determining whether you can build a collaborative working relationship. If you have difficulty working with the company representative, it may be an indicator of incompatibility. The right partner should be willing to adapt to your center's process and needs, not expect your center to accommodate a one-size-fits-all plan for claims processing and billing.

Use the evaluation list to carefully review the needs of your center against what the revenue management company can provide. Keep track of additional fees to determine whether the overall cost is unreasonable. Look for a business partner that does not break out and charge for every service separately. For example, the fee for the back-office service of electronic claims submission with basic accounts

Company Name:				
Services	Experience	Reputation	Fees	Impression
Credentialing				
Contract review				
Electronic claims				
Collection services				
Compliance audits				
Analytics				

Company Name:				
Services	Experience	Reputation	Fees	Impression
Credentialing				
Contract review				
Electronic claims				
Collection services				
Compliance audits				
Analytics				

Company Name:				
Services	Experience	Reputation	Fees	Impression
Credentialing				
Contract review				
Electronic claims				
Collection services				
Compliance audits				
Analytics				

Figure 3. Sample partner evaluation form.

receivable should fall within 3% to 8% of collections and should include financial reports at no additional charge.

Choose the company that is experienced, is service oriented, offers competitive rates, provides software and support services, and will be a good long-term partner but does not lock the center into a long-term agreement if the partnership doesn't work out as planned. Negotiate a service-oriented agreement that allows for a reasonable out clause without penalty and returns all data to the center if the partnership is dissolved.

The third and final step in choosing a revenue cycle management partner is verification of the contract and services rendered. You should never sign an agreement until you have read it carefully and have verified the following:

- Clarity of service definitions as negotiated
- Correctness of fees for contracted services
- Presence of a reasonable out clause without penalty
- Guarantee of service and performance levels
- Guarantee of compliance with the Health Insurance Portability and Accountability Act (HIPAA)
- Provision of certified coders in claims processing
- Data ownership by your urgent care center on contract termination
- Compliance and quality-assurance programs

Routinely review the fees and the quality of services rendered monthly. Develop a good working relationship with your management representative, and discuss any issue that your center encounters in the revenue cycle or problem that affects the cash flow of your center. Be available to exchange information about changes in regulatory, health plan contracts, and payment models. Be open to suggestions for improvement and encourage your partner to bring their expertise and ideas to your attention for discussion. Consider new lines of service to enhance the successful financial management of your center. This two-way dialogue will create a partnership that will improve your bottom line over time.

CONCLUSION

Urgent care centers carry the complete financial responsibility of providing patients with high-quality medical and diagnostic services. Any delays in payment for services can financially undermine a center's ability to provide care. Being proactive to manage the increasing complexities of the revenue cycle process, from patient registration to claims reimbursement, is critical to the center's financial success.

By choosing the right revenue cycle management partner, you will assist your center in managing the revenue cycle process, fulfill documentation and payment model requirements to supply consistent income, and deliver financial stability so that the center can continue providing quality medical services.

KEY POINTS

1. Revenue cycle management starts when a patient enters the facility for medical care and ends when services are paid for.
2. Successful management of patient registration is critical to the success of the revenue cycle management process.

3. Provide detailed training and uniform protocols for the registration staff to follow.
4. Use technology to verify patient eligibility, co-pays, and deductibles.
5. Accurate and complete medical documentation is a key component for charge capture, payment, and compliance.
6. Revenue cycle management requires attention to detail through consistent and systematic review of financial reports. Review monthly financial reports to evaluate the success of the revenue cycle process and management partnership.
7. Price isn't everything. Choose an experienced urgent care revenue management partner that is service oriented.
8. Read and carefully verify contractual services and fee structure before signing a partnership agreement.
9. Create a close working relationship with your management partner.
10. Hold your management partner accountable for missed metrics and poor service.

CHAPTER 25

Marketing Overview

Megan Lamy

MARKETING IS NOT JUST a matter of fulfilling a checklist of activities but is rather a process that requires much thought, analysis, creativity, implementation, and evaluation. The science of marketing is complex in that you are formulating and integrating a strategy across multiple delivery channels, an array of services and products, multiple business units, a large number of customers, and frequently varying customer goals—all of this within an ever-changing, competitive environment. Yet by applying the right marketing tools and processes, you'll be on your way to executing an effective marketing strategy to further your urgent care company. The order in which you approach this marketing process is important. Follow the sequence described in this chapter.

MARKETING ANALYSIS

An effective marketing strategy springs from a foundation of strong marketing analysis, including analyses of your customers, competition, and company. To determine how you are going to reach new customers, you must first determine who your targeted customers are, what the competition is offering, how they are targeting customers, and how your company should position itself in the marketplace.

Customer Analysis

Defining your target customers is one of the first steps in identifying your marketing strategy, which in turn will determine the marketing messages, campaigns, and channels you use. The urgent care industry is fortunate in that its services apply to a broad audience (adults, seniors, children and babies, professionals, families, and so forth). The challenge is that your marketing messages should be targeted and tailored specifically toward each of the various audiences. By segmenting your target market—that is, dividing it into subsets of customers with common needs or characteristics—you can better reach these various audiences with more targeted messages that match your company's benefits with their specific needs. Segmenting options to consider are segmenting by age, sex, geography, job function, industry, seniority, economic status (for discount programs), insurance plan type (such as Medicare), or customer life cycle. Market segmentation should be carefully considered for each individual urgent care clinic because the demographics, trends, and opportunities within each clinic's market can vary. So how do you determine who your targeted audiences are?

Internal Patient Data

If you have been in business for an extended time, then you may already have patient data to start answering this question. By analyzing past customer demographics and trends, you can begin to understand the types of customers who are frequenting your urgent care clinic, when or how often, and the value of these various audiences. This will not only give you an idea of your best type of existing customers to focus on but will also clue you in to potential customer segments that aren't visiting your clinic and can be added to the mix. If for some reason you do not have prior patient data to glean information from, or it is not in a format that can be automatically organized for analysis, you may have paper (or perhaps electronic) patient surveys that can be reviewed and assimilated for helpful information on patient demographics and trends. Alternatively, if you're still struggling to identify your customer prospects after failed attempts at these options, you can hire third-party organizations to perform demographic customer and prospect profiling, often using demographic overlays and a comprehensive database of US consumers to find prospects just like your best identified customers.

Market Analysis

During the process of choosing your urgent care clinic location, you probably performed a market analysis to understand whether the strengths, opportunities, attractiveness, and dynamics of your market outweighed the threats and weaknesses, and to make sure you were entering a sustainable market that allowed for market growth, profitability, resource channels, and other key success factors. By tapping into this research and expanding on it, you can better understand the potential customer bases and sources that are unique to your clinic's market. For instance, your clinic may be located within a college town, a city with a large Hispanic population, a retirement community, a downtown area surrounded by businesses and professionals, or a tourist hotspot, in which it makes sense for your clinic to target one (or some) of these specific audiences.

Competitive Analysis

Performing a competitive analysis allows you to determine the strengths and weaknesses of your market's competitors, develop any barriers that can prevent competition from entering your market, and identify the distinct advantages you have that should be promoted. It is critical to know the ins and outs of your competition when pursuing your own marketing initiatives. You must know what you're up against and how your services and value compare with those of other centers trying to earn new business or even steal your existing customers. A competitive analysis will also give you insight into creating the most effective and compelling marketing messages.

The simplest way to track all of the competition and their information is to complete a spreadsheet or some other thorough document that can be stored for easy access and updated regularly by your team. Recommended information to gather includes the following:

- Business name
- Address
- Proximity to your location
- Length of time in business
- Estimated market share
- Hours
- Services
- Website address
- Price comparisons
- Insurance accepted
- Staffing model (nurses, specialist physicians, primary-care physicians, emergency medical technicians, medical assistants, etc.)
- Unique offerings, programs, and value
- Marketing presence
- Strengths
- Weaknesses

By gathering and continually monitoring information on the competition, your company can better position itself ahead of them and aim its sights at being or becoming the urgent care leader in your market. Keep in mind that market leaders, who are consistently creating new industry and marketing concepts as well as unique service offerings, are also automatic targets for imitation. If you are the market leader or plan on being so, you must always be on the lookout for the next marketing progression, service improvement, or new addition to your business offerings that most likely doesn't exist yet. But if your company is behind the competition and their advantages are exceeding yours (which a competitive analysis should identify), then you should consider how your urgent care business, service, and marketing can become more competitive in the current market.

Company Analysis

Once you have identified your targeted customers and where the competition stands, it is time to evaluate your own company and how it can be best positioned in the minds of consumers. A company (or business) analysis is a discipline that identifies the changes to an organization that are necessary in order to achieve strategic goals. Although the topic of branding is covered in detail in Chapter 29, "Developing Your Brand," it is important to note here that a company analysis must involve the development of a brand promise for your organization. A *brand promise* is a detailed statement from the organization to customers identifying what values, characteristics, benefits, and behaviors consumers should expect from all interactions with the brand. Even though a brand promise is not typically distributed for external sources, it is a foundational commitment by your company to customers that should serve as an internal blueprint and steer every aspect of your business, including all of the marketing. The brand promise must be developed by or alongside the most senior leaders of your organization, because backing up this promise in every customer interaction will require complete organizational alignment and support and, quite possibly, some necessary organizational changes.

To arrive at one clear and concise sentence that boldly states what your customers can continually expect from your company (that is, your brand promise), you should consider the following specific questions:

- *How does your leadership team want the company to be positioned toward customers?* Conduct internal surveys among your leaders and team members, as well as interviews when necessary. This will give you insight into the collective brand values and competitive differentiators that your organization feels are the most important aspects of your brand.

- *What are your customers looking for in an urgent care company?* Send an external survey to existing customers who have opted in for further communication from you. You can also commission a focus group using people in the general community who match your targeted customers. It is preferable for the focus group to be run by a professional, third-party administrator.

- *Is your organization capable of delivering this desired brand?* Once the compiled results of these internal surveys, interviews, external surveys, and focus groups have been analyzed and coupled with the vision, mission, and values of your organization, you will have all of the necessary data and input required to create a strong and compelling brand promise. Now your leadership team must determine what organizational changes are necessary in order to deliver this promise without fail.

Note: Once you create a brand promise, you can take this a step further and develop your organization's *value proposition* and, if you truly have a unique competitive advantage in the industry, you can craft your *unique selling proposition*. Although these flow out of the brand promise and are important to articulate, they are not covered in depth in this chapter.

MARKETING PLANS AND GUIDES

After building your strong foundation of systematic analysis, it is time to develop your company's marketing strategy. This strategy will then drive your marketing messages, tactics, and campaigns. Outlining and documenting this strategy using the following plans and guides as tools will provide your marketing team with an organized overview of all the marketing components and how they will work together, as well as a game plan for tackling the various tactics your strategy has determined appropriate.

Marketing Budget

Before you can complete the marketing strategy, plans, and tactics, the marketing budget that your company will allocate toward all of its marketing efforts must be determined. Methods for determining how much of the overall budget should be allocated to marketing include the historical method (adding an increased percentage to the budget total used previously), the fixed percentage of sales method, the method based on marketing objectives, the method that uses industry averages, and the method that is a conglomerate of multiple methods. It will be up to your leadership team to determine the budget allocation method that is best for you and your current marketing goals. Keep in mind that this budget-allocation process should begin months before the calendar year that you are planning for so that your marketing budget can be determined and approved before the new year begins. As you tentatively plan your annual marketing budget breakouts in conjunction with documenting your marketing strategies and plans (after all, a marketing budget is the quantification of marketing plans), it is wise to make quarterly or even monthly commitments when you can, rather than annual commitments, so that your marketing budget can be adjusted based on results as you proceed. This is why it is important to track marketing costs as you go in order to analyze cost versus benefit.

Marketing and Sales Plans

In many industries, companies will typically develop both a marketing plan and a sales plan. The marketing plan, which contains much information from prior analysis, is an overview guide often composed of the following:

- ▶ An executive summary
- ▶ A situational and market analysis of several parameters, including
  - Targeted customers
  - The needs of those customers
  - Your competition
- ▶ A strengths, weaknesses, opportunities, and threats (SWOT) analysis for your company
- ▶ Your marketing objectives

- The marketing strategies, both short- and long-term and ranked in priority, that will achieve these objectives
- The tactics that will be executed under your marketing strategy

Your marketing objectives might be to maintain your existing base of customers but increase visits by the acquisition of new customers. An example of marketing strategies for these objectives would be outlining how you will use a positive patient experience and the promotion of new programs and services to maintain your existing customer base, and the various referral sources, community partnerships, and events you will target to expand your customer base.

In the sales plan, which is part of your overall marketing strategy, you focus on quantifying these objectives and the sales tactics that will be executed in order to achieve both specific, measurable results you've outlined and your overall marketing objective. Because of the overlapping nature of marketing and sales within the service-based urgent care industry, consider combining the marketing and sales plans into one document per region or representative. Further, deploy representatives who can successfully cover both marketing and sales within a given target market to maximize efficiency and better leverage community relationships.

Media and Advertising Plan

A media and advertising plan should be carefully developed once it has been determined that your budget allows for it and, more importantly, that it is a viable and cost-effective way to reach your targeted customer segments. For urgent care companies, most of the target markets are based on a defined geographic area surrounding a clinic location and may involve varying targeted customer segments if multiple locations exist. Because of the local nature of most urgent care companies and their marketing, mass media options (television, radio, billboard campaigns) are typically not the most worthwhile media options. It is best to implement localized media and advertising for your urgent care locations' target markets that have the most need and potential for increased business. Localized media examples include

- Local print publications targeting your chosen customer segments, such as
  - Parenting and family magazines
  - Printed college directories
  - Spanish-language publications
  - Newsletters for seniors
  - High school sports magazines
  - Newsletters for homeowners' associations or other neighborhood organizations
- Drive-time radio spots, preferably as part of a specific seasonal campaign, on local stations located within your target market only

- Outdoor signage that is in a prime location in relation to your clinic and target audience; this can sometimes be a more affordable option than additional building signage
- Direct mail campaigns like the service from the US Postal Service called Every Door Direct Mail, which is targeted at specific households on the basis of matching demographics, trends, and geographic location; see https://www.usps.com/business/every-door-direct-mail.htm

That being said, if you can leverage media buys across your markets from the same media partners that have been deemed effective (that is, the same parent radio station, publication, outdoor signage company, printing company), then you will be able to save on costs, allocate those funds elsewhere, and do more with your marketing budget. The same can be said about the opportunity to leverage paid media with a plan that capitalizes on nonpaid public relations opportunities.

A lot of additional detail and thought goes into creating a media plan. Consider these initial topics alone that must be addressed:

- *Which media channels are most appropriate for our targeted market segments?*
- *What is the reach, or total audience?*
- *What is the most effective frequency to use?* A good rule of thumb is to have a frequency of at least three times. It is much more effective to advertise frequently in smaller spaces for greater repetition and brand recognition than to have a one-time large, expensive ad.
- *How much money should be allocated in each medium?*
- *How cluttered is each of the desired media options?*
- *What is the overall impact of the media option as it relates to our customers?*
- *What is the best advertising size to cost ratio for each medium?*
- *What dates are most effective to secure?*
- *What are the best media channels for promoting seasonal campaigns and offers?*

And these are just some of the media plan considerations that need to be made! Creating a media plan is an involved task that requires media expertise and experience; it is also a time-consuming task because of the plethora of back-and-forth communication required with media representatives during both the creation and maintenance of the plan. However, if a media and advertising plan is done professionally and right, the time and significant costs involved in implementing it can reap large rewards for your company. If you do not have an employee on your team with a background in media, it would be in your best interest to consider partnering with a media specialist to help create this important plan and to educate your team on how it should be maintained.

Brand Standards Guide

A brand standards guide is an internal manual that outlines all of the dos and don'ts of the organization's brand identity, across a wide range of applications. Every organization should have a brand standards guide because it is essential to maintaining effective use of your brand components (logo, design, colors), enhancing the marketing efforts of your organization, avoiding misrepresentation of your brand, and ensuring that for consumers your brand (company) evokes trust, confidence, and professionalism. Brand standards guides can be simple, complex, or somewhere in between, but certain key information should be included:

- Your brand (company) description, which should correlate with and highlight your company's vision, mission, and values
- Your brand promise
- Acceptable and unacceptable usages of the brand and its symbols
- Specific element details: colors, designs, image styles, brand signature, accents, and so forth
- Typographic elements
- Messaging: tone, style, and guidelines for customer-segment communications
- Employee guidelines for customer interaction
- Templates for business documents, marketing collateral, signage, and electronic communication
- Reproduction guidelines for partnering vendors and agencies

Once you have compiled all of the key elements for your brand standards guide, finalized the design and details of the document, and obtained approval and buy-in from the company leaders, then it is time to distribute a copy (electronic or hard copy) of the guide to all company stakeholders, including employees. Delivery of the guide is best accompanied by brief brand standards training that reviews the importance of adhering to the guide and stresses the impact it has on how the company must operate and interact with customers. This guide will have the greatest impact on steering the professionalism, consistency, and effectiveness of your marketing and communications.

COMPELLING MARKETING MESSAGES AND COMMUNICATIONS

After performing analyses, creating a brand promise, and developing a brand standards guide, you have the basic components you need to start compiling and perfecting your marketing messages before formatting and deploying them. As you do so, keep in mind the following goals and recommendations.

Message-Development Goals

- Every message must adhere to the company's brand promise (which should already be aligned with the company's vision, mission, and values) and brand standards guide.

- Each message should be written with its relevance to the appropriate audience in mind and tailored toward the targeted customer segment.

- The marketing messages must grab your audience's attention, or your customers will never pay attention to the company information you are trying to distribute.

- The various messages should have a clear call to action and objective that must be easily identifiable to the audience.

- Your messaging must differentiate your company from the competition and position you ahead of them in the minds of the readers.

- Avoid using the passive voice or words that do not reflect confidence and trust (such as *maybe*, *try*, *could*, *hope*). Direct commands are ideal.

- Your messages are a reflection of your company, so they must be professional in nature, edited thoroughly for the removal of mistakes, and designed to impress.

Message-Formatting Recommendations

Collateral

There is a wide array of collateral formats that you can use to reach customers, so put careful thought into the format, size, and message length that is going to be most effective for your targeted audience. You can certainly focus on one targeted collateral piece per customer segment that speaks the messages you want them to receive and act on, but you must also balance the printing cost of tailoring all your collateral to specific segments. Be creative and consider options that allow you to get your non-segment-specific content out to all (for example, a trifold brochure), but include an insert or even a section for variable data printing to tailor a portion to targeted customer segments. If you feel it's worthwhile in the long run to print different collateral pieces specific to segments, then choose less-expensive options that can be easily updated and reproduced, such as a one-sided flyer that can be printed in-house versus a brochure that requires professional printing.

Design elements and formatting play a huge role when you are creating collateral because they have the power to grab and keep consumers' attention, separate out content into more digestible bites (or bullets), and greatly enhance the look and tone of pieces. In your brand standards guide, the design elements should already be invented and used consistently. In addition to the branding, messaging, and contact information in your collateral, be sure to include a trackable call to action so that you can measure the effectiveness of your collateral. Tracking examples include but are not limited to unique 1-800 tracking numbers, unique links to special website landing pages, coupon codes, and QR (Quick Response) codes, which are two-dimensional bar codes that allow customers to access digital information from printed materials.

Signage

Creating messages for marketing signage (whether it be a billboard, bus shelter sign, banner, or vehicle advertisement) is challenging because you have to convey your brand in an extremely succinct and memorable way (ideally in eight or fewer words) in hopes of building strong brand recognition. Two of the most important elements of sign messaging that you will not want to leave out are your company's logo and contact information, preferably branded (such as a unique-link landing page or a 1-800 tracking number).

Promos

Choosing effective promotional pieces (promos) for your marketing efforts is more challenging than it may seem. Although your promo items should align with your brand and service, they should be unique, attention-grabbing, useful, long-lasting (have a long shelf life), and relevant to your audience. Because there is usually not a lot of room to print on promo items, the company information you choose to include is critical. These pieces are used primarily for brand recognition and top-of-mind awareness, so you ideally want to include your company logo, contact info (a unique-link landing page and a phone number that preferably can be tracked), and your tag line if it is a strong one that helps clarify and identify your service. By focusing on a few highly effective promotional pieces and ordering them in bulk for multiple clinic locations, you will obtain economies of scale and can stretch your promotional dollar. You can also save on costs by wisely distributing promotional pieces: Choose the most effective item to give to your target customers instead of blanketing them with multiple costly promotional products that are not all likely to be saved.

LOCAL MARKETING: BUILDING CONTINUAL REFERRAL SOURCES

Local marketing is where the tactics outlined in your marketing and sales plan come into play. To realize the marketing objective of increasing visits by acquiring new customers, start building relationships and partnerships in the medical field, business world, and community that can become continual referral sources for your urgent care locations. The process of building and maintaining these referral source relationships is time-consuming and repetitive; your marketing team will soon begin to see which partnerships have the most potential to refer customers to your urgent care locations. By thoroughly documenting all of these referral source interactions in a sophisticated customer-relationship management program, your marketing employees will be able to analyze which types of relationships are proving to be the most worthwhile so that they can focus their attention most effectively.

Take some time to consider which of the following referral sources make the most sense for your team to target, what unique partnerships or referral programs you can develop for them, and which of your company benefits or offerings will resonate the most with each of these sources. Explore event and sponsorship opportunities that will provide significant value for your company on the basis of the time and costs involved. It is crucial that your marketing employees be trained in the areas of health-care law that specifically apply to marketing and sales so that they can adhere to these laws while seeking referrals.

- Medical field
  - Primary-care physicians and other appropriate specialists
  - Pharmacists
  - Hospitals
  - Urgent care competition with significantly shorter hours of operation
  - First responders

- Opportunities within businesses
  - Occupational medicine
  - Influenza vaccines
  - Events
  - Human resources recruiting (when fitting)

- Community
  - Schools (nurses, coaches, front-office staff, teachers, and principals)
  - Day-care centers
  - Senior centers
  - Hotels, apartments, and recreational vehicle centers
  - Residential homes (most efficiently targeted by media advertising and direct mail)

- Events
  - Communities and neighborhoods
  - Nonprofit organizations
  - Health walks and runs
  - Sports
  - Families (children, parents)
  - Seniors
  - Professional networking
  - Chamber of Commerce events (the effectiveness of chambers varies by city and region)

- Sponsorships
  - Sports leagues (professionals, amateur adults, and little leagues)
  - Events (see the preceding list)

ENHANCING CUSTOMER RELATIONSHIPS AND LOYALTY

As you continue your local marketing efforts in order to acquire new patients, you'll need to be continually thinking about how your company will enhance and add value to your center's relationships with both existing and new customers. How will your company develop and secure the loyalty of these patients? Here are some questions and examples to contemplate:

- In what ways can we create a more positive patient experience?
  - Stellar customer service
  - Service guarantee
  - Timeliness
  - Cleanliness
  - Discount program for qualifying patients
  - VIP program
  - Follow-up care

- What are additional convenience factors that will have customers coming back to our location versus a competing center?
  - Online check-in
  - Priority check-in
  - The ability to wait wherever you would like
  - Availability of appointments
  - Electronic records accessible at all your company's locations
  - Bills payable online

- What forms of communication will continue to positively solidify our brand in these customers' minds and educate them on additional available services?
  - Clinic signage
  - Discharge paperwork
  - Website
  - Call-backs
  - Advertising and media
  - Email campaigns
  - Direct mail

TRACKING RESULTS AND SOURCES OF SUCCESS

Tracking the quantifiable effectiveness of your marketing strategy and tactics is a must. By correlating efforts with actual results, you can improve marketing performance, draw support for marketing from the rest of the company, and allocate budgets more effectively. Setting up marketing analytics will all be in vain, however, if you do not analyze and act on the resulting data to improve marketing performance.

CONCLUSION

There are plenty of marketing tactics that your urgent care company can use, but these do not drive your marketing strategy. Instead, developing your company's marketing strategy upfront and on the foundation of analysis and budget is critical to efficient and effective marketing. This strategy will then drive your marketing messages, tactics, and campaigns. Outlining and breaking out this strategy within a defined marketing plan (and in many cases an advertising and media plan) will help your marketing team members schedule their time and tackle the various tactics that your strategy has determined are appropriate. Through these tactics you'll focus on reaching targeted new customers, developing customer loyalty, and creating continual referral sources. By tracking the results of these marketing efforts, you'll be able to identify the marketing channels that are successfully driving patient traffic and revenue growth, increasing return on investment, or meeting whatever goals that you are using to evaluate the success of your urgent care center.

KEY POINTS

1. The order in which you approach the marketing process is critical.
2. An effective marketing strategy springs from a foundation of strong marketing analysis of your targeted customers, your competition, and your company.
3. By segmenting your target market—that is, dividing it into subsets of customers with common needs or characteristics—you can better reach various audiences with more-targeted messages that match your company's benefits with their specific needs.
4. Performing a competitive analysis allows you to determine the strengths and weaknesses of your market's competitors, develop barriers that can prevent competition from entering your market, and identify the distinct advantages you have that should be promoted.
5. Spend the time necessary to create your company's brand promise (a detailed statement from the organization to customers that identifies what values, characteristics, benefits, and behaviors consumers should expect from all interactions with the brand) and your brand standards guide (an internal manual that outlines all of the dos and don'ts of the organization's brand identity, across a wide range of applications).
6. Develop a marketing and sales plan per region or representative. Deploy representatives who can successfully implement both the marketing and

sales tactics of this plan within a given target market in order to maximize efficiency and better leverage community relationships.

7. Implement localized media and advertising for your urgent care locations' target markets, specifically pursuing the markets that have the most need and potential for increased business.

8. Developing compelling marketing messages requires reflection of your brand promise and guide, relevance to your audience, an attention-grabbing factor, a clear call to action, differentiation, the avoidance of the passive voice, and professionalism.

9. Build relationships and partnerships in the medical field, business world, and community in order to establish continual referral sources for your urgent care locations. Nurture and enhance these customers' relationships and loyalty by creating a more positive, convenient patient experience and strategically implementing ongoing, branded communication.

10. Tracking the quantifiable effectiveness of your marketing strategy and tactics, which includes analyzing and acting on the resulting data to improve marketing performance, is a must.

CHAPTER 26

Consumer Engagement Using Social Media

Lisa Cintron

THE EVOLUTION OF MEDICAL PROVIDER AND PATIENT INTERACTION IN SOCIAL MEDIA

Social media has profoundly altered the way medical institutions, health-care providers, and urgent care clinics communicate with their audiences. Millions have made online sharing part of their everyday lives, creating new communication channels and challenges for industries of all kinds. If a brand is not on the social media bandwagon, it is missing out on an essential and fundamental method of connecting and communicating with its market.

Brand communication has come full circle. Before the emergence of radio or television, print and word-of-mouth marketing were the only advertising vehicles available. With each technological advance, the gap between the brand and the end consumer was widening until eventually brands were doing all the talking and the consumer was doing all the listening. Currently, commercials on radio, television, and now Internet sites are increasingly bold and obnoxious and delivered at higher and higher decibels. Consumers are bombarded with everything from billboards on roadways to signage on buses, subways, and gas pumps and in checkout lines at the grocery store. Consumers simply cannot get away from the bombardment of messages selling them something hundreds of times a day.

Enter social media, an apparently quieter and gentler mode of communication, spawned by groups consisting of friends and acquaintances supporting each other's mutual hobbies and interests. This was a way to keep in touch on a whole new level. Word-of-mouth marketing, which was in action primarily during social gatherings and around dinner tables, now had another venue and soon joined the online media blitz. Honest, uncensored online conversations were now possible, giving people the opportunity to review products, services, and medical providers and discuss everything from the best diaper to the presidential election.

Such conversations have quickly become the mainstay of the 21st century. By 2013, activities related to social media had made it into the everyday lives of millions and millions of people. These activities are changing the way marketing messages are crafted, shared, and delivered.

NARROWING THE GAP OF COMMUNICATION WITH SHARING AND ENGAGING

Social media has become a significant aspect of business development. It has altered the way individuals and businesses communicate about brands and how they conduct business. Social media is responsible for condensing corporate hierarchies and compressing the theory of "6 degrees of separation" down to about 4.74 degrees.[1]

Social media was not a corporate- or media-invented activity but was invented, invested in, and driven by the people. Hence, corporations, media outlets, and brands had to change the way they engaged and conducted business with their end consumers.

Today the Internet is nearly as dynamic as real life, and buyer behavior has shifted in response. Patients are smarter, savvier, and more informed about what they want and need. They educate themselves about medical issues and treatments and research medical providers before they decide on an office visit. Asking a physician a question online to make an informed medical decision has become the status quo for anyone who uses the Internet. With such tools in place, medical clinics and providers have the ability to position themselves at key points in the consumer decision-making process. Urgent care clinics and providers must fully integrate with the social scene in terms of search engines, social media, content, and blogging to take advantage of the times when the patient is searching for information.

Let's look at a timeline that demonstrates how much has changed since 2000.

CONSUMER BUYING AND DECISION-MAKING TIMELINE

Before the emergence of social media, consumer behavior was dictated by television, radio, and published media, through which information was disseminated to the public. Brands decided what they wanted the consumer to know about their products and services and crafted high-marketing-dollar campaigns to drive the message out.

The buying and decision-making timeline (Figure 1) shows us that brands literally created the buying cycle in an attempt to lead consumers to believe they needed or wanted the proffered products or services. Radio and television commercials, as well as print ads, guided this monumental task by reaching out and capturing the attention of buyers. However, though brands with huge marketing budgets could afford such media blitzes, smaller businesses with less-robust marketing budgets were often left in the dust. With the advent of social media,

---

1 Markoff J, Sengupta S. Separating you and me? 4.74 degrees, *New York Times*, 2011 November 21. Available from http://www.nytimes.com/2011/11/22/technology/between-you-and-me-4-74-degrees.html.

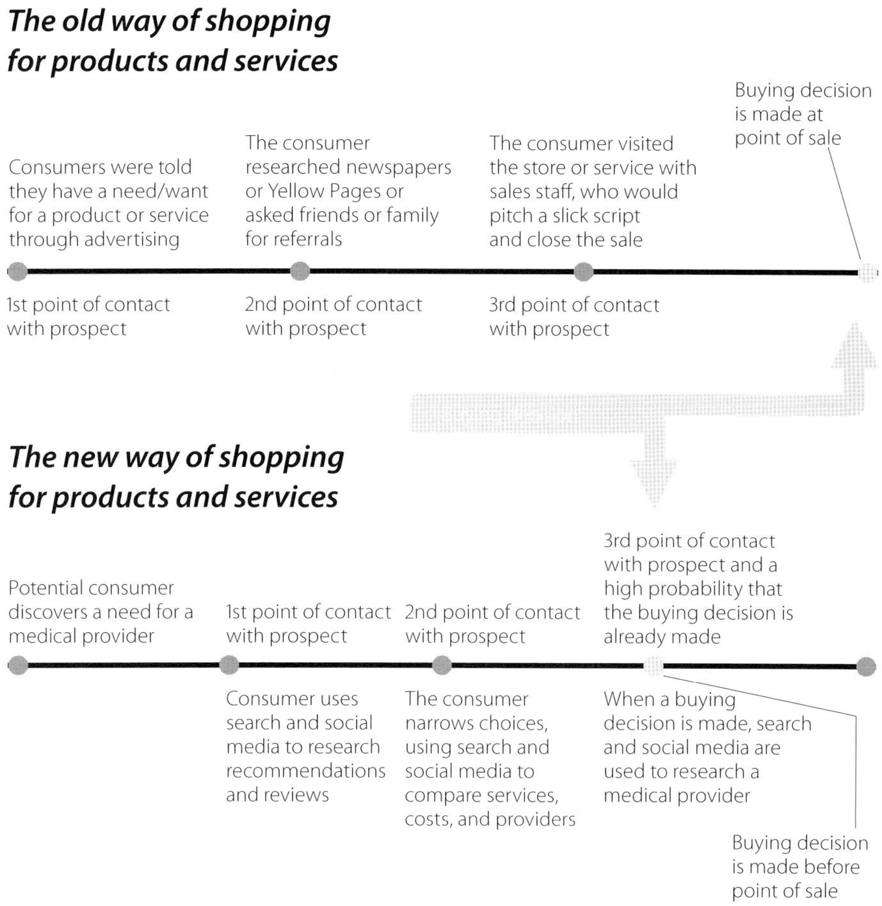

The old way of shopping for products and services

1st point of contact with prospect	2nd point of contact with prospect	3rd point of contact with prospect	
Consumers were told they have a need/want for a product or service through advertising	The consumer researched newspapers or Yellow Pages or asked friends or family for referrals	The consumer visited the store or service with sales staff, who would pitch a slick script and close the sale	Buying decision is made at point of sale

The new way of shopping for products and services

	1st point of contact with prospect	2nd point of contact with prospect	3rd point of contact with prospect and a high probability that the buying decision is already made
Potential consumer discovers a need for a medical provider	Consumer uses search and social media to research recommendations and reviews	The consumer narrows choices, using search and social media to compare services, costs, and providers	When a buying decision is made, search and social media are used to research a medical provider. Buying decision is made before point of sale

Figure 1. The consumer buying and decision-making timeline as it used to be versus in the age of social media.

small and medium enterprises now have just as much leverage as the big brands to capture market share. The days when only Fortune 500 companies dominated the airwaves and drove consumer behavior are most certainly over—or nearly so.

To position your urgent care center at key points on the buying and decision-making timeline, follow these 11 steps:

1. Define your target market and campaign goals.
   - Ask: Who are your existing patients?
   - Expand on your list of existing patients to include your ideal patient.
2. Create a website about your specialty and services with a good clean design and great content. The goals of your website are to provide a memorable first impression *and* to deliver attractive visual content that is educational.

3. Incorporate a blog into your website; blogs are activity hubs for content-sharing on social sites. Blog posts should be sharable content in that they are educational, inspirational, and thought-provoking. This is content that people want to share and link to.
4. Create accounts for the social media platforms you wish to use in your marketing campaign (Figure 2). Fully complete all profiles, histories, and timelines and upload photos and logos. In 2013 the top social media platforms were
   - Facebook
   - Twitter
   - LinkedIn
   - Google+
   - Pinterest
   - Instagram
   - Reddit
5. Add and link all social media accounts to your website, your blog, and to each other.

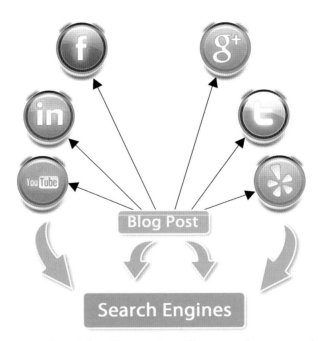

Figure 2. Structure of a social media campaign. All concepts from your website, blog, and user-generated social media content flow to and are used by search engines to index your website.

6. Add social media buttons to each page of your website as well as a social media action block to allow your website visitors to "like," "share," and "+1" your pages or pieces of content.
7. Announce your site to friends, family, and current patients and colleagues through all social media platforms and email. Ask them to "like," "tweet," "link," and "+1" your site. This will start building your network.
8. Continue to build your network by adding friends, contacts, and followers.
9. Create an editorial blogging calendar of creative and useful content ideas for your posts.
10. Create 10 to 15 blog posts at a time and add them to your editorial calendar. Most blogging content management systems have the ability to automate the submission and release of individual blog posts. The goal is to be consistent, adding at least two blog posts per week. Posts should
    - Be original and have unique content
    - Be in the range of 400 to 1500 words in length
    - Include video, photos, or audio podcasts
    - Link to outside sources to add value
11. Syndicate and share each blog post with all of your social media accounts.

Positioning is key. When the patient is ready to research a medical condition or medical provider, you want your information there to fulfill their need for due diligence. Therefore, a consistent presence on social media platforms is essential to capture the attention of potential patients during their decision-making process (Figure 3).

LEVERAGING SOCIAL MEDIA NETWORKS IN REFERRAL MARKETING

Unlike a direct network of friends, family, and colleagues, which is smaller and typically cited as representing only 1 degree of separation, a social media network is a much more diverse and larger system. On average, a Facebook user has approximately 130 friends separated by 2 degrees; that translates to a social network of about 10,000 friends for only 1 individual.[2] Social media tools have such an enormous reach that any blog post, article, or piece of content will literally reduplicate in a network thousands and potentially millions of times.

However, leveraging a network is much more than posting pieces of content and waiting for potential prospects to find them; it's about building relationships. The capacity to go back to the basics of human interaction will determine where the strength of a brand will lie.

---

2 Statista: Average number of Facebook friends of U.S. users in 2013, by age group, from Arbitron, Edison Research. Available from http://www.statista.com/statistics/232499/americans-who-use-social-networking-sites-several-times-per-day/.

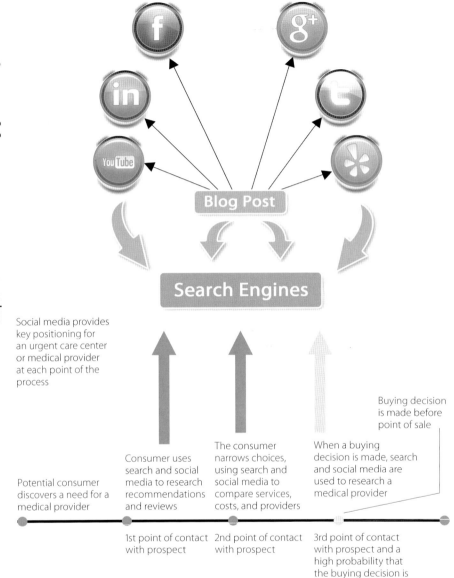

Figure 3. Fulfillment of consumer actions at key points of contact using social media and search engines.

LEVERAGING CONSUMER-GENERATED CONTENT THROUGH RELATIONSHIPS

Consumer-generated content is content written and posted by website visitors in response to a blog post, a comment, article, video, or anything that inspires them to comment on your brand, business, products, or services. Comments show up everywhere on the Internet—on websites, social media sites, and in forums—and can have tremendous value in positioning the search engines to help build a brand. Remember too that negative comments can be quite destructive if not addressed.

How can a brand build a stellar online reputation and avoid potentially destructive consumer-generated content? With a solid proactive system in place to handle consumer complaints and concerns before they get out of hand. A proactive system includes a customer service policy that is already ingrained in the DNA of the company, allowing its concepts to flow naturally into any online social media efforts and engage with the audience in a positive way.

How to Win Friends and Influence People, a book first published in 1936 by influential writer and motivational speaker Dale Carnegie, became one of the best-selling self-help books of all time. In it, Carnegie talks about building relationships to achieve financial success, which is just as important today as it was in the 1930s:

> 15 percent of one's financial success is due to one's technical knowledge and about 85 percent is due to skill in human engineering—to personality and the ability to lead people.[3]

Let's look at some of Carnegie's principles more closely to get a better idea of how relationship building can empower and facilitate a mutually beneficial relationship between a company and social media.

Principle 1: Show a Genuine Interest in Other People

Start with people, not technology. One of the barriers to entering the social media arena is that it takes time to cultivate and create meaningful relationships. Social media offers an abundance of tools for leveraging time and effort, but it is the interaction between the brand or medical provider and the potential patient that is important. When medical providers are deeply engaged with their audience because they truly care and are interested in providing the best services and information, people feel the caring behind the effort and are attracted to it.

Principle 2: Smile

Smiling is a simple, easy way to make a good first impression. How can you smile while you're sitting at your computer? Make sure the photos you upload show you when you're smiling, for one thing, instead of when you are frowning or looking offscreen instead of at the viewer. For another, when you're posting, sharing, and

---

3   Carnegie D. *How to Win Friends and Influence People*, New York, NY: Simon & Schuster, 2009.

engaging online, display an energy that is reflective of a smile, not a frown. A logo is not conducive to the cultivation of an honest and conversational relationship with human beings—with your audience. Frankly, even a photo of your dog can generate a certain amount of interest. For your urgent care center, include a photo of your supporting staff members looking pleased to be working with patients.

Joy, compassion, friendliness, and concern can be conveyed through a written message just as clearly as it can directly through a message spoken by one human being to another in the same room. Customer-service organizations have long taught that if you're on the telephone, it always helps to smile; though the customer on the other end can't see you, they can feel the smile radiate right through the phone lines. Infusing your social media campaigns with inspirational content is sure to provoke smiles as well. Take a look at Stride gum and its "Where the hell is Matt?" campaign, with more than 80 million views combined across three videos. These videos show Matt Harding dancing—joyously, if badly—with people of various native cultures in front of famous landmarks and sightseeing spots. Matt, who had uploaded his original video to YouTube in its early days to share his travels with friends and family, was probably as surprised as the rest of us when it went viral and reached millions of viewers.

Eventually, Stride offered Matt the opportunity to produce two more videos. Matt, however, insisted that the integrity of his original creation remain intact. To this end, the only branding message you see in Stride's videos is a logo discreetly placed on the screen when the credits roll and in the information section on YouTube. Stride easily achieved its goal of making people smile and encouraging a feel-good response to their brand and product. This campaign is considered one of the most memorable in social media history.

Principle 3: Remember, One's Name Is the Sweetest and Most Important Sound in Any Language

Carnegie says that a person's name is the sweetest and most important sound in any language, but in the age of social media, it's also the sweetest and most important *sight*.

Facebook has been the leader in using friends' names in posts and photos. One of the reasons people flocked to Facebook early on was for its photo-sharing and tagging capabilities. Now, with the ability to use face recognition and tag friends in comments and captions, the potential benefits are enormous. At this point, though we cannot hear our name audibly, we can see it highlighted in photos and comments.

Direct marketers have been using this technique for decades, and email marketers use it too. Direct mail and email often include a personal greeting such as "Dear Joe" or "Hello, Mrs. Smith." The mailing may go to a list of thousands, but each reader feels as if that email or that piece of snail mail has been sent personally to them. Such tactics have been proven to increase conversion rates exponentially.

Personalization is key in social media too. Addressing customers by name can have a big impact. One method is by using the @ sign before an individual's name so that they know a comment or a post is directed at them. This is an efficient way to target a specific person in an online conversation, and audiences appreciate the extra touch.

Principle 4: Be a Good Listener; Encourage Others to Talk About Themselves

Seek first to understand, then to be understood.

Social media can enhance a company's ability to pursue open-ended communication with its customer base. But the expectation should be to understand the customer first. One way to explain the intricacies of social media is to liken it to a social gathering or party, because the same kinds of behaviors—the ones that either draw people to each other or push them apart—are also inherent in social media transactions.

When a brand increases self-reference, it only promotes its products and services, so its viral capacity declines. In other words, when the company or brand talks exclusively about itself, its audience won't be interested in sharing its content, which reduces the reach of the message.

When implementing social media, you should aim a portion of the content at encouraging open-ended discussion, with the intention of creating a dialogue or reaction. Such dialogues take place between brand and consumer, and betweeen consumer and consumer. Conversations should include commenting, asking and answering, rating, reviewing, and promoting content.

Many companies have lofty goals of implementing a social media campaign. Yet many times when the audience does engage with a piece of content, the company chooses to walk away rather than respond. When the company shows no inclination to change this reaction, the audience soon feels undermined and undervalued—and then ceases to engage at all. Eventually, the social media campaign is aborted and deemed a failure.

Brands spend millions of dollars in market research to understand their customers. If a social media plan is executed consciously and with care, it can deliver a big bang for very few bucks. The critical piece is understanding that implementation requires knowing how to listen *and* respond. Additionally, social media can bolster the reputation of a company that has poor customer service. But again, for this type of engagement to be successful, it's the company's DNA that matters. When customers have a problem, issue, or complaint, they want to be heard; they want to know that someone is listening. Even if the problem can't be solved in the way the customers want or expect, listening to them can help defuse a potentially volatile situation. Social media can be used as a platform to encourage this type of two-way communication. Truly listening and engaging is sure to create a loyal customer following.

Principle 5: Interest People

The best way to interest other people is to talk about *them—their* interests. Truly relevant content can be identified only by understanding the interests, needs, and pain points of the consumer's social community. Participating and engaging requires regular interaction between brand and audience. It also requires awareness about what your audience is discussing on their pages and in their sphere of influence. Interesting content leads to engagement; engagement leads to social media and search engine results.

Principle 6: Make People Feel Important, But Do It Sincerely

Justin Bieber is a great example of this principle. He has a talent for making his fans feel important. Even before he was discovered and signed by Usher, he had almost single-handedly established a loyal following by using smart marketing techniques, including keeping his tween followers abreast of his everyday activities and uploading homemade videos of his school auditorium performances across the country. When his debut album came out, millions of fans lined up to buy it. Justin dedicated an entire year to gaining insight into his fans through active engagement. The fans responded by feeling that they were first in Bieber's heart and soul. The continued feedback appears to keep Bieber grounded and close to his devotees. His method has clearly made him an entertainer with one of the most loyal group of followers in the industry. Smart!

But you don't need to be Justin Bieber to make someone feel important. A business or brand should never forget that without their customers they wouldn't exist. The lesson to be learned from recent years is that a company should never be out of touch with its customer base. Maintaining a dialogue is the best way to stay relevant. Relevance keeps your customers feeling that they're the most important people in the world.

HOW SOCIAL MEDIA VENUES AFFECT SEARCH

In 2010, Google's Caffeine algorithm update put a new spin on the link between social media and search engines. Until then, the theory that the two were definitively linked was relatively unproven. With the Caffeine update, it can no longer be denied that social media has an impact on search. The link between social media and search is twofold:

- ▶ Social media sites act as feeder sites into other main sites, building a solid foundation of links that support and deliver page rank into main monetary sites. Although a valid point can be made that social media links are coded behind the scenes as "no-follow" (meaning that search engines won't monitor the pages carrying the links), that doesn't matter when we look at how sites increase their search rank by using only social media sites.

- ▶ High levels of social activity establish websites in search engine rankings. When a brand is engaged and offers valuable content to its readers, resultant signals to the search engines increase a website's authority in the ranking algorithm.

Use these three simple strategies to help boost search engine presence through social media:

- Employ keyword-rich titles and content.
- Employ keyword-rich alt text in images. (Alt text is coding that describes the images when a cursor hovers over them.)
- Add regular updates to trigger Google's Freshness algorithm for temporary increases in search engine rankings.

CONCLUSION

Is social media really advertising's holy grail, as it's touted to be? When approached in a consistent, organized, well-thought-out fashion, social media can deliver traffic and conversions. Social media is about investing time to build assets the way you might in real estate—by purchasing a number of "Internet properties" that will provide value to your business for many years to come. Social media is about fulfilling the needs of your consumers for information while educating them about your brand. It's about nurturing customer relationships, valuing those relationships, and delivering what your customers are searching for. It's about co-creating with customers and prospects to reach a mutually satisfying end: a win-win for everyone.

Finally, social media is the place where the 21st century meets the new generation to execute a new way of doing business.

KEY POINTS

1. Patients have changed the way they research medical conditions and medical practices, make decisions, and conduct due diligence. They are smarter, savvier, and more informed about what they want and need and about whom they are willing to have treat them.

2. Having a website is no longer optional; it is essential to be competitive regardless of the market. A website or blog also provides businesses and brands with a vehicle for participating in social media and becoming part of the online conversation.

3. Consumers and patients make their decisions much sooner and on the basis of more information than ever before. When patients are ready to make a decision on a medical provider, your urgent care center must already be in position in the search results by consistently engaging in online conversations.

4. Social media can provide enormous reach for any blog post, article, or piece of content and will literally reduplicate that content in a network thousands and potentially millions of times.

5. Make sure you have a customer or patient service policy as part of your social media strategy to help defuse any negative social media comments.

6. Social media is about a lot more than just posting information about you and your medical clinic. It's about building long-term customer relationships and engaging in ongoing conversations to produce loyal followers.

7. Apply the six main principles in Dale Carnegie's *How to Win Friends and Influence People* to your social media strategy to get positive results.

8. Social media and search are tightly linked. Brands highly engaged in social media outlets benefit from increased authority in search engine rankings.

9. Social media can affect search and increase website ranking in the search engines. Therefore, social media can help drive traffic to a website.

10. When considering the investment of time in social media, think of it as establishing a property position online where each one requires ongoing care and nurturing.

CHAPTER 27

Public Relations: A Tool for Success

Erin Terjesen

From remote rural towns to major metropolitan areas, the United States has seen explosive growth in the number of urgent care center openings since the early 2000s. Despite this increase, many urgent care centers and networks have been slow to include public relations (PR) in their collection of communication tools to position these centers as easy, fast, high-quality, and affordable solutions for nationwide health care.

Whether your vision is to operate an urgent care business as a single-location practice or as part of a multistate health provider network, using PR and best practices for working with the media are critical. Your urgent care center must establish awareness within the business and local communities, positioning its medical expertise and the range of solution-oriented health-care services that it can offer.

Using PR to gain local or national media attention is both a cost-effective and results-oriented practice that will build your business and brand, as well as help patients to distinguish your urgent care center from the competition. As a key element to your business operations, PR services can be managed in partnership with a sole PR practitioner or a PR agency, or with an internal full-time and media-trained resource.

The most critical goals for executing strategic PR efforts as part of an urgent care center's communications tool set include the opportunity to

- Establish or raise awareness of the urgent care center as an innovative and patient-friendly health-care delivery channel
- Promote the expertise and level of care patients will receive
- Position your urgent care center's medical leadership as subject-matter experts on medical or regulatory affairs

Every urgent care center is well equipped with state-of-the-art equipment and a talented, highly qualified staff, but if patients or potential patients do not know about the solutions, convenience, expertise, and customer service an urgent care center provides patients every day, the business may suffer if new patients are not seeking you out.

For urgent care practices, incorporating strategic, consistent, and properly supported PR efforts will provide exposure by writing and pitching news-related stories.

Whether you plan to use a full-time, in-house communications professional or a contracted PR agency partner, PR stories will be created with the sole purpose of creating interest on the part of local and national media outlets. Because urgent care medicine provides innovative health-care services through a trifecta of highly qualified providers, business management expertise, and superior customer service, a PR professional or agency is critical to helping build the right lists of media markets, editors, writers, and other outlets to get your message out there clearly and effectively.

Not only is PR free of the expense and sticker shock of traditional paid advertising, but it also establishes increased credibility with patients or prospective patients through objective third-party coverage.

WHAT DOES PUBLIC RELATIONS SUCCESS LOOK LIKE?

Outline a list of key objectives for what defines a successful PR campaign or communications initiative for your unique urgent care business, as well as a list of media outlets you would consider for speaking directly to your target markets. To get started, make a list of goals such as these:

- Bring new patients into your urgent care center by establishing key separators from competition (convenience, affordability, certified medical professionals, expanded services, technology, shorter waits or shorter door-to-doctor times, etc.) and keep existing patients coming back as repeat customers
- Highlight success stories of current patients' positive experiences
- Position urgent care medicine and the skilled, friendly staff as health-care experts (locally or nationally, depending on your business model)
- Build awareness of the full range of your urgent care center's services
- Localize national urgent care centers by making them more present and involved in local community events, publications, websites, and so on
- Promote a growing involvement in the local community through charitable partnerships, education, special localized promotions, and sponsorships

THE HUNGRY MEDIA

If you were to ask a panel of health-care, medical, or community writers, healthcare or lifestyle bloggers, or broadcast media representatives, most panel members would tell you that they rarely receive health-care stories and medical news from urgent care centers, and that the majority of such items that are pitched come from either hospitals with large in-house communications staff or massive PR agencies contracted with health-care-related giants such as pharmaceutical companies. Reporters are hungry for short, compelling, and community-focused stories, which is perfectly aligned with the urgent care center business model. This presents key opportunities for urgent care centers to step in and present their medical expertise, achievements, statistics, and unique services that the individual center or group of centers provides to their community.

Using best practices with any PR and media initiatives is critical to positioning your business effectively and securing the placement opportunities available across print, online, and broadcast media outlets. PR can be a very cost-effective use of marketing dollars if best practices are understood. To effectively present story ideas to reporters and media representatives and have the best chance of securing placement, it is important to remember some small insider tips that can make a big difference.

What Defines Media in Today's World?

The types of outlets that are considered to be media continue to evolve. From traditional multimedia such as print, which once included only magazines and newspapers, to television and radio of the broadcast world, to new media, such as socially powerful websites, highly influential bloggers, and social media destinations such as Facebook, Twitter, Google+, Pinterest, LinkedIn, and much more, each type of outlet requires communication in a distinct voice to a more personalized audience.

How to Talk the Talk: Using Media to Offer Your Target Market Real Solutions

It is critical that you take the time to understand who your prospective patients are, where they look when seeking health care, and what solutions they want.

The first question any PR professional should answer for every story or media pitch is "Why should I care?" This may sound simplistic, but writers, editors, and bloggers receive hundreds (if not thousands) of emails and pitches every day, so establishing the answer to that question early on is critical. Separate yourself from the pack by creating a hook in the headline of your press materials or subject line of your email that will not only catch a writer's attention but also (and most importantly) keep it, so they feel confident they are offering their readers, followers, viewers, or listeners tangible, easy-to-understand solutions.

In creating a calendar of media-targeted content, make sure your news is focused on solving problems or serving as a patient and/or community resource. Focus on needs that often go unmet for patients who need immediate medical attention, such as

- *Availability*   Do urgent care centers offer a larger range of flexible hours (evenings, weekends, walk-ins, etc.) at times when the offices of primary-care physicians tend to be closed?

- *Affordability*   How do the costs patients will experience at your urgent care center compare with those of hospital emergency departments in the same geographic area, both with and without health plan participation?
- *Location, location, location*   Where is your urgent care center located in relation to your target patient's demographics?

Determining What Is Newsworthy: Creating Your Own News

When you are so closely tied to the business or health-care practice side of your urgent care center, it may be difficult to see all the many newsworthy things going on. This is why an external PR partner or agency can offer a tremendous amount of perspective, strategy, and insight and can even create news when nothing outside of the ordinary is going on.

Working as a partner with urgent care centers, PR professionals should consider an expansive range of key areas for writing stories:

- The expertise of your medical staff as subject-matter experts and/or consumer health advocates
- The availability of state-of-the-art equipment
- Statistics on door-to-doctor time at your center in comparison with door-to-doctor time for many overcrowded urban emergency departments
- Achievements in customer service
- Rankings of customer satisfaction and rates of referral
- Medical compliance
- Key community or charitable partnerships
- Achievements, awards, or other forms of recognition
- Embracing technology, from check-in to check-out and beyond
- Hot public topics such as
  - Immunizations
  - Seasonal flu and available vaccinations
  - Sports or annual physicals
  - Overcrowding of emergency departments
  - Health-care accessibility and affordability, regardless of insurance

PUBLIC RELATIONS TACTICS

PR tactics involve a variety of activities, including the following:

- Creation of the "Why should I care?" hook and newsworthy story
- Researching and writing content for press releases

- Building a highly targeted media list of writers and outlets
- Establishing go-to relationships with reporters
- Choosing the best way to pitch each story
- Creating a range of pitches specific to each media category
- Conducting follow-ups to gauge interest; answer questions; provide photos, logos, and quotes; and schedule interviews with the appropriate subject-matter experts to round out the story

With the goal of raising awareness of your urgent care business practice, establishing relationships with key reporters and influencers is critical for securing relevant and repeat coverage. For example, positioning one of your urgent care physicians as a subject-matter expert or as a consumer health advocate could help solidify repeat media coverage. It is important to use the medical expertise offered inside the walls of your urgent care center and make it available to the world through media.

With the Internet exploding as the most influential, global, and real-time media outlet for communications, education, business, and social media, PR practitioners are partnering with urgent care center management more and more every day to harness its power in strategically beneficial ways. Devoting resources to both understanding and staying abreast of best practices is very imperative because the rules change every day.

The United States alone has more than 239 million Internet users (a number that accounts for almost 73% of the nation's population). Understandably, today's patients and consumers use the Internet to search for health-care providers, learn more about urgent care medicine and the services and benefits it provides, understand the convenience and high level of medical service offered by urgent care practices, explore locations that are in their local community, and read reviews of other patients' experiences at that urgent care practice center, something that earlier generations could not do. By promoting your urgent care center's medical talent and customer service online through media channels and review sites and by properly routing search-optimized press releases, urgent care providers have the opportunity to establish trust online with potential patients even before serving them or their families in person. Also, PR stories and articles offer instantaneous traffic to your business's website, which you have set up using best practices for search engine optimization.

The Internet and the main search engines such as Google, Yahoo!, AOL, and Bing are replacing traditional information sources such as phone directories. PR is a vehicle to get your business or medical experts featured through articles that can drastically boost your search potential and online presence.

Using communications professionals and consistent effort to establish your business in the community will provide the media a tangible team of business and medical experts to offer their readers, listeners, and followers. Urgent care center operators can be creative in educating the public about urgent care services, expertise, and practices. Establishing a clear message, being easy to find online, and speaking out as a community resource for health care can reduce the public's confusion and establish urgent care centers as an easy, high-quality, fast, and affordable solution.

Engage!

Using the media to execute strategic PR initiatives should be an integral tool to help establish your urgent care business in your local market(s) and be a communications vessel for growth. When media relationships are established and urgent care managers or PR representatives make themselves readily available to local media as medical experts, consumer advocates, and business resources, credibility is established. The best advice is not to wait for news to happen. Create it!

Get the Most out of Positive Patient Experiences

Unhappy or unsatisfied customers tend to promote their negative experiences 11 times more than happy, satisfied customers promote their positive experiences. Take action and get your happy customers to be your walking—or typing—billboards! Gather and promote positive customer experiences by encouraging patients to share their positive experiences on review sites such as Yelp and on social media sites such as Facebook, Twitter, and LinkedIn. Sharing the exposure of positive patient experiences positions an urgent care center for repeat visits and recommendation by word of mouth from the patient's perspective. For the media, highlighting achievements in patient satisfaction is newsworthy if your business or press release can include tangible statistics that tie into true patient health-care success stories.

SELECTING A PUBLIC RELATIONS AGENCY OR INDEPENDENT PRACTITIONER

With the variety of broadcast, print, online, and social marketing outlets considered to be media in today's world, distinguish your voice and message clearly and in a well-supported way. Because there are many levels of operations in an urgent care center, each business must decide who is the best available company representative to execute PR efforts with one unified voice. Whether you choose to contract with an independent PR practitioner or agency to represent you or instead use an internal communications management resource, this person or team must understand your business, your goals, and workday in order to create news, pitch it properly to the appropriate media, secure story placements, and be available to speak in times of both opportunity and crisis.

A PR professional or agency will be an integral partner, so you must ask key questions and discuss major points before deciding on your communications representation:

- Explore direct, results-oriented questions about your goals, your industry, your community, and your business.
- Ask how and why media is the most effective way to engage and reach a targeted audience of patients and prospective patients.
- Understand the range of services they can and will provide (PR only, or are additional marketing, training, and integrated social media support services available?).
- Gather and contact references from current or past clients to understand deliverables, availability, customer service, and return on investment achieved.
- Ask for details on previous campaigns executed, from the initial research and strategy to the final media placements and results.

Most PR professionals are trained in two key areas: (1) creating and securing news coverage and (2) serving as a company or client spokesperson. In addition to having a PR or media spokesperson ready to represent your urgent care practice in any situation, it is important that each urgent care center designate a business or operational resource as well as a medical resource to be knowledgeable, trained, and available to serve as a spokesperson. Each spokesperson should go through a detailed media training process and ultimately be available for interviews to represent the company and anticipate questions on a variety of key subject matters, core business objectives, and topics of emergency or crisis communications.

PR plays a critical role in preparing a company spokesperson or spokespeople for preparing for, anticipating, and fielding questions from the news media. Spokespeople or communications representatives must be trained, be able to think fast on their feet, and be able to eloquently speak to a variety of media outlets about many subject matters. Because of the large range of business and medical expertise that urgent care centers provide to patients on both a local and national scale, preparedness is key.

A qualified PR professional or internal representative will help you guide the PR efforts of your urgent care practice and serve as a resource to managing large-scale local, national, or global events (changes in laws or regulations, massive product recalls, etc.) as well as smaller yet still newsworthy events (such as sharing a patient's success story, talking about seasonal illnesses, or announcing a new hire). PR professionals and urgent care center managers should see everything as newsworthy and everything as an opportunity, from the big stories, such as the intricacies of how medical innovations and government regulations are changing our health-care climate, to the little ones, such as tips on how to treat a spider bite.

Because of the integration of PR with social media, the effectiveness of strategic PR efforts will continue to increase in popularity and necessity as urgent care center operators look for innovative ways to break through the communications clutter, distinguish the achievements and unique offerings of their business, increase the number of patients they are serving, and offer clear solutions to both current and potential patients where they predominantly spend their time—online. Before ever even consulting with a physician or nurse, most patients start their search for information and even consider making preemptive health-care decisions online. Media coverage helps patients find you through optimized links incorporated within the body of websites and blog articles, as well as through videos tagged with key search term content.

CONCLUSION

Careful selection of a PR agency or professional is a critical undertaking. Once you have made your selection, a methodical and consistent message and approach are key to raising awarenss and increasing patient volume. Additionally, use your PR agency or professional to handle crisis communication and to provide media training. Finally, coordinate your PR game plan with your social media strategy to achieve the best results.

KEY POINTS

1. Your urgent care center must establish awareness within a business and local community, positioning the medical expertise and range of solution-oriented health-care services it can offer.

2. Send out a request for proposals to a number of PR agencies to gauge their level of expertise about the industry. Evaluate their contacts and their past ability to secure media placement.

3. PR is an effective and inexpensive way to increase the public's awareness.

4. The most critical goals for executing strategic PR efforts as part of an urgent care center's communications tool set include the opportunity to raise awareness of, promote the expertise of, and position your urgent care center's medical leadership as subject-matter experts.

5. Use your PR agency to handle disaster communications and address negative publicity with an effective, well-thought-out crisis communication plan.

6. Integrate and coordinate your PR with social media strategy to reach as many consumers as possible.

7. Assign a spokesperson for your clinic and task the PR agency to provide media training.

8. The use of PR to drive awareness and increase patient volume is a slow, methodical process. Do not expect immediate results. It is important to start your PR strategy long before the doors of the clinic are open.

CHAPTER 28

Crisis Communications Management

Erin Terjesen

A CRISIS IS AN ELEVATED or significant threat to operations with potential negative consequences if not handled effectively. Emerging from a communication crisis with your urgent care business's reputation intact is both critical and possible.

Prevention is the key to living through a corporate communications crisis and emerging to tell the story. A crisis threatens an urgent care company's reputation, stature, and relations with key stakeholders, medical or business staffers, or patients. Escalation of an issue to a true crisis is typically the result of a management failure to respond appropriately to an issue, emergency, or accident in a timely manner and with the proper communication.

To manage your crisis, you can choose to let others (most likely less qualified than you) tell your story, or you can be prepared and willing to step in front of the microphone and control the message yourself.

Health-care-related organizations that respond proactively (that is, before a crisis develops) and appropriately to issues, accidents, or emergencies are far less likely to experience a crisis. Organizations that handle the situation well can actually enhance their reputations, strengthen their company's position, and even boost consumer trust and loyalty after a crisis is navigated or eliminated.

Urgent care organizations can minimize and mitigate their risks by clearly defining management controls and policies that govern issues such as ethics, equal opportunity, and workplace safety. Failure to address these issues appropriately or manage these risks increases the potential for an urgent care organization to experience a crisis.

Normally, only organizations that "don't get it" (fail to respond appropriately to a challenge) or that try to avoid issues by using a head-in-the-sand approach fail to communicate and ultimately reach the crisis stage.

But it is much easier to recognize a crisis than it is to prevent one. That is why teaming your urgent care leadership team with public relations (PR) and corporate communications professionals for a plan and a roadmap is critical to understanding how crises arise and to reducing risk.

IDENTIFYING THE THREAT

In the urgent care community, the threat a crisis imposes is the potential damage inflicted on an urgent care organization, its stakeholders, its patients, its staff, and its industry. A crisis can create three related threats, which are often interconnected: public safety, financial loss, and loss of reputation.

- *Public safety* In health care, accidents, defective products, and neglect of policies and procedures can result in risk of injury and potentially even loss of life.
- *Financial loss* Operational disruption causes a trickle-down effect of lost business opportunities, both immediately and long term, from changing consumer confidence.
- *Loss of reputation* All crises reflect negatively on an urgent care organization and threaten to tarnish the reputation of an urgent care company's customer service or medical expertise.

Effective crisis management handles threats sequentially: Public safety is the primary concern, because failure intensifies the damage from a crisis. After public safety has been remedied, reputation and financial concerns are considered because, ultimately, crisis management is designed to protect an urgent care center's business and its stakeholders from threats and reduce the impact of threats.

Crisis management is designed to prevent or lessen the damage a crisis can inflict on an urgent care organization, its stakeholders, and its patients. Crisis management consists of three phases:

- *Pre-crisis* Prevention and preparation
- *Crisis response* Response to a crisis by management or key representatives
- *Post-crisis* Exploration of ways to better anticipate and prepare for the next potential crisis, after fulfilling commitments made during the prior crisis for follow-up information

There are five key elements in crisis communications management:

- *Be prepared* Do not wait until something has gone awry before creating a communications plan.
- *Do not delay* Be ready to respond quickly and with confidence.
- *Practice candor* Be authentic and genuine in your response.
- *Be honest* Even if an executive, a business manager, or a member of the staff made a mistake, being honest is the fastest way to answer questions and regain trust.
- *Work together with media and your audience* Both groups can help you restore your organization's credibility and spread your message far, wide, and fast.

BE PREPARED

Plan for the best but prepare for the worst. Preparing the company for a crisis does not mean that something bad will happen to (or around) your urgent care business, but in our 24/7 world of communications, it is best not to find out about a problem from your customers or clients. Being prepared to address a challenge quickly in a crisis is the key to maintaining trust.

This remains true even as the media we use to communicate continue to evolve rapidly. Though traditional news media such as major newspapers, radio, and TV still play a big role in a crisis, social media's instantaneous and global delivery platforms have shifted the rules.

To be best prepared and play by these new rules, invest in professional communications resources as well as the time to strategically establish recognition of your urgent care practice or business, the expertise and high level of service it provides, and its accomplishments across all media channels.

RESPOND QUICKLY AND WITH AUTHENTICITY

Silence is not always golden. It can sometimes be perceived as fear or lack of a clear position. When it's your time to address tough issues and challenges, don't be afraid to communicate. From product recalls to corporate blunders, every business and every business leader makes mistakes. It is the organizations that can proactively and reactively acknowledge challenges sincerely and with clear steps moving forward to address the issue that typically come out best in a crisis.

ANTICIPATE TO AVOID: CRISIS PREVENTION AND PREPARATION

Crisis prevention involves seeking to reduce known risks that could lead to a crisis. This is part of an organization's risk-management program. Preparation involves creating the crisis-management plan, selecting and training the crisis-management team, and conducting exercises to test both your plan and the team. Urgent care organizations are better able to handle a crisis when they have a crisis-management plan that is updated at least once a year, have a designated crisis-management team or representative, conduct exercises to test the plan regularly, and prepare draft crisis responses that are based on assessed risk factors. The planning and preparation allow crisis teams to react quickly and to make effective decisions in real time.

CREATING A COMMUNICATIONS CRISIS-MANAGEMENT PLAN

Sending strategic and accurate messages during a crisis can minimize negative media attention and fear. An effective crisis communications plan considers the following:

- *What could go wrong?* From the trivial to the complex, what issues could arise that might escalate into a crisis? Asking yourself this question helps your urgent care practice or business identify what will be needed from a communications perspective as well as a business planning perspective. It also helps to educate your stakeholders, managers, and staff as to the types of issues that could turn into a crisis situation requiring activation of internal and external communications plans.

- *Who is in charge?* Identify your organization's key leaders, managers, or stakeholders, especially those who need to be involved in decisions or an immediate response. Roles and responsibilities should be clear. In advance of a crisis, name who has final approval of strategy, messages, and timing.

- *What is our strategy?* Two critical elements in any crisis response are immediacy and transparency. Urgent care centers or networks are unique because their business model incorporates not only the staffing you would see within a corporation but also highly specialized medical practitioners and staff that operate directly with consumers in a fast-paced work environment.

- *Who is our designated communications representative?* Whether you use an internal or external communications resource or team, review your list of anticipated "what could go wrong" problems and identify who is the most qualified, trained, and credible representative to address each of them to the media, customers, or both. In most cases, an urgent care communications crisis can challenge a trained professional or executive because of the high-stress environment that emerges instantaneously, so training and preparedness are critical.

THE IMPORTANCE OF A TRAINED, COMPOSED, AND PREPARED VOICE

A key component of crisis-team training is spokesperson training. With the help of a PR or communications professional, designated organization members must be prepared to talk to the news media during a crisis. Media training from a trained communications professional is critical and should be provided to key executives, company spokespeople, and even key physicians before a crisis hits. Here is a short list of best practices for speaking to the media:

- *Be decisive* Communicate your position clearly. Avoid saying "No comment" because this has a negative perception with consumers, who assume that it implies guilt or avoidance of the issue.

- *Be concise* Respond clearly to avoid any confusion or misconception. Avoid industry or professional jargon or overly technical terms.

- *Be confident on camera* A pleasant and professional demeanor is key. Avoid nervous habits like fidgeting, saying "um," and talking too quickly.

Always maintain eye contact (look directly at the camera) and speak directly to the person speaking to you.

- *Be informed and consistent*   Your spokesperson and all potential spokespeople should be briefed on the latest information and key message points. Situations can change fast, and if your spokesperson is not available, you need informed backup resources ready to step forward.

- *Anticipate potential questions*   Role-play your responses with communications professionals and members of your executive team to ensure you hit the key takeaway messages and eliminate hesitation that shows an uncertainty of your position.

- *Be proactive*   Managers and executives don't have to wait until a crisis hits to prepare drafts of communication materials to be used during a crisis. Use a communications professional to draft statements on behalf of executive leadership, key physicians, and management. Your organization may even consider purchasing dark domains that host webpages addressing your most anticipated crisis communications and that you activate only when needed. In these templates, blank spots can be filled in with key details once they are known. Whether your legal representation is internal or external, have a legal partner review and preapprove messaging to save time, confusion, and stress during a crisis.

A GLOBAL AUDIENCE: HOW SOCIAL MEDIA PLATFORMS HAVE SHIFTED THE RULES

The rise of social media means that online engagements and communications (both positive and negative) spread in an instant. If you don't fill the social media news gap, someone far less qualified probably will. This is why prevention and being proactive in your business practices and quality controls are important.

Social media is an incredibly powerful and useful tool to potentially identify warning signs that a crisis could be developing *before* it spirals out of control. Do not be afraid of social media, but instead arm yourself with experienced marketing and communications professionals who can strategically position your business across a recommended assortment of platforms to help industry partners, stakeholders, and customers stay informed and engaged.

Know Where You Sit

Stay informed of social media mentions of the urgent care industry, the name of your business, the names of key executives, and any key pharmaceutical or manufacturer partners. You can set up no-cost Google Alerts as well as tracking mentions on Twitter, Facebook, and other platforms. Assign an internal resource or external communications partner to manually search daily for any mention of your organization, key executives, or partners. In addition to checking via the major search engines, also search through the industry's leading blogs and news agency sites.

The Power of Video

Have an internal or external communications resource regularly check video-sharing sites like YouTube. Posted video can spark both positive and negative global attention in seconds. In 2007, video was posted that sparked attention about rats in a New York City KFC restaurant. Because the company acted swiftly to voluntarily post information and the video on their own website, very few people actually viewed the video on YouTube. Most people who saw the video did so from KFC's website. This is an example of why acting quickly, being transparent, and using your own business's website can be critical in a crisis, because your website is where most consumers will go first when a challenge emerges.

In addition to using your home page or a specific page of your site dedicated to news or crisis communications, also consider using industry and consumer blogs. The advantage of connected, relevant blogs is that they provide effective ways to share immediate, updated information about a developing situation or a situation that has already transpired —including but not limited to a company's position and, most important, mention of a plan to address the situation and move forward. Integrity and honesty help reestablish trust from the media, your industry, and your patients.

Blogs and other interconnected industry websites can be updated instantly. Once a blog's content has been posted or discovered, respond to questions, feedback, queries, or comments quickly, honestly, and in a time-sensitive manner. Silence and inactivity can be perceived as a lack of urgency or a lack of care.

CRISIS RESPONSE

Crisis response consists of two phases: (1) initial crisis response and (2) reputation repair and application of lessons learned.

Initial Response

Your initial response should be quick, accurate, and consistent.

- ▶ *Be quick* Aim to provide a response in the first hour after the crisis occurs. This is a huge argument for preparation so that your urgent care organization can tell your side of the story (the key points managers want to convey about the crisis to your stakeholders). Your quick response to a recently developed situation may not have much new information, but it positions your urgent care organization as a source and as being in control. Silence is too passive and invites others to control the story. An early response allows your organization to generate greater credibility than a slow response does. Crisis preparation makes it easier for crisis representatives to respond quickly and effectively.

- ▶ *Be accurate* Media and patients want accurate information about what happened and context for how an event may affect them. When events are moving quickly, the risk for inaccurate information is high and can make your organization look disorganized or inconsistent.

- ▶ *Be consistent*   Try to speak with a unified voice to maintain accuracy, even if this voice entails a variety of experts (medical, business, and communications). Make sure your spokespeople are briefed on the same information and the key messaging.

  Especially for urgent care organizations, quickness and accuracy play an important role in public safety. When public safety is a concern, people want to know what happened and how a situation is being addressed. Quick, effectively executed actions can also save your business money by preventing further damage and protecting reputations by showing that the organization is in control. But remember that speed is meaningless if the information is wrong. Inaccurate information can increase rather than decrease the threat to public safety. Select your distribution channels to reach your key stakeholders, management, or patients swiftly and effectively.

- ▶ *Speak to the right audience*   Crisis situations can be framed by media coverage, which means media can be the first audience considered. But a key advantage of social media and the Internet, email, text messaging, calling mobile phones, and so forth is the capacity to communicate in direct ways to each of your audiences. Take advantage of technology by defining in advance how best to reach your employees or staff members, stakeholders, patients, opinion leaders in your community, and the media. In today's world, consumers are trained to go to an organization's website first when news breaks (and media outlets will often link to websites in their online stories). Make sure you can quickly update your website, Facebook fan site, Twitter feed, and so on, to include news and information about the current situation. Fight reputation damage by arming your various audiences with the facts.

Reputation Repair and Application of Lessons Learned

After the crisis ends, the goal is to return to business as usual as quickly as possible, regaining the focus of the mission of your urgent care practice. At this point, the crisis is no longer management's primary focus, but it does still require evaluation. Reputation repair may be continued or initiated during this phase. It is also important to follow through with any communication promised by communication managers or representatives during the crisis, so you do not risk losing the trust of media, patients, or the general public. Also, your organization should release updates on the recovery process, investigation, and any corrective actions.

A crisis should be a learning experience. The crisis-management effort must be evaluated to see what is working and what needs improvement. Every urgent care company should continuously seek ways to improve prevention, preparation, and the organizational response.

Best practices after a crisis include the following:

- The delivery of all information promised to stakeholders as soon as the information is known
- Keeping stakeholders updated on recovery efforts, investigations, and corrective actions taken or planned
- Analysis of how the crisis-management plan was executed and ways to improve for the future

CONCLUSION

We all hope a crisis never befalls your urgent care organization, but it's a good idea to build up a bank of goodwill—acting honorably and transparently, communicating a sense of your values and the benefits you offer your employees, patients, and other key audiences, and showing a respectable level of service, expertise, and responsiveness. This strong brand positioning and establishment of experience helps people forgive more quickly when something goes wrong. If you pair a communications approach that engenders trust with a solid crisis communications plan, you should not panic when something goes awry. Instead, prepare to communicate with speed, accuracy, and confidence.

KEY POINTS

1. Preparation should be the rule, not the exception.
2. No organization is immune from a crisis, so do your best to prepare, train, empower, and anticipate.
3. Figure out the facts and decide how much of these facts should be communicated publicly.
4. Respond succinctly and with an expression of genuine concern for the impact the situation has had on patients, medical professionals, staff members, or stakeholders.
5. Effective crisis management can minimize damage and in some cases allow an urgent care organization to emerge stronger.
6. Execute best practices.
7. Be honest, because transparency creates trust.
8. Know your audiences, and know the best way to reach them quickly and effectively.
9. Embrace technology and social media; don't hide from it.
10. Be consistent to create a unified voice and inspire confidence.

CHAPTER 29

Developing Your Brand

Kat Smith

The success of any business depends in large part on the end user's ability to clearly distinguish one product from another in the marketplace and, on the basis of those distinctions, make a selection. Branding is the main tool used to distinguish your products from those of the competition. It's why millions of people wake up every day and order a Starbucks coffee. It's why your neighbor will only drive a Volvo. And it's a tool you can use to make your urgent care center the community go-to.

DEVELOPING YOUR BRAND

Why Brand?

The three main purposes of branding are product identification, repeat sales, and new sales. Product identification is the cornerstone and, of these three, the most important. If no one recognizes your product or service in the market, you will be hard pressed to make any repeat or new sales. Branding helps you to distinguish your products and services from all others in the marketplace. This is why the name *iPod* conjures up a myriad of musical images, but you might scratch your head in confusion if I brought up the name *Zune*.

A brand that has wide recognition and well-perceived quality is more likely to garner brand loyalty among consumers and in turn generate repeat sales. Having high brand awareness and a respected image is particularly beneficial when you want to introduce new products (and make new sales). For example, General Mills's Honey Nut Cheerios, which debuted in 1979, as a supporting product line to Cheerios, has since gone on to outsell the original and become the top-selling cereal in the United States.

Brand Identity

The outward expression of a brand is made up of many components, including its name, trademark, visual appearance, and communication style, all coming together to form a brand identity. Think about how you want the consumer to perceive your brand, because this identity will ultimately be built by you. Focus on authentic qualities and characteristics that you want to provide potential patients, and develop a brand promise that you can sustain and deliver.

Your brand name should be easy to remember and pronounce, should be classic (avoid the temptation to follow naming fads), and should have positive connotations. The most effective brand names are those that build a connection between the personality of the brand and the actual services being provided. Additionally, you should consider not just how your brand name sounds but also how it will look visually. Even the most talented of designers can only do so much with a poor brand name.

Part of your brand identity may qualify for trademark protection, which gives you the exclusive right to use it. Some examples are

- *Sounds*, such as the NBC chimes
- *Catch phrases*, such as Charles Schwab's "Ask Chuck," and MasterCard's "Priceless!"
- *Shapes*, such as the Coca-Cola bottle and BMW's dual-kidney grille
- *Decorative color or design*, such as the distinctive blue of Tiffany & Co. or the Burberry check pattern
- *Abbreviations*, such as Coke, NPR, or the Met

Trademark rights come from use rather than registration—though you will have to file an intent-to-use application with the US Patent and Trademark Office. Trademark protection typically lasts 10 years but operates on a use-it-or-lose-it basis. To learn more about obtaining and defending a trademark, go to www.uspto.gov or consult a lawyer specializing in intellectual property.

Visual Identity

The overall aesthetic look of your urgent care center's communications is known as its visual identity. To achieve an effective visual brand identity, use a consistent set of visual elements to create brand distinction. Visual elements may include specific typefaces, colors, and graphic elements.

Selecting your set of corporate typefaces may seem like a no-brainer, but there are several factors to consider. Remember you will be using these designated typefaces on all of your marketing materials, from a small promotional handout to a 14-by-48-foot billboard. Legibility is key. If you hire a designer to create your own custom typeface, be sure to ask that they include all relevant characters and symbols in the fonts that you may possibly use (for example, the symbol for a prescription, ℞).

Colors not only enhance the appearance of an item but also influence our behavior. You would be wise to consider the psychology of color when designing the palette for your marketing materials, because your color choices could be sending a specific message to the people who view them.

An owner must be sensitive to the color-sensitve emotional characteristics of the specific ethnicities of the communities they serve. In the United States, the following colors are often associated with certain qualities or emotions:

- *Red* is the color of passion and is tied to strong emotions like love, boldness, and life (think "blood"). Red is used often to symbolize an important alert or warning, which is why this color is so often used for emergency departments. Note that the American Red Cross and Johnson & Johnson will vigorously defend their respective trademarked red crosses.

- *Orange* is a bright color that pops. It denotes creativity and newness and can also symbolize ambition; fast-food chains and energy products regularly use it.

- *Yellow* is an attention grabber. It is often associated with warmth, energy, and cheerfulness. Because of its vibrancy, it is best used as an accent.

- *Green* has been closely associated with growth, wealth, luck, and safety. It is one of the easiest colors for the human eye to process and is often used for insurance plans and financial firms. Green is also associated with eco-friendly products. Note that the National Safety Council has a trademarked green cross.

- *Blue* is one of the most commonly used colors because it is often associated with trustworthiness, productivity, reliability, and responsibility. Blue is a good choice for businesses and has been the most popular color choice among banks. Be careful to stay away from the blue of Blue Cross.

- *Purple* was once a rare color and historically has been linked to royalty. Today it is still a color that is associated with power, wealth, and spirituality. It is often used in marketing campaigns targeting women.

- *White* symbolizes purity, cleanliness, and youthfulness. Modern and abstract white lends itself well to website designs and is now being used for clinics and hospitals to represent sterility.

- *Black* is the shade of authority and power. It is a sophisticated color used to convey elegance, exclusivity, and luxury. It is well suited for advertising designer goods, such as luxury vehicles.

- *Silver*, or gray, is usually associated with traditional and serious brands. Conservative in nature, it makes a good base color to provide more visibility for bolder accent colors.

Think about what kind of emotional response you want your patients to feel not only on first glance but also when they engage with your service. Colors, when properly used, can be powerful tools that not only entice your target audience but also benefit your overall marketing success, because they help distinguish between competing brands.

Graphical elements are often the first component people visualize when asked about a specific brand. Imagine the Nike swoosh, the golden arches of McDonald's, or the World Wildlife Fund's panda; these are all examples of a company's brand mark, or logo. The old adage "A picture is worth a thousand words" applies here because logos can quickly speak volumes about your business, your mission, and the services you offer. A well-designed symbol of your brand is a simple way for your target audience to easily distinguish your products from those of competing brands.

There are five elements you should strive for when entering the logo design process:

- *Simplicity*   This makes your logo more easily recognizable. Coco Chanel advised, "Always remove one thing before you leave the house." In Ludwig Mies van der Rohe's formulation, "Less is more." I tend to agree with this sentiment when it comes to logo design.

- *Memorability*   This is closely associated with simplicity; the simplest logos are often the most easily recognized. Think Nike, Mercedes, and Apple.

- *Timelessness*   Trends come and go. Your branding shouldn't. Although it is true that many brands have received facelifts over the years, the majority maintain the core elements that they originally launched with. Think General Electric or Ford.

- *Versatility*   An effective logo is one that can work across a variety of media and applications. Your logo should still be able communicate your message if it is printed in one color or reverse color, is the size of a billboard, or is as small as a stamp, and thus should be scalable vector art. Gradients and images do not work as logos.

- *Appropriateness*   Your logo should resonate with its intended audience. For example, although a whimsical typeface and color scheme might be appropriate for a nail salon, it would be far from appropriate for an urgent care center.

Brand Personality

You may remember the commercials about Macintosh (Mac) computers versus personal computers (PCs) that run Microsoft's Windows operating system, more formally known as the "Get a Mac" campaign, a series of 66 ads that Apple aired from 2006 to 2009. This award-winning campaign featured John Hodgman as the bumbling corporate PC and a young Justin Long as the cool, friendly, and composed Mac. The two actors brought the brands to life and were a perfect embodiment of how Apple and Microsoft were viewed by consumers at the time. Today these ads are still a great example of brand personality.

The personality that you create for your brand should be composed of a set of human characteristics to which your target audience can relate. There are numerous types of personalities and associated traits that you can assign to your brand. Table 1 outlines three brand personalities.

Table 1. Three Brand Personalities and Their Traits

The Nurturer	The Performer	The Executive
• Generous • Caring • Stable • Conscientious	• Fun • Playful • Spirited • Adventurous	• Assertive • Organized • Driven • Outspoken

When selecting a personality type and its accompanying traits, consider the emotional associations you want people to make when they think about your urgent care clinic. Understanding your brand's personality not only will help you craft the most appropriate messages but also will assist you in the selection of effective media and suitable partnerships.

The personality you pick will influence your brand's strategy at every touch point; it will help set the tone of your marketing communications, will influence your visual style and design, and may even affect your company's dress code. Ultimately, having a deep understanding of your brand's personality will enable you to deliver a consistent brand experience that resonates with your audience and leaves a lasting impression.

Brand Experience

The sensations, feelings, thoughts, and behavioral responses an individual has toward a brand's identity are known as the brand experience. The brand experience you deliver directly affects consumer satisfaction and loyalty.

Regardless of touch point, the experience of your brand is what matters most to your patients and consumers. Every member of your organization has an impact on the customer's experience and therefore on the brand. Your staff must understand and believe in your urgent care center's brand promise in order to deliver on it to every patient, every day.

Impressions count, and the last one you leave a patient with is most often the one that will stick. Experiences are incredibly powerful and will influence individual perceptions of a brand. Always deliver on your brand promise, or your brand will be redefined in the minds of your patients, because unfortunately a great logo won't make up for poor customer service.

Branding in the Digital Age

According to a BIA/Kelsey study, 97% of consumers research products and services online before buying local. In view of this statistic, you should develop a comprehensive and aggressive online branding strategy for your urgent care centers.

Effective online branding delivers the same experience you provide to users who engage with your brand offline. This means that when you supply content online, it aligns with the same brand standards you provide everywhere else.

Maintaining a consistent voice and message is just as important as carrying over your visual branding to the Internet.

Directories

Like water, your patients will take the path of least resistance. If your competition's urgent care center shows up online and yours doesn't, chances are you are going to miss out on potential patients. There are many online directories out there that you can request to be listed on, and some are even free.

As a first step, create a Google+ Local page for all your urgent care center locations. This will allow all your centers to be found on Google Search, Maps, Google+, and multiple mobile platforms. Not only will you show up across the Internet but you will also have the power to upload your contact information, hours, services, photos, and more. The more information you give people, the more likely they are to convert into patients. In addition, patients can leave reviews and feedback—and a positive review is the best form of advertisement.

Other directories you might consider include Yelp, Yahoo! Directory, and FindUrgentCare.com.

Social Networks

Facebook, Twitter, Google+, LinkedIn, YouTube, and Pinterest—the list of social networking sites is not a short one, but it is one you should pay attention to. Discovering where your target audience lives online is crucial because engaging with them online and turning them into fans is one of the best things you can do for your brand.

If you are just looking to dip your toes in the water of social networking, the best place to start is Facebook. Currently the number one social networking site in the world, Facebook is a valuable branding tool you can employ to reach your target audience. A study of social media usage indicates that Facebook users who "like" your page are 51% more likely to make a purchase and 60% more likely to recommend your brand once they become a fan of your Facebook page.

Another study, appearing in the *American Journal of Medical Quality*, suggests that hospitals with a large number of likes also receive higher marks for the quality of care they deliver compared with hospitals with fewer followers. Not surprisingly, the study also indicated that likes are positively associated with patient recommendations.

Before joining any social network, think about what content you wish to share with your followers. Your brand can take the approach of being a content curator or a content creator, or even a mix of both. You should also set a realistic goal for how often you will post content to your page. If you are the only one managing your accounts, you may wish to post as little as two times a week. In this case frequency is not nearly as important as consistency.

Social networking is about much more than sharing your own content; after all, just break down the term—it's networking on a social level. Engaging with your followers is an important part of this networking process. If they ask you a question online, answer it. If they leave you positive feedback, thank them. And if they should happen to leave a not-so-pleasant review, address the issue head on and then try to move the conversation offline.

The added bonus of maintaining a presence on a variety of social networks is that your urgent care center will return even more results when searched for online.

Company Blog

Creating your own original content for consumers to engage with and share is a crucial part of online branding, and starting a blog on your urgent care center's website is an easy way to do this. Blog entries can be relatively short and can cover a variety of topics that interest both you and your target audience.

Create an editorial calendar in advance, and plan to stick to it. If you elect to have a blog, it is important to update it regularly. Once you are steadily generating your own content, be sure to share it across your various social networks.

Tools of the Trade

Numerous tools are available online today that can help you measure and quantify the success of your online branding efforts. Here are a few that I recommend—and the best part is, they are all free:

Brandify

Brandify, at www.brandify.com, is an analytics tool that can help you gauge your business's online presence with its Brand Report Card. Brandify can provide insight into how your urgent care clinic shows up online and, on the basis of this information, offer guidance on how to enhance your social media presence, online listings, and search engine results.

Alexa, Google Analytics, and Quantcast

A leading provider of free, global web metrics, Alexa, at www.alexa.com, offers an easy way to discover the most successful sites on the web by keyword, category, or country. You can harness their analytics for competitive analysis, benchmarking, and market research. Google Analytics, at www.google.com/analytics/, provides similar analytic analysis for market research and keyword or phrase use. Similar to Alexa and Google Analytics, Quantcast, at www.quantcast.com, measures global site traffic. In addition they offer free audience composition reports, which can help you more easily identify the demographics and psychographics of your online visitors.

Google Alerts

When someone mentions your urgent care center on the web, Google Alerts, at www.google.com/alerts, will notify you via email and provide links to the reference sites, so you can see what is being said. This is an easy way to monitor and stay on top of your brand's buzz.

Bitly

Bitly, at bitly.com, is an excellent tool for tracking the links that you share across your various social media channels. It not only shortens standard links so that they are less cumbersome but also allows you to monitor in real time the frequency with which your links are clicked. This makes it an easy way to measure which topics are generating the greatest interest.

CONCLUSION

Creating a brand that resonates with consumers is not something that can take place overnight. It takes time, effort, and a lot of consideration. Set your brand goals and standards, and then stay consistent. Stay true to your brand's core identity when delivering patient care and services; a consistent experience will result in greater patient satisfaction, which leads to greater brand loyalty and a lifetime customer.

Yet your brand should adapt to change. It is easy to get caught up in the notion that everything must be perfect because this will be your brand forever. However, the most successful brands have survived in today's markets because they are consistently evolving with the times and, when necessary, rebranding themselves to remain relevant. Developing your urgent care center's brand should be a fun and rewarding experience, but it requires a thoughtful approach.

KEY POINTS

1. *Branding* distinguishes your products and services from all others in the marketplace.

2. Your *brand identity* is made up of many components, including a name, a trademark, visual appearance, and communication style.

3. An effective *visual identity* uses a consistent set of visual elements to create brand distinction and may include specific typefaces, colors, and graphic elements.

4. Five elements you should strive for when entering the *logo design* process: simplicity, memorability, timelessness, versatility, and appropriateness.

5. Select a unique set of traits to form your *brand personality*; this will help you craft appropriate messages, select effective media, and form suitable partnerships.

6. Your *brand experience* is what matters most to patients, and it must deliver your brand promise through all audience touch points, everywhere and always.

7. Your customers are online, and your brand should be too. Effective *online branding* should deliver the same experience you provide offline.

8. *Track and measure* your branding efforts. If you don't quantify what you are doing, you will never know whether you are flourishing or failing.

9. *Consistency* is a crucial component of branding. Brands that are consistent across all customer touch points leave a firm impression and are more easily recognized.

10. From time to time, you may need to *realign* and update the face of your brand to keep it current in the urgent care market.

CHAPTER 30

Metric-Driven Management: Harnessing Information in the Urgent Care Organization

Laurel Stoimenoff

NEARLY ALL URGENT CARE center operators will tell you that they have systems or processes in place to implement key metrics in their businesses, yet metrics are meaningless without an ongoing and disciplined approach to amass, monitor, disseminate, and take action on the information. Microsoft's Bill Gates summed it up perfectly when he said, "The most meaningful way to differentiate your company from your competitors, the best way to put distance between you and the crowd, is to do an outstanding job with information. How you gather, manage, and use information will determine whether you win or lose."[1] In other words, your work doesn't stop when your office manager hands you the data she's collected on a colorful spreadsheet. You won't excel in a sustained fashion until you have established processes in place to respond to any unfavorable variances or opportunities for improvement.

A well-designed management-control process is the engine that drives change and performance. Metrics, or key performance indicators (KPIs), are essential components of an organization's approach to its overall strategy for operational excellence and market success. The word *control* is often applied negatively. For example, few employees seek "control freaks" as bosses. But control is actually a disciplined and deliberate intervention that supports the organization's quest to achieve or exceed its business objectives.

Management control accompanied by the ongoing monitoring of KPIs should be dynamic, responsive, and inclusive. John Naisbitt, author of *Megatrends*, says that true power is not about "money in the hands of a few" but rather "information in the hands of many." Distribution can be selective, and not all information needs to be or should be shared at all levels; on the other hand, good leaders should keep in mind the adage "What gets measured gets managed" when it comes to sharing those items that might enable an individual's direct ability to influence an outcome.

---

1   Pearl M. Gaining a competitive advantage: a little difference makes all the difference. In: *Grow Globally: Opportunities for Your Middle-Market Company Around the World*. Hoboken, NJ: John Wiley & Sons; 2011.

THE BALANCED SCORECARD

Robert Kaplan and David Norton, authors of the best seller *The Balanced Scorecard* (1996)—as well as of *The Strategy-Focused Organization* (2000) and *Alignment: Using the Balanced Scorecard to Create Corporate Synergies* (2006)—address how an organization can implement scorecards to define what is important to the organization and then use "balanced scorecards" to achieve and refine its strategy. Scorecards are divided into four quadrants: finance, internal business processes, the customer, and learning and growth.

To *balance* a scorecard means ensuring that all four categories are addressed, as follows: The *financial* quadrant of the scorecard addresses those items most important to investors; the *customer* quadrant focuses on how the organization creates value for its market; both are considered external measures. The *internal business processes* and *learning and growth* quadrants, which look at how the organization develops talent and encourages innovation to prepare for the future, are internally focused measures. Again, by assessing all four aspects, one can create a balanced picture. Kaplan and Norton make the argument that too often metrics are strictly applied only to the financial concerns of the company, but that great companies use a more comprehensive approach to reach their strategies and goals. Determining what is most important to the organization and striving for a balance between internal and external considerations are the necessitating factors.

THE MANAGEMENT-CONTROL PROCESS

The process of defining what is important to an organization often begins with its strategic plan, mission, and vision. If an organization is going through an exponential growth phase, its metrics will undoubtedly be different from the metrics revealed if it is in the midst of a stabilization or turnaround period. With defined short-range and long-range objectives in place, goals and tactics can be established to be sure they are achieved.

Setting leadership processes that ensure alignment and clarity within the organization regarding its direction and the supportive roles of its employees is a critical tactic, or stage, of the strategic plan. Every stage of the control process should be aligned with specific metrics that support either prompt or proactive responses or course corrections. Start by defining those steps that must occur annually, quarterly, monthly, and daily. Remember, even if your organization's key leaders commit to a disciplined approach, it is doomed to failure if the management-control process is not supported and driven from the top down.

Each phase of the process also builds on the next (Figure 1), as in a communication and reporting plan, which focuses on the common themes of mission, vision, and strategy. At each stage of the management-control process, participants should have access to the data most essential to driving the agenda in their area. Organizations should employ the *knowledge pyramid* (Figure 2), which

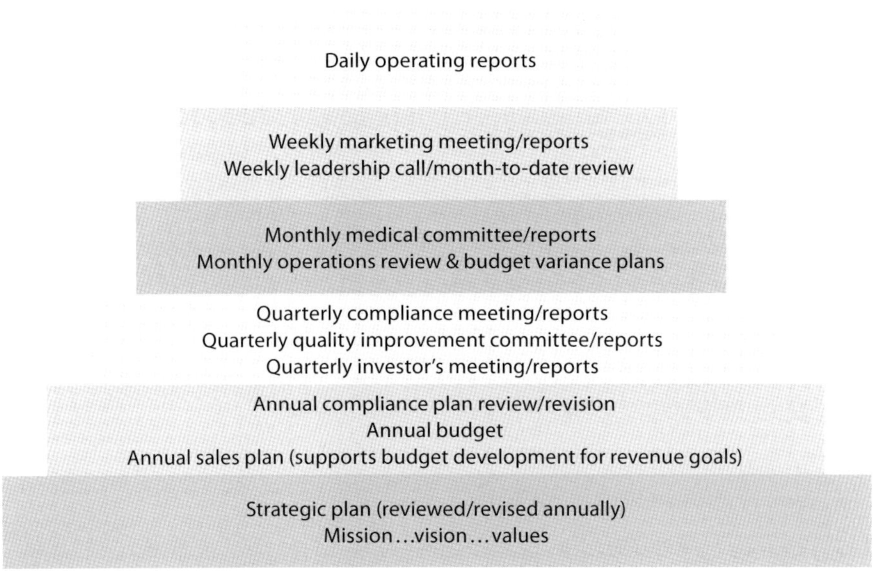

Daily operating reports
Weekly marketing meeting/reports
Weekly leadership call/month-to-date review
Monthly medical committee/reports
Monthly operations review & budget variance plans
Quarterly compliance meeting/reports
Quarterly quality improvement committee/reports
Quarterly investor's meeting/reports
Annual compliance plan review/revision
Annual budget
Annual sales plan (supports budget development for revenue goals)
Strategic plan (reviewed/revised annually)
Mission…vision…values

Figure 1. Example of an urgent care organization management-control process.

demonstrates the process by which data become information and information becomes knowledge. It is at the knowledge level that leadership makes good decisions.

Medical personnel are well aware of the conundrum presented by false positives and false negatives. The same principle is at work when reviewing data,

Decision Making
Synthesizing
Analyzing
Summarizing
Organizing
Collecting
Knowledge
Information
Data

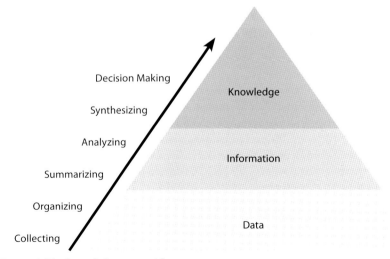

Figure 2. The knowledge pyramid.

in that only further knowledge allows us to truly determine whether action is necessary. Overreacting to metrics whose variances should have been predictable, such as a reduction in overall net revenue per visit during a month of a high number of flu shots or school physicals, can quickly erode the credibility and value of the process. In nearly all cases, if the causative factors associated with a variance aren't immediately evident, that variance is merely a symptom that merits additional investigation versus a knee-jerk response.

Once metrics and benchmarks are selected to accompany each segment of the management-control process, the next step is providing the necessary training to address

- How the data are gathered and reported
- When management can anticipate seeing the data
- What management can do to influence the data favorably
- Who is ultimately accountable for performance
- What the process is if the data do not conform to the standards

Computations to determine the appropriate metric for each level and process of the organization must be easily understood by those expected to respond to it. *Economic value added* (EVA) is a financial metric used to calculate the creation of shareholder value; it looks at profits after taking into consideration the cost of capital. It is calculated in four steps, as follows:

1. Calculate net operating profit after tax (NOPAT)
2. Calculate total invested capital (TC)
3. Determine the weighted average cost of capital (WACC)
4. Calculate: EVA = NOPAT − WACC% × TC

This metric is the gold standard when compared with others such as *net income* or *earnings per share*, but it is hardly a metric that an organization would want to share at the level of center manager. It is complex, and it would be nearly impossible for the center manager to implement meaningful actions to influence a metric whose derivation is a mystery. Selected metrics must be compelling and actionable by the recipient. In every business there are players and coaches. The coach's scorecard should be comprehensive; the expectation is that the coach knows what to react to and what to ignore. The coach also knows when to identify outliers that may soon become elevated to an organizational or team goal.

SETTING PRIORITIES

The 4 Disciplines of Execution: Achieving Your Wildly Important Goals, by Chris McChesney, Sean Covey, and Kim Huling (2012), is a practical management tool for achieving sustained results. It speaks of the lower-level battles that must be won to win the war—that is, to achieve the goals of the organization. What's important is to assess which battles have a direct correlation to the war being fought; the ones that don't aren't worth the focus. The authors state that teams must establish "wildly important goals" (WIGs) to concentrate their energies on what really matters to realize a goal. The reality is that most teams cannot effectively achieve more than two goals at a time. The message here is that the company may wish to win 10 battles in a year, but if human resources get stretched too thin, chances are good that employees will elect to make no change at all.

McChesney, Coving, and Huling advise that once your WIGs have been fixed, you should create "a compelling scoreboard." Employees need to know if they are on a winning path; without a compelling scoreboard in place, you run the risk of demotivating the team. For example, if your urgent care facility's current WIG is to decrease patient wait time, the metric of minutes from walk-in to triage or walk-in to provider might be selected, but as critical as the goal is, it is equally critical to present and keep it front and center to the team throughout the workday. Otherwise, it will quickly lose its status as a WIG.

Scoreboards that chart trends and are hung in the break room, success recognition, and spirited competition among urgent care centers make any metric more meaningful. The center manager of clinic A who argues that their wait time is longer because of high patient volume will likely jump on board when they see how internal processes have revealed that an even busier clinic B is eclipsing them on the scoreboard. This is when data become information, and information becomes a credible argument-buster.

DATA DISTRIBUTION

Producing WIG scoreboards does not mean that organizations should limit overall metric assessment. A disciplined approach identifies which metrics align with your WIGs as well as what information should be provided at each level of the organization. In addition to balanced WIG scoreboards, your assessment may determine that your center manager needs only a limited amount of information every day to influence the performance of the business unit, such as

- ▶ Total visits compared with the budget
- ▶ Missed over-the-counter collections
- ▶ Average charge per visit compared with the budget
- ▶ Staffing compared with the budget (calculated as full-time equivalents per patient visit)

Table 1 is a sample scoreboard. The clinic's WIGs are focused on improving cash collections and the patient experience, specifically door-to-door time. The organization has communicated these goals across all its clinics and created themes: Tomorrow's Cash Today and Every Moment Counts. Leadership ensures

Table 1. ABC Urgent Care 1st quarter WIGs

Clinic	Every Moment Counts— Door-to-Door Time Goal: 1 Hour or Less	Tomorrow's Cash Today	
		Clean Claims Success % Goal: 98%	% Correct Over-the-Counter Collections Goal: 98%
Central	1:02	87%	92%
Northeast	0:56	92%	89%
South	0:52	95%	98%

that every employee understands the goals and the measurements. Metrics are associated with each goal and are visible to all clinic personnel.

The urgent care center operator must explore and exploit the capabilities of the systems to produce actionable information and disseminate that information on an ability-to-impact versus a need-to-know basis. Leadership must remain cognizant of the day-to-day challenges associated with managing a busy urgent care center. *The 4 Disciplines of Execution* describes these challenges as the *whirlwind*, or the daily essential responsibilities that can interfere with meaningful change and improvement.

Complacency can also be a problem; it is often a manifestation of information overload. To avoid complacency, prioritize key performance indicators at each managerial level of the organization and add no more than two WIGs per team at any given time to effect meaningful and sustained change. Even if they are unaware that they are doing so, nonfinancial personnel may drive the financial performance of the organization if they are given the proper metrics.

USING METRICS TO IMPROVE PERFORMANCE

As for any quality-improvement model, once an opportunity for improvement is identified, a phased process is implemented. The phases are *plan, do, study,* and *act* (PDSA): plan the corrective action; implement the corrective action; study the corrective action (and associated metrics); and finally, take action by modifying the correction, or commit to it and operationalize it into the organization. This *metrics continuum* has more specifically been described as follows:

1. Defining the standards used to gauge success
2. Applying the standards through collection of relevant data
3. Evaluating the data collection results
4. Calibrating the business strategy or its execution

Metrics management is a dynamic process. Goals change along with the metrics on which the organization is focusing to achieve those fluid objectives. In our example of the clinic seeking door-to-door time of 1 hour or less, once that goal is achieved and proven sustainable, the next opportunity for improvement should be introduced with its own set of metrics. Door-to-door time may remain on the organizational dashboard or visible at the coach level while frontline employees are allowed to focus on the next battle needed to win the war. It is essential to avoid changing goals too quickly, so that employee fatigue doesn't set in as each new flavor of the week is presented. There are times where immediate corrective action is warranted, but such times should be the exception rather than part of a well-planned approach to ongoing improvement.

Example of a Corrective Action

Here is a process-and-profit improvement example using corrective action as measured by two simple metrics:

An urgent care center operator is concerned. Securing new patients into her established three clinics has not been a problem, as she has an excellent marketing representative who constantly finds ways to pursue new patient opportunities through schools, events, churches, and other referral venues. The problem is that the patients who come in to clinic A (one of her three clinics) for care don't seem to return, as indicated when the numbers are benchmarked against those of clinics B and C. Because all three clinics have been open for approximately the same 5-year period, it does not appear that the return patient percentage should be dramatically different.

The operator visits outlier clinic A to assess possible causative factors. She also visits the more successful sites to observe the patient experience throughout specific encounters. Her hypothesis is that clinic A's failure to secure the same percentage of return patients is due to the clinic's providing only adequate instead of memorable experiences. Our operator notes that clinic A staff members pride themselves on being very efficient but that their efficiency could be perceived as uncaring. She establishes a patient experience program as clinic A's wildly important goal. The program is themed Every Patient Counts! The metrics that will be used to determine its effectiveness are as follows:

- Percentage of established patients (goal: 63% when benchmarked against clinics B and C)
- Percentage of patient satisfaction scores of "highly likely or 5 out of 5" for the survey question "Would you return again to this urgent care center for care?" (goal: >90%)

Training is implemented and service checklists are created for each employee by job description. Front-office personnel have a different set of expectations from those of back-office medical assistants. Physicians have their own set of expectations, nuanced for their role in the care process.

The scoreboard is placed in the break room, and daily scores are noted, along with month-to-date aggregate scores. Our operator makes sure that successes are celebrated and that trended setbacks result in immediate action and intervention.

Feedback on surveys soon reveals a correlation between wait time and the likelihood that patients will return to clinic A in the future. Therefore, the urgent care center operator instigates an increased focus on the time it takes to triage and room patients. Once this step is implemented, survey scores soon start improving week after week, subsequently influencing the percentage of established patients. More patients begin to cite "friends and family" as their sources of information about the center and as influencers in their decision to seek care at clinic A. Six months later, clinic A's performance is exceeding that of clinics B and C. Clinic A becomes the new benchmark for service excellence.

METRIC SELECTION

There are numerous metric-selection opportunities in the urgent care setting depending on the area of interest. For example, metrics can be used to assess operations, financial performance, quality, the patient experience, the employee experience, and marketing and sales. The dos and don'ts of metric selection are outlined in Table 2.

When reviewing the metrics in Table 3, it is important to recognize that many are meaningless in isolation and hence are beneficial only when benchmarked against others. The examples provided are sample opportunities that may be appropriate for an urgent care setting, with the understanding that each organization must customize and focus its scorecard to align with its particular strategy.

For instance, an outlier provider on "Emergency department transfers per provider as a percentage of total patients seen by that provider" may merit some level of peer review to ensure that said transfers were appropriate and not an opportunity for training and development. Emergency department transfers in and of themselves are a normal part of doing business and good patient care. One could also review this metric on the basis of time. Are emergency department transfers within the organization increasing as a percentage of total patients during the last hour of operation? Transfer rates may simply be a manifestation of the acuity level of patients seeking after-hours care or a manifestation of a tired team ready to call it a day. Only a more detailed analysis of the variance will provide the answer.

Similarly, metrics that look at market share as the total number of patients served over a period of time per ZIP code and divided by the total population of that ZIP code are meaningless unless the operator is benchmarking one clinic against another or one time period against another.

Table 2. The Dos and Don'ts of Creating a Strategic Metric Plan

Do	Don't
► Tie the metric to the strategic planning process	► Limit metric development to senior executives; everyone in the organization should understand the process and contribute to it
► Make sure everyone in the organization understands what is being measured and why	
► Limit the number of metrics to optimize understanding and usefulness; focus on the truly crucial variables	► Treat metric development as a one-time event
► Use a graphic format to display results to ease recognition of trends, interrelationships, and outliers	► Wait for perfection of every detail
► Link metrics to reward systems when and where appropriate	► Introduce metrics only for compensation purposes
► Accept uncertainty about the future and anticipate some failures	► Underestimate the cause-and-effect relationship between your metric and the desired outcome
► Secure the commitment of senior management in the development and selection of measures and targets	

Adapted from Krentz SE, DeBoer AM, Preble SN. Staying on course with strategic metrics. *Healthcare Financial Management.*

Table 3. Metrics

Metric/Category	Calculation	Balance
Operations		
Visits/day	Total visits/total days	Finance
Staff efficiency	Total visits/total staff hours	Int bus processes
Provider efficiency	Provider visits/total provider hours	Int bus processes
Supply management	Total supply cost/visits	Int bus processes
Right staffing	Total profit/total ftes	Finance
Provider cost/visit	Total provider costs/total visits	Finance/int bus processes
Total labor cost/visit	All labor costs (including benefits)/total visits	Finance/int bus processes
Environment efficiency	Profit/facility square foot	Finance

(continued)

Table 3. Metrics (continued)

Metric/Category	Calculation	Balance
Time of service collections	Actual TOS collections/ correct TOS collections	Finance/ int bus processes
Clean claims	Clean claims submitted/total claims	Finance/ int bus processes
Provider visit revenue	Provider-generated net revenue/ provider visits	Finance
Nonprovider visit revenue	Nonprovider net revenue/ nonprovider visits	Finance
Internal resource utilization	Internal laboratory tests/visits	Int bus processes
Internal resource utilization	Internal radiology panels/visits	Int bus processes
Collections efficiency	Days sales outstanding (DSO) calculation	Int bus processes
Marketing		
Marketing effectiveness	% New patient growth year over year	Int bus processes
Website effectiveness	Total click-throughs to "register online"/ total web visits	Int bus processes
Market penetration	Patients served by ZIP code/ZIP code pop.	Int bus processes
The Employee Experience		
Onboarding	% Employees completing orientation in first 30 days	Learning & growth
Feedback	% Employees with current performance reviews	Learning & growth
Succession plan	% Employees under growth/development plans	Learning & growth
Engagement	Employee engagement survey tool	Learning & growth
Engagement	% Providers utilizing at least 50% of their CE benefit/year	Learning & growth
Compliance	% Employees completing annual mandatory training (HIPAA, safety, compliance, information control)	Learning & growth/ int bus processes
The Patient Experience		
Pt. satisfaction	Patients ranking "likelihood to return" a "5"/ total respondents	Customer
Throughput	Average door-to-door time	Customer
Follow-up calls within 24 hours	Total calls (or contacts) made/ total sick or injured patients on the prior day	Customer

(continued)

Table 3. Metrics (*continued*)

Metric/Category	Calculation	Balance
Quality/follow-up	Total results call-backs within 24 hrs of receipt/total results rec'd	Int bus processes
Quality/provider reads	Total initial radiology reads/final reads concurring with initial read	Learning & growth
Pt. Satisfaction	Net promoter score calculation*	Customer
Left without being seen (lwbs)	Patients who checked in but did not get care/total patients	Customer
Patient satisfaction	Return or established patients/total patients	Customer
Pt. Satisfaction	Patient complaints/total patients	Customer
Quality	Total ED transfers by provider/total provider patients	Learning & growth

* Net Promoter Scores (NPS) allow an organization to benchmark clinic versus clinic as well as organization versus other industries. NPS is based on a 0–10 scale and takes into account your organization's promoters (those who would score you as a "9" or "10" on "Likelihood to refer you to someone else" and "Likelihood to return") and your detractors (those scoring the same categories as 0–6). Those scoring 7's and 8's are considered passives, in that their experience was satisfactory but they are not loyal customers. Scoring is calculated as follows: Net Promoter Score = % Promoters – % Detractors.

CONCLUSION

Strategy drives your management-control process and the corresponding metrics used as the measuring stick to ensure that you remain on track. It is an approach that requires organizational buy-in and support at every level. With ongoing analysis, *leading indicators* are likely to emerge. Leading indicators have a high probability of predicting an outcome. As an example, patient ranking of the overall experience with the physician may end up being the most relevant indicator of overall patient satisfaction. In this case, patient ranking would be your leading indicator, worthy of the most intense scrutiny and prompt intervention when unfavorable variances occur. You may also find that some metrics have very little relevance at all to performance and may therefore elect to eliminate them from further review.

As you create an organizational scorecard, you may wish to weigh these leading indicators more heavily when generating an aggregate score on a company, a clinic, or a provider scorecard. You might employ color coding, which indicates whether the score's variance from goal was negative or positive. The key is not only to support the interpretation of data into information and, subsequently, into knowledge but also to coach and support the translation of that knowledge into *action* and *results*. Use the data to generate healthy competition among staff members, managers, and health-care providers, and *always* recognize and celebrate success. Execution of a disciplined management-control process in collaboration with the selection of the right dataset is sure to improve your organization on all levels. An efficient and quality-driven organization supported by both loyal patients and engaged employees makes it highly likely that your urgent care operation will flourish.

KEY POINTS

1. A well-designed management-control process is the engine that drives change and performance.
2. Metrics, or KPIs, are essential components of the organization's approach to its overall strategy for operational excellence and market success.
3. Urgent care organizations must determine what is most important and strive for a balance between internal and external considerations.
4. Balance comes from ensuring the metric scorecard addresses four major areas: finance, internal business processes, the customer, and learning and growth.
5. The process of defining what is important to an organization often begins with its strategic plan, mission, and vision. Once the organization has defined its short- and long-range objectives, it can establish the tactics needed to achieve it.
6. What is critical when determining the appropriate metric for each level of the organization or process is that the computation is easily understood by those expected to respond to it.
7. Urgent care center operators must explore and exploit the capabilities of their systems to produce actionable information and to disseminate that information on an ability-to-impact, not a need-to-know, basis.
8. Though metrics management is a dynamic process, it is essential to keep the focus from changing too quickly. Otherwise, employee fatigue will be inevitable and goals will be viewed as the flavor of the week.
9. Teams must establish their WIGs to concentrate their energies on what is truly important to achieve a goal. Most teams cannot effectively achieve more than two goals at a time.
10. Strategy drives your management-control process and the choice of corresponding metrics as the measuring stick to ensure you remain on track. With ongoing analysis, leading indicators are likely to emerge. Leading indicators have a high probability of predicting an outcome.

CHAPTER 31

Laboratory Overview

Tracy Patterson

ON-SITE LABORATORY TESTING IS frequently performed in urgent care centers and physician offices. Same-day testing during the patient visit can improve the care the patient receives and enhance the patient experience. Which tests the urgent care center performs should be determined by the needs of its patients and the effect the tests will have on patient care. Laboratory test regulations vary greatly, as do the costs associated with performing them, so careful planning is needed. Understanding the need (demand) for a test, how the test is regulated, and the total costs to perform the test is necessary to determine which laboratory tests the urgent care center will undertake.

The information in this chapter about Clinical Laboratory Improvement Amendments (CLIA) and Centers for Medicare & Medicaid Services (CMS) regulation is a summary. It does not include all regulations and requirements. Every state has an office for laboratory licensing and regulation. Requirements can vary, and states can impose separate licensing requirements and stricter guidelines than the federal government. State requirements are not explored in this chapter; to learn your state's specific requirements, contact your state offices (Table 1).

CLINICAL LABORATORY IMPROVEMENT AMENDMENTS

The CLIA of 1988 established quality standards for laboratory testing to ensure the accuracy, reliability, and timeliness of patient laboratory results. In 1992, the final CLIA regulations were published, specifying that requirements are based on the test performed and not on who performs the test or where the test is performed. In 2003, the Centers for Disease Control and Prevention and CMS published final CLIA quality systems laboratory regulations. CMS regulates all human laboratory testing (except research) performed in the United States.

Under CLIA, a laboratory is defined as "a facility that performs testing on materials derived from the human body for the purpose of providing information for the diagnosis, prevention, or treatment of any disease or impairment of, or assessment of the health of, human beings." Therefore, urgent care centers that

Table 1. Important CMS Websites and Links

State survey agency contacts	http://www.cms.gov/Regulations-and-Guidance/Legislation/CLIA/Downloads/CLIASA.pdf
List of approved accrediting organizations	http://www.cms.gov/Regulations-and-Guidance/Legislation/CLIA/Downloads/AOList.pdf
Categorization of tests	http://www.cms.gov/Regulations-and-Guidance/Legislation/CLIA/Categorization_of_Tests.html
CLIA regulations and Federal Register documents	http://www.cms.gov/Regulations-and-Guidance/Legislation/CLIA/CLIA_Regulations_and_Federal_Register_Documents.html
CME courses for laboratory directors of moderate-complexity laboratories	http://www.cms.gov/Regulations-and-Guidance/Legislation/CLIA/CME_Courses_for_Laboratory_Directors_of_Moderate_Complexity_Laboratories.html
Proficiency testing programs	http://www.cms.gov/Regulations-and-Guidance/Legislation/CLIA/Downloads/ptlist.pdf
CLIA certificate fee schedule	http://www.cms.gov/Regulations-and-Guidance/Legislation/CLIA/Downloads/CLIA_certificate_fee_schedule.pdf
Application for certification, CMS-116	http://www.cms.gov/Medicare/CMS-Forms/CMS-Forms/Downloads/CMS116.pdf
Tests that are granted waived status under the CLIA	http://www.cms.gov/Regulations-and-Guidance/Legislation/CLIA/downloads/waivetbl.pdf

Please note at the time this chapter was written, these links were active; this may change.
CLIA, Clinical Laboratory Improvement Amendments; CME, continuing medical education; CMS, Centers for Medicare & Medicaid Services.

perform only specimen collection and handling for transport to an outside laboratory do not qualify as laboratories under CLIA.

CLIA requires all facilities, regardless of whether payment is requested, that perform even one test (waived or nonwaived) to meet federal requirements. If your urgent care center performs tests for diagnostic purposes, it is considered a laboratory under CLIA and must obtain appropriate CLIA certification.

CLIA classifies laboratory testing according to four complexity levels: high; moderate; provider-performed microscopy ([PPM] a subset of moderate complexity); and waived testing. The majority of urgent care centers possess a moderate-complexity or waived-testing laboratory.

CERTIFICATE TYPES UNDER THE CLINICAL LABORATORY IMPROVEMENT AMENDMENTS

There are five certificate types available under CLIA. Each is effective for 2 years.

- *Certificate of waiver (COW)*   Issued to a laboratory that performs only waived tests

- *Certificate for PPM*   Issued to a laboratory in which the provider (physician or midlevel practitioner) performs microscopy procedures during the course of a patient's visit. Only certain microscopy procedures are included under this certificate, and they are categorized as being of moderate complexity.

- *Certificate of registration*   Issued to a laboratory that has applied for a certificate of compliance, allowing it to perform nonwaived (moderate- or high-complexity) testing until the laboratory is inspected for compliance with CLIA regulations

- *Certificate of compliance (COC)*   Issued to a laboratory that performs nonwaived (moderate- or high-complexity) testing once the state department of health conducts an inspection and finds the laboratory in compliance with CLIA regulations

- *Certificate of accreditation (COA)*   Issued to a laboratory that performs nonwaived (moderate- or high-complexity) testing on the basis of the laboratory's accreditation. There are six CMS-approved accreditation organizations: AABB, American Osteopathic Association, American Society of Histocompatibility and Immunogenetics, COLA (formerly known as the Commission on Office Laboratory Accreditation), College of American Pathologists, and the Joint Commission. When you apply for accreditation, you concurrently apply for a COA from CMS.

No matter how many categories you perform testing under, only one certificate is required; that certificate should be for the highest (most complex) category of testing you perform. Therefore, if you need a COC or COA because you are going to perform complete blood cell counts, you would not need to apply for a COW.

Although there are a few exceptions to the need for CLIA certification, the one that possibly applies to a urgent care center laboratory is the exemption for a state CMS-approved laboratory program. The two states with approved programs are Washington and New York. New York's program has only a partial exemption. To determine your laboratory requirements and requirements for exemption, contact the health department for your state.

Note: For all types of CLIA certification you must notify your CLIA representative within 30 days of any changes in ownership, name, location, or laboratory director. For high-complexity testing, technical supervisory changes also must be reported. A "change in ownership" is any change in ownership, not only a majority change.

SURVEYS

Laboratories that have COW or PPM certificates are not subject to routine surveys. CMS does, however, perform a small percentage of educational visits to COW or PPM laboratories. These visits can provide helpful information to staff members to help ensure quality, and they should be taken seriously. The following excerpt is taken from the letter that COW or PPM laboratories receive before a visit from CMS:

> It is our intent that the focus of these inspections be educational only; however, if any serious risk to human health remains uncorrected, we may have to pursue further action. We will also re-visit a small number of the laboratories that have problems to ensure they are providing good quality testing.

If your laboratory holds a COC or COA, you must meet all nonwaived testing requirements, and you are subject to every-other-year surveys. Surveys may be performed by CMS, a state surveyor, or the accreditation organization's surveyor, depending on the certificate type. COA laboratories must also meet the requirements of their accreditation organization. Additionally, if you have a COA, your laboratory may undergo a validation survey by CMS or a state surveyor; these surveys are used to validate the findings of a recently performed accreditation organization survey.

If CMS or the state office receives a complaint against your laboratory, you may undergo an unannounced survey (that is, undergo a survey without receiving advance notice), no matter your certificate type.

CERTIFICATION COSTS

A minimal certificate fee is payable every 2 years when you apply for a COW, certificate for PPM, COC, or COA. There are no other registration or compliance fees aside from the certificate fee for a COW or a PPM. If you apply for a COC, a one-time registration fee that covers the cost of the CLIA enrollment and a compliance fee that covers the cost of the initial inspection are required. After payment of registration and compliance fees, CMS sends out a certificate of registration. Once the inspection has been done and your laboratory has passed, and on payment of the certificate fee, CMS sends out a COC. Certificate and compliance fees are paid every 2 years after that.

A one-time registration fee for CLIA enrollment is required when applying for a COA. Once CMS receives verification from your accreditation organization of choice, CMS requires a certificate fee and a validation fee, on receipt of which it sends out your COA. As long as your laboratory remains compliant, certificate and validation fees are due every 2 years. Other fees, such as the survey fee, are set by and payable to your chosen organization of accreditation.

You can obtain more information concerning fee amounts from the CMS or CLIA websites or from state agencies. Compliance (survey) fee amounts can be obtained from state agencies or accreditation organizations.

No matter the certificate type, applications are submitted without payment. Once your accreditation organization or CMS processes the application, it issues a fee coupon for payment. After payment is received, your center's certificate will be mailed to you.

TESTING

All CLIA certificates have a 10-digit number. This number is used to identify and track your laboratory throughout its entire history. You cannot begin testing until you receive your certificate.

If you perform only waived tests and want to add PPM procedures or other nonwaived testing, or have a PPM and want to add other nonwaived testing, you must apply for the appropriate certificate and cannot begin testing until you have received the new certificate. If you have a COC or COA and want to add tests different from those on your current certificate, you must notify the state agency or the accreditation organization of the new testing before you begin this testing.

Note: In a change-of-ownership situation, there are pluses and minuses to changing the existing CLIA certificate or applying for a new certificate. As part of the acquisition planning, determine the direction you will take, because the application process for a new certificate should be completed by the time ownership and payer changes are made.

Although CLIA does not require written policies for waived testing personnel, you are required to ensure that testing and results are accurate and that manufacturer instructions are followed. Competency assessment of these testing personnel will help you meet the necessary criteria. All nonwaived testing personnel should be assessed for competency, no matter the certificate type. CMS has the following six criteria for assessment:

- ▶ Direct observations of routine patient test performance, including patient preparation (if applicable), specimen handling, processing, and testing
- ▶ Monitoring the recording and reporting of test results
- ▶ Review of intermediate test results or worksheets, quality-control records, proficiency testing (PT) results, and preventive maintenance records
- ▶ Direct observations of performance of instrument maintenance and function checks
- ▶ Assessment of test performance through the testing of previously analyzed specimens, internal blind testing samples, or external PT samples
- ▶ Assessment of problem-solving skills

In addition to these six criteria, CMS recommends that assessment of personnel for PPM procedures include the following questions:

- Is the test actually performed during the patient's visit?
- Is the correct microscope type used (limited to bright-field or phase contrast)?
- Is the patient specimen processed correctly and in a timely manner?
- Does the midlevel practitioner perform the test and report results according to the laboratory's procedure?

WAIVED TESTING

For waived testing, CLIA requires that you

- Enroll in CLIA and obtain a certificate
- Follow the manufacturer's instructions for the waived tests you are performing
- Notify CLIA if you wish to add tests
- Notify CLIA within 30 days if any changes in ownership, facility name, address, or director occur
- Pay the certificate fee every 2 years
- Permit inspections

Most of these requirements are administrative in nature, with the exception of following "the manufacturers' instructions for the waived tests you are performing." This requirement will require the most diligence by you and your staff and, along with good laboratory practices, should be the focus of any waived laboratory.

Each test product that you purchase should have an insert that lists the manufacturer's instructions. These instructions should be followed completely on every test. Both the testing personnel and the providers using the results should have an understanding of the manufacturer's instructions. Providers should pay special attention to the sections on intended use and testing limitations. Reviewing and training on the quick reference instructions alone is not adequate to meet the CLIA requirement.

When training your staff and establishing procedure, provide instruction (based on the manufacturers; instructions) on at least how to

- Monitor the expiration date of tests, reagents, and controls
- Perform maintenance checks of equipment
- Run quality-control checks as required

- Track storage and handling requirements, including temperature and humidity monitoring
- Train testing personnel on performing tests, reading results, and following laboratory procedure

Note: If the manufacturer's instructions include recommendations and suggestions, you are not obliged to follow these. However, doing so is considered good laboratory practice and is strongly recommended.

PROVIDER-PERFORMED MICROSCOPY

PPM, although considered nonwaived, does not have the same criteria as other nonwaived testing. Tests classified as PPM have the following criteria:

- The examination must be performed by a physician or a midlevel practitioner (nurse practitioner, physician assistant) during the patient visit on a specimen obtained from the provider's patient or a patient of the group practice.
- The procedure must be in the moderately complex category.
- The primary instrument for the test must be a microscope.
- The specimen must be labile; a delay in testing could compromise the accuracy of the test.
- Control materials are not available to monitor the entire testing process.
- Limited specimen handling is required.

Also, PPM laboratories count toward the five-laboratory limit of laboratory directors put in place for nonwaived laboratories.

NONWAIVED TESTING, MODERATE

Taking your laboratory from waived to nonwaived means significant changes. It is strongly recommended that you find resources with in-depth knowledge and experience in taking laboratories nonwaived. Major changes include the qualifications of the laboratory director, the addition of a technical consultant or clinical consultant, the need to perform PT, and an increase in your laboratory quality-control program.

There are pluses and minuses to having either the COA or COC to perform moderate-complexity tests. Costs, requirements, availability of resources, and approaches to inspections can vary, and all aspects should be reviewed before making your decision. Before deciding on your certificate type, review all your options and listen to recommendations from your state. Your accreditation organization may have additional criteria besides those of CMS and CLIA, so check with your organization for specifics. If you are a multistate urgent care center provider, you may want to go with an accreditation organization so as to remove any differences between states.

It is the laboratory director's responsibility to ensure that the laboratory develops and uses a *quality system* approach. This approach should provide for accurate tests and reliable results. In addition, the laboratory director will need to take an active role in the operations of the laboratory and be a resource to the testing personnel. Laboratory director's duties include but are not limited to the following:

- Ensuring that testing systems are of a quality appropriate to the patient population
- Ensuring the adequacy of facilities and conditions for testing that are safe for employees
- Ensuring that there are adequately educated and trained staff members to perform testing
- Reviewing test procedures and procedure manuals
- Ensuring that test procedures and laboratory practices, duties, and responsibilities are available in writing
- Ensuring that testing procedures are followed

CMS states that in a quality system approach,

the laboratory focuses on comprehensive and coordinated efforts to achieve accurate, reliable, and timely testing services. The quality system approach includes all of your laboratory's policies, processes, procedures, and resources needed to achieve consistent, high quality testing services. Integral to the quality system approach is quality assessment, which involves the following activities:

- Ongoing monitoring of each testing process used in your laboratory in order to identify errors or potential problems that could result in errors
- Taking corrective action
- Evaluating the corrective actions taken, to make sure that they were effective and will prevent recurrence

The laboratory director can perform the functions of the technical consultant and the clinical consultant, or these roles can be filled separately. The clinical consultant is generally responsible for ensuring that test reports contain the necessary information for interpretation and is available for consultation regarding results and their interpretation. The technical consultant is normally responsible for ensuring that

- Appropriate testing methods are used
- PT is completed per regulations
- Quality assessment is performed and quality programs are established
- Testing personnel are appropriately trained and can demonstrate competency
- Written policies and procedures are established
- Corrective action and remedial training occur when needed

Note: Although there are some exceptions, in general, laboratory directors of nonwaived laboratories are limited to overseeing five laboratories, whereas there is no limit on the number of waived laboratories that can be under the auspices of a laboratory director. When the laboratory director oversees both nonwaived and waived laboratories, the limitation applies only to the nonwaived laboratories.

PT is not required for any test that is waived but is required for some nonwaived testing. Those nonwaived tests that require PT are categorized by CMS as *regulated* analytes, and a list of them can be found on the CMS website. Tests that are waived and that are performed nonwaived may require PT even when their waived counterparts do not. PT is performed to evaluate the accuracy of testing being performed by your laboratory. It involves the testing of unknown samples, typically three times a year. After testing the PT samples in the same manner as your patient specimens, your laboratory reports its sample results back to your PT program. The program then grades the results using CLIA grading criteria and sends you the scores.

When you receive a failed test (under a passing score or a nonpassing score), review the PT testing and take corrective action. Repeated failing scores on a test may result in your laboratory's losing its ability to perform that particular test. There are many criteria for the performance of PT; look to your PT program provider for a full list of requirements and rules.

Note: PT is required not per site but instead per certificate. If you have multiple locations under the same certificate, the PT for the sites is combined.

THE NEED FOR AND COST OF LABORATORY TESTING

The first step in determining the type of laboratory testing you will perform in your urgent care center should be assessing the need for a particular test. Any testing, laboratory or otherwise, should meet criteria for medical necessity. The most common laboratory tests performed in an urgent care setting include

- Dipstick urinalysis, nonautomated or automated
- Fecal occult blood

- Pregnancy: urine test
- Glucose: blood test
- Point-of-care tests for group A β-hemolytic streptococci, influenza A and B, and mononucleosis
- Chemistry panels (waived and nonwaived)
- Complete blood cell counts (nonwaived)

As you choose your tests, including the particular brand of kit and analyzer, it is important to realize the full costs. To understand the impact of laboratory testing on your urgent care center, you should fully model its addition. Start by asking the following questions:

- Within my existing patient population, what is the demand for each test?
- Will the demand for a particular test change with on-site availability?
- Will a particular test increase my scope of care?
- Do I have the staff I need to perform testing?
- Will I need to hire or contract leadership to start or maintain my laboratory program?
- Do I need additional space in my facility to perform additional testing?
- Do I need to perform any modifications to my existing facility to perform additional laboratory testing?

Consider the following questions when selecting your point-of-care test kits:

- Does the box come with separate tests for controls, or do you have to use some of the patient testing kits?
- Are the controls sold separately?
- How quickly does the kit or control expire after being opened?
- When running controls, are they run monthly, per box, or per operator?
- Is the test easy to operate?
- How does the quality of the test compare to others of its type?
- What PT is required?
- What is the staff time needed to perform the test?
- Will this test alone or in conjunction with others change my staffing needs?

Note: You may want to consider negotiating directly with a particular manufacturer. You may receive better pricing with the commitment, and many manufacturers' products have similarities that would be beneficial when training your staff to perform the test.

For tests requiring the purchase of analyzers and equipment, consider these questions:

- What are the costs of required annual maintenance?
- What does my staff have to do to perform maintenance and fix errors?
- Is the manufacturer available for service the hours that my laboratory is open?
- Is service provided on-site?
- Does the manufacturer provide loaners when equipment is out for repair?
- How long is the warranty, and what does it cover?
- What PT is required?
- What reagents and supplies are needed to run the test?
- Does the test interface with my electronic health record?

HOW TO GET STARTED

Start with testing that is beneficial to the majority of your patients. Allow your staff to focus on performing the more commonly ordered tests and becoming experts. The cost difference between switching your certificate from COW to COC or COA compared with starting out with a COC or COA is minimal. For new urgent care centers, it makes sense to begin with COW and grow from there.

Note: With the prevalence of global or flat-rate reimbursement in urgent care, it is important to understand what laboratory testing is included in your global or flat rates.

CONCLUSION

Urgent care is defined by same-day diagnosis and treatment, and laboratory testing can play a significant role in meeting that definition and ensuring a successful urgent care center. Take your time and research the regulations, the available testing, and your patients' needs. Don't forget to ask questions and ask for help.

KEY POINTS

1. Having laboratory services as part of your urgent care center allows you to provide better patient care and a better patient experience.

2. Laboratory testing, even done once without payment, requires that you obtain a CLIA certificate. You must obtain your certificate before you begin testing.
3. There are four types of CLIA certificates; apply for the one that covers the highest level of laboratory service you plan to provide.
4. Contact your state office regarding CLIA. There may be additional state-specific requirements or limitations regarding laboratory testing. Some states require you to obtain a separate certificate or permit in addition to your CLIA certificate.
5. Visit CLIA at http://www.cms.gov/Regulations-and-Guidance/Legislation/CLIA/ for additional information, including forms and helpful links.
6. Know when and how you need to notify CMS about changes to your laboratory testing and staffing (laboratory director, and so on).
7. Using testing kits and equipment requires you to follow the manufacturer's instructions.
8. Moderately complex testing requirements are significantly greater than waived testing requirements and have significant costs associated with them. Weigh the benefits of moderate testing closely before making a change.
9. No matter your certificate type, adequate and periodic staff training is key. It will help you meet regulatory requirements and will also reduce repeat testing and waste associated with errors.
10. Perform a full analysis and model when determining which laboratory testing to perform. This includes patient demand, regulation requirements and costs, and costs to perform testing, both direct and indirect.

CHAPTER 32

Implementation of a Moderate-Complexity Clinical Laboratory

Lynn R. Glass

URGENT CARE CENTERS HAVE become an important component in health-care delivery, bridging the gap between the traditional physician practice and the emergency department.

Typically, an urgent care center treats patients who do not have serious illnesses or life-threatening injuries but do require immediate attention. Providing on-site laboratory testing affords added value and quality of service for the patient and timely results for the caregiver to provide evaluation, diagnosis, and treatment while the patient is on-site (Figure 1).

Implementation of laboratory testing is not a plug-and-play operation, however, and a timeline should be established to ensure that critical elements are not missed during the implementation process, causing delays in licensing, validation, and completion of go-live testing.

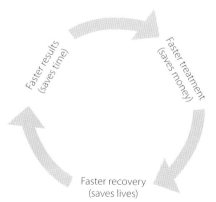

Figure 1. The value of on-site laboratory testing.

THREE MONTHS OUT...

Applying for Licensure

The Clinical Laboratory Improvement Amendments (CLIA) define a laboratory as "a facility that performs testing on materials derived from the human body for the purpose of providing information for the diagnosis, prevention, or treatment of any disease or impairment of, or assessment of the health of, human beings."

Every urgent care laboratory must have a CLIA license before patient testing begins. A license can be waived or nonwaived, but for the purposes of this timeline, the assumption is that you are establishing a nonwaived laboratory. You can download the CLIA application form, CMS-116, from the Centers for Medicare & Medicaid Services (CMS) website, www.cms.gov. Revisions to this form are made periodically; make sure that you submit the most recent form.

If only a CLIA application is warranted, submission may not be necessary 3 months before initiation of laboratory testing; however, there are often state-specific rules and regulations and separate state applications and designations to deal with. A listing of state offices with contact information can be found at www.cms.gov. States with additional licensure requirements may require up to 3 months for approval and scheduling of an on-site inspection before issuance of a license. Table 1 lists state-specific licensure and regulations requirements.

Negotiating Insurance Contracts

Medicare provides a clinical laboratory fee schedule that is revised and uploaded to the CMS website in November each year for the next year's allowable reimbursement. This fee schedule can be found at www.cms.gov.

You will have to negotiate insurance reimbursement for in-house laboratories individually with each carrier. Follow initial calls or other correspondence with insurance companies with a meeting with your region's insurance representative, not only to be credentialed with a contract agreement for patient visits and treatment but also to provide for reimbursement of laboratory testing. Most insurance companies will provide an exhibit or addendum with an in-house laboratory fee schedule; however, negotiations may be necessary to provide reimbursement for additional testing not on the typical list of allowable tests.

Some insurers offer global rates or fixed-rate schedules. You should research such arrangements to determine what testing is included in each of these fee schedule reimbursement types.

Contacting a Laboratory Equipment and Supply Distributor and a Technical Consultant

In the typical urgent care center, clinical laboratory testing includes point-of-care (POC) testing, defined as medical testing at or near the site of patient care, bringing tests conveniently and immediately to the patient, allowing for immediate evaluation and treatment.

Table 1. State-Specific Licensure and Regulations Requirements

State	Requirements for Testing	Exempt Tests
California	Laboratories offering only waived testing and/or microscopy performed by health-care providers do not need a state license, but they must register with the state health department and pay a small fee. (They must also have the proper CLIA certificate.) Nonwaived laboratories must obtain state licensure. State-licensed laboratories require licensed personnel for a number of testing functions. The personnel requirements for POLs performing moderate- and high-complexity testing are no more stringent than CLIA; however, clinical laboratories performing testing for the patients of six or more physicians must continue to staff the laboratory with licensed personnel such as registered nurses, physician assistants, and state-licensed medical technologists. The latter can perform testing in the specialties for which they are licensed in these laboratories. CME: 12 hours required	CLIA guidelines
Connecticut	Laboratories performing only waived testing do not need a state license. All moderate- and high-complexity laboratories must be licensed and surveyed by the state. The state is not CLIA-exempt and does not approve accrediting organizations for compliance with state regulations.	CLIA guidelines
Florida	Waived laboratories: state licensure not required Nonwaived laboratories: state licensure required Personnel: licensure for nonwaived laboratories with exceptions; laboratories with certain designations (as with a POL) do not require state-licensed medical technologists to perform testing	CLIA guidelines

(continued)

Table 1. State-Specific Licensure and Regulations Requirements (continued)

State	Requirements for Testing	Exempt Tests
Hawaii	Requires state licensure Personnel: required for nonwaived laboratories	CLIA guidelines
Louisiana	POLs are exempt from state licensure Personnel: licensure for nonwaived laboratories CME: required	CLIA guidelines
Maryland	Waived laboratories: state licensure required Nonwaived laboratories: state licensure required Personnel: CLIA guidelines	Cholesterol testing requires a permit for temporary or mobile laboratories; the number of testing events determines the permit fee
Massachusetts	State licensure required if physically testing in state, if specimens are collected in state, and if the physician collects and sends specimens outside of state	Capillary whole-blood cholesterol Capillary whole-blood glucose Capillary whole-blood hematocrit Capillary whole-blood hemoglobin Capillary whole-blood prothrombin time (INR) Complete UA with microscopy ESR Latex slide tests, qualitative (no dilutions required) Occult blood (stool) Pregnancy test (qualitative) Tape preparation for pinworm ova Serologic tests directly from swabs Sickle cell screening Throat culture, screening only (including bacitracin disc) Urine culture, screening only Wet smears (e.g., *Trichomonas*, yeast, KOH)
Montana	No state licensure CME: 14 hours required	CLIA guidelines

(continued)

Table 1. State-Specific Licensure and Regulations Requirements (continued)

State	Requirements for Testing	Exempt Tests
Nevada	State licensure required	CLIA guidelines
New Jersey	State licensure required for any laboratory performing tests other than the eight listed under exempt tests. New Jersey does not recognize all FDA-classified waived tests and recognizes only those listed in CLIA of 1988 with waived designation.	Blood glucose by FDA-approved home device Dipstick UA, nonautomated ESR, nonautomated Fecal occult blood Hemoglobin copper sulfate, nonautomated Ovulation test Spun hematocrit Urine pregnancy—visual color comparison
New York	Waived laboratories: eligible to apply for limited service laboratory application Nonwaived: must apply to the Physician Office Laboratory Evaluation Program for a CLIA number POL-CLIA/clinical-state New York CLIA exempt for other laboratory designations and are licensed through the Wadsworth Center	Special requirements for waived HIV testing
North Dakota	Personnel: need licensure CME: 20 hours/per contact hours required	CLIA guidelines
Oregon	No state licensure Personnel: licensure required Substances of Abuse registration is required	CLIA guidelines
Pennsylvania	State licensure required	CLIA guidelines (revised May 18, 2012)

(continued)

Table 1. State-Specific Licensure and Regulations Requirements (*continued*)

State	Requirements for Testing	Exempt Tests
Rhode Island	Waived laboratories: no state license required. Nonwaived laboratories: state licensure required. CME: 30 hours per 2 years for MTs, MLTs, cytotechnologists, histology technicians. Only licensed personnel can perform moderate-complexity testing.	CLIA guidelines
Tennessee	POL exempt from state licensure. Independent, hospitals, etc.: licensure required	CLIA guidelines
Washington	CLIA exempt; requires state licensure. All laboratories are required to have an MTS license. State licensing program is exempt from CLIA.	CLIA guidelines
West Virginia	Waived laboratories: no state license required. Nonwaived laboratories: state license required. Personnel: nonwaived laboratories require licensed personnel. CME: Nonwaived personnel are required to have 10 hours per year	CLIA guidelines

CLIA, Clinical Laboratory Improvement Amendments; CME, continuing medical education; ESR, erythrocyte sedimentation rate; FDA, (US) Food and Drug Administration; HIV, human immunodeficiency virus; INR, international normalized ratio; KOH, potassium hydroxide; MLT, medical laboratory technician; MT, medical technologist; MTS, medical testing site; POL, physician office laboratory; UA, urinalysis.

Most POC analyzers and test systems are sold through medical distributors, which can provide information on analyzers, test systems, ancillary equipment, supplies, and consumables.

A distributor sales representative may provide information on transportable, portable, or handheld instruments, or analyzers and equipment with a small footprint that can be housed at or near the site of patient specimen collection. A distributor will also have access to many manufacturers of rapid kit tests or may have private-label branded products they can provide at lower costs than national brands.

You should hire a qualified, licensed technical consultant with expertise in licensure, CLIA compliance, state regulatory concerns, integration of laboratory equipment, and ongoing compliance to ensure continued quality of testing. Consultants can be found locally, through accreditation organizations, or through nationally recognized consulting companies with expertise in this arena.

Selecting a Test Menu

Part of setting up the in-house laboratory is deciding what tests you will conduct there. Urgent care centers typically see the following conditions that may require laboratory testing:

- Bladder and urinary symptoms
- Coughs, colds, and influenza
- Ear and eye problems
- Muscle aches and pains
- Nausea, diarrhea, and vomiting
- Back, pelvic, and stomach pain
- Skin rashes, bruises, and bites
- Strep and sore throat
- Upper respiratory infections
- Shortness of breath and chest pain

Urgent care centers often use POC analyzers and rapid diagnostics because they offer timely results, have small footprints, and are generally easy for the laboratory staff members to use. Table 2 lists the most common tests offered by urgent care centers and the patient conditions most often encountered in urgent care for which such tests are helpful.

Maximize your test menu, taking into consideration your estimated volume of testing, patient population needs, and cost per test, to ensure a test menu that not only fits the needs of the patient population but also provides a financial foundation that makes the laboratory a revenue center and not a cost center.

Table 2. Medical Indications and Appropriate Testing

Test or Panel	Medical Indications	Tests Included
CBC count, automated differential	Fever, headache, malaise, fatigue, localized pain, bruising, infection, weakness, dizziness	WBC count, RBC count, Hgb, Hct, platelets, WBC automated cell differential
Chemistry panels (CMP, BMP, electrolyte, hepatic)[a]	Electrolyte and fluid imbalance, indications of abnormal kidney function, indications of abnormal liver function, symptoms of diabetes or chronic disease, protein abnormalities[a]	Sodium, potassium, chloride, CO_2, BUN, creatinine, glucose, calcium (total or ionized), ALT, AST, alkaline phosphatase, total bilirubin, direct bilirubin, total protein, albumin[a]
Lipid panel	Cardiovascular disease, pancreatitis, diabetes, chronic renal conditions, dyslipidemia and associated conditions (skin lesions), hyperthyroidism and hypothyroidism	Cholesterol, triglycerides, HDL (may also include calculated LDL, VLDL, and risk factor)
Urinalysis	Bladder and urinary infections, pelvic pain, blood in urine	pH, ketone, glucose, bilirubin, blood protein, urobilinogen, leukocytes, nitrites, specific gravity
Cardiac markers	Shortness of breath, chest pain	CKMB, troponin I, myoglobin, BNP, D-dimer
Glucose, HbA_{1c}	Diabetes, hypoglycemia, hyperglycemia	Glucose, HbA_{1c}
Group A β-hemolytic streptococci	Sore throat, fever, swollen lymph nodes, nasal draining, swollen glands, difficulty swallowing	Group A β-hemolytic streptococci
Influenza A and B	Fever, headache, chills, cough, sore throat, body aches	Influenza A and B
Mononucleosis	Fever, sore throat, swollen lymph nodes, swollen tonsils, chills, headache, fatigue, loss of appetite, pain in upper left abdomen	Mononucleosis

(continued)

Table 2. Medical Indications and Appropriate Testing (continued)

Test or Panel	Medical Indications	Tests Included
RSV	Cough, stuffy or runny nose, sore throat, earache, fever	RSV
Helicobacter pylori	Gastritis, burning abdominal pain, weight loss, loss of appetite, bloating, burping, nausea, vomiting, black tarry stools	*H. pylori*
Urine HCG	Pelvic pain, vaginal bleeding, normal pregnancy	Urine HCG
Occult blood	Stomach disorders, rectal bleeding, fecal impaction, gastroenteritis, vomiting, heartburn, diarrhea	Occult blood
Blood gases	Abnormal lung function, abnormal kidney function, indications of metabolic imbalance	pH, Po_2, Pco_2
Drugs of abuse	Ingestion of unknown medications, suspected drug use, presentation with disorientation	Amphetamine, barbiturates, methamphetamine, methadone, benzodiazepines, THC, cocaine, opiates, PCP, tricyclics, MDMA, methadone, oxycodone

[a]Chemistry panels may include various components of tests listed and various patient conditions to allow for medical necessity and coverage. ALT, alanine aminotransferase; AST, aspartate aminotransferase; BMP, basic metabolic panel; BNP, B-type natriuretic peptide; BUN, blood urea nitrogen; CBC, complete blood cell; CKMB, creatine kinase MB; CMP, comprehensive metabolic panel; Hct, hematocrit; HDL, high-density lipoprotein; HbA_{1c}, glycated hemoglobin A_{1c}; HCG, human chorionic gonadotropin; Hgb, hemoglobin; LDL, low-density lipoprotein; MDMA, 3,4-methylenedioxymethamphetamine; PCP, phencylidine; RBC, red blood cell; RSV, respiratory syncytial virus; THC, tetrahydrocannabinol; VLDL, very low density lipoprotein; WBC, white blood cell.

Selecting Analyzers, Test Systems, and Test Kits

When you have selected the test menu, you can select analyzers, test systems, and test kits that support the selected tests, meet the requirements of your laboratory license, are within the technical capabilities of your laboratory staff, and fit within the available space and specifications of your laboratory.

Most POC testing is typically performed with handheld or smaller stationary analyzers that require minimal training for laboratory staff members and fit the available space. When selecting laboratory test systems, consider analyzers and test systems that

- ▶ Provide appropriate test menus
- ▶ Provide adequate cost per test and time to test
- ▶ Fit within the physical space available
- ▶ Have acceptable specifications with regard to physical space, electricity, plumbing, ventilation, and Internet capability when warranted
- ▶ Provide adequate time to first test
- ▶ Ensure ease of use for laboratory personnel
- ▶ Require little or no maintenance
- ▶ Include a minimum 1-year warranty (for any items other than rapid kits)
- ▶ Require few additional consumables and supplies
- ▶ Support HL7 (Health Level 7 informatics) capability if needed for additional integration of a laboratory information system (LIS)

TWO MONTHS OUT...

Personnel and Laboratory Support Staff Members

Personnel requirements for waived testing are much less stringent than for testing performed in a moderately complex laboratory. In a laboratory performing moderately complex testing (Table 3), the following personnel are required:

- ▶ Laboratory director
- ▶ Clinical consultant
- ▶ Technical consultant
- ▶ Testing personnel

Contact the CLIA or state office in which the urgent care center will reside to determine if there are additional personnel requirements specific to that state that supersede the CLIA requirements.

Table 3. Personnel Requirements in the Moderately Complex Laboratory

Position	Requirements

Laboratory director	One of the following:
	• Licensed MD, DO, or DPM, *and* certified in anatomic or clinical pathology
	  • *or* laboratory training or experience consisting of 1 year directing or supervising nonwaived tests
	  • *or* since September 1, 1993, has earned at least 20 CME credits in laboratory practice addressing director responsibilities
	  • *or* training equivalent to 20 CME credits obtained during medical residency
	• Doctoral degree in laboratory science *and* certified by an HHS-approved board
	  • *or* 1 year of experience directing or supervising nonwaived testing
	• Master's degree in laboratory science *and* 1 year of laboratory training or experience *and* 1 year of experience supervising nonwaived testing
	• Bachelor's degree in laboratory science *and* 2 years of laboratory training or experience *and* 2 years of experience supervising nonwaived testing
	• Before February 28, 1992, qualified as director under state law or Medicare laboratory regulations

Technical consultant	One of the following: • Licensed MD, DO, or DPM, *and* certified in anatomic or clinical pathology • *or* 1 year of laboratory training or experience in nonwaived specialty or subspecialty of service • Doctoral, master's, or bachelor's degree in laboratory science *and* 1 year of laboratory training or experience in nonwaived specialty or subspecialty of service • Bachelor's degree in laboratory science *and* 2 years of laboratory training or experience in nonwaived specialty or subspecialty of service *Note:* "Training or experience" in specialties and subspecialties can be acquired concurrently.
Clinical consultant	• Licensed MD, DO, or DPM • Doctoral degree in laboratory science *and* board certified in specialty or subspecialty of service
Testing personnel	• Licensed MD, DO, or DPM • Doctoral, master's, bachelor's, or associate's degree in laboratory science • High school graduate or equivalent *and* completed military medical laboratory specialist (50-week) course • High school graduate or equivalent *and* documentation of training at the present facility for testing performed

CME, continuing medical education; DO, doctor of osteopathic medicine; DPM, doctor of podiatric medicine; HHS, (US) Department of Health and Human Services; MD, medical doctor.

Physicians who will act as laboratory director may be required to complete an online course to be deemed qualified for this position. These courses provide 20 or more continuing medical education credits that will satisfy the requirement. Several online courses are available; an outside consultant can provide information and assistance to enroll in this course. A course-completion certificate must be submitted to the CLIA and state agencies for proof of qualification. The physician acting as the laboratory director can, if qualified, also be named the clinical consultant in this type of setting.

Although under certain conditions and qualifications the laboratory director may act as the technical consultant, he or she may not qualify to perform this function, and an outside technical consultant may be hired for a minimum of 1 year, until the laboratory director gains the required 1 year of experience in the clinical laboratory setting. Some states require an outside technical consultant for a minimum of 1 year, per state-specific laboratory licensure and regulatory statutes; contact your state agency to determine if an outside technical consultant is required before submission of applications.

Testing personnel may be medical technologists (MTs), registered nurses (RNs), licensed practical nurses (LPNs), physician assistants (PAs), nurse practitioners (NPs), physicians, medical assistants, and staff members with a minimum of a high school diploma and evidence of training. Again, state-specific licensure and regulatory restrictions may apply; contact your state agency to determine qualifications necessary for testing personnel.

Testing personnel can be acquired through Internet-based recruitment; local newspaper advertising; contacts with other hospitals, clinics, and physician office laboratories (POLs); and medical- and laboratory-related periodicals. Review résumés, conduct phone and on-site interviews, and verify all credentials and references before hiring testing personnel. Generally, personnel should be identified and hired a month before beginning laboratory operations, to complete training and validation on analyzers and test systems.

Reagent and Analyzer Contracts

All contracts, including terms and conditions, reagent pricing agreements, service contracts and warranties, and leasing agreements, must be signed and in place at least 2 months before completion of laboratory setup, to ensure timely delivery of analyzers, supplies, consumables, and supplemental materials. Training slots are generally not scheduled until contract signatures are in place, and they normally are scheduled 2 months out from delivery and integration of analyzers. Failure to complete this process in a timely manner may delay delivery, installation, and training and, more importantly, may affect a go-live date for patient testing.

Once contracts are in place, compile orders for all reagents, consumables, supplies, and ancillary equipment you need, so that the delivery of all items can take place before delivery and integration of analyzers.

Laboratory Information Systems

An LIS integrates laboratory analyzers and provides an interface for transmission of test results from analyzers to a central server. The testing personnel can review results from a central monitor and compile one comprehensive test report combining results from all analyzers. The LIS can also be interfaced with the facility's electronic health record (EHR) system to provide paperless efficiency, with results stored cumulatively in patient files. The LIS can also provide cumulative quality-control results and summary files, maintenance files, and programs for additional data, such as linearity studies and calibration verification. LIS integration and training is normally performed on-site, and vendors usually require a minimum of 2 months in advance of actual integration to secure training slots for identified personnel.

Completion of Physical Site

If the urgent care center is new construction, or if major renovation must be completed for an existing space, coordination is essential to ensure that an adequate number of electrical outlets are present; that all specifications for Internet connections and for the electrical, water, heating, ventilation, and air-conditioning systems have been given to architects and contractors; and that adequate physical space and counter work areas are available for all analyzer and test systems. Additional state requirements may need to be addressed for specific building codes, drainage, and effluent studies. Failure to address these specifications can cause delays in the opening of your clinical laboratory.

ONE MONTH OUT...

Hire Personnel

One month before initiation of actual patient testing, personnel should be hired who can be available for delivery, installation, and training on all analyzers and test systems. Once training is completed, personnel will be responsible for validation of analyzers, integration of an LIS, and review of all policies, procedures, and quality-assessment (QA) plans, to ensure quality of testing and completeness of documentation review and retention policies.

Delivery, Training, and Validation of Analyzers

One month before implementation of actual patient testing, analyzers are delivered to the laboratory site. Depending on the complexity of the analyzer, training can be scheduled either at the laboratory site or off-site at a manufacturer's training facility. Documentation must be in the personnel files of all testing personnel, providing evidence of completion of training.

A service technician can come on-site to set up analyzers and perform maintenance checks. The manufacturer can also provide a technical specialist, who will provide initial or follow-up training and can guide the testing personnel through the validation process.

Validation must be performed on any moderately or highly complex analyzer. Validation may be required on analyzers and test systems that are deemed waived tests, if state-specific regulatory requirements are more stringent. Contact the CLIA and state agencies to ascertain whether more stringent state requirements are in place.

Per CLIA regulation 42 CFR 493.1253(b)(1):

Each laboratory that introduces an unmodified, FDA-cleared or approved test system must do the following before reporting patient test results:

(i) Demonstrate that it can obtain performance specifications comparable to those established by the manufacturer for the following performance characteristics:

(A) Accuracy.

(B) Precision.

(C) Reportable range of test results for the test system.

(ii) Verify that the manufacturer's reference intervals (normal values) are appropriate for the laboratory's patient population.

Accuracy is an indication that the method provides correct results, and can be verified by

- Testing reference materials
- Comparing results of tests performed by the laboratory against results of a reference method
- Comparing split-sample results with results obtained from a method that is known to provide clinically valid results

Precision is a measure of the reproducibility of results that is verified by assessing day-to-day, run-to-run, and within-run variation, as well as operator variance. This can be accomplished by

- Testing quality-control material in duplicate over time
- Repeat testing of known patient samples over time
- Repeat testing of calibration materials over time

Reportable range is an indication of the high and low values for a test obtainable on the system. This can be verified by

- Assaying low-, normal-, and high-value calibration of control materials
- Evaluating known samples of abnormal low, normal, and abnormal high values

Reference ranges, or normal patient values, can be provided by the manufacturer or can be found in published sources. Before using these ranges, verify that they apply to your patient population on the basis of demographic variables such as age, sex, and region. The laboratory should verify these reference ranges with an appropriate number of samples before using them in the final patient report.

Validation studies should be performed by testing personnel within the laboratory. Manufacturer technical specialists or outside consultants can guide the testing personnel through the process, but actual studies must be conducted by the personnel who will be performing patient testing. The laboratory director must review, accept, and sign off on final data reduction and reports before patient testing can begin.

Integration of the Laboratory Information System

Integration of the LIS should take place after all analyzers and test systems are in place and validation studies have been completed and approved.

For a routine LIS installation, a support specialist from the LIS manufacturer will travel to the site, set up the computer workstation and central server, connect all cable connections, and verify transmission of results, both through electronic transmission and through manual data entry. This process normally takes 2 to 5 days, depending on the complexity of the laboratory and the number of instruments to be interfaced. If the LIS will be further interfaced with an EHR or a reference laboratory server, additional time may be required on-site; however, this process is normally handled remotely in coordination with the EHR and reference laboratory information technology counterparts.

Validation of interface connections must be performed and documented for transmission of both patient and quality-control results before the system is deemed operational.

Policies and Procedures

Policies and procedures must be in place for all analyzers and test systems in the laboratory. These policies should include processes, documentation, and operation in pre-analytical, analytical, and post-analytical phases of testing.

Pre-analytical phase factors include but are not limited to

- Patient preparation
- Specimen collection and labeling
- Storage, preservation, and transport
- Processing and referral
- Specimen acceptability and rejection

Analytical phase factors include but are not limited to

- Maintenance
- Malfunctioning equipment
- Quality control

- Calibration and calibration verification
- Patient test management and performance
- Proficiency testing

Post-analytical phase factors include but are not limited to

- Review of results
- Critical values
- Corrective action
- Record retention

The laboratory director is ultimately responsible for the compilation of a complete policies and procedures manual, in addition to compiling assay-specific policies and procedures. A qualified outside technical consultant or consultant group can be hired to customize these manuals for the urgent care center, with final review and signature by the laboratory director.

Quality-Assessment Plan

A comprehensive and effective QA plan is essential to provide continued quality of service in the laboratory setting. *Quality assessment* is an ongoing review process that encompasses all facets of the laboratory's technical and nontechnical functions and all locations and sites where testing is performed. QA also extends to the laboratory's interactions with and responsibilities to patients, physicians, and other laboratories ordering tests, and the other nonlaboratory areas or departments of the facility of which it is a part.

QA plans monitor various indicators over time and identify errors or potential problems in the laboratory setting. Corrective action must take place to rectify any problems identified; this action includes identification and resolution of the problem and may include development of policies to correct the problem and prevent recurrence, counseling or retraining of personnel involved, and communication to other laboratory personnel and staff members as appropriate. All pertinent laboratory staff members must be involved in the assessment process and actively review of indicators, assessment of patient testing involved, corrective action, and follow-up to ensure that problems and errors do not occur in the future.

The laboratory director is ultimately responsible for the compilation of a complete QA plan. A qualified outside technical consultant or consultant group can be hired to customize this plan for the urgent care center, with the laboratory director responsible for final review and signing off.

Proficiency Testing

Proficiency testing is an external quality-assurance check and an assessment tool for determining regulatory compliance.

According to 42 CFR 493.801:

> Each laboratory must enroll in a proficiency testing...program that meets the criteria in subpart I...and is approved by HHS [the US Department of Health and Human Services]. The laboratory must enroll in an approved program or programs for each of the specialties or subspecialties for which it seeks certification. The laboratory must test the samples in the same manner as patients' specimens.

This regulation refers to nonwaived, regulated analytes; however, if state regulatory rules exist that are more stringent than CLIA, they supersede this regulatory standard, and additional enrollment in proficiency events may be warranted for additional analytes and tests considered waived and exempt from this requirement. Contact your state office to determine if additional proficiency enrollment is required.

A proof-of-enrollment letter must be obtained from the proficiency provider and must be made available to the inspector before implementation of any patient testing. Table 4 is a list of approved proficiency-testing providers.

Setup of Patient Draw Site

Patient samples can be collected in examination rooms, or a separate draw site can be set up for collection of specimens. If patient specimens are collected in an area where patient testing will be performed, care must be taken to conform to

Table 4. CLIA-Approved Proficiency-Testing Providers, 2013

AAFP-PT
11400 Tomahawk Creek Parkway
Leawood, KS 66211-2672
(800) 274-7911

Accutest, Inc.
PO Box 999
Westford, MA 01886
(800) 665-2575

American Association of Bioanalysts (AAB)
205 West Levee Street
Brownsville, TX 78520-5596
(800) 234-5315

American Proficiency Institute (API)
1159 Business Park Drive
Traverse City, MI 49686
(800) 333-0958

(continued)

Table 4. CLIA-Approved Proficiency-Testing Providers, 2013 (*continued*)

American Society for Clinical Pathology
8900 Keystone Crossing, suite 620
Indianapolis, IN 46240
(800) 267-2727, (317) 876-4169

California Thoracic Society (CTS)
575 Market Street, suite 2125
San Francisco, CA 94105
(415) 536-0287

The College of American Pathologists (CAP)—Surveys
325 Waukegan Road
Northfield, IL 60093-2750
(847) 832-7000

Commonwealth of Pennsylvania
Department of Health
Bureau of Laboratories
PO Box 500
Exton, PA 19341-0500
(610) 280-3464

External Comparative Evaluation for Laboratories (EXCEL)
College of American Pathologists
325 Waukegan Road
Northfield, IL 60093-2750
(800) 323-4040

Maryland Department of Health and Mental Hygiene
Office of Health Care Quality—Laboratory Care
Spring Grove Hospital Center
Bland Bryant Building
55 Wade Avenue
Catonsville, MD 21228
(410) 402-8029

Medical Laboratory Evaluation (MLE) Program
25 Massachusetts Avenue, NW, suite 700
Washington DC 20001-7401
(800) 338-2746, (202) 261-4500

New York State Department of Health
Governor Nelson A. Rockefeller State Plaza
PO Box 509
Albany, NY 12201-0509
(518) 474-8739

(*continued*)

Table 4. CLIA-Approved Proficiency-Testing Providers, 2013 (*continued*)

Puerto Rico Proficiency Testing Service
Public Health Laboratories of Puerto Rico
PO Box 70184
San Juan, Puerto Rico 00936-8184
(787) 274-6827

WSLH
Proficiency Testing Program
465 Henry Mall
Madison, WI 53706-1578
(800) 462-5261

CLIA, Clinical Laboratory Improvement Amendments.

Health Insurance Portability and Accountability Act (HIPAA) guidelines. Consider the following factors in determining placement of the draw station:

- All papers in the testing site containing pertinent patient information must not be visible to patients.

- Patients' documents must remain closed unless an additional notation must be made in a patient's record concerning specimen draw or collection.

- Any paper or label that contains patient information and that is not filed or secured in the laboratory must be shredded before discarding.

- Laboratory requisitions or encounter forms must be kept with testing personnel and at central company locations in each station.

- If screens are accessible for view by patients or others who may be in a laboratory or draw site, a cover must be placed over the screen or monitor to protect all patient information from view by these individuals.

Table 5 lists items and supplies needed for draw stations in addition to general laboratory supplies.

Preparation for Inspection Process

In states where only a CLIA license is required, the laboratory will receive a certificate of registration, which acts as a temporary license to begin testing. A CLIA inspection will be performed to review comprehensive laboratory operations within 11 months from issuance of this certificate, and if the laboratory is found to be compliant, a certificate of compliance or accreditation will be issued as the permanent license on file.

Table 5. General Supplies Needed in Clinical Laboratory Setup

- Adhesive bandage strips
- Alcohol prep pads
- Antifatigue mats
- Basic tool set
- Biohazard absorbent pads, 4″ × 4″
- Biohazard bags
- Biohazard labels
- Centrifuge, with designated rpm and number of tubes (normally 6)
- Clorox unscented bleach
- Cotton balls
- Cotton-tipped applicator sticks, 6″
- Countertop shield, for processing specimens
- Disinfectant cleaner for counters
- Distilled or deionized water
- Eye wash station (must have continuous flow to both eyes)
- Face shield
- Freezer (manual defrost)
- Gauze, 2″ × 2″
- Gauze, 4″ × 4″
- Gloves, powder free, latex, large
- Gloves, powder free, latex, medium
- Gloves, powder free, latex, small
- Gloves, powder free, nitrile, large
- Gloves, powder free, nitrile, medium
- Gloves, powder free, nitrile, small
- Glucola glucose drink
- Heel warmers
- KimWipes cleanup wipes
- Laboratory coats, large
- Laboratory coats, medium
- Laboratory coats, small
- Lancets
- Needle holders, disposable safety
- Needles, safety
- Paper tape
- Paper towels
- Parafilm flexible film, 2″ × 250′
- Pipette bulb
- Pipette tips for 10-µL to 200-µL adjustable pipette
- Pipette tips for 100-µL to 1000-µL adjustable pipette
- Pipettes, plastic transfer disposable, 5 mL
- Pipettor, micropipette, 10 µL to 200 µL, adjustable (dependent on testing performed)
- Pipettor, micropipette, 100 µL to 1000 µL, adjustable (dependent on testing performed)

(continued)

Table 5. General Supplies Needed in Clinical Laboratory Setup (*continued*)

- Plastic pour-over tubes for storage and transport of specimens
- Refrigerators
- Rocker for tubes
- Room-temperature thermometer and hygrometer
- Saline
- Sharps container
- Smelling salts
- Spill kits, biohazard
- Spill kits, chemical
- Test tube racks
- Thermometer, NIST, freezer, –30° to 0°C
- Thermometer, NIST, refrigerator, –5° to 15°C
- Timer
- Tourniquets
- Tube closures, 13 mm
- Tube closures, 16 mm
- Tubes, gold top (SST)
- Tubes, green top (lithium heparin)
- Tubes, lavender top (EDTA) K2 or K3
- Tubes, light blue top (sodium citrate)
- Tubes, plastic, 12 × 75 mm
- Urine container with screw cap
- Volumetric pipette, 1 mL (either glass or disposable)
- Volumetric pipette, 5 mL (dependent on testing performed)
- Wash bottle with cap, 16 oz
- Wooden applicator sticks, 6″

EDTA, ethylenediaminetetraacetic acid; NIST, National Institutes of Standards and Technology; SST, serum separator tube.

In states that require additional state licensure, it may be necessary for a surveyor to provide an on-site inspection before performance of any patient testing. All elements of the laboratory must be in place and accessible for the inspection, which will focus on the following categories:

▶ Personnel qualification documentation and training records

▶ Policies and procedures, and assay-specific policies

▶ Comprehensive QA plan

▶ Validation of all moderate-complexity analyzers

▶ Processes in place for sample collection, test requisition, and accessioning; supplemental logs and forms to ensure adequate tracking; and documentation throughout the testing process

- Quality-control processes
- Enrollment in proficiency testing
- Processes in place for patient test management and review of results
- Corrective action plans

CONCLUSION

A properly set-up and maintained in-house testing laboratory can be a vital tool in the urgent care setting to assist in timely evaluation, diagnosis, and treatment of its patients. This adds quality and value to both the patient and the practitioner providing treatment and allows for faster results, faster treatment, and ultimately faster recovery.

KEY POINTS

1. Any "facility that performs testing on materials derived from the human body for the purpose of providing information for the diagnosis, prevention, or treatment of any disease or impairment of, or assessment of the health of, human beings" must obtain a CLIA certificate before any patient testing, regardless of the complexity of the testing.

2. Laboratories should verify whether additional state regulatory standards apply and whether additional application for state licensure is warranted.

3. Personnel requirements vary by complexity of testing and by state; ensure that all personnel in the laboratory setting have documented credentials and applicable licensure.

4. Hire outside technical consulting assistance with increased levels of testing complexity to ensure optimal operation, lean operational practices, and ongoing compliance.

5. Optimize services by providing a test menu that supports the center's patient population, provides timely results, supports on-site diagnosis and treatment, and ultimately improves patient care.

6. Balance added value and improved quality of care with financial considerations relating to cost per test and overall profitability when assessing needs in the laboratory.

7. Negotiate insurance contracts well in advance of go-live laboratory operations or have flat fee schedules in place for immediate generation of revenue.

8. Purchase test systems that provide adequate data and supportive documentation for sensitivity, specificity, accuracy, and precision of results.

9. Be confident that the named laboratory director is aware of the responsibility to provide oversight for both personnel and laboratory operations for continued successful and compliant laboratory testing, or hire outside technical consulting support to fulfill this requirement.
10. Market the laboratory in the urgent care center as an opportunity for patients to be provided not only with immediate attention but also with greater quality of service through timely evaluation, diagnosis, and treatment.

CHAPTER 33

EMTALA in Urgent Care Medicine

Rachel A. Lindor

THE EMERGENCY MEDICAL TREATMENT AND ACTIVE LABOR ACT (EMTALA), commonly referred to as the "patient anti-dumping act," is designed to prevent hospitals and emergency departments (EDs) from refusing to treat patients who are unable to pay for their care. Enacted in 1986, EMTALA was inspired by a smattering of highly publicized cases in which patients with life-threatening conditions were turned away from EDs because they were uninsured.

Although EMTALA was originally designed to protect indigent patients who presented to EDs, its scope has expanded considerably since 1986. Currently, the provisions of EMTALA apply to all patients, regardless of insurance status, age, immigration status, or any other characteristic. In addition, the act's provisions apply to a number of clinical care sites, not only the traditional EDs that were originally targeted by the legislation. Identifying these additional sites is the first major focus of this chapter.

For health-care providers and institutions that *are* subject to EMTALA, the law can be broken into three main requirements. First, all patients must be given an appropriate medical screening exam designed to detect emergency medical conditions. Second, if an emergency medical condition is found, patients must be stabilized before being discharged or transferred. Third, if an emergency medical condition is found and the institution does not have the capabilities to stabilize the patient, the act requires both that the patient be transferred to a site that does have the necessary capabilities *and* that the site with the specialized capabilities accept that transfer as long as it has the capacity to do so. Additional details regarding these requirements are the second major focus of this chapter.

The requirements of EMTALA are enforced through three major avenues. First, the Centers for Medicare & Medicaid Services (CMS)—the federal agency that interprets and oversees EMTALA—receives and investigates claims for alleged EMTALA violations from state surveyors. In 2000, the last year in which EMTALA violations were internally reviewed, CMS received around 400 claims and found violations in about half of those, representing roughly 5% of hospitals with EDs. When CMS finds that a violation has occurred, the agency can begin the process of terminating a hospital's Medicare provider agreement. In almost all cases, the hospital submits a corrective action plan that details changes it will make to prevent future violations, thus putting a halt to the termination process and retaining its provider agreement.

In the second avenue for enforcement, CMS can authorize the Office of Inspector General (OIG) to further investigate the claims and impose sanctions on offenders. By statute, the OIG can assess penalties of up to $50,000 against offending physicians and hospitals. In most cases, however, the OIG attempts to enter into a settlement agreement with the hospital or physician. In the late 1990s, the last years to be studied, the OIG received about 100 claims per year from CMS and chose to investigate roughly 40% of these. Decisions to investigate were based on the severity of the allegations, the history of complaints against the hospital, and other considerations. Almost every hospital and physician investigated entered a settlement with the OIG that allowed them to pay an amount similar to that of a civil monetary penalty but without having to admit any wrongdoing.

The statute also gives individuals who are injured by alleged EMTALA violations the right to sue the offending hospital in civil court, which is the third avenue for EMTALA enforcement. There are few data regarding the incidence of EMTALA-related lawsuits, but many malpractice claims arising from EDs include both common law malpractice claims and allegations of EMTALA violations. The potential for private civil suits puts institutions at risk for much more significant financial liability than the government-imposed civil monetary penalties.

DOES EMTALA APPLY TO MY INSTITUTION?

EMTALA applies to "Medicare-participating hospitals and critical access hospitals" that have a "dedicated emergency department," and its requirements are triggered when a patient "comes to the emergency department."

The interpretation of EMTALA's terminology has changed significantly since the law's passage in 1985, largely because of the emergence of several tragic cases that highlighted the problems with EMTALA's requirements being applied too narrowly. For example, in one case a hospital refused to treat a pregnant woman in labor and with fetal distress because she presented to the hospital's labor and delivery unit rather than the ED, eventually resulting in the death of the baby.[1] In a later case, a hospital refused to treat a teenager who was bleeding to death outside the entrance of the ED, arguing that he had not "come to" the ED as the law reads.[2] The circumstances in these cases highlighted the ambiguities around the terminology of EMTALA and prompted CMS to issue multiple clarifications of its interpretation of the law, as summarized below.

- "Medicare-participating hospitals":
    Medicare-participating refers to hospitals that have entered into a provider agreement with the Medicare program, which allows them to

---

1   *McIntyre v. Schick*, 795 F. Supp. 777 (E. D. Va. 1992).
2   See, for example, Jeter J. Hospital blasted for not aiding teen. *Sun Sentinel*. May 20, 1998. Available from: http://articles.sun-sentinel.com/1998-05-20/news/9805190304_1_hospital-workers-emergency-room-police-officer.

accept payments from CMS for care provided to Medicare beneficiaries.[3] Almost all traditional hospitals participate in Medicare, though smaller private hospitals, subspecialty clinics, and urgent care practices often do not. Facilities should have very little confusion about whether they are "Medicare-participating."

Hospitals: EMTALA adopts the same definition outlined in the Social Security Act, which defines a hospital as an institution primarily engaged in providing care through physicians to inpatients.[4] *Inpatients* are further defined as those patients who are admitted to the hospital with the expectation that they will occupy a bed and stay for at least one night.[5]

▶ *Dedicated emergency department* was a term intentionally chosen to be broader than the idea of a formal, or named, ED so that institutions could not escape EMTALA obligations by renaming their services. Instead, CMS provides three descriptions for a facility that may be considered a dedicated ED, even if it does not claim to be one. By CMS's interpretation, a facility is considered a dedicated ED for the sake of EMTALA if it meets one or more of the following three criteria:

- It is licensed by the state as an emergency room or ED.
- It is "held out to the public" as a place that provides care for emergency medical conditions without requiring an appointment.
- It has seen at least one-third of its patients for emergency medical conditions without requiring that they have an appointment.

The first definition is quite clear. A facility should know if it is licensed. However, because most states do not license EDs separately from hospitals, this first definition accounts for the minority of dedicated EDs.

The second definition addresses facilities that are "held out" as EDs. In its regulations, CMS notes that it will consider a variety of factors when determining whether a facility meets this definition, including the name of the institution, posted signs, advertisements, or other means.[6] From this, it is clear that a site that calls itself an ED and advertises itself for emergency care will almost certainly be considered a "dedicated emergency department" for the purposes of EMTALA; it is less clear whether a site that calls itself an urgent care center or a "minute clinic" will be considered a distinct type of entity or whether it too will fall under the definition of a dedicated ED. Currently, CMS provides little additional guidance about its interpretation of this "held out" definition, leaving it to be subjectively determined on a case-by-case basis.

The third definition designates facilities as "dedicated emergency departments" if one-third of their patients are seen for emergency medical conditions on an unscheduled basis. Whether a facility meets this

3   42 Code of Federal Regulations § 489.24(b).
4   42 United States Code § 1395x.
5   42 Code of Federal Regulations § 489.24(b).
6   42 Code of Federal Regulations § 489.24(b).

definition is based on a sample of patient records taken from the previous year. Specifically, state surveyors are instructed to look at 20 to 50 patient records that involve presenting complaints or diagnoses that are associated with emergency medical conditions.[7] It is easy to see how the sampling method might result in an overestimation of the proportion of visits for emergency conditions and thus an overly broad designation of dedicated EDs. Therefore, this definition creates some uncertainty for institutions that see anywhere near one-third of their patients for emergency conditions on an unscheduled basis, especially if there is a significant variation in their census from year to year.

It is worth noting again that only Medicare-participating hospitals are bound by EMTALA. Facilities that are not Medicare-participating, regardless of whether they meet any or all of the three definitions under discussion, are not required to comply with EMTALA. Likewise, freestanding EDs or urgent care centers not associated with a hospital, as defined by CMS, are not bound by EMTALA, even if they meet one or more of the definitions of a dedicated ED.

▶ *Come to the emergency department:* Not surprisingly, determining whether a patient has "come to the emergency department" and thus triggered the EMTALA requirements is more complex than the simple language of the statute would imply. After a Chicago teenager was left bleeding near the entrance of an ED, CMS changed its interpretation of this phrase to include the areas surrounding the hospital proper. Specifically, the agency adopted the "250-yard rule." Under this rule, patients are deemed to have come to the ED if they are on the hospital's campus, defined as hospital property within 250 yards of the hospital's main building.[8] "Hospital property" in this rule includes not only the hospital buildings on the main hospital campus but also the campus's roadways, sidewalks, and parking lots.[9]

Another question arises when patients present to facilities that are owned and operated by a Medicare-participating hospital but are off the campus of the main hospital. If patients present at these locations, are the providers at the facility required to comply with EMTALA just because its parent hospital has a dedicated ED? In the case of a facility that meets at least one of the three definitions of a dedicated ED *and* is owned or operated by a Medicare-participating hospital, the answer is yes. Simply being located off the main hospital campus does not exempt these qualifying facilities. In the case of a facility that does not qualify

---

7   Centers for Medicaid & Medicare Services. State operations manual, appendix V—interpretive guidelines—responsibilities of Medicare participating hospitals in emergency cases. Revised July 2010.
8   42 Code of Federal Regulations § 489.24(b).
9   42 Code of Federal Regulations § 413.65(b).

as a dedicated ED, regardless of whether it is owned or operated by a Medicare-participating hospital, the answer is no.

This approach to off-campus facilities represents a change from earlier CMS proposals. In the past, CMS required all off-campus facilities that were owned and operated by a Medicare-participating hospital to fulfill the requirements of EMTALA. Given the difficulties this created for facilities not equipped to handle emergency medical conditions, CMS changed its proposal in 2010 to exempt these facilities.

Another related issue involves the obligations of facilities that qualify as dedicated EDs but are only open part time. Because these are often located in rural or underserved areas, CMS modified the obligations of these facilities to be less demanding in order to reduce the risk that these facilities would close because of EMTALA regulations. Under current policy, hospitals that offer emergency medical services on a part-time basis are required to comply with EMTALA only when their dedicated EDs are open. When a dedicated ED is closed, the hospital is no longer bound by EMTALA and may refer patients on as appropriate.

Notably, all Medicare-participating facilities, even those that are not obligated to follow EMTALA requirements, still have an obligation under Medicare's conditions of participation to put procedures in place to deal with patients who present with emergency medical problems.[10] Such procedures may be as simple as directing employees to provide the level of care the facility is capable of providing or calling an ambulance to transport the patient to a more appropriate facility, but they must be in place in all Medicare-participating facilities.

WHAT IS REQUIRED TO COMPLY WITH EMTALA?

EMTALA can be broken down into three main requirements and a number of secondary administrative requirements. The three main requirements include an obligation to

- Provide a medical screening exam
- Stabilize patients with emergency medical conditions
- Transfer patients only when medically necessary and accept medically necessary transfers

Medical Screening Exam

Hospitals subject to EMTALA are required to perform an "appropriate medical screening examination."[11] Although there are no specific steps mandated as part of this screening exam, the statute does require that it be designed to determine whether an emergency medical condition exists.[12] This prevents hospitals from using simple questionnaires or superficial evaluations to meet the nominal requirements of EMTALA while circumventing its underlying purpose.

---

10   42 Code of Federal Regulations § 482.12(f)(3).
11   42 Code of Federal Regulations § 489.24(a)(i).
12   42 Code of Federal Regulations § 489.24(a)(i).

The statute expressly limits a hospital's screening obligations to those that are "within the capability of the hospital's emergency department." This includes the ancillary services that are routinely available to providers in the ED. However, it does *not* place an obligation on dedicated EDs to have the capabilities to screen for every type of emergency medical condition.

Past CMS advisory letters, citations, and litigation suggest that the following are important elements, all of which must be documented, for an appropriate medical screening examination:

- A complete log of patients, with the disposition of their cases
- A record of the triage process and its conclusions
- A record of vital signs
- A record of the patient's history of the problem
- Results of the physical exam
- Use of any appropriate ancillary testing or on-call physicians
- A repeat record of vital signs at discharge or transfer[13]

The statute also calls for the screening examination to be conducted by a health-care provider who is trained to deal with emergency situations.[14] This provider does not have to be a physician but must be specifically designated for this role by hospital policies. Though the use of nonphysician providers for this role is allowed by EMTALA, any decisions made by those providers will ultimately be ascribed to the physicians on duty.

Many cases have been litigated concerning the meaning of the term *appropriate* in the phrase "appropriate medical screening examination." In view of the legislative history of the statute, most courts have interpreted this term to refer to an exam that is applied relatively uniformly to paying and nonpaying patients alike, not necessarily one that is well designed or thorough. Courts have not generally interpreted minor deviations from standard screening procedures to be evidence of disparate treatment unless there was other evidence of an improper financial motive in the case. Because it is not possible to outline the appropriate screening steps that should be taken for each type of potential patient, the determination of appropriateness is made on a case-by-case basis.

It is important to note that the medical screening exam just described is not the same as the medical triage performed when patients first enter an ED or similar site. Rather, triage can be thought of as a very brief process designed to determine which patients are in need of rapid access to a full medical screening examination. Increasingly, facilities that are subject to EMTALA are using the triage process to redirect patients with nonemergency conditions to more

---

13   Moy MM. *EMTALA Answer Book 2012*. New York: CCH; 2012.
14   42 Code of Federal Regulations § 489.24(a)(i).

appropriate sources of care. This may improve some aspects of patient flow, but any choice to use such a policy must be carefully weighed against the risks; reliance on the triage process rather than a full medical screening exam opens the door for liability under EMTALA if any patients who are sent elsewhere are later harmed by an emergency condition that was not detected by the triage process. If an appropriate medical screening exam is performed by qualified personnel and no emergency medical condition is detected, the ED's EMTALA obligations have been met.

Stabilization

EMTALA's second major requirement, stabilization, is mandatory only if the medical screening examination detects an emergency medical condition. More detailed definitions of the terms *stabilization* and *emergency medical condition* are necessary for a full understanding of his requirement.

The EMTALA statute defines an emergency medical condition both generically and as it relates specifically to pregnant women. In general, an emergency medical condition is one that is of sufficient severity that a lack of medical attention could be expected to result in one of three things: the serious jeopardy to the health of the individual, the serious impairment of bodily functions, or the serious dysfunction of any body part. Notably, CMS specifically includes symptoms of severe psychiatric problems or substance abuse as emergency medical conditions. For pregnant women in active labor, an emergency medical condition is present if the health of the woman or unborn child is in serious jeopardy, there is not enough time to safely transfer the patient to another hospital before delivery, or the transfer may threaten the health or safety of the mother or unborn child.

Although these examples provide some insight into CMS's expectations for health-care providers, they afford little guidance in individual patient encounters. The meanings of *serious* jeopardy, impairment, and dysfunction remain almost entirely subjective. Some patients present with signs and symptoms that obviously meet these descriptions, and others present with minor complaints that clearly do not qualify. But most patients fall somewhere in between. In these cases, it is best for providers to err on the side of caution and properly stabilize patients who land in this middle ground.

The statute's definition of *stabilized* also introduces a large element of subjectivity. By statute, *stabilized* means that "no material deterioration of the condition is likely, within reasonable medical probability, to result from or occur during the transfer of the individual from a facility." A health-care provider who determines that a patient's condition is stable enough for discharge does not necessarily violate EMTALA even if the patient's condition deteriorates soon after discharge. As long as the provider's decision was based on a reasonable determination that deterioration was unlikely, the provider has met the EMTALA obligations.

The stabilization requirement can be met in one of three ways: by stabilizing the emergency medical condition, by admitting the patient for further treatment as an inpatient, or by transferring the patient to a different hospital. By statute, dedicated EDs must provide whatever stabilizing treatment is necessary "within the capabilities of the staff and facilities available at the hospital," including that of on-call physicians. If the ED does not have the capabilities to stabilize a particular patient, it must transfer the patient to a different hospital that does, assuming that the benefits of doing so outweigh the risks. In other words, EMTALA does not require that dedicated EDs all have the same capabilities, but it does require them to use the resources they have and to transfer patients when it is medically warranted.

Transfers

EMTALA's third major requirement calls for appropriate transfers. The transfer requirement is composed of two separate obligations: to transfer patients out of an ED when it is medically necessary (as already discussed) and, for hospitals with specialized capabilities, to accept those transfers. Because urgent care providers are rarely, if ever, expected to receive unstable patients from outside institutions, this section focuses instead on situations in which it is appropriate to transfer patients to outside hospitals and the necessary procedural requirements for doing so.

There are only two situations in which it is appropriate to transfer an unstable patient under EMTALA. First, a patient may be transferred if the patient requests a transfer. This option is suitable only if the patient has been informed about both the risks of a transfer and the hospital's obligations to treat. In this case, the patient must sign a written request that acknowledges being informed about both of these things and must still want to be transferred.

Second, physicians or other qualified personnel may certify patients for transfer if the providers determine that the benefits of the transfer outweigh the risks. A written summary of the risks and benefits that were considered in the transfer decision is required. If a physician is available, this process must be completed by the physician. If there is no physician available, this process may be completed by personnel who are qualified under hospital bylaws or formal policies. In these cases, the nonphysician personnel must still consult a physician to cosign the certification before transfer.

Once the decision to transfer is made, there are four key elements of an appropriate EMTALA transfer:

▶ The ED must provide whatever medical treatment it has the capacity to provide in order to minimize the risks to the patient's health during the transfer.

▶ The ED must send the receiving facility copies of all of the relevant medical records available at the time of transfer, as well as any relevant records that become available after the transfer.

▶ The transfer must be carried out by qualified personnel and with appropriate equipment; giving the patient directions to a different hospital and allowing a family member to drive the patient there does not suffice.

- ▶ The receiving facility must have agreed to accept the transfer and must have the necessary resources and personnel to treat the patient.

In addition to the screening, stabilization, and transfer requirements, facilities that are subject to EMTALA must also follow a number of administrative requirements, including the following:

- ▶ Creating an EMTALA compliance policy
- ▶ Setting policies that explicitly state which providers are qualified to perform the medical screening exam
- ▶ Establishing a list of on-call physicians and procedures for reaching them as necessary
- ▶ Posting signs that inform the public about the applicable EMTALA requirements
- ▶ Keeping a log of all patients who come to the ED and storing records of all transfers for at least 5 years[15]

CONCLUSION

An urgent care center is subject to EMTALA if it meets the definition of a Medicare-participating hospital or critical-access hospital *and* qualifies as a dedicated ED by one of three specific definitions. These facilities have a duty to provide an appropriate medical screening exam to all patients, to stabilize patients who are found to have an emergency medical condition, and to transfer patients who cannot be stabilized by the facility. There are a number of other requisite administrative duties as well.

Although the law remains nebulous about exactly which providers it applies to, the precise criteria for the performance of a medical screening exam, and how severe a patient's condition must be before stabilization is required, a good rule of thumb is to follow not only the letter but also the intent of the law, because EMTALA is clearly designed to protect patients from being neglected or denied care for financial reasons. If a patient needs care, providing that care is always a safe choice.

KEY POINTS

1. The provisions of EMTALA apply to all patients, regardless of insurance status, age, immigration status, or any other characteristics. In addition, the act's provisions apply to a number of clinical care sites, not only the traditional EDs that were originally targeted by the legislation.

---

15 Government Accountability Office. Emergency care: EMTALA implementation and enforcement issues. June 22, 2001. GAO-01-747. Available from: http://www.gao.gov/products/GAO-01-747.

2. For those health-care providers and institutions that *are* subject to EMTALA, the law can be divided into three main requirements:
   - All patients must be given an appropriate medical screening exam designed to detect emergency medical conditions.
   - If an emergency medical condition is found, the patient must be stabilized before being discharged or transferred.
   - If an emergency medical condition is found and the institution does not have the capabilities to stabilize the patient, the act requires both that the patient be transferred to a site that does have the necessary capabilities and that the site with the specialized capabilities accept that transfer as long as it has the capacity to do so.
3. EMTALA requirements are enforced through three major avenues:
   - CMS: When CMS finds that a violation occurred, the agency can begin the process of terminating a hospital's Medicare provider agreement.
   - CMS can authorize the OIG to further investigate the claims and impose sanctions on offenders. By statute, the OIG can assess penalties of up to $50,000 against offending physicians and hospitals.
   - The statute also gives individuals injured by alleged EMTALA violations the right to sue the offending hospital in civil court.
4. By CMS's interpretation, any facility that meets one or more of the following three criteria is a dedicated ED for the sake of EMTALA:
   - The facility is licensed by the state as an emergency room or ED.
   - The facility is "held out to the public" as a place that provides care for emergency medical conditions without requiring an appointment.
   - The facility sees at least one-third of its patients for emergency medical conditions without requiring an appointment.
5. Only Medicare-participating hospitals are bound by EMTALA. Facilities that are not Medicare-participating, regardless of whether they meet any or all of the three definitions above, are not required to comply with EMTALA.
6. Likewise, freestanding EDs or urgent care centers not associated with a hospital, as defined by EMTALA, are not bound by EMTALA, even if they meet one or more of the definitions of a dedicated ED.
7. When patients present to facilities that are owned and operated by a Medicare-participating hospital but are off the campus of the main hospital, EMTALA applies if the facility meets at least one of the three definitions of a dedicated ED *and* is owned or operated by a Medicare-participating hospital. Simply being located off the main hospital campus does not exempt these qualifying facilities.

8. In the case of a facility that does not qualify as a dedicated ED, regardless of whether it is owned or operated by a Medicare-participating hospital, EMTALA does not apply.

9. Institutions subject to EMTALA are required to perform an "appropriate medical screening examination" to determine whether an emergency medical condition exists.

10. The screening examination must be conducted by a health-care provider who is trained to deal with emergency situations. This provider does not have to be a physician but must be a provider specifically designated for this role by policy.

CHAPTER 34

Engaging Accountable Care Organizations in Urgent Care Centers

John Harris

What Is an Accountable Care Organization?

An accountable care organization (ACO) is an organization of health-care providers that is responsible, both clinically and financially, for the care of patients across settings, from physician offices to acute care to long-term care facilities.

ACO contracts reward providers for improving the quality of care and lowering the total cost of care. ACOs are loosely managed, with no gatekeeper referral or preauthorization requirements.

The major ACO program today is the Medicare Shared Savings Program (MSSP). Many commercial insurers are also pursuing ACO programs to reward providers for improving care quality and lowering costs.

MSSP ACOs are either of the following:

- Physician-only ACOs—group practices, networks of individual practices (individual practice associations), or selected federally qualified health centers and rural health centers

- Hospital–physician ACOs—either hospitals and physicians in partnership or hospitals with employed physicians

ACO entities must

- Have a formal legal structure

- Make a 3-year commitment to the program

- Have a minimum of 5000 beneficiaries

Beneficiary Assignment

Medicare assigns beneficiaries to an ACO by looking at the ACO's network of physicians and determining what Medicare beneficiaries received the plurality of their primary care from these physicians in the prior year. At year end, Medicare determines where these beneficiaries received their care in the contract year and reconciles assignments and payments.

Shared Savings

If the ACO achieves a specified minimum savings level (from 3.9% less than expected costs for the smallest ACOs down to 2% for the largest), all savings are shared between the ACO and MSSP from the first dollar. The ACO can receive up to 50% of the savings it achieves. There is no requirement to take on financial risk for the first 3 years, although ACOs that are able to do so can achieve a higher rate of savings.

Quality of Care

The share of savings received by the ACO is adjusted according to performance on quality measures. To maximize its share of savings, the ACO must measure performance on 33 quality measures. In year 1, credit is given for reporting on each measure. In years 2 and 3, actual performance on these measures counts. There is also a financial incentive for the use of electronic health records, although these are not mandatory.

Data Sharing

Patients' clinical data are shared within the ACO unless patients opt out.

Cost Tracking

ACOs receive quarterly reports on the aggregate costs of providing care for their patients. All Medicare Part A and Part B costs are accrued to the ACO's tally. Services are paid for at Medicare provider rates. ACOs also receive detailed claims data to monitor care and identify opportunities for improvement.

Accountable care organizations (acos) are provider organizations that agree to exert extra effort to improve the quality and lower the costs of care, and to be rewarded financially if they do so. As of January 2014, there are more than 400 ACOs caring for 25 million Medicare beneficiaries, or about 40% of all beneficiaries. ACO presence varies by local markets; some markets have no ACOs, whereas in others, ACOs care for 50% of all Medicare beneficiaries.

Centers for Medicare & Medicaid Services leaders see ACOs as a historic opportunity to obtain authentic change because they make possible

- Better care for individuals
- Better health for populations
- Lower per capita cost

It is generally agreed that to be successful, ACOs must be able to

- Manage chronic conditions effectively
- Avoid unnecessary inpatient admissions
- Reduce post–acute care costs
- Engage patients
- Have electronic health records or alternative ways to track and improve quality scores
- Use care guidelines and evidence-based medicine
- Provide patient-centered medical care, possibly through a patient-centered medical home
- Manage end-of-life care

WHY SHOULD ACCOUNTABLE CARE ORGANIZATIONS BE INTERESTED IN URGENT CARE CENTERS?

Urgent care centers can help ACOs reduce the total costs of patient care, improve accessibility of care and patient-satisfaction indicators, and possibly increase ACO market share.

Reducing Total Costs of Care

ACOs need to drive down the total cost of care for the Medicare patients allocated to their physicians, in order to achieve savings that can be shared among participants. Because all care for ACO enrollees is paid for at standard Medicare rates, the best way for ACOs to drive down costs is by decreasing use of services or substituting a less-expensive form of care.

One possible area of substitution is the emergency department (ED). ED visits are an extremely expensive form of care, and visit volumes have grown rapidly; in the decade ending in 2008, the rate of ED visits grew at twice the rate of the US population.[1] ACOs may be able to achieve savings by substituting less-expensive urgent care center visits for a portion of ED visits.

The difference in cost between an urgent care visit and an ED visit *for the same diagnosis* ranges from $228 to $583.[2,3] Substituting urgent care visits for ED visits that are not truly emergencies could help ACOs reduce population health costs. The population over age 65 makes about 500 ED visits per 1000 population per year.[4] A recent study found that 59% of all ambulatory ED visits are potentially preventable.[5] Using the savings-per-visit figures already discussed, an ACO with 20,000 enrollees could save $655,000 to $1,749,000 by diverting 30% of its ED visits to urgent care.

The feasibility of such a diversion strategy is demonstrated by the experience of Anthem Blue Cross and Blue Shield in Virginia. The organization was able to reduce its ED visits by 14% *in 1 year* among members who were part of a patient-education initiative aimed at diverting ED visits to urgent care centers.[6]

In California, where the high rate of managed-care enrollment has resulted in physician groups' providing capitated rates, some multispecialty group practices have established their own urgent care centers to serve their patients while holding down costs. Even when these practices operate at a loss, they can still reduce the capitated patient cost to the group by reducing use of the ED.[7]

Improving Accessibility of Care and Patient-Satisfaction Indicators

By improving accessibility of after-hours care and making care immediately available in the daytime for minor problems, urgent care centers can help ACOs increase patient satisfaction. This can have a positive impact on an ACO's quality score, which in turn will affect the amount of savings it can retain.

Given the right partners, ACOs may be glad to avoid having to arrange for their own after-hours coverage. A threatened shortage of primary care physicians (PCPs), combined with the increasing demands that quality measurement

1. American College of Emergency Physicians. How overcrowding affects your access to emergency care. n.d. Available from: http://www.acep.org/Content.aspx?id=25906&terms=overcrowding.
2. Weinick R, Burns R, Mehrotra A. Many emergency department visits could be managed at urgent care centers and retail clinics. *Health Aff (Millwood)*. 2010;29:9:1630–6.
3. Mehrotra A, Liu H, Adams JL, et al. Comparing costs and quality of care at retail clinics with that of other medical settings for 3 common illnesses. *Ann Intern Med*. 2009;151:321–8.
4. Centers for Disease Control and Prevention. National hospital ambulatory medical care survey: 2010 emergency department summary tables. Available from: http://www.cdc.gov/nchs/data/ahcd/nhamcs_emergency/2010_ed_web_tables.pdf.
5. Sadownick S, Ray N. Population-based measures of ambulatory care quality: potentially preventable visits and emergency department visits. Medpac. October 5, 2012. Available from http://www.medpac.gov/transcripts/1012_presentation_ppv.pdf.
6. WellPoint, Inc. Emergency room interventions using Google Maps and education empower consumers to choose ER alternatives for non-emergency conditions. June 23, 2011. Available from: http://ir.wellpoint.com/phoenix.zhtml?c=130104&p=irol-newsArticle&ID=1579424&highlight.
7. Weinick R, Betancourt R. No appointment needed: the resurgence of urgent care. California HealthCare Foundation. September 2007.

and other initiatives place on PCPs, could make it difficult for ACOs to find the resources required.

Diverting nonemergency visits from EDs to urgent care centers can also have a positive impact on quality of care and patient satisfaction in EDs. The length of an ED visit has increased to 4 hours in recent years.[8] Fewer ED visits means reduced backlogs and waiting time and potentially higher satisfaction scores.

Of course, the ACO will benefit from using urgent care centers as part of their care network only if patients are referred back to their ACO PCP, along with relevant medical record information.

Involving Urgent Care Primary-Care Physicians

Urgent care centers are playing a growing role in competition between hospitals; about 25% of urgent care centers are hospital-sponsored. When a hospital sponsors an urgent care center, a hospital–physician ACO may well want to involve the PCPs in its hospital-sponsored urgent care center, to keep patients within its network.

When this chapter was written in 2014, there were approximately 6500 urgent care centers, and about one-quarter of those opened since 2011. Further growth is projected. Urgent care center physicians are an increasing proportion of the primary-care resources available in many communities. By signing up urgent care center PCPs as part of their network, ACOs can increase enrollees, spread overhead costs, and lower their required rate of minimum savings.

With more than 35 urgent care centers for every ACO as of April 2013, there would appear to be a buyer's market for ACOs, even if the ratio is halved as more ACOs are initiated.

WHY SHOULD URGENT CARE CENTERS BE INTERESTED IN ACCOUNTABLE CARE ORGANIZATIONS?

Urgent care centers have the potential to increase patient volume by working with ACOs, while maintaining their current form of practice. Assuming that an ACO with 20,000 enrollees would eventually be able to divert 30% of *Medicare* (patients 65 years and older) ED visits to urgent care, that ACO would generate about 3000 urgent care visits per year from this diversion, or about $648,000 in gross revenues. Net revenues could be considerably less with a Medicare flat-rate payment, if no procedures are carved out.[9] These figures could grow rapidly by 2025 as the population over age 65 doubles.[10] There could well be additional visit diversion from the younger patients of physicians working within an ACO; as

---

8 Press G. 2010 emergency department pulse report. Available from: http://www.pressganey.com/newsLanding/10-09-19/Emergency_Department_Pulse_Report_2010.aspx.
9 Based on $216 per urgent care visit (from Weinick R, Betancourt R. No appointment needed).
10 Center for Workforce Studies. Physician shortages to worsen without increases in residency training. Association of American Medical Colleges. Available from: https://www.aamc.org/download/150584/data/physician_shortages_factsheet.pdf.

history shows with managed care, when a care pattern is established in one population, physicians will tend to apply it to other populations as well.

Active participation as members of an ACO could also allow the PCPs at an urgent care center to participate in the sharing of ACO cost savings; this has the potential to generate an additional income stream for the urgent care center.

Taking a proactive role in developing an involvement with ACOs could also be a defensive move for urgent care centers. Without active participation by urgent care centers, some ACOs may choose to establish their own after-hours services. This could actually reduce the number of patients available to urgent care centers, a major threat when the number and size of centers is growing.

STRATEGIC ACCOUNTABLE CARE ORGANIZATION OPTIONS FOR URGENT CARE CENTERS

Urgent care centers have a number of possible strategic options in relation to ACOs.

Option 1:
Be a Participating Accountable Care Organization Provider

An urgent care center can participate in an ACO as a contracted provider, with Medicare beneficiaries allocated to the ACO, based on care provided by the urgent care center's PCPs. The urgent care center and ACO would need to decide whether the urgent care center would

- Become the PCP of patients it now cares for episodically
- Refer urgent care center patients to PCPs in the ACO for care of chronic conditions, and so forth, which the ACO might prefer

If the decision were made to have the urgent care center become a PCP within the ACO, the urgent care center would need to provide the care required to conform to the ACO quality-of-care measures (Tables 1 and 2), including those involving ongoing care of patients with chronic conditions. If it did not, the ACO could suffer from a reduction in the program savings it could share. Indeed, some ACOs may determine how savings will be shared within the ACO at least in part on the basis of how well individual physicians perform on these measures.

Urgent care centers that are owned by a hospital with an ACO are likely to be included within the ACO.

Option 1 Pros

The option of being an ACO provider could lead ACOs to actively encourage patients to use the urgent care center for after-hours care. The urgent care center could become the official after-hours coverage system for the ACO, and the ACO's on-call service could refer patients to the urgent care center. This option would also eliminate the possibility that the urgent care center would lose patients to an ACO that decides to provide its own after-hours care solutions.

Table 1. ACO Quality-of-Care Measures—General

Patient and Caregiver Experience (7 Measures, Scored as 2)	Care Coordination (6 Scored Measures)	Preventive Health (8 Scored Measures)
• Getting timely appointments and information • How well your physician communicates • Patients' rating of their physicians • Access to specialists • Health promotion and education • Shared decision making • Health status or functional status	• 30-day readmissions • Admissions: COPD, CHF • Percentage of primary-care physicians with EHR incentive payments • Medication reconciliation after discharge • Falls screening	• Influenza immunization • Pneumococcal vaccination • Adult weight screening and follow-up • Tobacco use assessment and tobacco cessation intervention • Depression screening • Colorectal cancer screening • Mammography • Portion of adults aged 18 years and older who have had their blood pressure measured within the preceding 2 years

ACO, accountable care organization; CHF, chronic heart failure; COPD, chronic obstructive pulmonary disease; EHR, electronic health record.

Source: Medicare. Available from: http://www.cms.gov/Medicare/Medicare-Fee-for-Service-Payment/sharedsavingsprogram/Quality_Measures_Standards.html.

Option 1 Cons

If the urgent care center becomes a PCP for patients it now cares for episodically, this option would fundamentally change the nature of the care provided by the urgent care center to more of a neighborhood care center. Depending on whether or not the urgent care center already has physician relationship support services in place, it might also require a significant investment in the systems required to act as a *good partner* to the ACO (see below) and to provide ongoing care of patients with chronic conditions.

Although urgent care centers that choose to participate with a single ACO and have patients attributed to that ACO can still provide urgent care to other ACOs' patients, the other ACOs may be less willing to partner with the urgent care center in the way described below.

Option 2: Be a Good Partner

Urgent care centers can seek to obtain some of the benefits of option 1 without its possible drawbacks by serving as an after-hours resource for one or more ACOs without being a participating ACO provider. This would be in some ways similar

Table 2. ACO Quality-of-Care Measures for Care of At-Risk Populations

- Patients with diabetes mellitus (scored as a single measure, all or none)
  - HbA_{1c} control (<18%)
  - LDL control (<100 mg/dL)
  - Blood pressure >140/90 mmHg
  - Tobacco nonuse
  - Aspirin use: Daily use for patients with diabetes and cardiovascular disease
  - HbA_{1c} poor control (>9%)
- Patients with hypertension
  - Blood pressure control documented in plan of care
- Patients with ischemic vascular disease
  - Complete lipid profile and LDL control (<100 mg/dL)
  - Use of aspirin or antithrombolytic
- Patients with heart failure
  - Beta-blocker therapy for left ventricular systolic dysfunction
- Patients with coronary artery disease
  - Drug therapy for lowering LDL cholesterol
  - Angiotensin-converting enzyme inhibitor or angiotensin therapy

ACO, accountable care organization; HbA_{1c}, glycated hemoglobin A_{1c}; LDL, low-density lipoprotein.
Source: Medicare. Available from: http://www.cms.gov/Medicare/Medicare-Fee-for-Service-Payment/sharedsavingsprogram/Quality_Measures_Standards.html.

to relationships that urgent care centers may currently have with individual PCPs who refer to them for after-hours care.

By playing well with ACOs, the urgent care center could receive incremental volume increases, resulting from ACO efforts to divert patients from EDs and provide for after-hours care. Urgent care centers that make an effort to help ACOs manage their cost of care, while communicating well with ACO providers, will be seen as good partners. Specifics include the following:

▶ Referring patients back to their ACO physicians for follow-up

▶ Integrating the flow of patient information, so that the ACO receives a full picture of the patient's encounter with a minimum of effort. ACO providers would want to receive history notes for the visit, laboratory tests, and imaging results (including digital images); information on medications prescribed; and notes on recommended follow-up.

▶ Supporting ACO quality-of-care goals, both by providing top-notch customer service (to maximize the ACO's ratings) and by sharing the data required for ACO quality measures in care coordination, preventive health, and at-risk populations (supporting the ACO in achieving full credit for care provided)

Option 2 Pros
The option of partnering with an ACO could well result in increased patient volume for the urgent care center. It might give the urgent care center greater flexibility than option 1 in working with multiple ACOs, allowing the investment of effort required to be amortized over multiple ACO relationships. In addition, by improving continuity of care for the urgent care center's patients, this option could create a virtuous circle, where patients who are increasingly satisfied make greater use of the urgent care center.

For those urgent care centers that already work collaboratively with community physicians, this option could be relatively straightforward to achieve. NOW Care, for example, makes sure that PCPs get a chart back the day after they see the patient.[11]

Option 2 Cons
For those urgent care centers that are not as far down the path to collaboration with community physicians, significant effort and some cash investment would be required to integrate the flow of information to ACOs. All urgent care centers would have to invest effort to collect and share the data required for relevant ACO quality measures. It is also possible that because it is not an official part of an ACO, the urgent care center could get shut out of providing after-hours care for one or more ACOs.

Option 3: Wait and See
Because MSSP ACO providers can't directly control where their patients receive care, an urgent care center could choose to ignore the existence of ACOs and simply continue its current way of operating, maximizing customer satisfaction, and relating to community physicians. Whether or not it chooses to work with ACOs, the urgent care center will still have its Medicare contract.

Commercial ACOs could evolve into models that discourage the use of certain providers. However, this is not likely to have an adverse effect on urgent care centers. Insurers are unlikely to disincentivize their use because the alternative to using an urgent care facility might well be the more expensive ED.

Option 3 Pros
The wait-and-see option is an easy strategy, requiring no investment, no negotiations, and no additional effort.

Option 3 Cons
The extent of disadvantages resulting from this option will depend on the individual market. In a market with a significant ACO presence, there are proportional risks to an individual urgent care center that pursues this strategy. The ACOs may develop formal or less-formal relationships with other urgent care centers, attempting to direct patients to them and causing a loss of volume for any urgent

---
11 Weinick R, Betancourt R. No appointment needed.

Table 3. Impacts of ACO Strategy Selected on Urgent Care Centers

Strategy	Positive Impacts		Negative Impacts	
	Potential Volume Increase	Potential Incentive Revenue	Investment/ Effort	Practice Style Changes Required?
Be a participating ACO provider	+++	++	+++	+++
Be a good partner	++	+	++	++
Wait and see	+	+	+	+

ACO, accountable care organization.

care center that chooses to ignore their existence. The ACOs could also develop their own after-hours care mechanism, in effect shutting urgent care centers out. If ACOs have a small market presence and appear likely to continue to have a small presence, these risks will be much less significant.

CONCLUSION

Urgent care centers have several options (Table 3) in how they respond to ACOs, with many variants possible.

Each urgent care center has to consider its unique market and the way in which it prefers to do business. How many ACOs does the market include, and are they led by physicians or instead by a health system? How competitive is the urgent care environment? What is the mix of independent versus hospital-owned urgent care centers?

In considering strategy with regard to ACOs, urgent care centers will also want to consider the ways in which ACOs evolve in the coming years. They could vanish from the scene—a failed experiment—with providers reluctant to renew in year 4. In that year Medicare will rebase the level from which savings must be achieved (which will then be lower), and it is also likely to require a higher *rate* of savings. Alternatively, effective ACOs could gain market share and exert greater control over care. Finally, effective ACOs could decide to move to a Medicare Advantage plan model, for a more financially sustainable long-term future.

KEY POINTS

1. An ACO is responsible for all aspects, both clinical and financial, of the patient's care, encompassing everything from outpatient to acute to subacute care.

2. There are two types of ACOs: physician-only ACOs and hospital–physician ACOs.

3. The goal of an ACO is to lower the cost and improve the care delivered to the patient.
4. Owners of urgent care centers have a variety of options for how to participate with an ACO. Options should be thoroughly explored with an eye toward the future inasmuch as the decision could have significant repercussions.
5. Urgent care centers should consider joining an ACO to help lower the on-demand cost of care for the ACO's population of patients.
6. An urgent care center, if set up properly, could also participate as a PCP and be assigned a population of patients to manage.
7. If an urgent care center elects to participate with an ACO, the operator of the center must ensure that it can deliver on the care, the reporting, and the sharing of patient records back to the patient's PCP.

CHAPTER 35

Urgent Care Imaging and Interpretation

Tim Hogan

THE RADIOLOGY DEPARTMENT OF an urgent care center plays an important role in the diagnosis and treatment of illness and injury. The department should be designed to provide accurate, efficient, and timely radiology service to its clinical providers and patients. Equipment, workflow, and interpretation are some of the major considerations in designing a radiology department.

Radiology is a branch of health sciences that uses imaging to identify injuries and to diagnose and treat diseases inside the body. The acquisition of the images is usually performed by the radiology technologist. The images are first interpreted by the on-site clinician (*primary interpretation*). Most urgent care centers have their studies overread by a board-certified radiologist for patient safety and quality assurance. The radiologist then completes the study with a *final interpretation* in the form of a report, which is transmitted back to the clinician with the timeliness and quality that meet the needs of each specific clinic and patient. This report becomes a permanent part of the patient's health record.

Understanding which equipment best accommodates your clinic's needs requires understanding of all of the equipment options available and an understanding of the needs of your facility. Most often, only a few different modalities are used in urgent care centers—x-ray, ultrasound, and, in some larger centers, computed tomography (CT). Each of those modalities has different types. Within x-ray there are computed radiography (CR) and digital radiography (DR). With ultrasound there are traditional two-dimensional (2-D) ultrasound, three-dimensional (3-D) ultrasound, and Doppler ultrasound systems. CT machines come in single-slice, multislice, and dual-source multislice models.

To set up your radiology department in a way that achieves excellent patient care in an efficient and cost-effective manner, you must consider your information technology systems, your electronic health record system, the radiology modalities you will use, your teleradiology provider's technology, and your interpretation protocol. Here is one efficient process used by many urgent care centers:

1. The patient is initially processed and evaluated.
2. When indicated, images are obtained.
3. After the images are available, the on-site clinician returns to the patient after reading the images.
4. The physician (who is not the on-site clinician) uses the information gathered during this sequence to create an impression and thus a preliminary diagnosis.
5. All of the information about the patient that is gathered by the on-site clinician, including the preliminary diagnosis, becomes part of the case that is presented to the radiologist for final interpretation.

X-RAY EQUIPMENT

Although some urgent care centers still use plain film systems, medical imaging professionals increasingly require digital imaging.

There are two basic types of digital x-ray scanning equipment: CR and DR. Both produce high-quality images in less time than traditional plain films, and each has features that may be advantageous. When deciding between CR and DR systems, you should understand the differences and similarities between the two types of systems with regard to costs, workflow, and current patient demographics and volume.

Computed radiography typically refers to cassette-based technology that uses a scanning mechanism to extract information from the exposed cassette. In DR, sometimes referred to as cassetteless, the latent image is transferred directly from a detector to a system monitor without the need for a reader mechanism. The similarities between CR and DR technology are primarily in the digital format of the resulting image. Both CR and DR image formats can be stored in a digital picture archiving and communication system (PACS), and the appearance of the digital images can be manipulated with proper software.

DR has reshaped the field of medical imaging and continues to evolve with new image-processing and image-manipulation techniques. Although there continues to be considerable interest in both CR and DR modalities, DR may offer improved workflow for routine procedures because of the elimination of cassette manipulation and processing, as well as a greater capacity to limit radiation exposure.

ULTRASOUND

Ultrasound is a noninvasive medical test using high-frequency sound waves to visualize soft-tissue structures in the body. Ultrasound is used to help diagnose a variety of conditions and to assess the condition of soft-tissue organs after injury or illness. It is also used for obstetrics and gynecology, cardiology, and cancer detection and to improve the accuracy of certain diagnostic and therapeutic procedures. The main advantage of ultrasound is that certain structures can be observed without using radiation. Ultrasound can also be done much faster than x-rays or other radiographic techniques.

A traditional 2-D ultrasound system has seven basic parts:

- *Transducer probe* The transducer probe is the main part of the ultrasound machine, the part that emits the sound waves and receives the echoes. The transducer probe has a sound-absorbing substance to eliminate background reflections from the probe itself. Transducer probes come in many shapes and sizes. The shape of the probe determines its field of view; the frequency of emitted sound waves determines how deep the sound waves penetrate and the resolution of the image.

- *Central processing unit (CPU)* The CPU contains the microprocessor, memory, amplifiers, and the power supply for the microprocessor and the transducer probe. The CPU sends electrical currents to the transducer probe to emit sound waves, and also receives the electrical pulses from the probes that were created from the returning echoes. The CPU does all of the calculations involved in processing the data and forms the image on the monitor. The CPU can also store the processed data and image on disk.

- *Transducer pulse controls* The transducer pulse controls allow the ultrasonographer to set and change the amplitude, frequency, and duration of the ultrasound pulses emitted by the transducer probe and to set the scan mode of the machine.

- *Display* A basic monitor displays the images from the ultrasound data processed by the CPU.

- *Keyboard and pointing device* The keyboard and pointing device are used to input data and take measurements from the display.

- *Disk storage device* Acquired images can be stored on a disk drive or on removable media.

- *Printer* A printer is available to print the image from the displayed data.

There are three basic types of ultrasound machines: traditional 2-D systems, 3-D systems, and Doppler systems.

- 3-D ultrasound systems produce 3-D images of the soft tissue. With a 3-D system, several 2-D images are acquired by moving probes across a section of the body surface or rotating inserted probes. The 2-D scans are combined by software to form 3-D images.

- 3-D ultrasound imaging lets the ultrasonographer get a better look at the organ being examined. It is most commonly used for early detection of cancerous and benign tumors (examining the prostate gland for early detection of tumors, looking for masses in the colon and rectum, detecting breast lesions for possible biopsies); visualizing a fetus to assess its development, especially for observing abnormal development of the face and limbs; and visualizing blood flow in various organs or in a fetus.

- Doppler ultrasound is based on the Doppler effect. When an object reflecting the ultrasound waves is moving, it changes the frequency of the echoes, thus creating a higher frequency if it is moving toward the probe and a lower frequency if it is moving away from the probe. How much the frequency is changed depends on how fast the object is moving. Doppler ultrasound measures the change in frequency of the echoes to calculate how fast an object is moving. Doppler ultrasound is used mostly for cardiology studies and to measure the rate of blood flow through the heart and major arteries.

After you evaluate the different types of ultrasound machines and the different brands and features, the decision of which machine to use depends on the number and types of patients you expect to see.

COMPUTED TOMOGRAPHY

CT combines a series of x-ray views taken from many different angles, using algorithms to create cross-sectional images of the bones and soft tissues inside the body. Although this imaging technology is becoming more common throughout the medical community, it is not popular in urgent care settings because CT systems are expensive to own and operate; furthermore, reimbursement for urgent care centers to use CT scanning is shrinking.

However, if your urgent care center has the appropriate demand for a CT scanner, then you need to understand the costs and benefits of CT. A CT scan is particularly well suited to quickly examining people who may have internal injuries from car accidents or other types of trauma. A CT scan can be used to visualize nearly all parts of the body. CT is acquired in the axial plane, with coronal and sagittal images produced by computer reconstruction. Radiocontrast agents are often used with CT for enhanced delineation of the anatomy. CT scans can gather and process much more data than x-rays, but CT exposes the patient to more harmful radiation.

Conventional Scanners

The conventional CT scanner was first put into service in the 1970s. At the time, these scanners were revolutionary. This was before wireless technology, so large cables were attached to one end of the rotation tube. To avoid tangling these cables, the CT scanner had to be rotated in reverse after each picture rotation. This resulted in a longer scanning time.

Spiral Scanners

Spiral CT scanners were introduced in the late 1980s. Spiral scanners rotate continuously in one direction while the patient is moved through the scanning ring. The increase in scanning speed of the spiral CT scanner enables thinner picture slices of the area being scanned, which produces better images and helps the radiologist more easily make a diagnosis.

Multislice Scanners

The multislice scanner, introduced in 1998, captures multiple image slices during the rotation of the CT x-ray tube, shortening the time needed to complete CT scans compared with the spiral scanner. The image slices captured by the multislice scanners are also thinner than those produced with the spiral scanner. Improvements since 1998 have led to dual-source CT scanners that allow even thinner slices and more images. This boosts the scanner's ability to produce clear data that can be manipulated with modern 3-D software to create spectacular images of the heart, veins, and arteries.

ARCHIVING IMAGES

Urgent care centers and other medical imaging facilities are required to store radiographic images. In larger facilities, images are stored in a PACS, which provides economical storage of and convenient access to images from multiple modalities. Electronic images and reports are transmitted digitally using the digital imaging and communications in medicine (DICOM) file standard and transmission protocol; this eliminates the need to manually file, retrieve, or transport film jackets. Nonimage data, such as scanned documents, can be incorporated using standard formats, once encapsulated in a DICOM file.

A PACS consists of four major components: the imaging modalities, a secured network for the transmission of patient information, workstations for interpreting and reviewing images, and archives for the storage and retrieval of images and reports. Combined with available and emerging web technology, a PACS has the ability to deliver timely and efficient access to images, interpretations, and related data. A PACS breaks down the physical and time barriers associated with traditional film-based image retrieval, distribution, and display.

In the United States, a PACS is classified as a medical device and is regulated by the US Food and Drug Administration. There are many systems and solutions available for storing images that are not officially a PACS. Many x-ray systems' teleradiology operating platforms allow for the storage and retrieval of images, reports, and other worksheets but are not necessarily promoted as a PACS. They are often referred to as image viewers instead. Not all image viewers are diagnostic quality.

The downside of a PACS is its cost. An urgent care center usually cannot afford its own PACS. One alternative is to contract with an Internet-based PACS company that will allow you access to its PACS for a per-study charge. This is fine if it's your only way to access stored images. The most common way that an urgent care center stores images is in its own x-ray system and at an off-site backup location. The use of an Internet- or cloud-based facility is an off-site option but might be expensive. An affordable alternative to off-site storage is to buy a simple external storage drive and back up your patient images each day, transporting the backup drive off-site at closing time. This way you have on-site access through your x-ray system and off-site storage too.

RADIATION SAFETY

All policies and procedures for the x-ray department should be in writing. You need to be aware of your state's regulations and guidelines for safe equipment operation and maintenance, as well as the required competencies for x-ray technicians. In general, these services are regulated by a state health department.

The amount of radiation used in most examinations is small, and the benefits greatly outweigh the risks. Patients should be assured that properly conducted imaging carries minimal risks and that imaging is done only when clinically indicated.

IMAGE INTERPRETATION

The type of image interpretation done varies with the situation.

- *Primary interpretation* The primary interpretation of images is done by the practitioner who is with the patient. In an urgent care setting, this is the diagnosis that is given by the physician, nurse practitioner, physician assistant, or other health-care provider who is on-site with the patient, talking with them, touching them, and looking at the images. This impression is an important part of the information transmitted to the radiologist. The primary read can be a preliminary report or a final report. It is a final report only if the on-site physician does not have it overread by a certified radiologist.

- *Preliminary report* The preliminary report mentions all emergency findings in detail. It also contains brief information about nonacute findings that may or may not be a part of the emergency. This report is shorter than a final report because it is intended to provide enough information to an emergency physician without too much other information. Most emergency physicians want a short report; after all, it's an emergency. They don't want to spend time reading details about nonemergency findings. However, it's important that a preliminary report include a brief description of findings so that the health-care provider can tell the patient to expect additional information from the final report, which will always follow a preliminary report. Preliminary reports are typically used at night for emergency cases and are always followed by a final report the next morning.

- *Final report*   This is a complete radiologic report. This report includes all findings, acute and nonacute, in detail. For example, in a preliminary report there might be mention of a small nodule in a lung exam. The final report will mention its exact location and size. The final report is used for billing purposes and becomes a permanent part of the patient's health record.
- *Overread*   This is a report that is produced by a board-certified radiologist. The report concerns a complete study. A complete study should include patient demographic information, a thorough patient history, the reason for the exam, the primary interpretation, and the images. An overread is a final report.

Utility of Radiology Overreads

Just as you buckle your seat belt every time you get in a car or wear a helmet every time you ride a motorcycle, even though you have no expectation of having an accident, so you should have every radiology study overread by a radiologist.

It only takes one mistake or oversight to injure a patient, and this can create a huge problem for your clinic and the provider. It is a fallacy to assume that only difficult studies should be overread by a radiologist. Have 100% of your studies overread by a board-certified radiologist, because not doing so is a common reason for medical malpractice lawsuits in the urgent care industry.

If a lawsuit comes about because of a missed finding, and the study was overread by a certified radiologist, then the liability is borne by that radiologist. Many malpractice insurance providers offer discounts to those who have all studies overread by a certified radiologist. Having a radiologist overread improves overall quality of patient care, reduces your malpractice vulnerability, and possibly reduces medical malpractice premiums.

Choosing a Radiology Provider

Choosing a radiology provider to overread your studies is an important decision. Select one with a business model that meets the needs of your urgent care clinic. A case study is more than just a set of images; it includes pertinent information from the examination of the patient. Therefore, it is important to find a provider with an operating platform that offers a simple electronic method of sending additional information with the images. Most local radiology groups are not properly equipped to provide an overread service; they may not have an operating platform that enables you to provide the radiologist with the entire case study. A teleradiology company is much more likely to offer the right service for your clinic.

Most teleradiology companies have software that allows technicians to push the images and DICOM header information (patient demographics) all in one step. Then the technician logs in to a website where they can find a list of their patients. From there they can select a patient and input the additional information (reason for exam, history, and preliminary diagnosis).

Check references. Ask your potential radiology provider to give you references from other customers of theirs who are in your state and have a clinic similar to yours. Clinics in your own state are likely to be using the same pool of radiologists as you and thus can provide a reference relevant to the service that you should expect. Ask the references about turnaround times, access to speaking with a radiologist when necessary, and downtime. You should ask the radiology provider for a demonstration of the ordering process, and you should request curricula vitae of the radiologists. Here are some important questions to ask your potential radiologists:

- *Do your radiologists have certification from the American Board of Radiology?* If they aren't board certified, there may be complications for reimbursement.
- *Are your radiologists physically located in the United States?*
- *Is the connection between our urgent care center and your server a secure connection?* The Health Insurance Portability and Accountability Act (HIPAA) requires that all patient data be transmitted in a secure manner.
- *Is your workflow electronic and online, or is it based on faxing information back and forth?* A modern radiology or teleradiology company should have a simple-to-use electronic method of communicating pertinent information about the case.
- *When necessary, can a clinician have a verbal consult directly with a radiologist?* If the system is working properly and the on-site clinician's information is effectively conveyed in the case study, then verbal communication is usually not necessary. However, in some rare cases, it is necessary and there must be some easy way to arrange a verbal consult.
- *Are reports typed rather than handwritten?* Not everybody's handwriting is legible all of the time.
- *How do we get the report?* Your radiology provider should be able to fax it and have it available online, and you should be able to save it as an electronic file.

CONCLUSION

Effective communication is a critical component of diagnostic imaging. Quality patient care can be achieved only when study results are conveyed in a timely manner to the on-site clinician. An effective radiology workflow should be timely, should support the efficient flow of pertinent information, and should be reliable.

Circumstances unique to a particular clinical scenario may influence the methods of communication between interpreting physicians and referring clinicians. Timely receipt of the report depends on the workflow system that delivers it. Responsibility for the exchange of patient information relevant to the study falls on both the ordering physician and interpreting radiologist. The ordering clinician plays a role in obtaining the findings by leading the process of gathering and communicating information about the case.

If possible, all prior reports and images should be available for review and comparison with the current study. A request for imaging should include relevant clinical information, a working diagnosis, and pertinent clinical signs and symptoms. Such communication helps the radiologist to prepare a report that is most useful and meaningful to the on-site clinician. Your radiology workflow system must facilitate adding prior studies without much effort—some systems can be set up to search automatically for prior studies.

Proper design and operation of the radiology department will improve the quality of patient care, improve efficiency, and ultimately improve your value to the community and investors. The effectiveness and efficiency of your radiology workflow are the result of facility design, network design, and the workflow of the radiologists. When all parts of the puzzle are carefully planned and executed, you will have a productive and meaningful department.

With the understanding that a study includes images and information, it's important to develop an internal workflow in your urgent care center that facilitates the flow of this information. It is also important that the software that the radiologists use be designed to facilitate the flow of information. The radiologist will need patients' medical histories and preliminary diagnoses, so it's important to be sure that your workflow makes the on-site physician's notes available when additional information is submitted to the radiologist.

KEY POINTS

1. Equipment, workflow, and interpretation are key factors in operating a radiology department that flows smoothly and produces good results.

2. When deciding between CR and DR systems, you should understand the differences and similarities between the two types of systems with regard to costs, workflow, and your expected patient volume.

3. The main advantage of ultrasound is that certain structures can be observed without using radiation. Ultrasound can also be done much faster than x-rays or other radiographic techniques.

4. CT can gather and process much more data than x-rays. However, CT exposes the patient to more radiation than x-rays do.

5. Images, demographic information, additional history, the reason for the exam, and the preliminary diagnosis are all part of a radiology case.

6. Responsibility for the exchange of patient information relevant to the study falls on both the ordering physician and interpreting radiologist. The ordering clinician plays a role in obtaining the findings by leading the process of gathering and communicating information about the case.

7. Many x-ray systems and teleradiology operating platforms allow for the storage and retrieval of images, reports, and other worksheets but are not necessarily promoted as PACSs and are often referred to as image viewers.

8. An affordable alternative to off-site storage is to buy a simple external storage drive and back up your patients' images each day for off-site storage.

9. Many malpractice insurance providers will offer discounts to those who have all studies overread by a certified radiologist.

CHAPTER 36

Virtual Care

Ian Vasquez

Telemedicine and telehealth have long been perceived as an emerging space in health care, one characterized by high technology and niche applications. Before 2010, much of the buzz within telemedicine was the result of grant-funded pilot programs that concentrated on military, rural-health, and acute specialty-care applications. Telestroke, telepsychology, tele-ICU, and remote patient monitoring were the most commonly discussed systems and services in an evolving industry that was once perceived as being on the fringe of health care.

A dramatic shift began around 2010. Telemedicine is extending health-care access to US consumers in need of routine episodic care. Numerous services are now available (with new and different entrants every day) offering telephonic or online video chat consultations (e-visits) with medical providers that result in a diagnosis and possibly a prescription. Patients who access the service from home or a remote medical kiosk are able to forgo a traditional office visit for many common ailments that necessitate a generic prescription or a medication refill.

Many virtual-care services are the result of recently formed start-up ventures focused on an exclusively telemedicine business model. Increasingly, however, primary-care clinics, physician-management groups, accountable care organizations, and health systems are launching services or assessing how to approach the virtual-care space to extend their traditional medical offerings.

Adoption of such services among employers with self-funded health insurance has outpaced broader consumer adoption thus far. However, as consumer awareness grows and the availability and variety of such services increase, the competitive landscape for the traditional urgent care center will be inexorably shifted by competition from virtual-care providers. You should therefore have a thorough understanding of what virtual-care services are, how they are potentially competing for your clinic's patients, and whether virtual care is an appropriate offering in your business. You should assess regulatory concerns, compliance with the Health Insurance Portability and Accountability Act (HIPAA), technology requirements, and reimbursements before launching virtual services.

KEY VIRTUAL-CARE INFLUENCES

Until recently, virtual care was challenged by a number of obstacles (Figure 1):

▶ The regulatory environment was uncertain and the malpractice risk was forbidding. Providing care for traditional medical needs in a non-traditional approach raises an appropriate level of caution in the highly litigious, highly regulated health-care industry. The lack of telemedicine experience and track record within the malpractice insurance industry meant there was a limited number of carriers willing to underwrite telemedicine policies.

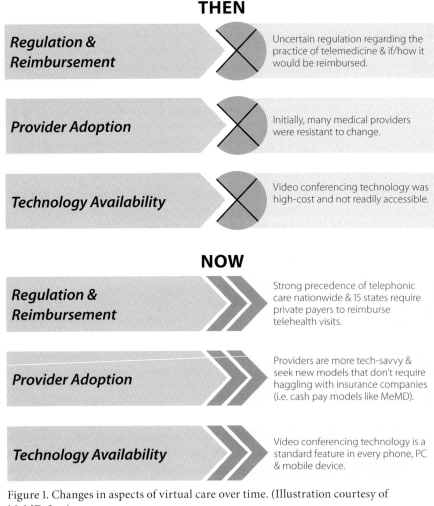

Figure 1. Changes in aspects of virtual care over time. (Illustration courtesy of MeMD, Inc.)

- Reimbursement was not favorable or clear. Payers were focused on creating and managing narrow networks to control cost in the traditional managed-care model. Experimentation with new access points for care was limited mostly to retail medicine (a new but still brick-and-mortar approach). The conversation in the boardroom of at least one of the nation's largest insurers for which I consulted focused on how to emulate the Apple Store in health care. No one had yet considered that perhaps it was the iTunes model we should be looking at.
- Technology remained expensive and difficult to access. Hard as it is to recall now, there was a time before FaceTime, Skype, and affordable webcam-equipped smartphones.
- Consumers were unaware and unaffected. With few pioneers in the space, consumers were unaware that virtual-care services were available. On top of scant awareness, American health-care consumers remained largely insulated from the underlying costs of accessing care in any modality.

Today, things are changing. Virtual-care solutions are becoming available that target routine ailments of regular people using commonly available web technology. Six factors stand out that are driving the movement to telemedicine care:

1. Videoconferencing technology and access to the web are now commonplace for all socioeconomic brackets. Virtually every laptop and mobile device comes with a webcam pre-installed, and the cost of network access to have these devices always online has fallen dramatically. Indeed, the digital divide appears to be closing at a pace previously unimaginable, by virtue of the availability of affordable smartphones and mobile devices. A 2012 Nielsen survey found that 58% of consumers aged 25 to 34 years with incomes ranging from $15,000 to $35,000 per year own smartphones (Figure 2).

2. A supply market now exists for medical malpractice insurance covering telemedicine. A sufficient variety of both admitted and, more commonly, nonadmitted carriers can now supply policies that cover telemedicine encounters. Some carriers can provide policies on a per-encounter pricing basis that aligns well with the urgent care model.

3. State regulators are beginning to require payers to reimburse for telemedicine visits, and many private insurers are voluntarily doing so as a way to reduce costs and improve outcomes. As of 2013, 42 states provided some form of reimbursement for telehealth services through their Medicaid program. Fifteen states (California, Colorado, Georgia, Hawaii, Kentucky, Louisiana, Maine, Massachusetts, Michigan, New Hampshire, Oklahoma, Oregon, Texas, Vermont, Virginia) have some form of mandate requiring payers to reimburse for telemedicine visits, and such legislation is in process in more states (Figure 3).

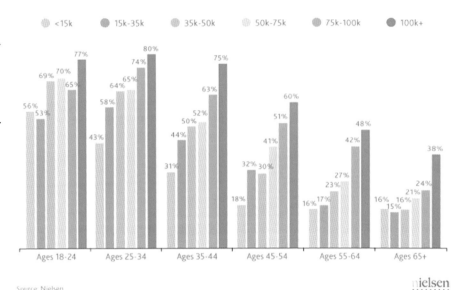

Figure 2. The prevalence of smartphone ownership by age and income. (From Nielsen, at http://www.nielsen.com/us/en/newswire/2012/survey-new-u-s-smartphone-growth-by-age-and-income.html, with permission.)

4. Health-care providers are becoming more familiar with telemedicine encounters. As the network of physicians engaging in virtual-care solutions grows and the community of health-care providers becomes increasingly adept at the use of technology in both the delivery and management of health care, the community at large has become increasingly open to virtual-care encounters.

5. Overall health-care costs continue to spiral higher. The Patient Protection and Affordable Care Act has the potential to compound the cost problem in the near term, given its expansion of guaranteed benefits and access to insurance, so the financial motive for cost-saving strategies that telemedicine can deliver continues to become more compelling.

In particular, large employers with self-funded health insurance plans have been the most creative and willing to experiment with innovations. Large employers have been the first to adopt wellness programs and are increasingly extending virtual-care services via telephonic access to physicians in order to reduce unnecessary use of emergency departments.

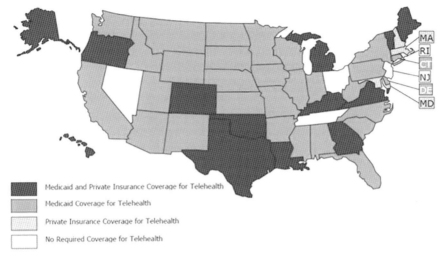

Figure 3. Availability of health-insurance coverage for telehealth. (From the National Conferences of State Legislatures, at http://www.ncsl.org/issues-research/health/state-coverage-for-telehealth-services.aspx, with permission.)

6. Consumers are becoming less insulated from the true cost of accessing health care and are therefore becoming more engaged in finding the most affordable and convenient options. Employer-based health coverage is moving toward high-deductible health savings account plans that shift more of the initial health-care costs to the consumer. The Henry J. Kaiser Family Foundation's 2012 Annual Employer Health Benefits Survey found that 31% of employers offering health insurance include a high-deductible plan. In 2010, only 15% offered high-deductible plans. This rapid pace of adoption promises to continue as employers become increasingly emboldened to seek change, given continued double-digit inflation in health insurance premiums.

Consumer-driven health plan designs, as they're commonly called, reduce the extent to which consumers are sheltered from the first-dollar expense of accessing health services. Because this places a greater part of the initial burden on the plan member, consumers are becoming increasingly engaged in seeking affordable options that may fall outside their traditional mental model for health care (Figure 4).

VIRTUAL-CARE USE CASES

What are some real-world examples of virtual care in action? Because of their focus on convenience and affordability, most virtual-care models are available in an on-demand format. In other words, one can request a virtual-care visit

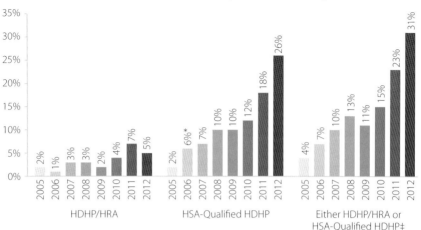

Figure 4. Distribution of various consumer-driven health plan designs among employers. HDHP, high-deductible health plan; HRA, health reimbursement account; HSA, health savings account. (From the Henry J. Kaiser Family Foundation, at http://kff.org/report-section/ehbs-2012-section-8/, with permission.)

without an appointment. In some models, however, appointments are expected and preferred.

Some models are facilitated and some are nonfacilitated, meaning that in some cases there is a nonclinician or a lower-cost clinician, such as a medical assistant or registered nurse, who first interacts with the patient. These individuals converse with the patient and confirm that the patient's condition and medical issue is appropriate for the type of virtual-care service being offered. The facilitator can also perform initial triage tasks such as confirming biometrics and vital statistics. Facilitators complete their tasks before the patient speaks with a physician or health-care provider with prescriptive authority (such as a nurse practitioner or physician's assistant). They may also be available during and after the completion of an encounter for troubleshooting issues, facilitating use of technology devices, and handling follow-up issues such as ensuring that prescriptions get to the appropriate pharmacy.

Virtual care has two common modalities: telephonic consultation and web-based video chat. There is very little specific guidance from any medical boards on which is preferable, but intuitively many conclude that a video-enabled option provides a better means for emulating a traditional office encounter and meeting the standard of care. That said, there are many conditions for which a video chat does not necessarily enhance the provider's ability to provide care (for example, a routine encounter to refill a prescription for a patient managing a previously diagnosed chronic condition).

Finally, virtual-care services must contemplate referral outlets. There will be occasions when patients access virtual care and have potentially serious or life-threatening issues that require an in-person exam. Virtual-care services should have previously identified points of care to which they will refer such patients (Figure 5).

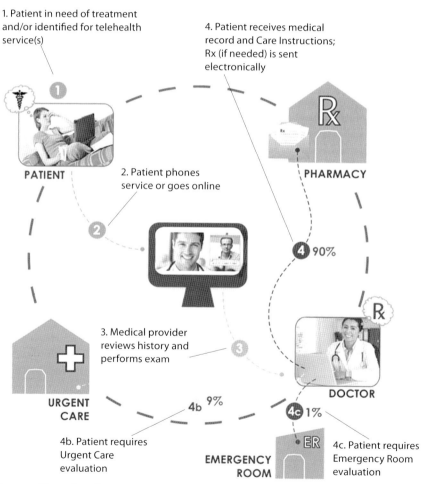

Figure 5. The order of events in a typical virtual-care encounter. (Illustration courtesy of MeMD, Inc.)

Use Case: E-Visits

E-visits allow providers to complete the same interview and diagnosis that occur in a traditional office visit using the web and videoconference technology. Routine ailments that commonly drive urgent care visits, such as upper respiratory infections, urinary tract infections, and minor abrasions, can be treated via e-visits.

E-visits enable providers to treat patients wherever their license allows them to legally do so. A provider in California, for example, can therefore expand the potential pool of customers to all of California's 37 million residents instead of only those within a 3- to 5-mile radius. E-visits can also be an option for expatriates seeking an opinion from a US health-care provider.

Use Case: Follow-Up Care

Urgent care patients do not often follow up with their urgent care clinic or provider after an office encounter. Customers of an urgent care clinic are often cost-conscious and time-conscious. Provided that a patient's condition is not worsening, the cost and drive time associated with a follow-up visit are prohibitive to pursuing a follow-up encounter.

Urgent care centers that offer e-visits for follow-up can do so at a lower cost and in significantly less time for both patient and health-care provider. Even cost-conscious consumers appreciate greater personal attention and more convenient access.

Use Case: Virtual Worksite Health Care

Large employers are rapidly adopting wellness strategies in an attempt to control rising health insurance premiums. Providing care at the worksite or through directly contracted health-care providers has become an increasingly popular approach to controlling costs. Therefore, worksite clinics, where employees can access basic primary care and sometimes occupational medicine, are one of the fastest-growing trends in employer-based health care. A 2008 Watson Wyatt study[1] concluded that nearly one-third of all large companies had or were considering a worksite clinic for their businesses. However, the high up-front investment and fixed overhead costs of a worksite clinic remain a major barrier to employers interested in this approach.

Leveraging telemedicine e-visits, urgent care centers can join networks that staff virtual worksite clinics. Employees can obtain access to physicians for the same ailments they would in a traditional worksite clinic at a dramatically lower cost to employers, and employers benefit from reduced absenteeism and increased employee satisfaction.

---

1   Watson Wyatt Worldwide. Companies not fully tapping potential of onsite health centers [press release]. March 19, 2008. Available from: http://www.hr.com/en/communities/companies-not-fully-tapping-potential-of-onsite-he_fe1dtykm.html. Accessed February 24, 2014.

Use Case: Worksite Wellness

Wellness programs are also on a rapid rise within employer-based health benefits. The current standard for employer wellness programs is establishing a population baseline through, in part, having all employees complete a health-risk assessment questionnaire and a biometric screening. The questionnaire provides the individual employee feedback on their personal risk factors on the basis of their self-reported behavioral choices and biometrics (height, weight, and so forth). A biometric screening provides verified measurements of height, weight, and blood pressure, as well as basic blood-panel information (cholesterol level, blood sugar level, and glycated hemoglobin A_{1c} level).

Taken together, these baseline assessments help identify individuals considered to be at risk for more serious chronic conditions such as heart disease and diabetes mellitus. At-risk employees are encouraged to take advantage of additional resources provided by the employer, such as health coaching or disease-management programs. Employers are provided the deidentified baseline information to understand how their group compares with the general population and what strategies for interventions best suit their employee base.

Employers are now looking for health-care providers to be involved in the review of employee health-risk assessments and biometric screen results and in the development of personal pathways for at-risk employees. One approach of virtual-care services is to deliver a web-based face-to-face review of employees' risk factors with a health-care provider.

KEY CONSIDERATIONS WHEN PLANNING TO PROVIDE VIRTUAL CARE

Urgent care centers and providers must be cognizant of the myriad risk factors, legal considerations (which vary considerably by state), and technological challenges associated with practicing telemedicine. It would be ill-advised, for example, for a clinic to simply use video calling to chat with patients and call that a telemedicine e-visit. Such an approach would almost certainly be in violation of HIPAA, the Health Information Technology for Economic and Clinical Health (HITECH) Act, and state medical board regulations.

Informed Consent Requirement

Some states require obtaining informed consent from patients before a telemedicine encounter. There are numerous criteria to evaluate each state's telemedicine regulations, and this is one of them. For example, the Texas Administrative Code Title 22, Part 9, of the Texas Medical Board Rules (probably one of the most complicated), says:

> Physicians who use telemedicine medical services must, prior to providing services, give their patients notice regarding telemedicine medical services, including the risks and benefits of being treated via telemedicine, how to

receive follow-up care or assistance in the event of an adverse reaction to the treatment or in the event of an inability to communicate as a result of a technological or equipment failure.

Compliance with HIPAA and the HITECH Act

The entire software setup and provision of service must ensure the privacy and security of patient data. This includes technical requirements such as encrypting data feeds, electronically logging who accesses medical records, and instituting password-strength and password-expiration policies. It also includes process requirements, such as preventing inappropriate disclosure of personal health information to noncovered entities.

Here are just a few examples of conclusions that have been commonly accepted as requirements under HIPAA. These are for illustrative purpose only and by no means constitute a comprehensive list:

- Electronic communications over the Internet must be encrypted from point to point to prevent interception.

- A password policy must exist that sets a standard for minimum password complexity requirements and password expirations.

- A patient must be made aware that they can request a report on everyone who has accessed their record electronically. The information technology (IT) system must be able to provide such a report by logging electronic access of patient records, and the HIPAA privacy office for the organization must be available and responsive to a patient's request for such a report.

- All vendors (and subcontractors to vendors) involved in supporting the IT solution should be contracted via a HIPAA business associates agreement.

- There should be no record of the communication between provider and patient left on the computer workstation for potential others to view. This is a common concern regarding using stand-alone video calling—the fact that conversation logs are left on the computer and the web.

Again, there are many other issues involved in HIPAA compliance. These are just a few of the more commonly accepted principles. The main point is that it is important to work with technology vendors that have an understanding of HIPAA compliance and that bear the responsibility with you of ensuring compliance.

Malpractice Coverage

Not all malpractice policies currently cover telemedicine. Urgent care providers should be certain that their policy covers telemedicine or should purchase a separate policy that specifically covers telemedicine visits.

Telehealth Platform

Various telemedicine solutions and providers are now available for urgent care providers to subscribe to or partner with. Some solutions even offer to cover the medical malpractice insurance associated with telemedicine visits. Urgent care clinic owners and providers would be well advised to make a thorough review of their state's telemedicine regulations and available solution providers before launching their e-practice.

Reimbursement

Some states require Medicaid and private insurers in the state to cover some telehealth services at parity with an in-office encounter. As of this writing, those states include California, Colorado, Georgia, Hawaii, Kentucky, Louisiana, Maine, Massachusetts, Michigan, New Hampshire, Oklahoma, Oregon, Texas, Vermont, and Virginia. A critical area for research (particularly because it is constantly evolving) is to determine what's covered in the states where your clinics are operating.

Cannibalization

Many urgent care center owners I've spoken with were initially concerned about cannibalizing their current patient base. They worried that patients who came to their office today would see them only online if given the option. If the reimbursement received via virtual care is less than the total revenue associated with an in-office visit, the concern becomes that reimbursing virtual care will create the net effect of reducing revenues. But consider these points:

- ▶ Patients are going to be given the option of virtual care whether or not a particular urgent care center offers it. The number of service providers is increasing daily. More importantly, many major health systems are going to offer virtual-care services to consumers soon if they are not already doing so. Thus, an urgent care clinic cannot prevent its customers from having access to virtual care. A practice can choose whether to compete in the virtual-care space or lose patients to virtual-care providers.

- ▶ The number of patients that a clinic can treat via virtual care is dramatically greater than the potential pool of patients that typically live within a 3-mile radius of the clinic. Providers can treat patients anywhere in the state where they are licensed, having the effect of increasing the potential patient base by orders of magnitude.

- ▶ Virtual care is a means to providing a differentiated service that will likely funnel more patients through a clinic's doors. By providing greater access to encounters with your clinic's medical staff, the business has additional opportunities to identify services that should be rendered in the clinic, explain them to the patient, and schedule an in-office follow-up.

STEPS TO TAKE WHEN CONSIDERING VIRTUAL CARE

1. Study the regulations in your state. Some of the resources provided in the "Helpful Resources" box can assist, but there is no substitute for reading your state's regulations on telemedicine.

2. Evaluate partners or service providers. It is often best not to reinvent the wheel, especially when it can be faster, more affordable, and more effective to partner in an emerging space. The technology solution, regulatory compliance, and even the provider network are all areas in which a vendor may bring a good solution to the table. The marketplace within the virtual-care arena is competitive enough that you should consider leveraging services or at least minimally assess what vendors are doing. Research them.

3. Examine the reimbursement potential in your market. The state in which your clinic operates may require payers to reimburse for virtual-care services that you could offer at parity with traditional encounters. Even if the state does not require it, payers in your market may be voluntarily reimbursing for telemedicine encounters. Reach out to them and find out what is allowed in your markets.

4. Clearly define your use case for virtual care, and logically work through the entire patient experience to identify what structures you will need in place. What happens if a patient's prescription does not get to the pharmacy? What happens if they have an adverse reaction in the middle of the

Helpful Resources

Trade Associations

- American Telemedicine Association: www.americantelemed.org
- Center for Telehealth and e-Health Law: ctel.org
- mHealth Summit: www.mhealthsummit.org
- HIMSS (Healthcare Information and Management Systems Society): www.himss.org

Research

- InMedica: in-medica.com
- FierceHealth IT: www.fiercehealthit.com
- California HealthCare Foundation: www.chcf.org

night? How will the patient receive a record of their encounter, discharge instructions, and provider notes? By having a solid understanding of all of the variations that may occur for the services you will offer, the requirements for people, processes, and technology will become clear.

5. Ensure that your technology solution is easy to use and is compliant with HIPAA and the HITECH Act. This is best done by evaluating technology partners who bear responsibility for ensuring compliance.

KEY POINTS

1. Virtual care is here for real and is not going away. It changes the competitive landscape for urgent care centers. Every urgent care center owner should have a clear strategy for understanding how to differentiate and compete against virtual-care services offered in their market and should potentially leverage virtual care as an extension of the services that their urgent care clinic offers.

2. Thoroughly investigate what solutions and partners are available to you that best fit your desired virtual-care services. It is often best not to reinvent the wheel.

3. Be aware of telemedicine regulations in the medical board rules of the states in which your clinics operate. They vary significantly by state.

4. Leverage the analysis done by policy experts and influencers in the space. Organizations such as the Center for Telehealth and e-Health Law and the American Telemedicine Association can be very helpful.

5. Be wary of the age of publications. Telemedicine regulation and state-specific details are changing incredibly quickly.

6. Be aware of the IT requirements imposed by HIPAA and the HITECH Act. Enforcement of these regulations and the penalties imposed are becoming more real. In most cases it is best to avoid cobbling together disparate technologies that are not delivered as a solution intended for health care.

7. Approach clinical quality in at least as rigorous a manner as you would in a traditional office encounter. Avoid the perception that virtual care is low-risk or low-quality because of its focus on low-acuity medical issues. Because it is a newer practice within medicine, it is as important as ever to focus on high-quality care that would withstand a rigorous third-party review.

8. Clearly define which use case your entity will provide, and focus on clarifying the value proposition and service offering for that application.

9. Check with payers and your state on the reimbursements for virtual-care encounters. They will vary by the state, the payer, and the use case.

10. Make virtual care part of your continued area of study. Nearly every health system and provider organization is considering virtual care of some kind. The number of potential new competitors in the virtual-care space is a multiple of the number of potential new competitors in urgent care and retail medicine. In addition, the technologies available, regulatory environment, and reimbursement environment are changing rapidly. Owners of urgent care centers should therefore study the virtual-care space with the same frequency and interest with which they would watch for a competitor opening a new clinic within a few blocks from their center.

CHAPTER 37

Setting Up a Health-Care Compliance Program

Tracy Patterson

Does your urgent care center need a compliance program? Yes. Until a few years ago, the development and implementation of a compliance program was voluntary. With the Patient Protection and Affordable Care Act of 2010 and the Health Care and Education Reconciliation Act of 2010 (2010 Health Care Reform), however, Congress mandated that providers, suppliers, and physicians adopt a compliance program. Even without the 2010 Health Care Reform's requirements, having an effective compliance program is just smart business. As a leader of your organization, you, along with others, should ensure that processes are in place to guide and support proper conduct. A compliance program doesn't automatically guarantee that all fraud or abuse will be eliminated, but an effective program will establish an environment that promotes prevention, detection, and resolution of misconduct, thereby reducing your risk for both.

Implementing and maintaining a compliance program requires a significant commitment of your organization's time and resources. Your program should match the size of your organization and the services you provide. Borrowing from another entity or purchasing a canned program and placing it on your intranet is not enough. Your program must be more than a written document; it must be an integral part of your organization's everyday existence. Per US Federal Sentencing Guidelines § 8B2.1(a)(2),

> To have an effective compliance and ethics program…an organization shall: (1) exercise due diligence to prevent and detect criminal conduct; and (2) otherwise promote an organizational culture that encourages ethical conduct and a commitment to compliance with the law.

2010 HEALTH CARE REFORM

The 2010 Health Care Reform is divided into two sections—one for nursing facilities and one for all other providers and suppliers. The more detailed of the two is the nursing facility section, which contains an implementation timeline. A time frame for all other providers and suppliers was not established as part of the regulation and was instead left to the discretion of the US Department of Health and Human Services (HHS).

The 2010 Health Care Reform detailed the following timeline for nursing facilities:

- By December 31, 2011, the secretary must have established and implemented a quality-assurance and performance-improvement (QAPI) program. Within 1 year, following the proclamation of the QAPI program regulations, nursing facilities must have submitted a plan to HHS to meet program standards.
- By March 23, 2012, the secretary of HHS, working with the Office of Inspector General (OIG), must have published regulations for "an effective compliance program" for nursing facility operating organizations.
- By March 23, 2013, nursing facilities must have put in operation a compliance program that meets the act's criteria.
- By March 23, 2013, the HHS secretary must have completed an evaluation of the compliance programs that nursing facilities have been required to establish.
- After March 23, 2013 (time frame not defined), the secretary must submit an evaluation report to Congress with recommendations on changes to the regulatory requirements for nursing facility compliance programs.

For nursing facilities, the 2010 Health Care Reform specified certain required components of a compliance program that include the following:

- Compliance standards and procedures for employees and other agents "that are reasonably capable of reducing the prospect" of criminal, civil, and administrative law violations regarding Medicare and Medicaid
- The assignment of overall compliance program oversight to "high-level personnel" with "sufficient resources and authority" to ensure such compliance
- The exercise of "due care" not to delegate "substantial discretionary authority" to individuals whom the nursing facility knew or should have known had a "propensity to engage in criminal, civil, or administrative violations"
- The effective communication of compliance standards and procedures to all employees and agents, including training programs or published materials
- The adoption of reasonable monitoring and auditing systems designed to detect compliance violations by employees and other agents and a mechanism that employees and agents can use to report violations without fear of retribution

- ▶ The consistent enforcement of appropriate disciplinary mechanisms, including for failure to detect an offense

- ▶ After detection of an offense, reasonable responses include steps to prevent further similar offenses, including any modifications to the compliance program

- ▶ The periodic reassessment of its compliance program to identify modifications necessary to reflect changes within the nursing facility organization and its facilities

Note: Although the criteria were not published by the deadlines above, the requirement to have a compliance program still exists. Nursing facilities must continue to develop and update their compliance programs despite the missing guidance. Other providers should also stay abreast of the nursing facility requirements, because similarities are likely to exist among them.

The 2010 Health Care Reform also contains compliance program requirements for all other health-care providers and suppliers. It requires that such providers and suppliers, as a condition of enrollment, establish a compliance program that contains core elements established by HHS. However, these requirements are largely undefined, and there is no specific implementation timeline. One could expect that HHS will continue to follow OIG guidance and the previously published elements for a compliance program. "All other health-care providers and suppliers" is a broad group that includes many industry sectors with organizations of different sizes. It is most likely that HHS's requirements will be implemented by industry sectors and will have variations depending on the size of the provider or supplier.

PUBLISHED GUIDANCES ON COMPLIANCE PROGRAMS

The Compliance Program Guidance for Medicare Fee-for-Service Contractors notes:

> In order to receive "credit" for good corporate behavior, the Federal Sentencing Guidelines require that organizational defendants exercise due diligence in the design and implementation of a compliance program intended to detect and deter fraud, waste and abuse. The Federal Sentencing Guidelines Manual at § 8A1.2, Application Note (k), sets forth seven steps that any compliance program must incorporate in order to demonstrate the due diligence element. These seven steps have been included in the various guidelines developed by the OIG and other compliance program authorities, and are believed to be the minimum requirement for an effective compliance program.

Since at least 2004, the OIG has issued multiple voluntary compliance program guidances that have been derived from or have a foundation in the Federal Sentencing Guidelines' seven elements for an effective compliance program. The 2012 Federal Sentencing Guidelines Manual, along with those of prior years, published criteria for an effective compliance and ethics program. The Centers for Medicare & Medicaid Services (CMS) published the Compliance Program Guidance for Medicare Fee-for-Service Contractors in March 2005, also similar to the Federal Sentencing Guidelines.

In 2000, as part of providing guidelines for a voluntary compliance program, the OIG stated that an effective compliance program for small practices should, at a minimum, have the ability to

- Conduct internal monitoring and auditing
- Implement compliance and practice standards
- Designate a compliance officer or contact
- Conduct appropriate training and education
- Respond appropriately to detected offenses and develop corrective action
- Develop open lines of communication
- Enforce disciplinary standards through well-publicized guidelines

As part of the CMS 2005 Compliance Program Guidance, seven key components of an effective compliance plan are defined as follows:

- Written policies and procedures
- The designation of a compliance officer and a compliance committee
- The conducting of effective training and education
- Development of effective lines of communication
- Auditing and monitoring
- Enforcement through publicized disciplinary guidelines and policies dealing with ineligible persons
- Response to detected offenses, development of corrective action initiatives, and reporting of said offenses and action initiatives to government authorities

As of March 2013, according to the OIG website, the "Seven Fundamental Elements of an Effective Compliance Program" are

- Implementing written policies, procedures, and standards of conduct
- Designating a compliance officer and compliance committee

- Conducting effective training and education
- Developing effective lines of communication
- Conducting internal monitoring and auditing
- Enforcing standards through well-publicized disciplinary guidelines
- Responding promptly to detected offenses and undertaking corrective action

Reviewing these publications can help guide you through the process of developing your compliance program. This will demonstrate your plan's commitment to ethical and legal business conduct, consider the recurring requirements of all the guidances, which highlight their importance. Your compliance plan should cover each of these topics in detail.

RISK ASSESSMENT

To include information relevant to your organization, you first must perform a risk assessment. The OIG has developed a list of four risk areas for small practices to consider as part of their compliance program development:

- Coding and billing
- Reasonable and necessary services
- Documentation
- Improper inducements, kickbacks, and self-referrals

For example, as part of your risk assessment you should consider how you handle durable medical equipment. Do you stock and bill direct or do you use a third-party closet arrangement? What are the compliance risks with each?

With your risk assessment in hand, you can begin to develop your compliance program.

COMPLIANCE PROGRAM COMPONENTS

Written Standards, Policies, and Procedures

Your compliance program should have written standards, including comprehensive policies and procedures, a code of conduct, summaries of key federal and state laws, and specific requirements by functional area (such as billing) that guide your organization and its employees on a day-to-day basis. They should be easily understood by, and posted and distributed to, all employees, as well as suppliers, agents, and contractors.

These written documents should be developed by your compliance officer or committee. To develop them, your organization will need to access additional resources, such as subject-matter experts and legal counsel. If you are new to compliance and are struggling with where to start, you may want to purchase

Key Laws

Want to know more about key health care laws? This list from the OIG provides some of the laws you might want to learn more about.

False Claims Act
Statute: 31 USC §§ 3729–3733

Anti-Kickback Statute
Statute: 42 USC § 1320a–7b(b)
Safe Harbor Regulations: 42 CFR § 1001.952

Physician Self-Referral Law
Statute: 42 USC § 1395nn
Regulations: 42 CFR §§ 411.350–.389

Exclusion Authorities
Statutes: 42 USC §§ 1320a–7, 1320c–5
Regulations: 42 CFR pts. 1001 (OIG) and 1002 (state agencies)

Civil Monetary Penalties Law
Statute: 42 USC § 1320a–7a
Regulations: 42 CFR pt. 1003

Criminal Health Care Fraud Statute
Statute: 18 USC §§ 1347, 1349

Resources

2012 Federal Sentencing Guidelines Manual
www.ussc.gov/Guidelines/2012_Guidelines/Manual_PDF/index.cfm

2011 Federal Sentencing Guidelines Manual
Effective Compliance and Ethics Program
www.ussc.gov/Guidelines/2011_Guidelines/Manual_HTML/8b2_1.htm

Federal Register, volume 65, number 194, Thursday, October 5, 2000, Notices
OIG Compliance Program for Individual and Small Group Physician Practices
oig.hhs.gov/authorities/docs/physician.pdf

OIG's Health Care Fraud Prevention and Enforcement Action Team Provider Compliance Training
oig.hhs.gov/compliance/provider-compliance-training/index.asp

HIPAA privacy and security rules:
www.hhs.gov/ocr/privacy/index.html
www.cms.gov/HIPAAGenInfo/

CMS physician self-referral law ("Stark law") information
www.cms.gov/PhysicianSelfReferral/

CMS physician self-referral law advisory opinions library
www.cms.gov/PhysicianSelfReferral/95_advisory_opinions.asp

OIG's Provider Self-Disclosure Protocol
oig.hhs.gov/fraud/selfdisclosure.asp

OIG's Compliance Program Guidance
oig.hhs.gov/fraud/complianceguidance.asp

Corporate Responsibility and Corporate Compliance: A Resource for Health Care Boards of Directors
http://oig.hhs.gov/fraud/docs/complianceguidance/040203CorpRespRsceGuide.pdf

OIG's health care fraud prevention and enforcement action team provider compliance training
oig.hhs.gov/compliance/provider-compliance-training/index.asp

OIG's recommended compliance resources
oig.hhs.gov/compliance/provider-compliance-training/files/ListofComplianceResourcesHandoutBR508r1.pdf

---

CFR, Code of Federal Regulations; CMS, Centers for Medicare & Medicaid Services; HIPAA, Health Insurance Portability and Accountability Act; OIG, Office of Inspector General; USC, United States Code.

---

a program with generic policies and procedures. The key to using a generic program is to make sure it comes from a reputable source and then use the content as a starting point; serious review and modification will be necessary to customize a program that fits your organization and is effective. Some key items to include in your written standards and policies and procedures are

- ▶ Duties of all employees, including additional requirements of the management team in promoting compliance and responding to complaints of noncompliance
- ▶ Employee training requirements, including the how, when, and what

- Incorporation of compliance into employee performance reviews
- Requirements for background checks and employment criteria
- Policy on disciplinary actions for noncompliance
- Audit requirements, including auditor skills, and how and to whom results will be shared
- Policy on how the compliance team will communicate with other key areas, including legal, billing, auditing, and human resources
- Policy on record retention required under law or payer agreements
- Procedures for reporting noncompliance, including the how and to whom
- Responsibilities of the compliance officer and compliance committee
- Specific policies on coding and billing; reasonable and necessary services; documentation; and improper inducement, kickbacks, and self-referrals

Just like other policies and procedures, your compliance program and documents should be easy to understand and written at the appropriate reading level for your workforce. If your workforce includes employees who speak English as their second language, you may need to provide documents in another language.

Compliance Officer and Compliance Committee

Every department and function needs a leader, and compliance is no different. Someone, or a group of someones, needs to manage and monitor your compliance program. This compliance "someone" should report directly to your owner, governing body, or chief executive officer. Reports should occur monthly or quarterly and on an as-needed basis. As part of managing the program, the compliance officer is responsible for adapting the plan as your organization changes. The compliance officer's main responsibilities should include educating employees about compliance, enforcing the compliance plan, investigating compliance issues and complaints, auditing the business for compliance, and instituting corrective action when needed. This officer will not know everything and should be provided resources like compliance education and access to experts. Care should be taken to allow your compliance officer independence with a reporting structure free from conflicts of interest. The smaller your organization, the harder this may become; therefore, reporting structure is one such area where seeking specific advice may be warranted.

Training and Education

All of your employees, including long-term temporary employees, health-care providers, officers, and board members, require training. You may also have a need to train nonemployees, such as independent contractors and vendors. Attendance at training sessions should be mandatory, and written acknowledgments should be obtained from all attendees. Written tests and feedback are great ways to ensure that your training programs are effective, by demonstrating retention and understanding. Most organizations and urgent care centers have a diverse workforce with a variety of educational backgrounds and experience; hence, one educational format may not be enough. Your compliance program should educate your employees on your standards of conduct and compliance with regulatory requirements and then further educate them on compliance issues related to their specific job functions. Your training should be periodic, and initial training should occur as close to the hire date as possible. It is not enough to train only once; add annual training that focuses on key points, new developments, and changes.

You will have to ensure that everyone in a management position is comfortable speaking about and enforcing the compliance program, especially the parts of the plan that apply to their specific areas and functions. All employees must understand that adherence is mandatory and disciplinary action will be taken for violations.

Using examples relevant to an employee's daily tasks is an effective technique for teaching compliance topics. If you do not know where to start, a variety of compliance materials and videos are available that are geared to the ambulatory care setting. These materials make excellent additions to your compliance program. Using posters, newsletters, and intranet communications spreads the message and keeps compliance front and center.

Open Lines of Communication

It's not enough to have a compliance plan and designate a compliance officer. You must also disseminate information to your employees and create an open-door policy that allows them to communicate with you. Provide the following:

- Anonymity for reporting and asking questions, when possible
- Protection from retaliation when making a good-faith report
- Confidentiality, whenever possible
- Multiple points of reporting, such as a compliance officer, compliance staff members, supervisors and managers, and a compliance hotline
- Multiple methods of reporting, such as telephone, email, drop box or internal mail, and face-to-face

Maintain a detailed log of all reports of noncompliance, even those that turn out to be false. Track the complaints by type and look for trends.

Monitoring and Auditing

Your compliance plan should catch issues before they get out of hand. The only way to accomplish this is to have regular and periodic audits *and*, when issues are found, to follow up on those audits after implementing corresponding corrective action, to determine whether the issues have been resolved. Make sure that your audits are conducted by a qualified auditor, who should have the necessary expertise in federal and state requirements and commercial and private payer rules. You may have to go outside your organization to find the right auditor. Auditors should be independent of any management team and provide written reports to the compliance officer or compliance committee for review.

Two important audit functions include the review of all billing practices and a claim audit. Billing practices should be reviewed to determine if they are current and complete in regard to payer contract requirements, regulations, and generally relied-on standards (that is, up-to-date Current Procedural Terminology codes).

For claim audits, determine whether your center will perform a retrospective or concurrent review. The type of review you conduct will affect the actions you take after review, including notifications and repayments. For either review type, the audit should determine whether

- ► Bills are accurately coded and reflect the services rendered
- ► Documentation is being completed correctly
- ► Services are reasonable and necessary
- ► Any incentives for unnecessary services exist

Benchmark your audits over time; trends in audits can be more telling than a single finding. Audits should be done annually, at a minimum, and audits throughout the year of new health-care providers and other staff members are important for catching issues early. When you are performing a chart audit, each health-care provider should have at least 5 to 10 charts audited; a bigger sample size is typically better. When issues are identified, repeat claim and chart audits should be completed after corrective action has been taken, to ensure effectiveness of changes.

Don't let your compliance plan get dusty; periodic evaluations are a must for assessing its effectiveness. If you see the same issues over and over, something must be addressed. Exit interviews are excellent tools for monitoring your organization's conduct. Ask the exiting employee about any violations they observed of the compliance plan, statutes, regulations, and payer requirements.

Enforcement and "Publicized" Guidelines

To be effective, your compliance program must outline the disciplinary actions for those who violate it. This includes not only actual violations but also the failure to detect violations when routine observation and job performance would reasonably expose a potential issue.

Although some flexibility is needed for mitigating circumstances, consequences should be consistent and appropriate to the nature of the violation. Disciplinary actions for violations may vary for intent, amount of financial harm, or number of occurrences; if you do vary disciplinary action, this information should be included in your policy. Depending on the requirement and corresponding violation, disciplinary actions could include verbal and written reprimands, probation, suspension, and termination. Those violations for which there is zero tolerance should also be detailed in your policy. For guidelines to be "well publicized," specific disciplinary standards must be included in employee training and written in the compliance plan and policies.

Written policies and procedures require a reasonable background investigation to determine whether potential employees have ever been criminally convicted or suspended or excluded from participation in a federal program. When subcontractors are used, consider requiring them to have a compliance program, including your minimum requirements for background checks. If they are independent contractors and don't have a formal compliance program or background check, you should have a written policy and procedure for including them in yours. Background checks shouldn't stop once someone is hired; conduct periodic reviews of your employees. If a violation is found in a periodic background check, remove the employee from sensitive work until corrective action or disciplinary action has been accomplished.

Response and Corrective Action Regarding a Detected Offense

An effective compliance program that monitors, audits, and maintains open lines of communication will in time be called on to handle a complaint or detect a possible violation. Hopefully, such a complaint or violation turns out to be nothing, but you should be prepared to investigate immediately and take corrective action if a violation has actually occurred. Depending on the situation, corrective action may include modifying a practice, returning an overpayment, or reporting to a government agency.

The worst thing you can do is establish a compliance program and then ignore its findings. Therefore, in your written policies and procedures include the following:

- How investigations will be handled
- Time requirements for investigating, including closing the investigation
- When to turn the investigation over to an outside resource
- When and how authorities should be notified

CONCLUSION

If you don't have a compliance program, or it has been a while since you have reviewed your program, start now. It takes time to develop a program and train your staff, but it also takes time to create a culture of compliance. There is no need to wait until CMS publishes implementation regulations to begin this process.

The OIG's training website lists the following "Five Practical Tips for Creating a Culture of Compliance":

- Make compliance plans a priority now.
- Know your fraud and abuse risk areas.
- Manage your financial relationships.
- Just because your competitor is doing something doesn't mean you can or should.
- When in doubt, ask for help.

KEY POINTS

1. Don't wait until it's too late. If you don't have an effective compliance program, start the process of implementing one immediately.
2. Stay alert. Review applicable health-care laws and payer requirements. Become part of the compliance community and stay up-to-date on developments.
3. Pay now so that you don't pay more later. Dedicate the necessary time and resources to develop an effective program and a culture of compliance.
4. Know your business. Perform a risk assessment and include all seven components of the Federal Sentencing Guidelines into your program.
5. Put everything in writing (code of conduct, policies and procedures, training programs, audit procedures).
6. Document and keep appropriate records (training records, audit results, reports of noncompliance).
7. Provide training and education to your employees, repeatedly. Make compliance an important part of your culture and part of your employees' daily tasks.
8. Be a leader; lead by example.
9. Ignorance is not an excuse. Do your homework, identify resources, and ask for help.
10. And because it can't be said enough, don't wait—start today.

CHAPTER 38

Audits by Managed-Care Organizations and Regulatory Agencies

Damaris L. Medina

THE CURRENT ECONOMIC CLIMATE has motivated an increase in attempts by government agencies and private payers to investigate coding and supporting documentation. The escalating pressure on both government and commercial payers to decrease costs will inevitably result in an increase in audit activity on payments to physicians and urgent care centers to recoup costs.

Government payers lead the charge, with the government allocating hundreds of millions of dollars to programs specifically designed to recover payments. These programs, through their multiple forms, are designed in coordination to perform several functions:

▶ Identify billing outliers through data-mining and coding algorithms

▶ Audit and investigate outliers or coding areas subject to high error rates

▶ Recover improper payments

▶ Assess civil and criminal penalties for payments that resulted from fraud

According to its own statistics, in 2012 the government allocated at least $600 million to recovering payments made to Medicare fee-for-service contractors.[1] That same year, *the government recovered more than $4 billion* from a number of sources related to audits, investigations, and civil and criminal penalties.

In the first half of 2013, the government reported expected recoveries of over $3.8 billion, consisting of over $521 million in audit receivables and approximately $3.28 billion in investigative receivables.[2] On June 6, 2013, the Centers for

---

1   FDepartment of Health and Human Services and the Department of Justice Health Care Fraud and Abuse Control Program Annual Report for Fiscal Year 2012.
2   Office of Inspector General. Semiannual report to Congress. October 2012–March 2013. Available from: http://oig.hhs.gov/reports-and-publications/archives/semiannual/2013/SAR-S13-Final.pdf. Accessed February 24, 2014.

Medicare & Medicaid Services (CMS) announced that the administration was responsible for the recoupment of more than $14.9 billion in health-care fraud recoveries in the last 4 years, compared with $6.7 billion in the prior 4-year period. This increase in recoupment has been largely aided by tools authorized by the Patient Protection and Affordable Care Act. In view of that phenomenal return on investment, the trend of increased government audit activity is likely to continue.

Although most government audits historically were limited to hospital payments, both government and commercial payers are beginning to turn their attention to Medicare Part B payments, specifically evaluation and management (E&M) services billed for urgent care. In September 2012, CMS announced that the recovery audit contractor (RAC) program would begin auditing claims that contain higher-level Current Procedural Terminology (CPT) codes for E&M services—specifically CPT codes 99214 and 99215. The audits of these codes were precipitated by a report that the US Department of Health and Human Services Office of Inspector General (OIG) issued in May 2012 titled "Coding Trends of Medicare Evaluation and Management Services." The report found that among physicians who consistently billed the higher-level E&M codes, 19.8% were internists, 12.2% were family physicians, and 9.9% were emergency physicians. These target specialties form the backbone of urgent care. Although the audit process was scheduled to begin in only one of the four RAC regions, it is expected to be expanded to the other three RAC regions.[3] In late 2013, CMS announced another auditing program focusing on E&M CPT codes 99214 and 99215, called the supplemental medical review contractor (SMRC) program.

Commercial payers are following the government's lead. Commercial payers commonly focus on particular code groups or particular issues. The identification of the higher levels of E&M services by the government as an issue area is expected to prompt commercial payers to increase their scrutiny of these codes. Many commercial payers reported an increase in post-payment audits by the end of 2012. The same trend was expected to be reported for the end of 2013.

The threat of external-payer audits to urgent care is tangible, and the amounts at stake are significant. Penalties for improper payments due to fraud include treble damages and civil penalties of $11,000 per claim. It is no longer enough for urgent care centers to concentrate their efforts on getting properly reimbursed for their services. Urgent care centers must be prepared to defend against efforts at recoupment of overpayments by both government and commercial payers. Thus, preparation and management strategies for external audits must be part of every urgent care center's business plan.

---

3   The audit process was started in RAC Region C, which is made up of the following states in addition to the US Virgin Islands and Puerto Rico: Alabama, Arkansas, Colorado, Florida, Georgia, Louisiana, Mississippi, New Mexico, North Carolina, Oklahoma, South Carolina, Tennessee, Texas, Virginia, and West Virginia.

TYPES OF AUDITS

The first step toward implementing a strategy to manage and prepare for external audits is to understand the types of auditing tools that are available to payers. There are three general types of audits:

- Commercial-payer audits
- Government-payer audits
- Audits and investigations by the US Department of Justice (DOJ) and the OIG

Audits by Commercial Payers

As audit activity increases in the public-payer sphere, commercial audit activity is following suit. Commercial payers seem to be focusing on medical necessity, legibility of records, and the appropriate use of E&M codes.

Commercial payers use a number of different methods to identify audit targets. Some sophisticated carriers use software that detects anomalies in billing patterns and identifies billing-pattern outliers. Your center may be identified as an outlier if your billing patterns differ from those of your peers. Some carriers have entire departments dedicated to studying billing patterns and implementing and conducting audit procedures for claims that are identified as a result of these studies. Other carriers contract third parties to handle these functions, including the actual audit of claims.

Regardless of the method used or the type of commercial payer initiating the audit, audits by commercial payers begin in a similar way—a time-sensitive request for medical records is made for past services. The circumstances under which an audit may be initiated are often delineated in the contract between the payer and the provider.

Commercial insurers also have been using informal reviews as a preliminary step before initiating a formal audit. At times an informal review may come in the form of a request for a review of records for the purpose of utilization review. The circumstances under which a commercial payer may request an informal review may also be delineated in the contract between the payer and the provider.

Audits by Government Payers

Audits of Medicare Claims

Audits by Medicare Administrative Contractors
Medicare administrative contractors (MACs) perform targeted claims reviews for specific problems identified by the Comprehensive Error Rate Testing (CERT) program. The CERT program randomly selects approximately 50,000 claims

submitted to MACs per reporting period. MACs request records from providers to determine compliance with CMS rules. If the documentation is not compliant, or if no information is received from the provider, overpayment notices are sent demanding adjustments for claims that have been found to be overpaid (or, in some circumstances, underpaid).

Audits by Recovery Audit Contractors
The RAC program began as part of a program under the Medicare Modernization Act of 2003. Because of its success, it became a permanent nationwide program under the Tax Relief and Health Care Act of 2006. Under the program, the government contracts with four regional RACs, who are responsible for reviewing claims on a post-payment basis within their assigned region. RACs receive data from CMS containing information for claims within their region. They are tasked with reviewing the data using proprietary data-mining methodology. In exchange for their work, RACs receive a contingency fee of a certain percentage of any identified improper payments.

There are three types of RAC audits:

- *Automated reviews*   Automated reviews are conducted by using proprietary data-mining methodologies. Data-mining methodologies identify improper payments without a review of medical records. If an urgent care center is subject to an automated review, it will simply receive a demand for payment.

- *Complex reviews*   In complex reviews, RACs identify claims having a high probability of error through their data-mining methodology. After these claims have been identified, RACs request medical records for review.

- *Semi-automated reviews*   Semi-automated reviews begin as automated reviews and progress to the level of complex reviews once more severe issues are identified.

Some RAC reviews are permitted to extrapolate the negative results of an audit to all other claims within a similar review period.

Audits by Zone Integrity Program Contractors
Seven regional zone integrity program contractors (ZPICs) are replacing program safeguard contractors. ZPICs are tasked with performing data analysis aimed at identifying potential problem areas, investigating potential fraud, and developing fraud cases for civil and criminal referral to the OIG and the DOJ.

Audits by Supplemental Medical Review Contractors
In 2013, CMS announced yet another auditing program: SMRC audits. CMS contracted with StrategicHealthSolutions, LLC, to audit Medicare Part A and Part B claims for improper payments. These audits have begun, with providers already receiving requests for medical records. StrategicHealthSolutions'

website lists E&M services (focused on CPT codes 99214 and 99215) as one of its areas of current medical review.[4]

Audits of Medicaid Claims

Audits Under the Medicaid Integrity Program

The Medicaid Integrity Program was created by the Deficit Reduction Act of 2005. It is the first-ever national strategy to detect fraud and abuse in federal and state Medicaid programs. It provides oversight and assistance to state Medicaid programs. Medicaid integrity contractors (MICs) perform audits of state Medicaid programs.

MICs are divided into three types:

- *Review MICs*   Analyze claims data to identify payment vulnerabilities
- *Audit MICs*   Conduct post-payment audits of documentation to identify overpayments
- *Education MICs*   Educate providers as needed, on the basis of issues discovered by the program

Payment Error Rate Measurement

The Payment Error Rate Measurement (PERM) program is used to measure improper payments in the Medicaid program. Each state is reviewed once every 3 years on a 17-state rotation. The PERM program also relies on independent contractors, who review and audit claims for improper payments. The target issues are eligibility and high-dollar overpayments.

Medicaid Recovery Audit Contractor

Medicaid RAC programs began in 2012 on a state-by-state basis. Each program has latitude in its own design and in determining which issues it wishes to target with the audits.

Audits and Investigations by the Office of Inspector and the Department of Justice

Investigations by the OIG or the DOJ can be initiated in several ways. They may be the result of any of the audit vehicles already described here, including commercial audits. If fraud is suspected, they may be initiated because of a sealed whistle-blower action, or they may be precipitated collaterally by a provider's relationship with an entity that is under investigation.

In 2012, a chain of urgent care facilities settled a case for $10 million on the basis of claims brought to the DOJ by a whistle-blower who was a former employee of the facilities. The allegations against the urgent care chain were related to

---

4   Although the program is purportedly designed to work on both Medicare and Medicaid claims, the current activity seems to be solely related to Medicare claims.

upcoding of urgent care services as well as billing for unnecessary allergy, H1N1 influenza virus, and respiratory panel testing.

OIG and DOJ investigations usually begin with a subpoena. A subpoena is a request for documents inclusive of, but not limited to, medical records. Subpoenas request email, other communications, and documents related to what are often numerous categories outlined in the subpoena.

PREPARING FOR AN AUDIT

Because of the success of the federal funding efforts, and because of commercial payers' increased audit activity, urgent care centers should invest in tools that will prepare them for what may be an inevitable event. One of the most useful tools in preparing for an audit is a comprehensive compliance program (see Chapter 37, "Setting Up a Health-Care Compliance Program"). A compliance program makes sure that there is a written policy for an urgent care center to follow in addressing issues that are commonly the centerpiece of both commercial and government audits.

A well-executed compliance program will address issues such as coding and billing practices, internal coding and documentation auditing, training programs, and procedures for dealing with overpayments and refunds. It should address potential employment issues such as discrimination and sexual harassment, and it should assign a compliance officer or other resource to address the training in, execution of, and ongoing compliance with the program. The program should also include a Health Insurance Portability and Accountability Act (HIPAA) policy and manual, and a written document retention policy.] Finally, even those urgent care centers that use outside billing companies must have their own compliance program, separate and apart from the billing company's program. This is because having a billing company does not transfer liability for coding errors away from the provider.

As part of or in addition to a compliance program, the following best practices are instrumental in keeping your urgent care center audit-ready:

▶ Identify a point person or team (this should be your compliance officer or compliance committee) to be responsible for audit-preparedness activities.

▶ Assess your urgent care center's risk areas by analyzing your utilization of procedure codes and modifiers in comparison with other similar centers. Software products exist to help you do this, or you can do it online on the CMS website.

▶ Monitor the CMS website for updates, reports, and materials related to audit activity, including CERT findings. Monitoring CMS audit activity will keep you up-to-date on audit target areas, which will help you identify potential risk areas within your center.

▶ Conduct periodic self-audits. You should contract with a third-party claims audit expert to conduct an external review of claims. Audits may be used in a variety of ways to ensure your center's compliance. Auditors can conduct a review of claims to ensure the sufficiency of documentation, as well as for the purpose of benchmarking your utilization of codes in comparison with your peers. Involving outside legal counsel in these audits may provide you with the ability to maintain the confidentiality of audit results through attorney–client privilege.

RESPONDING TO AUDITS

The keys to responding to audits from either commercial or government payers are readiness and a cooperative approach with the auditing entity. Except in the case of an audit occurring in the criminal realm, audits (by commercial or government payers) follow a similar process, and the response considerations are similar.

Response to Commercial-Payer and Government-Payer Audits

Most audits are initiated by a letter requesting documentation or medical records for particular claims.[5] On receipt of a request for documentation, the first step is to make sure that the letter is routed to the correct individual within the organization. The correct individual is often the compliance officer, or an alternative individual previously identified in the policies and procedures of the urgent care center's compliance program.

Once the letter is in the right hands, the urgent care center must identify the source and type of the audit. The name of the auditing agency should be apparent on the face of the letter. If the type of audit is not clear from the letter, the auditing agency should be contacted to make that determination.

Once the source and type of the audit have been determined, a center may consider whether to engage an attorney to handle the audit. This decision will depend on a number of factors, including the scope of the audit and the potential financial liability associated with the audit. In the event of a criminal audit, it is always advisable to contact an attorney. It may also be advisable to engage an attorney if the financial risk associated with an adverse finding is significant. The source and type of audit may be indicative as to the significance of the financial risk, because some types of audits allow for the extrapolation of adverse results of a limited audit to an expanded universe of claims. Finally, it is imperative to contact legal counsel if at any stage in the process you suspect potential fraud or abuse. Legal counsel may also be helpful in managing the specific requirements of different audits, because the requirements for audits can change often.

---

5   RAC automated reviews are initiated by a demand for payment without a request for documentation.

Perhaps the most important rule in responding to audits is to be aware of deadlines and to respond in a timely manner, or seek written extensions if a response within the prescribed period is not possible. In several types of audits, failure to respond in a timely manner to an audit may affect the disposition of the audit. It may also affect your right to appeal the findings of the audit.

Once the documentation in response to the letter request has been prepared and organized, you should analyze why your group is being audited. There may be legitimate reasons for your center's higher acuity rates or higher utilization of specific E&M or procedure codes. These issues may be addressed in advance with the inclusion of a cover letter. You may also want to include information related to your compliance program, policies, and procedures in your cover letter.

After receipt of the audit report, or while you await a response, you should undertake your own analysis of the claims at issue. Depending on the severity of the audit, it may be advisable to engage an outside coding expert to perform a separate analysis of the claims being audited, to determine if there are coding discrepancies. This analysis is helpful in determining whether to engage in the available appeals process. It is also advisable if extrapolation is evident. In the face of extrapolation, the organization should consider whether to analyze all claims in the claims universe to challenge extrapolation.

The appeals process may differ depending on the auditing entity. Most audits have several levels of appeal. It may be necessary to go through several levels, especially in the context of urgent care billing, because of the difficulty in urgent care coding. Furthermore, you should never assume that denials are correct. You should refer to your own independent analysis of the claims in determining whether to engage in the appeals process.

Response to Criminal Audits, Investigations, and Subpoenas From the Office of Inspector General

Criminal investigations or audits, or audits or investigations initiated by the OIG, should be handled in a very different manner. In the context of investigations or audits initiated by the OIG, groups will often first learn of them through a subpoena. As already noted, it is imperative that the group makes sure that a subpoena is routed to legal counsel that is experienced in handling government audits. Skilled legal counsel will ensure that there are an analysis and review of the subpoena and the requested materials, that they obtain a narrowing of the request if possible, that the response timeline is being met, that litigation hold letters are in place, that insurance coverage is addressed (if applicable), and that internal and external communication strategies are in place to best protect providers.

After the subpoena is received, legal counsel will advise the provider of the scope and breadth of the search for documents requested by the subpoena. It is important to make a diligent search for responsive documents because even the inadvertent nondisclosure of evidence can result in serious civil and criminal consequences. This is especially true today, when documents exist in several electronic forms within numerous electronic repositories.

Subpoenas now request electronically stored information as a matter of course. These requests make all electronic sources of data subject to search. These sources can include desktop computers, shared servers, smartphones, and even tablets. Information stored in these sources lasts forever. Forensic searches for data can uncover email, text messages, or documents that users thought they had permanently deleted. Therefore, it is increasingly important that urgent care centers and their employees be cognizant and careful of what they write or communicate through electronic means.

On receipt of a subpoena, an urgent care center must immediately preserve all information and suspend all deletion. The alteration or deletion of information after receipt of a subpoena, even if inadvertent, can result in civil spoliation or in criminal charges for obstruction of justice. A comprehensive written document-retention policy in a group's compliance program will facilitate the document search process and will protect a group from the possibility of the inadvertent deletion of data.

CONCLUSION

Perhaps the best defense against an audit is when the physician or allied-health professional documents the file. There is no substitute for a well-documented file; it increases reimbursement and protects against questions about services rendered.

KEY POINTS

1. Both government and commercial payers are seeking to recoup overpayments through audits.

2. Recent audit activity includes audits of the medical necessity of certain procedures performed in the urgent care setting and utilization of E&M codes frequently billed by urgent care centers.

3. Urgent care centers must have a general understanding of the numerous audit programs and auditing agencies in order to assess their risk for audits.

4. One of the most useful tools in preparing for an audit is having a comprehensive compliance program.

5. Identify a point person or team to be responsible for audit-preparedness activities in your urgent care center.

6. Assess your urgent care center's risk areas by analyzing your utilization of procedure codes and modifiers in comparison with other similar centers.

7. Monitor the CMS website for updates, reports, and materials related to audit activity, including CERT findings.

8. Conduct periodic self-audits. You should contract with a third-party claims audit expert to conduct an external review of claims.

9. On receipt of a request for documentation, the first step is to make sure that the letter is routed to the correct individual within the organization.

10. Once the letter is in the right hands, the urgent care center must identify the source and type of the audit.

11. Once the source and type of the audit have been determined, a center may consider whether to engage outside legal counsel to handle the audit.

12. Perhaps the most important rule in responding to audits is to be aware of deadlines and to respond in a timely manner, or seek extensions if a response within the prescribed period is not possible.

13. Once the documentation in response to the letter request has been prepared and organized, you should analyze why your group is being audited.

14. You should never assume that denials are correct. You should refer to your own independent analysis of the claims in determining whether to engage in the appeals process.

15. Criminal investigations or audits, as well as audits or investigations initiated by the OIG, should be handled in a very different manner. In the context of investigations or audits initiated by the OIG, groups must engage outside legal counsel to handle all aspects of the investigation, including response to subpoenas.

CHAPTER 39

Ensuring Patient Safety

John Shufeldt

IF ALL ELSE FAILS, patient safety needs to be the one constant—the one common denominator—by which the urgent care industry is recognized. Assuming this focus on patient safety is so important, the follow-up question we must therefore ask is whether we, as an industry, are spending enough time, money, and resources to ensure that we meet this objective.

First, we must recognize that urgent care medicine is by nature a high-risk undertaking. Generally, patients who present for services are generally not well suited to select the treatment modality or location most appropriate for their particular complaint, and thus many conditions and injuries exceed the level of service and care available at a particular facility. This is not to say that the provider cannot diagnose the condition and effectively treat the patient. Rather, it simply points to the need for the available resources, both human and equipment, that are necessary for the patient's immediate and ongoing care.

Urgent care medicine is more challenging than emergency medicine because it is akin to finding the proverbial needle in the haystack, and because emergency department (ED) providers generally have access to the resources to diagnose and treat the patient, as well as access to consultants and ancillary staff members to whom they can turn for assistance.

Moreover, in the ED, emergency physicians and their teams are trained to think "worst first," where everyone walking in is assumed to have a life-threatening condition until it is proven otherwise. Because an urgent care provider can treat hundreds of minor illnesses before facing a patient who may be very, or even indeterminately, ill, the ED's belief system does not carry over into the urgent care practice. This fact speaks to the need for maintaining a high level of awareness, even after hours of seeing patients, to ensure that the subtle spinal epidural abscess masquerading as mechanical musculoskeletal pain does not slip through undiagnosed.

Most patients with medical issues who end up in litigation or with adverse outcomes do not present screaming, "Look at me, I have XXXX," but they present exactly the way thousands of other patients with minor conditions present, perhaps save for one small nuanced laboratory test finding, historical nugget, or physical exam finding.

Other patient safety misadventures are always possible as well, including missed laboratory or imaging findings, inappropriate or absent informed consent, and acute care events that occur when staff members are untrained, poorly trained, or unaccustomed to caring for the critically ill.

COMMON SUBTLE CONDITIONS PRESENTING IN THE URGENT CARE CENTER

The practice of urgent care medicine is difficult. Obtaining patients' medical histories and performing thorough physical exams are only two absolutely crucial aspects of such practice. Without the typical benefits of long-term relationships, time, and unlimited diagnostics, our assessments and decisions must be made rapidly, relying on, and being comfortable with, imperfect and incomplete information gathered and synthesized just as quickly.

Medical providers can miss the diagnosis and still perform above the standard of care. What gets us in trouble is failing to chart evidence in the medical record that the missed diagnosis was considered and then discussed with the patient. Although it is true that patients often refuse further evaluation or testing—it is their right to do so—negative outcomes can be avoided and the provider can be absolved if patients have been given adequate information on which to base consent and if the discussion has been documented in the record.

Many types of medical misadventures can be considered rare, yet they do happen. Here are some examples of red flags and diagnoses for which urgent care providers need to maintain a high level of suspicion and that require immediate attention:

Vital Signs

- *Abnormal vital signs*   Adult patients with unexplained tachycardia, tachypnea, or borderline blood pressure. Likewise, hyperthermia and hypothermia are potential ominous signs of sepsis.

Neurologic

- *Subarachnoid hemorrhage*   Patients describing "the worst headache of their life" (as reported in the medical notes) and with a pain level of 9 to 10 on the pain scale. Imaging and lumbar puncture or direct referral to the nearest ED is warranted, as compared with the diagnosis of "a migraine."

- *Cavernous sinus thrombosis*   Patients presenting with a history of sinusitis and with a current worsening headache and possible visual changes require examination of the retina to look for increased intracranial hemorrhage and participation in a discussion of that possible diagnosis.

- *Meningitis*   Patients presenting with headache and fever, with or without a stiff neck, should participate in a discussion about the necessity for a lumbar puncture.

- *Acute angle closure glaucoma*   Patients presenting with a red, painful eye that goes undetected (hence, not discussed) because the provider instead focuses primarily on the patient's complaint of headache
- *Loss of visual fields*   Although patients with retinal detachment, central retinal artery or vein occlusion, and visual field loss secondary to a stroke are seen relatively rarely in the urgent care center, and they usually present with symptoms that most providers do not miss, their condition is time-sensitive and must be immediately addressed.

Chest

- *Chest pain*   In the majority of cases, patients who present with chest pain do not turn out to have a serious condition. The challenge, of course, is identifying the exception that proves the rule.
- *Pulmonary embolus*   Patients presenting with abnormal vital signs and having the potential for a pulmonary embolus (cancer, long travel, fracture, and so on), should have their Wells criteria documented and should be engaged in a thorough discussion so that they can provide informed consent.
- *Acute myocardial infarction*   Subtle patient presentations of acute myocardial infarction, particularly in women, are the norm, as are diagnoses in young patients under the age of 40 years. Electrocardiograms (ECGs), documented risk scores for thrombolysis in myocardial infarction, and discussions providing enough detail to allow for informed consent are imperative.
- *Dissecting aneurysm*   Patients rarely present to urgent care with the unusual, but not unheard of, complaint that often expresses as back pain or "tearing" pain. Such symptoms require blood pressure documentation (of both arms) and an ECG. If you suspect a dissecting aneurysm, it is imperative that you have a thorough discussion that includes treatment options, so that the patient can provide informed consent.

Abdomen

- *Ischemic bowel*   Ischemic bowel is an example of a condition in which the patient's pain is out of proportion to exam findings, and is seen typically in older patients or those who use cocaine or methamphetamine. The patient can become very ill very quickly and require immediate intervention. Check stool guaiac and vital signs.
- *Appendicitis*   Because the presentation for acute appendicitis can be initially benign, patients with even the smallest amount of tenderness or rebound and who still have an appendix should be given information on treatment options so that they can provide informed consent.

Genitourinary

- *Testicular torsion*   Males presenting with acute testicular pain, even if recurrent, should have an ultrasound to ensure that blood flow to the testicle is adequate, because torsion is a time-sensitive condition that must be evaluated expeditiously to save the testicle.

- *Ruptured ectopic pregnancy*   Women with positive pregnancy test findings and lower quadrant abdominal pain must immediately undergo ultrasound.

- *Ovarian torsion*   In females with acute onset of pelvic pain, the diagnosis of torsion is time-sensitive; action must be taken immediately to save the ovary.

Other

- *Tendon injuries*   Generally, penetrating wounds are the cause of tendon injuries, which are easily missed. Be on the watch for tendon injuries particularly in patients who present with clenched-fist injuries, in which the tendon may be lacerated, presenting a risk for serious infection.

- *Foreign bodies*   Other than button battery ingestion, missed foreign bodies do not pose a significant life threat, yet they are still a cause of malpractice suits.

- *Growth plate fractures*   In children, extremity injuries and tenderness or swelling localized to the growth plate, even in the presence of normal findings on x-rays, require splinting and further evaluation.

- *Lung nodules*   The legal literature is replete with cases of patients who present with a benign condition that requires a chest x-ray and then return a few years later with hemoptysis and receive a diagnosis of lung cancer—only to find out that the lesion was present on the radiograph from years earlier. This example underscores the fact that all x-rays should be overread by a radiologist.

Take-Home Points

- Keep your guard up.
- Take the time to document thoroughly.
- Discuss the patient's health issues and options with them thoroughly and document the discussion, and then document the patient's granting of informed consent.
- Write down your differential diagnoses—particularly for any life-threatening issues.

INFORMED CONSENT

Former US Supreme Court Justice Benjamin Cardozo wrote: "Every human being of adult years and sound mind has the right to determine what shall be done with his own body." Today, that simple statement remains the basis behind the concept of informed consent in health care.

Historically, physicians suggested treatment, performed procedures, and generally administered care in a paternalistic manner, with little if any patient involvement. Currently, the Supreme Court recognizes that every person has "a constitutionally protected liberty interest in refusing unwanted medical treatment," even if such a refusal can result in death.[1]

Understanding informed consent is of vital importance in urgent care medicine, particularly because our encounters with many patients are one-off and do not allow the establishment of meaningful rapport with clinic staff members or physicians.

Patient Competency

To give binding informed consent, the patient must be *competent*. In most states, the age of majority, or the age required to give informed consent, is 18 years. Parents or legal guardians are generally required to give consent for the medical treatment of minors. There are, however, some exceptions to this rule. In most states, marriage, and even pregnancy, can convey an emancipated status on minors, which means they can consent to their own treatment, as can minors with emergency conditions. Generally, common law and statutory law have held that physicians who provide emergency care for children without prior consent do so legally.

Parents who are minors themselves can give consent for the treatment of their minor children. As a matter of public policy, many states have also enacted laws under which a minor can consent to treatment for sexually transmitted diseases and mental health conditions, as well as other conditions, including substance abuse and injuries sustained because of domestic violence.

For a person who has reached the age of majority, competency can be defined as the ability to reason appropriately and act reasonably when provided with appropriate information by a health-care professional. Competency must always be assessed and documented in the medical record.

Disclosure of Appropriate Information

Once competency has been assessed, the provider must weigh what constitutes the correct amount of information to tell the patient in order for them to make an informed decision. Different states have different standards as to what constitutes "appropriate" informed consent. Some states use a *reasonable physician standard*—that is, what a reasonably prudent physician would

---

1   Cruzan v. Director, Missouri Department of Health, 497 US 261 (1990).

disclose in a similar situation. Other states use a *reasonable patient standard*—what a reasonable patient would want to know about the risks and benefits of a procedure prior to giving consent. In certain rare circumstances, physicians can claim that disclosing the treatment's risk may unreasonably bias the patient's decision, and that full disclosure may not be in the best interest of the patient.

Types of Informed Consent

The three types of informed consent are *general*, *specific*, and *implied*.

- *General consent* is obtained when patients enter an urgent care clinic. By signing a general consent form, patients signify that they are willing to undergo a history-taking and basic evaluation, including a limited battery of tests.

- *Specific consent* must be obtained prior to a patient's undergoing more invasive procedures or riskier or more expensive tests. Ideally, the physician should discuss *and* document said discussion with the patient about the specific indications for a certain procedure. The risks, benefits, and approximate cost of the procedure, any alternative procedures, and the risks or therapeutic and diagnostic challenges associated with not performing the procedure also need to be disclosed.

- *Implied consent* is applicable in certain emergency situations. In these instances, doing what is best for the patient is paramount. When the situation is so critical that there is no time to obtain consent, or if the patient is unable to give consent because of their condition, the assumption is made that a reasonably competent person in a similar situation would consent to treatment. For an emergency-implied consent to be valid, the patient or a surrogate must be unable—*not* unwilling—to give consent.

RIGHT TO REFUSE CARE

Courts have protected the patient's right to refuse medical care. The circumstances surrounding a competent person's decision to refuse treatment must be evaluated on an individual basis, however. The Supreme Court has opined that the patient's refusal must be weighed against "preservation of life, prevention of suicide, maintenance of the ethical integrity of the medical profession, and protection of innocent third parties."[2] If, for example, a patient has intentionally taken an overdose of prescription medication in an effort to end their own life, the patient would not be allowed to refuse life-saving measures.

If a patient is competent to refuse care and chooses not to initiate or continue a certain treatment regimen, the provider must document the discussion about the potential for an adverse outcome, up to and including the risk of death. Many patients who initially refuse appropriate medical treatment simply do not

---

2   *Mack v. Mack*, 329 Md. 188, 618 A.2d 744 (1993).

understand the nature of the procedure or the potential for such an adverse outcome. It is also important to allow the patient to change their mind and continue treatment, or provide other alternatives for their care. Refusing a specific procedure does not mean that the patient is refusing *all* forms of care.

In some situations, parents may refuse appropriate medical care for a child. If their refusal jeopardizes the child's life, however, physicians in some states can take temporary protective custody of the child under the state's child abuse laws. In general, a parent cannot refuse life-saving therapy for a child on the grounds of moral, ethical, or religious beliefs.

Obtaining informed consent in the urgent care setting is a crucial step in every patient interaction. Appropriate discussion and documentation protects not only the physician but also the patient. Being able to determine the course of one's care is a constitutionally protected right that ultimately encourages a more patient-centered approach to health care.

LABORATORY AND IMAGING FOLLOW-UP OR MISSED RADIOLOGY INTERPRETATIONS

The legal literature is replete with cases in which providers failed to follow up on laboratory findings or imaging results. It often happens like this: A provider orders a chem 7 (tests for levels of blood urea nitrogen, carbon dioxide, creatinine, glucose, serum chloride, serum potassium, and serum sodium) for a patient reporting urinary frequency. The ordering provider goes on vacation for a week and is gone when the laboratory results are faxed or emailed back. The serum sodium level is reported as 115 mmol/L. Three days later, the patient has a seizure, loses his airway, and ultimately dies, secondary to the hyponatremia that caused the seizure. Although the clinic has a policy about reviewing all laboratory tests, the provider who ordered it was gone and the covering provider happened to be a part-time locum tenens.

Or consider this misadventure of missed radiology findings: A patient presents with a cough and a fever. A chest x-ray does not reveal an infiltrate, and the patient is sent home with a diagnosis of bronchitis. A year goes by and the patient begins to cough up blood. A large lesion is discovered, which ultimately turns out to be lung cancer. In the course of the current physician evaluation, old films are obtained. The one performed at the urgent care facility a year previously actually reveals a small nodular density in the same exact area as the cancer.

There is an old adage: "If you don't take a temperature, you can't find the fever." Or, put another way, do not order a test if you will not want to work up any aberrant results. Medicolegally speaking, sometimes it is better *not* to order the test. If you do order a test or image, make sure you follow up and document the result, inform the patient of the results of the work-up and necessary follow-up, and document your communication with the patient in the medical record.

CRITICAL CARE EVENTS IN THE URGENT CARE CENTER

As already mentioned, urgent care centers are inundated with numerous patients presenting with minor issues. Occasionally, someone comes in very ill or becomes very ill once they arrive. In these situations, every second counts. Preparation for this eventuality is critical for both the patient and the well-being of your center.

When unexpected events happen, people look for someone to blame. An inadequate response at the urgent care center could be grounds for a wrongful death suit if the patient ultimately dies.

Before your center opens for the first time, and monthly thereafter, it is therefore advisable to run mock codes in your center. At the very least, work through tabletop discussions of "what if" scenarios. Such a practice will keep your constantly rotating front-office and back-office staff members oriented to their roles during an emergency. Do not forget to post signs at the front-office and back-office desks outlining the steps to take during a crisis, as follows.

Front-Office Tasks

1. Identify sick patients (pale, sweaty, short of breath, not communicating, altered mental status, severe pain, or bleeding) and get assistance from the back office.
2. Get the provider's attention immediately, even if they are in an exam room.
3. Ask the health-care provider if 911 should be called.
4. If the answer is yes, call 911 and provide information on the clinic cross streets, address, and specific building location, all of which is posted by the counter.
5. If you are not needed in the back, then once 911 has been dispatched, prop the front doors open, clear the path, and wait outside to direct the emergency crew into the center.
6. Tell patients waiting to be seen that there is an emergency, apologize for the wait, and inform them that they will be treated soon.

Back-Office Tasks

1. Check the code cart or emergency equipment tray at the beginning of every shift.
2. Respond to front-office requests for help with a "sick patient."
3. Notify the health-care provider if they are not already aware of the situation.
4. Ask the health-care provider again if 911 is needed. If so, direct the front office to call 911.

5. Bring a code cart or equipment and an oxygen tank into the room.
6. Anticipate needs (get an Ambu bag, mask, oxygen tubing, and other necessary items ready)

Health-Care Provider Tasks

1. Respond to calls for assistance even if you have to leave an exam room or procedure.
2. Quickly assess the patient (airway, breathing, circulation, and disability [ABCD]) to determine whether there is a need for a 911 call.
3. If the patient is tachypneic or hypoxic, give them oxygen via a face mask. If they have a weak pulse, raise their legs and set up for a normal saline infusion using a large-bore intravenous drip if available.
4. If the patient's mental status is altered, check their blood sugar level.
5. Support the patient until the emergency crew arrives.

Simply discussing these points and posting these tasks helps remind everyone what to do in case of an emergency. Although you may be well trained to handle and expect emergencies, not everyone has the kind of background or experience that makes them feel comfortable responding when such situations occur.

Using Checklists and Care Paths

In highly stressful or busy times, processes break down and staff members revert to training and "muscle memory." That is why checklists and repeated practice are necessary. The general public does not differentiate between the capabilities of an urgent care center versus an ED. Arguing that "we are only an urgent care center" during a trial is sure to be a nonstarter for the jury if there is an easily preventable bad outcome.

Take-Home Points

- Public expectation and the standard of care for urgent care centers is that they can handle emergencies (at least initially).
- Urgent care staff members must be trained for their roles during emergencies.
- Urgent care centers should have monthly mock codes or tabletop discussions on what to do in case of an emergency.
- Do no harm. You do not need to necessarily "save" patients (although saving them helps). You *do* need to respond appropriately and in a timely manner to patients who are experiencing an emergency.

IMPROVING PATIENT SAFETY AND PREVENTING MALPRACTICE IN YOUR CENTER

Discharge Instructions

Lack of proper discharge instructions is a common cause of urgent care malpractice. Consider this example: A patient gets sent home with the diagnosis of a urinary tract infection. The written instructions advise the patient to drink plenty of fluids and to follow up with her primary-care provider in 7 to 10 days for a repeat urinalysis. The patient starts the antibiotics, which she believes may be making her vomit; ultimately, she keeps the medication down about 50% of the time. In the interim, she becomes dehydrated and develops flank pain and an elevated temperature. By the time she realizes that it may not be the medication causing her problems, she has Gram-negative sepsis from pyelonephritis, is very dehydrated, and goes into renal failure. She ultimately develops renal insufficiency—all of this from a simple urinary tract infection. If the discharge instructions had been more specific, as follows, the outcome of the resulting lawsuit would have been much different:

- Get a repeat exam with your provider or back here in 1 to 2 days.
- Return immediately or go to the ED if your condition is worse or no better by the second day.
- If you cannot keep your medication down or stop producing your usual amount of urine, return or go to the ED *immediately*.

These instructions give the patient a very clear idea of what to watch for.

Laboratory and X-Ray Results

Not following up on laboratory results is a large source of malpractice litigation in all primary-care practices. For example, on Thursday, a 40-year-old man presents with a fever, swollen lymph glands, and an enlarged spleen. He is examined, and the health-care provider orders a simple blood cell count for a suspected viral illness. Ultimately, he is sent home with the admonition to take acetaminophen, drink plenty of fluids, and rest. The results of his complete blood cell count come back: He has a hemoglobin level of 9 g/dL, a platelet count of 15,000/µL, and an absolute neutrophil count of 150/µL. These extremely significant laboratory findings are missed by the back-office technician and sit on the desk of the health-care provider for the entire weekend. On Monday, the health-care provider on duty sees these results, correctly interprets them as worrisome for acute lymphoblastic leukemia, and calls the patient back—only to learn that he died the preceding day because of overwhelming sepsis.

Take-home point: *All laboratory results must be reviewed by a health-care provider and entered in the chart; the patient must be called back even if laboratory results are interpreted as normal.*

Radiology Overreads

Not having all x-rays overread by a board-certified radiologist is another common reason for medical malpractice in the urgent care setting. For example, a 48-year-old nonsmoker presents with blunt chest wall trauma from a motor vehicle accident. The health-care provider orders a chest x-ray and reviews the films for signs of rib or clavicle fractures, pneumothorax, and widened mediastinum, and correctly determines that none of these findings are present. The patient is discharged with pain medication and appropriate instructions. Six months later, the patient goes to his primary-care physician with weight loss, cough, fatigue, and hemoptysis, and ultimately receives a diagnosis of small cell lung cancer. The films taken 6 months earlier during the visit for blunt chest trauma reveal a mass on the patient's lung that ultimately proves to be the cancer. The health-care provider had been so intent on looking for trauma that they missed the rather subtle shadow in the superior lobe. All x-rays taken in an urgent care center must be reviewed by a board-certified radiologist. Some centers, in order to save money, only send out "high-risk" films for review. This is akin to saying you'll wear a helmet only on the days you think you might crash your motorcycle. No one misses the "high-risk" films. The misses occur on the "easy" films for which findings can appear incidental but in reality are extremely serious.

Service Recovery

Not addressing patient complaints in a timely manner is a frequent inciting event for eventual malpractice claims. The bottom line is that angry patients sue health-care providers. Therefore, keeping the patient happy is a great mantra to use in encouraging staff members to act professionally and courteously. When that fails and an angry patient contacts you complaining about care or service received at your practice, swallow your pride, listen, and make it right. When you do this, two things happen: First, you maintain the relationship with that patient, and they tell others about the lengths you went to ensure their happiness, but second—most importantly—the patient's anger is diffused, so they are less likely to pursue a legal remedy.

Informed Consent

It is worth repeating that failure to provide and document discussions with patients that lead to their granting of informed consent, particularly when the patient does not want to have a test performed or to be sent to the ED, is a common source for malpractice suits. Consider the 55-year-old man presenting alone with atypical chest and shoulder pain. This patient has normal findings on electrocardiography, normal troponin levels, and normal findings for his chest x-ray. Despite the normal results, the health-care provider correctly tells the patient that a further work-up is needed and recommends transfer to the ED. The patient refuses, however, and ultimately goes home and dies because of an acute myocardial infarction. The health-care provider has written "Go to the ED for further work-up" in the chart. The family sues, arguing that had the patient known the grave danger in which he was placing himself, he would have followed the provider's recommendation and gone to the ED. The family is ultimately awarded a high seven-figure amount. If the health-care provider had simply taken the time to write something like the following, then both the practice and the health-care provider would have been saved from financial ruin:

> I explained the fact that he is at risk for a heart attack and needs to go immediately to the ED for further work-up and monitoring. Understanding the risk of death or serious illness, the patient, who is competent and verbalizes understanding of the risks, is refusing to go to the ED....

That simple paragraph would have taken only a short time to write by hand, or seconds to click into place, if there was a macro for such a comment in the electronic medical record software.

Care Paths

Instituting protocols, or standing orders, for potentially high-risk conditions should be an imperative. Good providers make simple mistakes when busy or stressed, and the use of standing orders has been shown to prevent medical misadventures, ultimately lower the cost of health care, and make practices more efficient.

Poor Hiring Practices

Hiring rude or inadequately trained staff members and health-care providers is a guaranteed inciting event for medical malpractice. Health-care providers or staff members who do not know the center's policies are often rude to patients and other staff members, or are negativity-mongers who have no business working in health care. Not only will they predispose your clinic to malpractice suits but they will also chase off good team members who do not want to work in that kind of unsupportive environment.

Documentation

Poor, illegible, or inadequate documentation is typically the final nail in the coffin when trying to defend care that may border on the substandard. Many medical malpractice suits turn on documentation. Poor handwriting, scant documentation, and lack of documentation of the pertinent negatives are the basis for ultimately deciding the outcome of the case.

Callbacks

Performing callbacks to patients or their families (as appropriate) serves as an early warning detector to identify patients who have complaints about the service, are not getting better, or have not scheduled their follow-up visits. Patients love callbacks, interpreting this simple phone call as an indicator that you actually do care about them. It is the ultimate win-win-win. The patients appreciate them, the callbacks prevent unnecessary suits, and the staff members receive positive affirmation from grateful patients.

CONCLUSION

Patient safety in the urgent care center is a given in the eyes of our patients, our communities, and the payers. With requisite diligence, great customer service, and some simple tools, the reputation for quality care in our industry is absolutely achievable.

KEY POINTS

1. Urgent care medicine is a high-risk business because of the subtle presentation of some dangerous illnesses.
2. Educate your staff members and health-care providers about the potential high-risk misses.
3. Obtain and document appropriate informed consent.
4. Run mock codes and mock critical events so that your staff members become accustomed to working together in an emergency.
5. Post emergency "responsibility lists" in appropriate spots.
6. Have a system in place to ensure that laboratory and radiology reports receive appropriate follow-up.
7. Have all x-rays overread.
8. Use care paths and checklists to ensure that nothing is missed.
9. Document and provide thorough discharge instructions for every patient.
10. Practice service recovery to ensure that patients remain happy and satisfied with your care and service.

CHAPTER 40

Implementing Occupational Medicine

Laurel Stoimenoff

The decision to integrate occupational medicine (OM) services into the urgent care setting is one that requires planning and preparation. Although care of injuries and the provision of support services such as urinary drug screens (UDSs) seem to be the logical next steps when adding services and new revenue streams, these also come with nuances that the operational, marketing, and clinical teams must be prepared to address. The after-hours and weekend access to urgent care services is attractive to patients and employers alike. Urgent care center operatrors must do their homework to ensure that entering the occupational medicine arena is a strategic and planned activity likely to produce not only new revenue *but also* positive earnings.

OM has been a specialty of the American Board of Preventive Medicine since 1979. It can be defined as a "specialty field of medicine concerned with the assessment, maintenance, restoration, and improvement of the health of the worker through the application of the principles of preventive medicine, emergency medical care, rehabilitation, and environmental medicine."[1] Although OM is a recognized specialty, many primary-care and urgent care physicians are highly successful in serving employers and the workforce.

WORKERS' COMPENSATION

Workers' compensation is the insurance coverage required by the US government to provide benefits to employees who become injured or ill on the job. Employer insurance costs are a product of the risk associated with the type of business (construction versus a call center), historical claims, and the total gross payroll. Workers' compensation is administered by the individual states by the US Department of Labor's Office of Workers' Compensation Programs (www.dol.gov/dol/topic/workcomp). Regulations vary from state to state, and the Department of Labor website provides links to regulations and fee schedules for each one. Insurance typically covers medical care and vocational rehabilitation, and provides a benefit for lost wages. Some states allow employers to *direct* care to specific

---

1   Felton JS. *Occupational Medical Management.* Boston, MA: Little, Brown; 1990;19.

providers or networks. This directed care may have some limitations and applies to only a finite number of visits before the patient has a choice as to where to seek care. Directed care can either be an opportunity (if you have relationships with employers) or a barrier to patients attempting to access your center for care (if you are not an employer-selected provider). In general, a setting in which patients can choose their own providers may represent a more favorable regulatory environment for the urgent care center operatror because the business-to-consumer marketing tends to be the type most often practiced by the industry. Injured or ill workers may already be familiar with the urgent care setting in the neighborhood for care of non-work-related injuries, so it is a logical choice when they are injured on the job. Conversely, the injured worker is a clear opportunity to transition a workers' compensation patient into a loyal urgent care patient if the patient experience is exceptional.

MARKET ASSESSMENT

The Urgent Care Association of America's 2012 Benchmarking Survey[2] concluded that slightly less than 8% of respondents' urgent care center visits were related to workers' compensation. The survey also showed that respondents reported their urgent care centers provide predominantly *illness*-related care versus *injury*-related care when reviewing the top 15 combined work-related and non-work-related ICD-9 (*International Statistical Classification of Diseases*, 9th revision) codes, yet the US Bureau of Labor Statistics (BLS) reported over 2.9 million recordable work-related injuries for 2011:

- ▶ >340,000 related to sprains and strains
- ▶ >182,000 attributed to injuries to the back
- ▶ >225,000 involving slips, trips, and falls

The BLS also provides links and contact information so that the urgent care center operatror can evaluate the market potential within their own state(s) on the basis of the number and types of injuries and illnesses. Although safety programs and risk managers are experiencing good success reducing or eliminating injuries in the workplace, workplace injuries remain a very viable and often under-pursued opportunity in many markets. Workers and employers are interested in eliminating time off from work. Geographically convenient urgent care centers sensitive to employers' costs associated with injuries and lost employee productivity are well positioned to establish relationships that can result in ongoing patient volume. Additionally, urgent care centers and employers both benefit when a worker's follow-up care can be scheduled during slower times of the day, allowing for no-waiting care for the employee and reduced downtime in the urgent care clinic.

Evaluation of market competition is essential when developing any program, and OM is no exception. Employers value long-standing relationships if they are

---

2 Urgent Care Association of America. 2012 urgent care benchmarking report. Available from: http://www.ucaoa.org/orderreports.php. Accessed February 19, 2014.

confident they are receiving quality services by a provider who is also delivering that care cost-effectively and with attention to the employer's needs. Altering that referral relationship could prove challenging unless the urgent care center can identify opportunities to address unmet needs. Many OM providers offer care during standard business hours Monday through Friday despite the fact that many businesses operate with multiple shifts, 7 days a week. This presents the opportunity for the urgent care clinic to save the employer money related to after-hours and weekend injury care delivered in the emergency department for lack of an alternative. The "one-stop shop" offered by many urgent care centers saves employers lost wages when care is delivered efficiently. A single visit that includes access to laboratory services, radiology, contract services, medical care, and even physical therapy, combined with a single point of contact or employer liaison, can be a compelling differentiator.

Reimbursement for workers' compensation varies by state and regionally. State fee schedules should be investigated, as should the presence of local and national networks that may pay global or discounted fees. The industry is replete with networks and organizations providing support services, including bill review and utilization management. Networks tend to offer discounts for services, so the urgent care center operatror should understand the ultimate payment prior to agreeing to participate. Additionally, there are "silent PPOs" (preferred provider organizations) in which health-care providers may unknowingly agree in a contract to allow the contracting entity to lease the network to other networks or payers. A provider may then be surprised when a discount is taken from the anticipated reimbursement because the claim was processed through an organization with which the provider has no direct contractual relationship.

Care of the injured worker requires additional documentation, additional communication, and increased work for urgent care staff members regarding referrals, authorization, and other activities. The operator must be confident that reimbursement will be fair and account for the resources that will undoubtedly be applied to administering and caring for the injured worker.

INTERNAL ASSESSMENT

If the external environment is promising and the urgent care center operatror wishes to move forward with implementation planning for an OM program, they will then have to assess the internal environment—including the competencies of their staff members and health-care providers, physical environment, equipment, laboratory capabilities, clinical capabilities, medical records, information systems, and communications. The provision of workers' compensation services can easily bring increased costs associated with specialized clinical expertise, staff and provider training, additional documentation related to specific state or employer forms, and increased staff communication time for attaining authorizations and supporting referrals. An option would be to simply provide less complex services, such as UDSs and contract services (e.g., US Department of

Transportation [DOT] physicals), but operators must then recognize that they are giving up the most profitable component of care, which is the injury or illness visit and associated follow-up care. The Urgent Care Association of America has an excellent Occupational Medicine Skills Assessment tool posted on its website (www.ucaoa.org) that may also support the internal evaluation of clinical readiness and assist in the determination of the most appropriate entry level for the scope of care.

Hospital-owned urgent care centers often enter the OM sector because the system can also benefit from OM revenue associated with ancillary services such as radiology, physical and occupational therapy, and affiliated medical specialties. The stand-alone independent urgent care center operatror must evaluate the market opportunity and financial impact on the basis of only their internal scope of services, although the collaboration and referral relationships that naturally occur with other market providers can provide valuable networking opportunities.

Space must also be considered when pursuing a new service line. Because the majority of workers' compensation claims relate to injuries versus illnesses, some urgent care centers establish separate entrances and reception areas for "well" patients versus sick patients. There may be some secondary benefits associated with the separation if the center chooses to offer scheduled appointments for follow-ups, because it is then less evident that a worker is being taken back for care as a priority over a nonemergency walk-in urgent care patient. Space considerations also need to be made for special services such as audiometric testing booths if they will be required by patients or contracts.

SCOPE OF CARE

On the basis of the assessment of the market and employer and insurer needs, the urgent care center operatror must determine the level of service to provide and, if there are multiple sites, what level of service to provide at each location. If multiple locations exist in a reasonable geographic area, some services could be referred to the centralized occupational center of excellence, with basic services being provided at other sites. Basic services include injury care, on-site laboratory studies, sample collection for UDSs, pulmonary function testing, and imaging. Additional services supportive of an OM program include breath alcohol testing, audiology testing, DOT physicals, testing for respirator fit, and the administration of vaccines such as those for measles, mumps, and rubella and for hepatitis A and B Breath alcohol testing and audiometry equipment require specialized and equipment-specific training that must be considered when determining the services that the center will provide. Medical review officer services may be provided by the center itself if a provider has gone through the training and certification, or the services are typically available through the laboratories contracted with the urgent care center. The DOT defines a medical review officer as "a person who is a licensed physician and who is responsible for receiving and reviewing laboratory results generated by an employer's drug testing program and evaluating medical explanations for certain drug test results."[3]

PHYSICAL THERAPY

An April 2010 survey conducted by CorVel[4] concluded that 77% of all workers' compensation cases result in a referral to physical therapy. Each referral resulted in an average of 11 to 15 therapy visits, and therapy costs accounted for 20% of the total cost of the claim. Although this statistic includes both surgical and non-surgical cases, the role physical therapy plays in care of the injured worker is significant. A focused rehabilitation plan can return the worker to function more quickly. Therapists are skilled at putting together work-conditioning programs if a patient faces challenges in returning to their existing job or must be conditioned for a new role. Select therapists have special training in the performance of functional capacity examinations, which are 4- to 8-hour sessions of testing with the goal of objectively evaluating a patient's functional levels benchmarked against norms. A comprehensive report is included as part of the examination. Just as in independent medical examinations, the evaluating therapist has typically not been involved in the patient's care, to eliminate the potential for bias.

The urgent care center operatror entering the market should establish referral relationships with therapists who have expertise working with injured workers and are willing to offer same-day or next-day appointments. Alternatively, with an average volume of 10 to 12 new patient therapy referrals per week or more, some urgent care center operatrors have elected to provide the service in-house. Whether the urgent care center operatror elects to outsource therapy referrals or include therapy services in-house, a collaborative role with an experienced therapist who recognizes the nuances associated with the care of the injured worker is essential.

WELLNESS

Health-care reform is shifting care toward population health, and employers are focusing more attention on wellness as they analyze costs associated with absenteeism and presenteeism (employees coming to work in less than 100% health). Both the absent and the less-than-optimal "present" employee negatively impact productivity. In a 2010 study,[5] the BLS estimated that 3% to 5% of an employer's workforce was absent on any given day; another survey[6] suggested that the cost of absenteeism represented 35% of an employer's total payroll. Urgent care cen-

---

3   US Department of Transportation. Medical review officers. Washington DC: US Department of Transportation. Available from: www.dot.gov/odapc/mro. Accessed February 25, 2014.
4   CorVel Corporation. Physical therapy survey report. Available from: www.corvel.com/media/37209/compInsights_Physical_Therapy.pdf. Accessed February 13, 2014.
5   US Bureau of Labor Statistics. Absences from work of employed full-time wage and salary workers by occupation and industry. Available from: www.bls.gov/cps/cpsaat47.htm. Accessed February 13, 2014.
6   Mercer. Survey on the total impact of employee absences. Portland, OR: Mercer; June 2010. Available from: http://www.mercer.com/articles/global-health-perspective-archives.

ters have an opportunity to fortify employer relationships by expanding existing injury and illness services to overall employee wellness. The services can be as simple as conducting on-site health and biometric screenings once or twice a year or as extensive as programs on smoking cessation, employee health counseling, and proper nutrition and weight loss. Urgent care centers caring for an employer's workforce have the opportunity to explore services where they might provide greater value.

ON-SITE SERVICES

A 2011 survey of employer-sponsored health plans conducted by Mercer[7] revealed that 27% of employers with 500 or more employees offer an on-site medical clinic for occupational health services and 15% offer a clinic for primary care. Employers are acknowledging the productivity losses associated with lost work time, and the convenience of on-site health clinics allows the employer to provide a valued employee benefit while improving the health of the workforce. Early intervention associated with work-related injuries is simplified, with the potential to greatly reduce costs associated with work-related injuries. Urgent care centers have the opportunity to serve employers by setting up clinics that are supported by the more comprehensive services and capabilities of the local urgent care center. This extension of the urgent care practice can be expanded to caring for the workforce and their families after hours. Most employer-based clinics restrict the benefit to their employees, although some do extend the benefit to spouses and dependents.

WHAT DO EMPLOYERS WANT?

Most urgent care physicians excel at providing quality care to their patients in a service-oriented environment. This linear physician–patient relationship is where most centers flourish. The election to pursue the OM patient adds the employer as a new customer into the relationship, along with a series of additional personnel who are part of a team responsible for ensuring favorable clinical and functional outcomes as well as prompt return to work at the least cost. This team's success is measured by reducing the costs associated with claims. Reducing claims means faster return to work and decreased costs associated with care delivery. The BLS reports that of the 2.9 million reportable work injuries in 2011, over 908,000 resulted in an average of 8 days away from work. Although injured workers' benefits vary significantly by state, it is incumbent on urgent care personnel to work collaboratively with adjusters, case managers, and others involved in the case to manage the costs associated with the claim. The processes and documentation associated with the care often differ from the norm of the commercially insured patient, so the potential for a patient to become lost in the system is elevated as a risk. Employer complaints often relate to a perception that

---

7   Mercer. National survey of employer-sponsored health plans: 2011 survey report. Portland, OR: Mercer; 2012. Available from: http://www.mercer.com/articles/global-health-perspective-archives.

the physician or other health-care provider isn't sensitive to the employer's needs, particularly when those needs involve returning the injured worker to work. Employers offering light-duty options want to know what the worker can and cannot do. Providing specific restrictions and then allowing the employer to determine whether it can or cannot accommodate the worker places the urgent care clinic in a much more favorable light.

Many employers have policies and algorithms delineating how they want care provided to their injured workers. Urgent care clinics should have a mechanism, electronic or otherwise, for storing and referencing customized employer profiles. Information that may assist the urgent care provider in meeting the employer's needs includes the following:

- ▶ The company's name and address; and the best contact's name, phone number, email address, and fax number
- ▶ Regarding the employer's workers' compensation insurance company: name, address, phone number, and fax number
- ▶ The company's preference for returning workers to the workplace, whether it offers light duty, and the best mode of communication
- ▶ Drug screening, non-DOT 5- or 10-panel
- ▶ Drug screening, DOT
- ▶ Urine collection:
    - Only including preferred laboratory, or
    - Full-service UDSs and medical review officer services
- ▶ Are UDSs to be initiated at pre-employment or when a job is offered? Are they accident-related? Random? Other?
- ▶ Other services requested, such as pulmonary function testing, tuberculosis screening, hepatitis B immunizations, tetanus vaccines, and chest x-rays
- ▶ Audiometric screening or testing
- ▶ Negotiated costs for services requested

Employers ultimately want communication. They have concerns when workers are not compliant with the established plan of care. No-shows and cancellations can be red-flag behavior, and it is important to keep key employer contacts informed of risk behaviors. Although the majority of injured workers are genuinely committed to returning to work and function promptly, there is the potential to take advantage of a system unless the care team is vigilant and quick to identify those who may see an opportunity for secondary gain. The urgent care physician, as the initial provider of care to the worker, will engender employer loyalty if they also choose to play an integral role in supporting case management. Health care unfortunately can be delivered in silos (i.e., segregated parts of organizations), and there is no room for silos or uncoordinated care in the care of the injured worker.

REFERRALS

Urgent care centers are accustomed to making referrals to area specialists and ancillary services. Meeting the needs of the employer and the injured worker may generate an elevated urgency for prompt care delivery, often leading operators to designate referral coordination as a key position responsibility to a single individual or team. Lost work time is costly, and there is evidence that early intervention has a favorable impact on outcomes. Providers benefitting from urgent care referrals should be held to performance standards, including ready access. Medical specialists should agree to fast-track patients or risk losing the referral relationship, because the urgent care setting will be judged not only by the care it delivers but also by its ability to support the adjusters and case managers in ensuring prompt care, favorable outcomes, reduced or no lost work time, and ultimately claim closure. Recipients of referrals must also recognize the need to communicate findings promptly as well as report any detected risk behaviors. Many best-in-class clinicians think of the patient as their sole customer and strongly advocate on behalf of that customer. Although these caregivers may be excellent and reputable clinically, they may not be best for handling the injured-worker referral. Balancing the desires and needs of the employee *and* the employer is an art, and not all clinicians are artists.

OCCUPATIONAL MEDICINE AND THE HEALTH INSURANCE PORTABILITY AND ACCOUNTABILITY ACT

Medical providers are often under the impression that all parts of the Health Insurance Portability and Accountability Act of 1996 (HIPAA) apply when the benefits are covered through a workers' compensation claim. It is true that all health plans and medical providers are required to adhere to the privacy requirements mandated under HIPAA; workers' compensation, however, is *not* a health plan. Insurers, employers, and workers' compensation administrators legitimately need information in order to process a claim, provide disability evaluations, facilitate and evaluate the worker's ability to return to work, provide utilization review, comply with state reporting regulations, and investigate fraud. Covered entities therefore have greater freedom in sharing information with insurers, third-party administrators, and employers within reason and without authorization from the patient. It is equally important to recognize that covered entities remain subject to minimum necessary disclosures in order to receive payment or support the services cited above. Protected health information may be shared, but should also be limited in accordance with the regulations in Section 45 of the Code of Federal Regulations, 164.512(l). It is essential to restrict disclosures to only the information associated with the work-related injury. Urgent care clinics that maintain a single patient-specific medical record for work-related and non-work-related visits run the risk of innocently but inappropriately disclosing protected health information not associated with the work-related visit to an employer. Separate medical records may therefore be the best solution to mitigate risks associated with privacy violations.

DEPARTMENT OF TRANSPORTATION PHYSICALS AND OTHER PHYSICALS

Urgent care centers often advertise their ability to provide DOT physicals. According to the DOT, the physical examination "is conducted by a licensed medical 'examiner.' The term includes, but is not limited to, doctors of medicine (MD), doctors of osteopathy (DO), physician assistants (PA), advanced practice nurses (APN), and doctors of chiropractic (DC)."[8] The medical examination report is good for up to 24 months, depending on the medical examiner's assessment. The process of performing the examination can be a relatively routine service for an urgent care center, although the responsibility is great.

The National Registry of Certified Medical Examiners is a federal program that has recently established "requirements for healthcare professionals who perform physical qualification examinations for truck and bus drivers."[9] In order to become a certified medical examiner listed in the national registry, the medical provider must complete training and pass an examination through the Federal Motor Carrier Safety Administration's physical qualification standards. The national registry is visible to individuals seeking examination as well as to the general public. Effective May 21, 2014, physicians will be required to obtain certification in order to provide DOT physicals, as required by Section 391.41 of the Federal Motor Carrier Safety Regulations.

Some centers have also elected to provide flight physicals and provide the valuable service of determining the mental and physical fitness of pilots, air traffic controllers, and other aviation industry employees. To offer this service the center must have available an aviation medical examiner (AME) who is certified and listed in the national registry. AME certification requires substantial initial training and demonstration of competency, refresher training every 3 years, and attendance at an AME seminar every 6 years. Information is available at www.faa.gov.

---

8   Federal Motor Carrier Safety Administration. The DOT medical exam and CMV certification. Washington DC: US Department of Transportation. Available from: http://www.fmcsa.dot.gov/rules-regulations/topics/medical/aboutDOTexam.htm. Accessed February 25, 2014.
9   Federal Motor Carrier Safety Administration. Frequently asked questions: What is the National Registry of Certified Medical Examiners (National Registry)? Washington DC: US Department of Transportation. Available from: http://nrcme.fmcsa.dot.gov/about_faqs.aspx. Accessed February 25, 2014.

Independent medical examinations (IMEs) are comprehensive evaluations of patients by a medical provider who is completely independent and unbiased. In order to perform the IME, the physician or other health-care provider cannot have been involved in the care of the patient. This examination may not be a good fit for the urgent care environment in that the examinations are scheduled and involve a significant time commitment related to preview of medical records and prior tests, a comprehensive history (medical, social, vocational), a physical examination that may include an assessment of impairment, evaluation of the current treatment plan, and documentation of all findings. The examiner typically has special training related to impairment ratings, assessment skills, and documentation of findings. Although this type of examination would be atypical in the urgent care environment, it is not inconceivable to provide this type of service if physician and staffing resources are adequate. Provision of the service could enhance the credibility of the center as a destination for care of the injured worker.

MARKETING

While developing the OM program, you should also be developing your marketing plan. On the basis of the selected scope of services, urgent care center operatrors must determine the level of care and the target employer group they intend to serve. An employer who operates a business 24/7 is most often looking for a medical provider who also provides 24-hour access. Employer relationships are often cultivated over time, but customized service and the ability to serve both the patient and the employer help develop these loyal partnerships. Operators and sales teams must immerse themselves in the OM community, its professional associations, and its culture. The percentage of revenue obtained from workers' compensation tends to be small for the majority of urgent care clinics because they elect to not dedicate adequate resources to its development. The sales cycle can be lengthy, and resources and sales plans must be dedicated to retaining existing clients while also pursuing new business. Personnel should have a presence at local associations that cater to self-insured employers, case managers, claims adjusters, and other professional or trade groups involved in the industry. The annual marketing plan should target sectors (e.g., construction, hospitality, municipalities) and establish detailed plans for each in collaboration with clinical and operational leadership. Providing services to public sectors typically requires the urgent care center to submit a response to a request for proposals, which is likely to consume considerable time and resources. Operators must carefully choose how to balance the potential for new business with the costs associated in its pursuit. A single clinic in a large metropolitan area will be challenged to serve a large regional employer but can be a valued service for local restaurants and other small businesses. Setting realistic growth goals that are based on the urgent care center's selected level of specialized clinical skills, practice scope, geographic access, hours of operation, and wait times and on other employer needs will assist the marketing team in establishing equally realistic customer targets.

CONCLUSION

Many successful urgent care clinics had their genesis serving employers and the workers' compensation market, but industry surveys tell us that the majority of urgent care clinics focus most resources on the commercial market. Although additional resources are likely to be necessary to commit to shifting the urgent care center's payer mix to a greater percentage of this business sector, it can be a successful business strategy with proper planning and a well-executed implementation plan. A culture shift across the entire team is essential as the employer becomes a key customer in addition to the patient.

KEY POINTS

1. The election to add or increase the role of OM for the urgent care center requires the commitment of human and capital resources. Urgent care providers who do not plan and execute properly may realize new revenue but negative profit.

2. Evaluate your state's regulations regarding the ability to access injured workers. Are employers allowed to direct care to providers and networks of their choice, or do patients have the right to choose where they seek care?

3. Choosing to provide UDSs and other contract services may bring additional revenue, but the most profitable aspect of OM is the care of the injured or ill worker and the associated follow-up care.

4. Workers' compensation is not a health plan, and thus HIPAA does not apply as it does when the patient has either commercial or government-provided insurance. Employers have a legitimate need for information. Urgent care personnel can protect themselves by offering the *minimum necessary information*, securing a patient release, and maintaining separate medical records for work-related injuries and non-work-related visits.

5. Hospital-owned urgent care clinics also benefit from associated revenue inherent in caring for injured workers (imaging, laboratory, specialty referrals), but independent urgent care centers must ensure that entering the market is a viable option for their practice on the basis of their individual scope of services.

6. Time is of the essence in OM. Early intervention results in lower costs of claims and less time lost from work. The urgent care clinic must not only ensure ready access to its services and follow-up appointments but also refer to those specialty providers, ancillaries, and therapy practices that also offer prompt appointments and care.

7. Effective May 2014, medical providers will have to be certified to provide DOT physicals and be listed in the DOT's national registry.

8. Growing OM can be a slow process because employers, case managers, and claims adjusters have long-standing loyalties. Seek opportunities to address unmet needs, reduce the total cost of claims, and differentiate your center from the competition. Excellent communication and prompt care is a great start.

9. Create employer profiles within the urgent care center to ensure that the worker is being cared for in compliance with the employer's wishes.

10. Most employers offer some level of modified or light-duty work for injured workers. Most patients should be returned to work with restrictions noted, if any. Allow the employer to determine whether the patient must be taken off work because of an inability to accommodate the restrictions.

CHAPTER 41

Measuring and Improving Patient Satisfaction

Sybil Yeaman

PATIENT-SATISFACTION SURVEYS HAVE BEEN successfully used for decades by health-care providers to capture data on the quality of medical care and to evaluate improvements in the patient experience that they provide. Over the years, study results have demonstrated that as health-care providers improve patient satisfaction, they also improve patient outcomes. Armed with the knowledge that outcomes are linked to patient satisfaction, government programs and health plans now require hospitals and more health-care providers to conduct consistent patient-satisfaction surveys. As patient satisfaction increases and outcomes improve, risk for adverse events decreases and the cost of medical care goes down. Everyone benefits, starting with the patient. Thus government programs, health plans, and health-care providers will all continue to seek to define, meet, and exceed patient expectations.

Matching the increased focus on patient satisfaction and demand for better performance, there is a growing demand for improved quality in the survey process itself. Simple short-form questionnaires are now being replaced with more complex patient-satisfaction surveys. These newer questionnaires are designed to better evaluate the patient experience on both a physical and cognitive level.

THE VALUE OF PATIENT-SATISFACTION SURVEYS

Although measuring patient satisfaction is not yet a requirement for urgent care facilities, surveys should still be conducted consistently by all centers to facilitate continuous improvement practices in patients' care experiences and staff performance. Use of patient-satisfaction surveys to improve the patient experience will help with the following:

- ▶ Maximization of patient satisfaction
- ▶ Development of patient loyalty
- ▶ Improvement in patient outcomes
- ▶ Increases in volume through referrals

- Increases in marketplace trust
- Improvement in contracting and reimbursement
- Decreases in malpractice risk
- Increases in competitive advantage

There are many additional benefits that can accrue from the use of patient-satisfaction surveys; in addition to improving the patient experience, use of such surveys may facilitate increases in urgent care center market share in an increasingly competitive medical marketplace. Urgent care providers should consider that every satisfied patient who receives care in their facility will become part of their center's future bottom line and a source of increased business development. When patients share their positive care experience with others, they market the urgent care center more effectively than almost any form of advertisement can. Each patient is a referral source to encourage family and friends to seek care in your facility, rather than in the facility of a competitor. Importantly, the opposite is true for every negative patient experience that takes place in your facility. Negative patient experiences are so damaging because patients tend to share negative experiences more often than positive experiences, and with more people. This translates into financial loss from decreased future patient volume and increased business for your competitors.

Health-care plans or managed-care organizations (MCOs) compete with each other for members in an increasingly competitive environment, just as urgent care centers compete in their medical marketplace. Patient satisfaction and increasing market share are as important to MCOs as they are to other medical facilities. Thus, if urgent care centers consistently collect patient survey data and demonstrate improvement in patient satisfaction, such facilities will gain a competitive advantage for MCO contract opportunities and when negotiating reimbursement rates.

Consistent focus on resolving issues in patient satisfaction and improving the patient experience will lower the risk of malpractice lawsuits. It is widely accepted that the quality of the relationship between patients and health-care providers is a key issue in lawsuits. Good patient relationships are built on effective communication by health-care providers. Analysis of patient-satisfaction survey data to pinpoint any breakdown in communication will, in turn, enhance the patient experience, improve outcomes, and help protect the urgent care center from lawsuits.

STRUCTURE AND PURPOSE OF PATIENT-SATISFACTION SURVEYS

Early Surveys

Initially, patient-satisfaction surveys were rather random, were short, and focused primarily on satisfaction with the following:

- Convenience of facility location
- Waiting times
- Medical provider care
- Overall quality of care
- Billing services

As health-care providers responded to survey data and adopted new patient care initiatives, the patient experience improved; responses included developing more comfortable waiting areas, ensuring shorter waiting times, and improving quality of care. Responses to survey data resulted in new and higher standards of care for all health-care providers and facilities to meet patient expectations.

Recent Surveys

When research data demonstrated that outcomes improved with increased patient satisfaction, more health-care providers began to conduct patient-satisfaction surveys. They soon noted that additional benefits of patient satisfaction and improved outcomes include increased patient volume and facility growth. Similarly, health plans found that improvements in outcomes resulted in additional benefits such as improved cost control and higher profit margins, as well as market share growth. Therefore, health plans began to put increased emphasis on gathering outcomes data as well as conducting patient-satisfaction surveys. Over time, new questions were added to patient-satisfaction surveys to delve deeper into patients' perceived needs, to get more feedback about all patient encounters, and to analyze what was needed to improve outcomes. New questions focused on the following:

- Staff courtesy and respect
- Wait times in waiting area and examination rooms
- Comfort of waiting area and examination rooms
- Physician communication skills
- Physician competence
- Treatment planning and discharge instructions
- Follow-up telephone calls
- Staff professionalism

Ongoing Survey Demands

Data collection and reporting regarding outcomes and quality of care are no longer optional in many medical care settings. The Centers for Medicare & Medicaid Services (CMS) rolled out value-based purchasing in hospitals, as well as the pay-for-reporting programs in certain medical specialties. Health insurance plans are under pressure from federal legislation and government programs to demonstrate health plan quality and are increasing efforts to link outcomes to reimbursement by initiating higher pay for better outcomes as well as pay-for-performance programs.

Urgent care centers, although not yet directly affected by CMS reporting requirements, should expect to eventually be included in the federally mandated Physician Quality Reporting System initiatives,[1] because government programs, health insurance plans, and the health-care consumer are all demanding transparency, higher standards of care, and proof of improvement in quality of care. Large health insurance plans and MCOs have the resources to hire experts and implement patient-satisfaction survey programs, but small to midsized independent urgent care centers and medical practices are at a disadvantage because of tight operating margins and limited resources. Fortunately, technological advances offer solutions that are more cost-effective, improve staff efficiency, and provide accurate survey data collection, reporting, and analysis for quality improvement. These innovative data-gathering and data-measuring technologies minimize hassle and provide reliable survey findings. Options for collecting patient survey data include the following:

- Paper-and-pen data collection at check-out
- Check-out area computer or tablet kiosk
- Mailed surveys with return envelopes
- Follow-up surveys by telephone by facility staff or a survey service
- Online surveys that patients access from a link within an email received after their office visit
- Other outsourced survey services

Although some patient surveys and accompanying databases have been developed for medical groups, such as the American Medical Group Association standardized survey of patient satisfaction, most questionnaires and databases were developed for health insurance plans and hospitals. The most highly recognized of these are the National Committee for Quality Assurance survey used as part of its Healthcare Effectiveness Data and Information Set (HEDIS) quality care standards, and the Consumer Assessment of Healthcare Providers and Systems (CAHPS) survey database,[2,3] which was developed cooperatively

---

1 Centers for Medicare & Medicaid Services. Physician Quality Reporting System. Baltimore, MD: Centers for Medicare & Medicaid Services. Available from: http://www.cms.gov/Medicare/Quality-Initiatives-Patient-Assessment-Instruments/PQRS/index.html. Accessed February 25, 2014.

2 Agency for Healthcare Research & Quality. About the CAHPS Database. March 2011. Available from: https://cahps.ahrq.gov/cahps-database/about/index.html. Accessed February 25, 2014.

3 Agency for Healthcare Research & Quality. Appendix E. Definition of composites, ratings, and individual items. In 2013 chartbook: what consumers say about their experiences with their health plans and medical care. March 2011. Available from: https://www.cahpsdatabase.ahrq.gov/files/2013CAHPSHealthPlanChartbook.pdf. Accessed February 25, 2014.

with the Agency for Healthcare Research & Quality, RAND Corporation, RTI International, and Harvard University. The CAHPS database, a free web-based database used on a voluntary basis, was developed to standardize and evaluate patients' experiences with their health-care provider and their medical facility encounter.

Demand is intensifying for participation of additional medical-specialty care providers and facilities in patient-satisfaction surveys and measurement of quality improvement. Health insurance plan and hospital-based questionnaires and databases are undergoing customization for specific medical groups and practices, such as the CG-CAHPS, which is the CAHPS Clinician & Group survey database. Further pressure is applied by groups such as the American Board of Medical Specialties, which requires patient and peer surveys as part of maintenance of certification for their member diplomates.

Urgent care centers may be required to report survey results in the near future, possibly using the CG-CAHPS survey database or a similar tool. Whether submission is voluntary or required, submitted urgent care center survey data will become part of a growing national repository. This repository of patient survey data is primarily intended as a tool to compare satisfaction and quality of care results to national and regional averages by practice site, specialty, and region. Data will most likely be studied and then used by government health care plans and other health insurance plans to create a point of reference for measurement of patient care quality in pay-for-outcomes and pay-for-performance programs.

PATIENT-SATISFACTION SURVEY DATA BASICS

Because of increasing demand for proof of patient satisfaction and outcomes improvement, patient-satisfaction surveys are now a top priority. Survey questions are continually under development with the goal of capturing data about the many aspects of patient experiences, including cognitive and emotional reactions during and resulting from health-care encounters.

Volume

Whether an urgent care center develops and utilizes its own patient-satisfaction survey or uses a standardized outsourced form or an online data survey system, it is important to collect a sufficient volume of patient surveys to make the data statistically valid.

Here are some examples:

- ▶ A small urgent care center with limited resources that uses its own survey and staff could gather patient survey data from at least 10% of the patients treated by a provider on a quarterly basis.

- ▶ A midsized urgent care group or large urgent care company may outsource its patient surveys to gather a larger sample of patient data without interfering with staff functionality.

- Hospitals and health insurance plans may seek to gather patient-satisfaction survey data from all patient and member encounters.

Questionnaires

To get the most out of patient-satisfaction questionnaires, urgent care centers must set timelines to routinely gather patient survey data, specifying volume or percentages of surveys needed and following consistent data collection methods.

The questionnaires should include questions that probe the patient's medical experience as well as the patient's cognitive and emotional reactions during their encounter in the urgent care center. Here are some examples:

- Surveys about the waiting area experience should include questions about wait times, comfort of the waiting area, and courtesy of the registrations staff.
- Surveys of the medical examination experience should include questions about wait time in the examination area, physician competence and ability to communicate, and pain control.
- Surveys of the overall facility experience should include queries about convenience, cleanliness, expectations, and overall staff courtesy and respect.

Analysis

There are many methods for processing and evaluating patient survey data. Analysis can be as simple as counting the frequency of each patient's response for each provider and comparing it with previous survey and peers' results. Top-of-the-scale positive survey results can be compared with the bottom-of-the-scale negative results to help determine how well the urgent care center is functioning and what patients' perceptions are of how well medical staff members are treating patients during their urgent care encounter. More complex questionnaires obviously allow for more detailed data analysis. Gathering a higher volume of surveys and more patient data allows for deeper "dives" for enhanced analyses of variations in data that can result in more nuanced suggestions for quality control and improvement in patient satisfaction as well as outcomes. Here are some examples:

- An in-depth survey and analysis report can provide additional comparisons of the patient experience by age and education level. Age and education are just two factors that can affect a patient's needs, perspective, and perceived urgent care experience.
- An in-depth survey and analysis report will also allow administrative personnel to evaluate specific work areas, such as the waiting area, examination rooms, laboratory space, and check-out area. Collection of these data can help to pinpoint which work areas need quality improvements and which work groups need quality-of-care training.

IMPROVING PATIENT SATISFACTION

Improving patient satisfaction means improving the patient's experience both physically as they receive medical treatment and emotionally as they receive medical care (emotional support) from facility staff. It is important to consider that the patient's medical treatment may meet their expectations but their perceived emotional needs may not have been met. Perceived emotional support from urgent care center personnel creates great value in the patient care experience. Medical treatment can be bought at any urgent care center, but medical care has to be given. One is purchased, and the other is priceless.

Commitment to improving the patient's experience has to start administratively from the top before it can move down to become part of the urgent care center's culture. The commitment to quality improvement starts with owners and the medical director as patient-satisfaction reports are reviewed, analyzed, and discussed. Although the administrative team members who make such commitments are not necessarily the same team members who fulfill the commitments, the administration must construct the plan and lead the charge.

Plans for enhancing patient experience at your urgent care center should be specific, measurable, and implemented within a specific period of time. The time period could be as simple as within the next calendar quarter, and the measurement may be improvements in results of next quarter's patient survey. It is important to understand that such action plans determined by the leadership take time and ongoing commitment to incorporate into an appropriate aspect of center operation in addition to cooperation and collaboration of all center staff members.

Improving Medical Treatment Areas and the Patient Physical Experience

The easiest component to address in improving the patient's experience is the quality and physical comfort of the physical facilities within the urgent care center.

Waiting Area

The patient experience starts when the patient, often accompanied by family members or a friend, enters the urgent care center waiting area. The following items can make a difference.

- Floors and carpeting: routinely cleaned throughout the day
- Good lighting without glare
- Artwork on the walls
- Varied seating areas:
  - Single seating for individuals
  - Group seating for families and friends

- ► Television
- ► Educational or public health reading materials
- ► Patient bathrooms: cleaned and disinfected throughout the day
- ► Children's play area
  - Separate television for children
  - Routinely cleaned and disinfected throughout the day
  - Reading materials available

Registration Area

- ► Open registration area
- ► Uncluttered desk and surrounding area
- ► Well lit without glare

Triage and Examination Area

- ► Clean floors and counter areas
- ► Rooms disinfected after every patient
- ► Well lit without glare
- ► Hooks for coats, purses, and backpacks
- ► Current reading materials

Laboratory

- ► Clean floors and counter
- ► Well lit without glare
- ► Safety precautions in place
- ► Hooks for coats, purses, and backpacks

Radiology

- ► Clean floors and counter
- ► Lockers, shelves, or hooks for coats, purses, and backpacks, whichever are appropriate
- ► Safety precautions posted

Check-Out Area

- ► Open check-out area
- ► Clean floors and desk
- ► Well lit without glare

Improving Medical Care Areas and the Patient Emotional Experience

Although many urgent care centers provide a clean and well-lit medical facility, improving the patient experience requires additional considerations. These added touches will enhance the comfort of the patient's encounter:

Waiting Area

- Warm lighting
- Warm color schemes for walls, floors, and furniture
- Comfortable chairs
- Soft music
- Comfortable temperature
- Short waiting time—satisfaction decreases as wait time increases

Registration Area

- Warm lighting—no glare
- Warm color schemes as above
- Setup that maintains privacy during conversations with center staff members

Triage and Examination Area

- Pain control
- Anxiety management
- Warm color schemes
- Comfortable chairs
- Comfortable room temperature
- Setup that maintains privacy during conversations with center staff members
- Blankets available when appropriate
- Short waiting time—satisfaction decreases as wait time increases

Laboratory Area

- Warm colors
- Uncluttered counters
- Short wait time

Radiology Area

- Private changing area

Check-Out Area

- Warm colors
- Warm lighting
- Comfortable chairs
- Setup that maintains privacy during conversations with center staff

Positive Staff Members: A Primary Factor in a Positive Patient Experience

An urgent care center can make great strides in improving the comfort of their patients and provide the highest-quality medical treatment, yet will fail to improve the patient experience if the center staff members are discourteous, appear rushed, or do not demonstrate empathy and respect. Thus, it is extremely important for commitment to quality improvement to begin with the center owner and the medical director because they dictate the company culture. A positive and healthy culture is the glue that holds all patient quality improvements together and provides each patient with a highly satisfactory experience.

A Positive Culture

The relationship between administration and center staff members lays the groundwork for development of a culture of caring and highly performing professionals. When a caring and positive attitude is firmly demonstrated by management toward the staff, then the relationships among center staff members can flourish, which in turn creates trust and a positive attitude. This trust and positive culture is then transmitted to and experienced by the patients in every area of the center. This positive attitude creates a level of medical caring that cannot be bought or be taught. It is the priceless element that allows the urgent care center to meet patient needs on every level.

Attitude

Just as a positive and caring attitude is transmitted to fellow employees and patients, negative attitudes and unprofessionalism by center management transmit negativity to staff members and patients alike. It is therefore important to maintain zero tolerance for negative behavior. Everyone has a bad day, but an ongoing negative attitude must be addressed. Rudeness or curtness toward patients cannot be tolerated. However, the management team is responsible for ensuring that center staff members are not overworked or consistently rushed to complete tasks in an unreasonable period of time; such conditions, if present on a chronic basis, may cause staff members to appear rude or discourteous. Staff members who are efficient may be highly regarded, but efficiency cannot come at the expense of caring and a personal touch with patients. Patients sense the positive or negative culture of the center, which significantly affects how they feel about the medical treatment and care they receive.

Communication

Communication is the most critical component of the patient encounter; therefore, it's not surprising that poor communication or inadequate communication skills usually rank the highest on the list of causes for poor patient experiences for both medical treatment and medical care. This is especially true when physicians fail to communicate well with patients. Poor physician communication skills are often interpreted by patients as lack of empathy or lack of respect. Fortunately, scripts can be provided to the staff and good communication skills can be developed with training and practice. Implementing staff communication-training programs and awareness training will improve the patient experience, especially for physicians. When a physician communicates well with patients, the positive interaction demonstrates caring and builds a relationship of trust. Good physician communication is reinforced by good staff communication, especially about the patient treatment plan, and together these arenas of communication result in increased patient compliance and better outcomes. Better outcomes decrease malpractice exposure, and the positive experience converts the patient into a referral source for family and friends in the community.

Courtesy and Respect

Demonstration of courtesy and respect toward patients starts when the patient enters the center and interacts with staff members in the registration area and ends when the patient goes to the check-out area. These staff positions require well-trained employees who not only understand the complexities of health plan coverage, deductibles, and co-pays but who also are very courteous professionals. Reviewing insurance coverage and requesting payment is never pleasant, and it is even more trying when patients are in pain and possibly angry about the cost of medical treatment. Paying more for the right professionals in these often overlooked positions will be profitable in the long term via increased patient referrals. Courtesy and respect should be shown by all staff members through little courtesies and good manners such as knocking before entering the examination room, introducing themselves in all situations, active listening, checking on patient comfort, reassuring anxious patients, and thanking patients for waiting.

Staffing

Although finding highly skilled medical staff is difficult in a competitive marketplace, releasing uncaring staff and health-care providers who are consistently detrimental to the patient experience will be financially more profitable for the center in the long run. Also, such practices demonstrate management's commitment to establishing a caring and positive culture. Removing one or two negative staff members and replacing them with positive employees will go a long way toward establishing and maintaining a caring and positive professional team and culture.

Empathy

Empathy and kindness toward patients during medical treatment are key when patients are anxious and in pain. Provision of support for medical staff to spend time providing encouragement, paying attention to pain needs, or taking a moment to comfort a patient is part of management's responsibility and commitment to delivering a positive experience to every patient. Awareness and sensitivity training programs to attune staff members to the varying needs of diverse patients will greatly improve patient care. The same level of care for some patients may not be acceptable to other patients; for instance, older patients are often more sensitive to cold and may get cold quickly during treatment. Train staff members to check often on the comfort of elderly patients and offer additional layers for warmth in triage and in the examination room.

Listening

Taking time to really listen is an important part of the patient experience and of communication practice. When staff members listen to the patient's complaints and document them in the chart, the patient feels that they are being heard and not simply rushed through the process so that staff members can move on to the next patient. The physician's role in listening to the patient is even more important. During face-to-face encounters with physicians, even for short periods, patients should feel reassured that they are being heard. Eye contact as well as sitting down is important in patient communication, demonstrating that the physician is really listening to what is being said and is waiting for all the details in order to make the right medical decisions and provide the correct treatment.

MAINTAINING PATIENT SATISFACTION

Maintenance of ongoing patient satisfaction is, in fact, a commitment to continue improving the patient experience. As patient survey scores and their analyses improve, the quest for better patient experiences and outcomes should continue. It is essential to resist the temptation to become satisfied with the patient care status quo and stop the momentum of continuous improvement. Instead, celebrate improvements and reward the staff, but keep building on momentum, setting new objectives, and patient surveys as a foundation of center growth and development.

CONCLUSION

Patient-satisfaction surveys are an effective method for data capture and analysis of data about the quality of urgent care from the patient's perspective. Urgent care centers are not required to conduct patient-satisfaction surveys, but such surveys are a valuable tool for improvement of the patient experience. With the availability of online survey tools and outsourcing, an urgent care center has many options in addition to traditional telephone or print surveys. Even small cosmetic changes to improve patient comfort or reducing wait times by a few minutes can make a positive impact on the patient experience.

Responding to patient survey results and making adjustments to medical treatment and care will improve the patient experience and also build patient loyalty and trust in the marketplace. This translates into referrals and center growth. Patient-satisfaction surveys are an excellent addition to every center's quality-assurance program.

KEY POINTS

1. As health-care providers improve patient satisfaction, patient outcomes also improve. Patient-satisfaction surveys are an excellent tool for analysis of urgent care center patient encounters and subsequent improvement in patient experiences.

2. Improving the patient experience will turn every satisfied patient into a source of referrals of family and friends.

3. Health insurance plans are under pressure to improve outcomes and lower medical costs. Urgent care centers that collect current satisfaction survey data will gain an advantage when seeking MCO contract opportunities and negotiating reimbursement rates.

4. Urgent care centers are not obligated to meet CMS reporting requirements, but they should expect such requirements in the future as proof of higher standards of care and improved outcomes are incorporated into government and MCO contractual agreements.

5. Patient-satisfaction surveys should be conducted regularly and include sufficient volume to ensure production of statistically significant data.

6. Patient questionnaires should include questions that probe both the patient's physical experience during medical treatment and the patient's emotional experience during medical care.

7. Commitment to improvements in the patient experience must be initiated administratively from the top down to become part of urgent care centers' culture.

8. Improvements in aesthetics and comfort levels of the medical treatment areas enhance the patient experience.

9. A positive culture and caring employee attitudes are transmitted to patients and positively affect their overall perception of their medical treatment, care, and outcomes.

10. Celebrate improvements in patient satisfaction and outcomes with the center staff, but never become complacent. Constantly build momentum for continuous quality-of-care improvement as part of the center's culture.

CHAPTER 42

Evaluation and Management of Coding and Documentation

Sybil Yeaman

PROFICIENCY IN SELECTING THE appropriate level of evaluation and management (E&M) codes and thorough documentation regarding medical necessity of services in patient medical records generate correct reimbursement, facilitate compliance with regulatory guidelines, and lower malpractice risks. Inappropriate coding and lack of supporting documentation in medical records put medical providers at risk for consistent underpayments or audits for recoupment of overpayments, and higher malpractice risks. Information about E&M coding and documentation is provided here only for education purposes. Readers should always refer to American Medical Association (AMA), Centers for Medicare & Medicaid Services (CMS), and health insurance plan guidelines for specific coding and documentation requirements.

E&M codes were established in 1995, yet correct coding is still a challenge because of the complexities incorporated into the coding process for purposes of determining medical necessity and level of code for services rendered.

MEDICAL NECESSITY

Prior to the late 20th century, medical providers personally determined the medical necessity of the services they provided to their patients. Reimbursement came directly from their patients in a monetary or barter remuneration system. The increasing popularity of purchased health insurance coverage in the late 20th century generated a growing business of health insurance plans, which provided coverage for member services. To control costs, health plans began to define medical necessity to determine which medical claims to pay and which to deny. When payments were linked to medical necessity, conflicts and complexity regarding the definition and appropriate levels of reimbursement came to the fore, and they remain ongoing issues.

With reimbursement linked to medical necessity, physicians no longer determine medical necessity based solely on their individual professional opinion. Government medical programs (i.e., the CMS), individual state regulators, and health insurance plans have each defined medical necessity for their own needs and carry financial risk for determination of what is medically necessary. Our system of medical coding and accompanying reimbursement rates are based on predetermined medically necessary levels of health care provided by health-care providers and documented in the medical record. Five E&M levels for new patients and five for established patients each begin with minimal services and escalate to more complex services. Relative value units (RVUs) are assigned to each escalating level of service as part of a resource-based relative value system; the designated value for each level arises from calculation of the numbers of units of medical services provided, anticipated expense for the practice (facility), and the level of medical decision making and risk. These RVUs are in turn used to establish provider reimbursement rates. Higher E&M levels indicate more complex medical care and result in a higher RVU reimbursement.

EVALUATION AND MANAGEMENT CODE DEFINITIONS

Because E&M codes are the foundation for establishment of medical necessity, the appropriate level of care, and provider reimbursement rates, it is essential to understand commonly used terminology and details in distinctions of specific terms according to E&M guidelines. Before choosing E&M codes, medical providers need to know the following definitions based on the AMA guidelines developed by their Current Procedural Terminology (CPT) editorial panel:

- *Body areas*   The following body areas are recognized for sites of examination:
  - Head and face
  - Neck
  - Chest, breasts, and axillae
  - Abdomen
  - Back
  - Genitalia, groin, and buttocks
  - Each extremity

- *Chief complaint* consists of a concise statement describing the symptoms, problem, condition, diagnosis, or other factor underlying the rationale for the encounter (usually stated in the patient's words).

- *Concurrent* care describes provision of similar services to the same patient by more than one physician on the same day.

- *Contributory factors* are components of E&M services that are not key factors and are not provided in every patient encounter but are nevertheless important E&M services.

- *Counseling* is defined as face-to-face discussion with a patient or family member concerning one or more factors about diagnostic results, prognosis, risks versus benefits of various treatment or management options, instructions for treatment, compliance encouragement, risk reduction, and patient and family education.

- ▶ *Components*   Descriptors for the levels of E&M services recognize seven components.
    - *History, examination, and medical decision making* are key components.
    - *Counseling, the coordination of care, and the nature of the presenting problem* are contributing components.
    - *Time* is defined as face-to-face time for the office visit.
- ▶ *Family history* is a review of medical events in the patient's family, including significant information about the health or cause of illness of immediate family members, specific diseases related to the chief complaint, history of the present illness, and a review of systems.
- ▶ *History of present illness* is a chronologic description of the development of the patient's present illness from the first sign or symptom to the present presenting problem.
- ▶ *Three key components of E&M services* are history, examination, and medical decision making.
- ▶ *Levels of E&M services* include examinations, evaluations, treatments, conferences with or about patients, preventive pediatric or adult health services, and similar medical services.
- ▶ *Medical screening* includes the medical history, physical examination, and medical decision making required to determine the need or location for appropriate care of the patient.
- ▶ *Presenting problem* is a disease, condition, injury, symptom, sign, or other reasons for the encounter, with or without a diagnosis established at the time of the encounter. There are five types of presenting problems:
    - *Minimal problems* do not require the presence of a physician, but the encounter is under physician (on-site) supervision.
    - A *self-limited or minor problem* runs a defined course, is not likely to alter health status, or has a good prognosis.
    - *Low-severity problems* have low risk of morbidity, and there is the expectation of full recovery without functional impairment.
    - A *moderate-severity problem* carries moderate risk of morbidity without treatment and uncertain prognosis or probability of prolonged functional impairment.
    - *High severity* indicates high to extremely high risk of morbidity without treatment and moderate to high risk of mortality without treatment or high probability of severe, prolonged functional impairment.

- *Organ systems* The following examination organ systems are recognized:
  - Eyes
  - Cardiovascular
  - Ears, nose, mouth, throat
  - Respiratory
  - Gastrointestinal
  - Musculoskeletal
  - Skin
  - Neurologic
  - Psychiatric
  - Hematologic, lymphatic, and immunologic

- *Past history* is defined as a review of a patient's past experience with illnesses, injuries, and treatment, including major illnesses, injuries, operations and hospitalizations, current medications, allergies, immunizations and dietary status.

- *Review of systems* is obtained through a series of questions seeking to identify signs or symptoms that the patient may be experiencing or has experienced, to facilitate differential diagnosis and determine what specific tests, if any, are needed. Following are the 14 elements of systems review:
  - Constitutional symptoms
  - Eyes
  - Ears, nose, mouth, and throat
  - Cardiovascular
  - Respiratory
  - Gastrointestinal
  - Genitourinary
  - Musculoskeletal
  - Integumentary (skin and breast)
  - Neurologic
  - Psychiatric
  - Endocrine
  - Hematologic and lymphatic
  - Allergic and immunologic

- *Social history* includes past and current activities such as marital and living status, current and past employment, drug and alcohol use, education level, sexual history, and relevant social factors.

- *Time* is defined as face-to-face time for office visits.

- *Transfer of care* occurs when a physician who is providing management for some or all of the patient's problems relinquishes responsibility to another physician who explicitly accepts responsibility.

- There are four types of examination.
  - *Problem-focused:* Limited examination of affected body area(s) or organ system(s)
  - *Expanded problem-focused:* Limited examination of affected body area(s) or organ system(s) and other symptomatic or related organ systems
  - *Detailed:* Extended examination of affected body area(s) and other symptomatic or related organ system(s)
  - *Comprehensive:* General multisystem examination or complete examination of a single organ system

EVALUATION AND MANAGEMENT LEVELS OF SERVICE

Guidelines for E&M services include wide variations in skill, work, time, responsibility, and medical knowledge required for the prevention or diagnosis and treatment of illness or injury. Because the level of work and time to acquire the initial history, conduct the examination, and compile treatment data for a new patient are different from the level of service required for established patients, office and outpatient services are different for a new patient than they are for an established patient. There are five levels of service for new patients and five for established patients. *Note that* although levels of new patient and established patient service may look similar, they are not interchangeable.

A new patient is one who has not received professional services from the physician or another physician of the exact same specialty and subspecialty who belongs to the same group practice within the last 3 years (Table 1). An established patient is one who has received professional services from the physician or another physician of the exact same specialty and subspecialty who belongs to the same group practice within the past 3 years (Table 2).

Table 1. New Patient Service Level

Code	Description
99201	Problem-focused medical history and physical examination with straightforward medical decision making
99202	Expanded problem-focused medical history and physical examination with straightforward medical decision making
99203	Detailed medical history and physical examination with low-complexity medical decision making
99204	Comprehensive medical history and physical examination with moderately complex medical decision making
99205	Comprehensive medical history and physical examination with complex medical decision making

Table 2. Established Patient Service Level

Code	Description
99211	Minimal encounter, which does not require the physician, but with supervising physician on-site
99212	Problem-focused medical history and physical examination with straightforward medical decision making
99213	Expanded problem-focused medical history and physical examination with medical decision making of low complexity
99214	Detailed medical history and physical examination with moderately complex medical decision making
99215	Comprehensive medical history and physical examination with complex medical decision making

Putting It All Together

Most patients who seek care in an urgent care center are new patients and present with straightforward to moderately complex health risk issues (Table 3). Patients who present with complex and highly acute illness or injury would be assigned E&M code level 99205 and often require transportation to a hospital facility for ongoing medical care after stabilization.

Sample Scenarios of E&M Coding Levels and Medical Decision Making

▶ *99201*   Straightforward medical decision making, minimal risk
  - The patient presents with a minor problem.
  - The medical history and physical examination are limited to the affected area or a related organ system.

Table 3. Straightforward to Moderately Complex Health or Risk Issues

Code	Description
99201	Problem-focused medical history and physical examination with straightforward medical decision making
99202	Expanded problem-focused medical history and physical examination with straightforward medical decision making
99203	Detailed medical history and physical examination with medical decision making of low complexity
99204	Comprehensive medical history and physical examination with moderately complex medical decision making
99205	Comprehensive medical history and physical examination with complex medical decision making

- The medical history and physical examination reveal no other chronic conditions or other problems.
- The patient may receive a diagnostic x-ray or laboratory test.
- The condition is diagnosed, and treatment is managed with over-the-counter drugs.
- The prognosis is full recovery.

▶ *99202* Straightforward medical decision making with minimal risk
- The patient presents with a minor problem.
- The medical history and physical examination are limited to the affected area and related organ systems.
- The medical history and physical examination may reveal a controlled chronic condition or other problem(s).
- The patient undergoes diagnostic x-ray or laboratory tests.
- The condition is diagnosed, and the patient is treated and given a treatment plan and possibly a prescription.
- The prognosis is good.

▶ *99203* Medical decision making of low complexity with low risk
- The patient presents with two minor problems or minor uncomplicated injury.
- The medical history and physical examination are detailed and extend to related or symptomatic organ systems.
- The medical history and physical examination may reveal stable chronic condition(s) or previous problem(s).
- The patient undergoes diagnostic x-ray, laboratory tests, and superficial needle or skin biopsies.
- The patient may require simple abrasion and laceration repairs or removal of a foreign body.
- The condition is diagnosed, and the patient is treated and may require superficial dressings, a treatment plan, and prescription management.
- The patient is referred to a primary-care physician or instructed to return to the urgent care center for follow-up care.
- The prognosis is good.

▶ *99204* Moderately complex medical decision making with moderate risk
- The patient presents with a mild chronic illness, new acute problem, or acute injury.
- The patient undergoes extensive diagnostic radiography, laboratory testing, or needle or incision biopsy.
- The patient requires laceration repair, splinting, foreign body removal, or intravenous treatment.
- The condition is diagnosed, and the patient requires minor procedures, treatment, or prescription management.
- The patient is referred to a specialist for ongoing medical care.

- The prognosis is uncertain, with the possibility of some residual functional impairment.

▶ *99205* Highly complex medical decision making with high risk (also see the description of 99291). The patient presents with one or more severe chronic illnesses or a severe injury.
- The patient presents with a medical threat to life or bodily function or with abrupt neurologic changes.
- The patient receives treatment to monitor and stabilize conditions or injuries.
- The patient is transported to the closest hospital for ongoing medical care.
- The prognosis is severe and includes prolonged functional impairment.

▶ *99291, critical care (first 30–74 minutes)* The physician may consider use of this level of services in place of code 99205 for patients who present with a critical illness or injury that impairs one or more vital organ systems and presents a high probability of imminent or life-threatening deterioration of the patient's condition. Critical care involves highly complex decision making to assess, manipulate, and support vital system functions for prevention of further life-threatening deterioration of the patient's condition. (Code 99292 may be used in addition to 99291 for each additional 30 minutes of critical care.)

MEDICAL DOCUMENTATION

Medical documentation consists of more than simply recording a patient's complaint and medical services provided to resolve the presenting problem(s). It also involves documentation of the medical provider's medical judgment and decision making at the time of care and supports the medical necessity of the services and tests provided.

Many medical providers do not provide sufficient documentation, especially regarding history and medical decision making, because they do not realize the actual importance of the medical record until their medical insurance claims are denied and require supporting documentation for the appeals process or until they are involved with a malpractice case that questions their medical judgment and quality of patient care. Consider the following examples:

▶ When claims for services or tests provided are denied by a health insurance plan, medical documentation is required to support codes used in that claim and to facilitate the appeals process. Lack of supporting documentation results in denied appeals and denied compensation.

▶ When medical necessity of services is questioned by a health insurance plan or quality-management committee, medical documentation is needed to validate the medical necessity of the services provided. Lack of documentation may lead to denied appeals, cancellation of contractual relationships, and denied reimbursement.

▶ When the physician's medical judgment and patient care are questioned by an adversarial attorney, the medical record is required to support the physician's medical decision making and to demonstrate appropriateness of services provided. Lack of supporting documentation leaves an opening for misinterpretation of patient care quality and appropriateness.

These examples show how taking the time to document everything in each patient chart consistently and thoroughly to demonstrate medical judgment, medical necessity, and the appropriateness of provided services helps to protect the medical provider and the financial stability of the urgent care center.

The following CMS guidelines for documentation of basic medical record information clarify expectations as to what information to include in medical records:

▶ Medical records should be complete, legible, and understandable to others reviewing the chart, not just to the provider who wrote the entry.

▶ Documentation of each patient encounter should include the following:
  - The date of service
  - A reason for the encounter
  - An appropriate medical history in relation to the patient's chief complaint
  - A physical examination in relation to the patient's chief complaint
  - Reasons for and results of x-rays, laboratory tests, and other ancillary services
  - A review of other ancillary services used to determine pathology or other symptoms as appropriate
  - An assessment of the patient's condition
  - A plan for the patient's care

▶ Past and present diagnoses should be accessible to the treating and/or consulting physician.

▶ Relevant health risk factors should be identified.

▶ The patient's progress (including response to treatment), change in treatment, change in diagnosis, and patient noncompliance should be documented.

▶ The written plan should include treatments and medications (including frequency and dose), referrals and consultations, patient and family education, and specific instructions for follow-up.

▶ Documentation should support the intensity of patient evaluation and treatment, including the thought process and complexity of medical decision making, and consideration of chronic conditions treated at the time of service or on an ongoing basis.

▶ All entries in the medical record should be dated and authenticated (tied to the actual patient).

Another method for evaluation of the comprehensiveness of your center's medical records is to self-evaluate like an auditor. An auditor usually looks for the following documentation:

▶ Why was the patient seen?

▶ What did the patient describe as their problem(s)?

▶ Did the patient have other chronic problems?

▶ What extent of examination was needed?

▶ What extent of examination was performed?

▶ What did the examination reveal?

▶ What other services or tests were ordered?

▶ Were results of ancillary services and tests reviewed?

▶ What did each of the services and tests reveal?

▶ What were the diagnosis and prognosis?

▶ Were other chronic conditions taken into consideration?

▶ What treatment plan was the patient given?

▶ What referrals for additional care were given?

▶ What counseling was provided?

▶ Was the appropriate code chosen?

▶ Were the services medically necessary?

▶ Is the chart documentation legible and understandable to individuals other than the health-care provider writing the entry?

If documentation in the medical records is appropriate considering those questions, then it will most likely support the claims of the medical provider in any appeals process for reimbursement issues, as well as the appropriateness of the medical decision making and medical care under legal scrutiny.

Documentation Tips

▶ Always document clearly and legibly, or the medical record will be open to variable retrospective interpretation by an auditor or plaintiff's attorney.

- Indicate the patient's chief complaint at every visit. Verify the medical assistant's documentation of the chief complaint, especially for established patients. If there is no complaint or inaccurate data such as "patient f/u" are indicated as the chief complaint, then there is no clear reason for the encounter. Ensure that the chief complaint documented by the health-care provider matches the complaint documented by the medical assistant.
- Always verify whether a patient is a new or established patient at the beginning of the exam. Incorrect coding can result in incorrect payment or denial of claims. Remember that the encounter can be for a new injury even if the patient is an established patient.
- Always document review of the patient's medical history, family and social history, review of vital signs, and past or present pertinent information gathered by the medical staff prior to your examination. If such review is not noted in the medical record, the assumption is that the data were gathered but never reviewed.
- Always document the examination of affected area(s) and related organ systems and the process of medical decision making. Remember that if it is not documented, readers of medical records assume that it didn't happen.
- Always write orders for ancillary services and testing, then document your review of the results. A plaintiff's attorney can use lack of documentation to prove negligence.
- Always consider radiology overreads on x-rays for patients presenting with moderate-risk to high-risk pathologies. Missed pathology, whether related or unrelated to the presenting problem, can result in higher risk of patient morbidity or mortality without treatment.
- Always review patient data and documentation gathered and documented by the medical support staff. The medical provider is ultimately responsible for accuracy of the medical record.
- Always be clear and concise when documenting instructions regarding referrals for follow-up or ongoing care with primary-care providers or specialists. This demonstrates clarity of instructions and reinforcement of the importance of follow-up care as part of the treatment plan.
- Always provide only medically necessary reviews of systems, ancillary services, and testing. Providing additional services to raise acuity can create claims and appeals issues that hold up reimbursements.
- Always document everything in the medical record in a professional manner. What you write is part of the permanent medical record and will be read by others. If you are documenting retrospectively, add the date, the time, and your signature to the addendum.

- Always code on the basis of findings from the patient's medical history, physical exam, and complexity of medical decision making. *Undercoding* (using codes for lower-complexity services than indicated by the patient's actual condition) cheats you and the center of rightful reimbursement. In addition, it presents a falsely low acuity of the patient population to the health plan. *Overcoding* (using codes for higher-complexity services than indicated by the patient's actual condition) may initiate an audit.
- It is a requirement for the physician provider to be on-site at the urgent care center for any "incident to" services provided and documented by medical staff and billed under their identification numbers.
- Always complete, sign, and date documentation in the medical record on the date of service. Never amend or adjust previous medical documentation at a later date to cover up an error or an incomplete medical record. There is no legal defense for this.
- Always review health insurance plan contracts to make sure you understand and agree with coding and reimbursement guidelines before signing a contract or contract renewal. Taking the time to review utilization and negotiate for higher E&M reimbursement, even an incremental amount for each code, can improve the financial stability of the center.
- Always review reasons for claim denial. Denied claims can often be a warning of a coding and/or documentation issue.
- Always use a certified procedural coder who is experienced in urgent care coding. Routine review of coding and documentation will catch issues before they turn into large numbers of denials and time-consuming appeals.
- Always make an internal or external annual chart review a part of the center's compliance program. Chart reviews will help you catch coding and documentation issues before they result in an audit or legal issues.

Coding Specific to Urgent Care

- *CPT code S9083*   Global fee for urgent care centers. This is used when the center is contracted on a flat-rate or global-fee basis. In such cases, all services performed in the center are bundled into this code unless a carve-out has been negotiated. *Note:* Medicare does not reimburse any S-codes.
- *CPT code S9088*   This is defined as services provided in an urgent care center and is used in conjunction with an E&M code. It is not a stand-alone code. The individual responsible for billing should know which payer contracts will reimburse for this code and should bill appropriately.

Payers may expect the provider to code the encounter using the appropriate E&M methodology but pay the same global fee no matter the code. It is important to educate the providers that they still must document and code appropriately inasmuch as future flat-rate compensation will likely be based on the level of care previously provided to that particular health insurance plan's patients.

Urgent care providers who want to provide primary care should do so using a separate taxpayer identification number, but keep in mind that some payers may not be willing to contract for both services at the same place of service. Also, if a payer classified the care provided as urgent care, the payer may require that the patient pay the higher co-pay even if you consider the care to be primary in nature.

CONCLUSION

E&M coding and reimbursement levels are based on medical necessity and a combination of anticipated services, skills required, cost to practice, risk coverage, and medical knowledge required to provide patient services. Documentation in the medical record represents the level of medical decision making, services provided, and patient risk, and supports the level of coding. Together, the appropriate medical record coding and supporting claims documentation provide consistent financial reimbursement and lower malpractice risk for the urgent care center.

KEY POINTS

1. Accurate coding and appropriate medical record and claims documentation will help ensure timely claims processing, correct reimbursement, and lower malpractice risk.

2. The current coding system and health-care reimbursement are linked to medical necessity, so medical necessity is no longer determined solely at the physician's discretion. It is determined also by health insurance plans and by state and federal lawmakers.

3. Taking the time to know and understand the AMA definitions and CPT guidelines for E&M levels is essential to correct and accurate coding.

4. Be sure to document clearly, legibly, and professionally, because other medical providers and health professionals will have access to medical records.

5. Critical care, evaluation and management code 99291, may be used in place of code 99205 or 99215 when a patient presents with a critical illness or injury that requires vital system support to prevent further life-threatening deterioration of the patient's condition.

6. All coding must be supported by medical necessity. Additional review of systems or ancillary services to upcode to a higher E&M level will only result in claim denials and possible audits.

7. Downcoding to cover inadequate documentation habits lowers reimbursement and undermines financial stability of the urgent care center.

8. Many medical providers underdocument the medical history and medical decision-making areas of the medical record, resulting in lower reimbursements and higher malpractice risk.

9. Routine external or internal chart review will help center management personnel catch coding and documentation problems before they become an issue.

10. Employ an experienced certified coder on staff to oversee coding and documentation, or ensure that your billing company contractually guarantees use of a certified coder who is contractually guaranteed by your outside billing company or revenue cycle management company.

CHAPTER 43

Additional Services in Urgent Care

Natasha N. Deonarain

The traditional scope of urgent care ranges from ambulatory medical services typified by those provided in a family practitioner's office to those provided in a hospital emergency department. Since entering the healthcare market, urgent care clinics have evolved into much-needed access points for cost-effective health care. In addition to treating problems such as coughs, colds, and urinary tract infections, many urgent care centers now offer additional services such as medical aesthetics, occupational medicine, and substance abuse treatment to generate additional revenue. As cost shifting continued, patients became more consumer-oriented when paying out of pocket, and practices became increasingly cash-based. There are still significant opportunities for urgent care owners to add ancillary services or products to their core business strategy, effectively capitalizing on these trends.

This chapter focuses on the key issues to consider when deciding to add services or products to your urgent care facility, including aligning vision and values, changing outlook, performing research and planning, creating a strong management team, and solidifying financial structure. This chapter offers a few creative suggestions for additional services and products.

Urgent care clinic owners often look first at the financial bottom line when making decisions, but the potential financial upside may distract rather than enhance the core business strategy. Although generating positive cash flow is desirable and necessary, the most important determinant of success will be the degree to which an additional service or product can become integral to the organization. Careful strategizing before implementation protects your financial bottom line and is the best route to reach long-term success.

ELEMENTS OF A SUCCESSFUL BUSINESS STRATEGY

Aligning Vision and Values

Successful urgent care centers, just like any other business, require careful planning; unfortunately, many owners fail to plan. According to Jack Welch, former chairman and chief executive officer of General Electric, "Good business leaders create a vision, articulate the vision, passionately own the vision, and relentlessly drive it to completion."[1] Here are a few questions to consider:

- ▶ Do you know what you want to see as the future for your urgent care center?
- ▶ How does your choice of services or products align with that vision?
- ▶ Do you strongly believe in your choices, and why?

Time spent answering these questions first will determine the success of those services or products sold at your facilities. For example, if Dr. XYZ wants to set up an urgent care clinic, her core business strategy must include a scope of service. Patients will see medical providers on a walk-in basis for care of acute conditions such as trauma, infections, or pain. The staffing model should include support staff and providers (physicians, nurse practitioners, or physician assistants) trained in urgent care medicine. Dr. XYZ's vision of what this urgent care center will be in 5, 10, or 15 years may stop here; in other words, urgent care medicine is all that she may want to provide with this particular business model.

What if Dr. XYZ wants to do more? How should she choose which services or products to include in the practice? Decisions based solely on financial reasoning are likely to fail. Aligning choices with vision and values will produce a more positive outcome.

For instance, say Dr. XYZ has been approached by a local chiropractor who wants to work at an urgent care center. The chiropractor is willing to sublease space inside the urgent care center. Indeed, there are additional exam rooms available at the back of the facility, and he decides that he can generate additional revenue by renting this space. Unfortunately, Dr. XYZ was trained in a traditional allopathic medical model. In the past she called chiropractors, acupuncturists, massage therapists, and naturopaths "quacks" in front of her patients. What is likely to happen with the relationship between Dr. XYZ and the chiropractor? Even if the chiropractor is successful, pays his rent on time, and brings his own clientele to the center, the alignment of chiropractic services inside this center is at odds with Dr. XYZ's personal value system. In addition, Dr. XYZ doesn't seem to have a vision for the center. She began simply with the desire to run an urgent care clinic, and then added rehabilitative services in her back exam rooms.

Over time, Dr. XYZ may begin to actively discourage her patients from seeing chiropractors, forgetting that there is one down the hall. She may simply provide them with pain medications, telling them they will heal because this is how she was trained. Dr. XYZ may be unwilling to learn more from the chiropractor because she doesn't really believe in those types of services.

It is also likely that Dr. XYZ's medical staff members will keep to themselves and believe that they should remain separate from the chiropractor and his staff. Patients may become confused when they ask about other services available in

---

1   Welch J, Welch S. *Winning.* New York: HarperBusiness; 2005.

the clinic. It may become apparent to them that Dr. XYZ doesn't agree with their desire to use chiropractic services, and they may eventually feel like they're doing so against their physician's wishes.

Any or all of these factors may or may not come into play in this scenario, but at the heart of the entire decision lies the fact that Dr. XYZ has not aligned her vision with her values. In the long run, despite a cordial relationship with the chiropractor, she loses business synergy and the added benefit of increased cash flow through mutual patient satisfaction and repeat visits to the urgent care center that might have been possible with the addition of chiropractic services. Members of both staffs will likely become distanced and may not support each other. Staff members are often invaluable confidants of patients at discharge and can encourage them to seek wellness services in ways that physicians don't have time to do, given today's bureaucratic pressures. Dr. XYZ does not understand that such synergy is crucial to successful business relationships.

Aligning your vision before adding services or products is a key first step during the planning stages. What are your values? What do you see as necessary in the patient care continuum, and which other providers or products would fit well with your overall vision? Spend the extra time being honest so that you have the ability to wisely choose a best fit for your organization. Services or products provided in alignment with vision and values result in an integrated operation, passionate staff culture, and patients who will generate referrals as you enjoy growing profits.

Changing Outlooks

Physicians are notorious as terrible business owners. Michael E. Gerber states in his book *The E-Myth Physician: Why Most Medical Practices Don't Work and What to Do About It* that "learning how to be a [d]octor does not prepare you to develop a successful medical practice. Knowing how a practice works best has little to do with knowing how a [d]octor works best."[2] The crux of this problem is the fact that physicians have trouble working with systems. They are better as detail people. When it comes to making a decision of how to best add service or product lines, the urgent care center owner should adopt two fundamental but seemingly incongruous outlooks. First, the new service or product must be viewed as integrable with the rest of the center and must be treated as such to ensure that the whole operation works as one system. Second, it must be supported as if it were a *separate* business, using dedicated resources to launch and operate it. This includes varying elements of staffing, space, supplies, and management. The urgent care center owner must therefore shift between paying attention to the details of a separate business entity and integrating the new service or product into the system.

Dr. XYZ would like to dispense medications as part of the urgent care practice. This particular choice involves adding both a service and product to her

---

2   Gerber ME. *The E-Myth Physician: Why Most Medical Practices Don't Work and What to Do About It.* New York, NY: HarperBusiness; 2004:xii.

core business. What outlook will ensure success of this additional service and product?

First, all staff members must be trained to view the *service* of dispensing medication as an integral part of a patient encounter, not as an afterthought. In other words, when Dr. XYZ decides to include medication dispensing as an additional service, she should train her staff to *expect* that every patient who gets a prescription obtains the medication from the clinic supply. For the purposes of strategy success, beginning with an inclusive rather than exclusive outlook will help staff members understand that patients can save time, energy, and money when they buy a medication at the center. The outlook that Dr. XYZ has toward her new service and product will directly affect the outlook of staff members and in turn will dramatically affect the long-term success of the project. Concurrently, Dr. XYZ must view the medication-dispensing service as a *separate* business inside the urgent care center, meaning that she should dedicate management and other needed staff members when feasible to ensure that the dispensing process is implemented and then runs smoothly and correctly. In contrast to these suggestions, many urgent care center owners often talk to a sales representative about an exciting new product or service and immediately call their office manager and say excitedly, "Have this set up by Monday morning so we can get going!" This is a sure path to failure. The ability to view a new service or products as separate yet integrated is what turns physicians into successful business owners.

RESEARCH AND PLANNING

Once you have decided that additional services or products align with your vision and have examined strategy details, the next step is research. Two areas on which to focus are market and regulatory analyses. Note that marketing your service or product inside your facility (internal marketing) is equally important to external marketing.

Market Research

A common method of environmental analysis for a given product or service involves creation of a SWOT matrix (Table 1). This structured planning tool represents analysis of strengths, weaknesses, opportunities, and threats for implementation of a given product or service, as well as analysis of external factors which may impact achievement of overall objectives. In Table 1, Dr. XYZ examines the effect of organizational characteristics of the organization and environment on her proposed medication-dispensing project. Focus on a SWOT analysis as part of market research helps owners determine multiple objectives and may be useful for future planning. Collection and analysis of such meaningful information facilitates decisions as to whether the benefits for a given project outweigh the risks.

Regulatory Research

State and federal regulation affects creative urgent care business models. For instance, in Arizona, urgent care practice is licensed by the state's department of

Table 1. SWOT Matrix—Medication Dispensing

	Strengths	Weaknesses
Internal (characteristics of the organization)	• Convenient for patients • Cost-effective for patients • Saves patients time and energy • Encourages repeat customers • Improves reputation of center • Generates additional revenue • Fits with continuum of care for urgent care services	• Potential risk of medication-dispensing error • Service is dependent on patient volumes and type of presenting diseases • Unable to stock more expensive medications because of lower sales volumes compared with larger pharmacies • At risk for expiring inventory because of lower turnover
	Opportunities	Threats
External (characteristics of the environment)	• Competitor urgent care does not have a similar service • No pharmacy within 5–7 miles • Older patient population that requires multiple medications within target service area	• Regulatory pressures and changes • Larger pharmacy chains in the immediate target market • Disruption in supply because of unexpected factors • Lack of control over manufacturers' costs • Inventory cost may become prohibitive • Demand for medications may wane as patients seek other options

SWOT: strengths, weaknesses, opportunities, and threats.

health. Arizona state rules currently do not allow providers to commingle different services inside the same facility if those services are owned by separate corporate entities.

In this scenario, Dr. XYZ would like to sublease space to a physical therapist who owns and operates his own company, and she wants to keep her company separate from that of the physical therapist. The physical therapist's patients would enter the facility through the same front door as Dr. XYZ's patients but check in at a different front-office counter. They would be told to wait inside the same waiting room as Dr. XYZ's patients. This situation would be prohibited in Arizona because the physical therapist and Dr. XYZ own two separate corporate entities but their patients share doorways and waiting-room space. The only way Dr. XYZ would be able to operate different types of services inside the urgent care center would be to own a corporate entity that provides both urgent care and physical therapy services. The physical therapist would have to become an employee of Dr. XYZ's company. The department of health would require separate waiting rooms and doorways, one for urgent care and one for physical therapy patients.

Another regulatory issue is federal Stark law, which places limitations on certain physician referrals. In brief, a physician may not refer certain "designated health services" for Medicare or Medicaid patients if the physician or immediate family member has a financial interest in or relationship to the referral entity. If the corporation owns all services inside the urgent care facility and bills under a single tax identification number or employer identification number, generally the Stark law does not apply. However, urgent care center owners should consult an attorney for specific advice on the Stark law and other state or federal regulations when considering addition of services or products.

Marketing Plan

Marketing is key to generating repeat business; however, many owners only focus on marketing outside their actual facility. *Internal marketing* refers to how you plan to sell additional services or products to the patients who have already come for an urgent care appointment or visit. This is often called *cross-marketing* or *upselling*, and represents opportunities and means for customers to purchase items or services in addition to the one they originally intended, before arriving at the facility, to purchase.

Using Dr. XYZ's medication-dispensing service as an example again, how do patients in the waiting room know that they will have the option to purchase medication after their provider visit? Dr. XYZ may use posters or TV ads in the waiting room and exam rooms, thereby informing patients that such a service is available. She may train staff members to mention that availability of the additional service for the convenience of patients. She may place a medication-dispensing kiosk in the waiting room rather than in the back office, so that waiting patients see others buying medication after their visit, prompting inquiry about those same options.

Further, Dr. XYZ should not underestimate the power of her staff members as internal marketers. Testimonials or encouragement from staff members are invaluable, especially recommendations of additional services such as chiropractic care, massage therapy, acupuncture, or medical spa treatments. This is one way in which team engagement, integration, and marketing skills synergize to boost overall revenues for the entire practice by presenting creative health-care choices to urgent care center patients.

MANAGEMENT STRUCTURE

A very common mistake that many urgent care owners make, especially in tough economic times, is to add the management of additional services or products to the job duties of an already-stressed office manager and yet expect things to run smoothly. To avoid this pitfall, careful management planning prior to purchase and setup is necessary.

Dedicating staff for your new project does not have to add cost. By incorporating the steps outlined in this chapter, planning for efficiency will result in efficiency. The first thing you may want to do is answer a few questions with your office manager to help guide development of a proposed management structure. Here are a few points to consider:

- ▸ Who will be in charge of setting up the service or product line?
- ▸ Who will work with vendors, obtain pricing, make decisions, and see them through to implementation?
- ▸ Does this leader have the time and necessary skills to do what you would like, or would someone else be more qualified?
- ▸ Who will take the lead on checking supplies and managing inventory?
- ▸ What chain of command will be used?
- ▸ Who will be held responsible for ensuring smooth operation?
- ▸ Who will help market the product or service internally to other providers and staff?
- ▸ Are the proposed delegates willing and qualified to undertake such a project?

Once a proposed management structure has been outlined, check in with your office manager again and assess things honestly. Does the manager look apprehensive, stressed, or unwilling to start this project? Can you discuss things openly? If you don't take time to also evaluate these more subtle cues, your project may never take off because a key individual is not yet fully engaged.

Slowing down during the initial stages of planning, allocating staff resources carefully, and adopting an outlook that your additional service or product line is very much its own business while still being an important component of the entire organization will improve your long-term chances of success and make your investment worthwhile.

FINANCIAL STRUCTURE

Warren Buffett said in a letter to shareholders in 2001, "Bad things aren't obvious when times are good. After all, you only find out who's swimming naked when the tide goes out." When it comes to deciding which services or products to add to your urgent care center, it's easy to get caught up in believing that you can't go wrong, especially after the sales representative leaves your office. If you want to avoid exposure, spending a little time on a financial plan will minimize risk. Here are three basic areas on which to focus, each of which is discussed in this section:

- ▸ Start-up costs: Determine the amount of investment money needed for the project.
- ▸ Break-even point: Find the point where revenue equals expenses.

- Unique billing issues: Investigate issues that surround billing for healthcare services, which are different than for urgent care.

Start-Up Costs

Initiating any business venture requires an initial capital outlay. Let's continue with the example of Dr. XYZ's medication-dispensing project. She may require specialized dispensing equipment, office supplies, initial medication stock, additional staffing, locked cabinets, computers, and other items. She will also require enough cash on hand to float the project (i.e., pay debt obligations or use as working capital). Dr. XYZ may want to create a spreadsheet reflecting minimum and maximum sales projections for the first few months to give her a good idea of best-case and worst-case scenarios and delineate the time required to break even.

Break-Even Point

The break-even point is reached when revenue equals expenses. Dr. XYZ estimates that it will take approximately 2 months to reach the break-even point, after which any increase in daily prescription sales generates profit. Many factors can affect the break-even point, including fluctuating patient volume, operating costs, and changes in supply costs or delivery turnaround times; these factors should be considered during careful financial analysis of start-up costs and time to the break-even point.

Billing Issues

Additional health-care services that fall under state or federal regulation, such as physical therapy, occupational medicine, chiropractic practice, or laboratory testing, may affect billing practices and billing cycles. For example, if you are considering the addition of physical therapy or chiropractic services and will accept health insurance plans, it is wise to make sure that your billing department is familiar with billing practices for these services. The nuances of medical billing vary for rehabilitative, chiropractic, and urgent care. Health insurance plans will often outsource these claims to third-party administrators. Thus, your clinic may need separate billing departments, each specializing in a particular service provided within the urgent care center. Spending extra time and effort in advance of adding new services to examine unique billing issues will eliminate or at least reduce rejected claims.

CREATIVE IDEAS FOR ADDITIONAL SERVICES IN URGENT CARE

As discussed in this chapter, the addition of services or products toward development of a more comprehensive business model can improve your reputation with patients and generate revenue. If planned and implemented correctly, these models can be lucrative, especially as we enter an era of "retail medicine" in which patients expect more for every health-care dollar spent.

Following are a few suggestions, grouped according to characteristics. If you are expanding services or products, you should consider sticking within a particular group to enhance visibility and sales around a particular strategic model.

Rehabilitative Services

In a rehabilitative services model, the urgent care provider fixes the initial medical problem and then refers a patient for rehabilitation. Types of conditions may include ligamentous injury or sprains, muscle strains, joint inflammation, and even nerve entrapment syndromes. The urgent care provider can treat a patient with back strain with acute pain medication, and then refer them to a physical therapist or chiropractor at the same facility. Adding massage therapists, medical acupuncturists, neuromuscular experts, or kinesthesiologists may also be considered.

Wellness Services and Products

Patients are no longer happy with quick fixes. Today, they want options for becoming well and maintaining wellness. Although the core business model of urgent care offers a quick fix, wellness services can create a refreshing model in which patients *want* to see their physician. Additional services such as nutrition counseling, weight-loss counseling, weight-loss support groups, exercise consulting, bioidentical hormone management, anti-aging product sales or anti-aging services, or nutraceutical or vitamin supplement sales serve to capitalize on these demands.

Aesthetic Services and Products

In the past, it might have seemed strange to add medical spa or even spa-type services at an urgent care center. However, the addition of staff members who can perform Botox injections, collagen injections, facials, laser hair removal, and massage therapy and can handle sales of medical-grade skin products can change the image of urgent care to include an element of pampering.

Alternative Services

Although many practices previously categorized as alternative are now becoming mainstream (e.g., acupuncture and traditional massage therapy), other Eastern modalities may be lucrative in today's marketplace. These services may include Reiki, Shiatsu, deep-tissue or joint massage, reflexology, craniosacral therapy, acupressure, healing touch or vibrational modalities, magnet therapy, and light therapy. There is room to expand alternative treatments in urgent care centers as demand grows for more than traditional prescriptions for patient problems.

Orthopedic and Pain-Management Services

In a business model that incorporates orthopedic services and pain-management services, additional providers may include orthopedic, chiropractic, physiatry, or podiatry specialists within the urgent care center, as well as pain-management experts. Urgent care centers will become increasingly popular as patients are saddled with the direct costs of health care. Expensive emergency department care is no longer an option. Trauma-related disorders are among the top five most expensive medical conditions in the United States. Consider adding point-of-service acute and follow-up care, interventional and noninterventional pain management, or rehabilitation.

Chronic Pain–Management Services

For some, the suggestion of adding management services for chronic pain may be a tough one to consider because of the stigma attached to it in urgent care and emergency medical practice. The chronic use of opioids has escalated since the 1990s, costing the United States approximately $560 to $635 billion annually. The addition of providers who specialize in chronic pain management may contribute to alleviation of this problem. Often, patients are willing to pay out of pocket for addiction treatment because it so profoundly affects their lives. Help for these problems represents a much-needed community service but may also be a lucrative endeavor for the practice.

CONCLUSION

Your business is only as strong as its weakest link. When owners consider whether to add a new service or product line for an urgent care center, they often look only at the financial bottom line. The most important determinants of success, however, will be how well the new project becomes engaged with the entire organization, and the attitudes held by each person at the center. Appropriate strategy development begins by aligning the owner's vision and values with careful analysis of management and team structure, and involves promotion of high levels of collaboration as a key to overall success.

KEY POINTS

1. *Aligning vision and values*   You must first believe in your product or service line before you are able to sell it.
2. *Changing outlooks*   View your additional service as a separate business that is concurrently an integral part of the overall organization.
3. *Long-term viewpoint*   Beware of following the latest trend in service or product hype.
4. *Research and planning*   Spend time on market research and planning, and carefully consider state and federal regulations.
5. *Scalability*   Begin small but plan big. Make sure you have room to expand.
6. *Management structure*   Delineate carefully your key players.
7. *Financial structure*   Carefully examine start-up costs, the break-even point, and unique billing issues.

8. *Monthly performance reviews*   Share key data with all staff members on a regular basis and create new goals for success as needed.
9. *Cautious risk taking*   Understand that any new venture comes with risk, and plan accordingly.
10. *Celebrating success milestones*   Recognize and celebrate team efforts and organizational milestones on a frequent basis.

CHAPTER 44

Integrative Medicine

Marty Martin

INTEGRATIVE MEDICINE (IM), THE evolutionary movement of complementary and alternative medicine (CAM), is growing in popularity in all types of health-care settings. This chapter is one of the first explorations—if not *the* first—of how CAM services might be integrated into the urgent care setting. The Affordable Care Act has served as a catalyst for a focus not only on wellness and preventive health but also on alternative delivery models like accountable care organizations. This chapter outlines the view that CAM and IM should have their own place within all urgent care centers, and it highlights 10 urgent care centers across the United States that have made CAM part of their business models. Allow these illustrations to serve as inspiration, a basis for a best practice, or simply a demonstration of today's reality that CAM can be successfully incorporated into urgent care if we are willing to travel the more innovative route.

Before describing how such an integration can be undertaken, we must first define CAM. According to the National Center on Complementary and Alternative Medicine of the National Institutes of Health, CAM includes "...those medical systems, professions, practices, interventions, modalities, therapies, applications, theories, or claims that are currently not part of the dominant or conventional medical system."[1]

Specific CAM practices include natural products (most of which are regulated as *dietary supplements*); mind–body practices like yoga, tai chi, and meditation; manipulation and body-based medicine, including chiropractic and massage therapy; energy medicine (e.g., Reiki); and whole systems of healing like naturopathy, homeopathy, traditional Chinese medicine, and Ayurveda. But even if you do not provide any of these CAM modalities, your urgent care center can still embrace an IM perspective.

---

1 National Institutes of Health. Alternative Medicine. Expanding medical horizons: a report to the National Institutes of Health of alternative medical systems and practices in the United States. Washington DC: US Government Printing Office; 1994 [Publication No. 017-040-00053770].

INTEGRATING COMPLEMENTARY AND ALTERNATIVE MEDICINE INTO YOUR URGENT CARE CENTER

Providing specific modalities such as acupuncture or homeopathy in your center is one approach to employing CAM practices. There is another approach, however, one which dates back to George Engel's biopsychosocial model (1913–1999) of illness and disease and embraces tools such as assessment, treatment, and health promotion, the underlying core characteristics of CAM.

Business Plan

Views expressed about CAM often end up as ideological debates rather than attempts to see CAM from a business perspective. In the field of urgent care, as in any area of business, a good plan must address four basic questions:

- Is there a growing market for this service?
- Is there a way to make sustainable revenue from this service?
- Is there a way to differentiate your business from others in the same industry?
- Are there any risks to providing or not providing this service?

You may be surprised to learn that the answer is yes to all four questions, as illustrated in the following examples from actual urgent care centers. Use these questions as a guide, and allow your responses to help you make a strategic decision about whether including CAM in your center is the right thing to do.

Is There a Growing Market for This Service?

There is definitively a market for CAM services. Table 1 lists some facts about the CAM market that are of particular interest to the urgent care industry. To date, no study has determined the prevalence of CAM use specifically among patients who use urgent care centers. By extension, however, Gulla and Singer found that slightly more than half (56%) of emergency department (ED) patients have used CAM treatments, with the majority using massage, chiropractic services, and herbs. Given that half of ED patients have worked with CAM therapies, it is safe to assume that at least half of all urgent care center patients have also used CAM, particularly because of the lower level of acuity of urgent care compared with EDs.[2]

Ayers discusses the importance of targeting specific demographic groups in general and of serving middle- and upper-income families as an urgent care

---

2   Gulla J, Singer AJ. Use of alternative therapies among emergency department patients. *Ann Emerg Med*. 2000;33:226–8.

Table 1. CAM Market Facts

- Two-thirds (68%) of the US population has used CAM services within the past 12 months.[a,b]
- Women and highly educated individuals are more likely to use CAM.[b]
- Individuals with higher incomes are more likely to use CAM.[c]
- Americans spend more than $27 billion annually on CAM treatments, most of which are out-of-pocket expenses.[d]
- In a 12-month period, 38 million adults visited a CAM practitioner, totaling about 354 million visits.[e]

[a] MacLennan AH, Wilson DH, Taylor AW. The escalating cost and prevalence of alternative medicine. *Prev Med*. 2002;35:166–73.
[b] Ni H, Simile C, Hardy AM. Utilization of complementary and alternative medicine by United States adults: results from the 1999 National Health Interview Survey. *Med Care*. 2002;40:353–8.
[c] Wooton JC, Sparber A. Surveys of complementary and alternative medicine: Part I: General trends and demographic groups. *J Altern Complement Med*. 2001;76:251–3.
[d] Institute of Medicine of the National Academies. *Complementary and Alternative Medicine in the United States*. Washington DC: National Academies Press; 2005:35.
[e] Weider M. NCCAM 2007 CAM spending report: review, implications, and call for comments. *Natural Medicine Journal*. 2009;1:1–3.
CAM, complementary and alternative medicine.

---

center operator. Oddly enough, the demographics between CAM and urgent care overlap,[3] as shown in Table 1.

The psychology of individual health-consumer decision making and help-seeking behavior is the driver of these facts. Specifically, individuals increasingly value a more holistic orientation to their own health and well-being. In addition, they are more concerned about the short- and long-term side effects of all types of medication, in particular pain medication. Accordingly, in the "2010 Complementary and Alternative Medicine Survey of Hospitals: Summary of Results," jointly published by the Samueli Institute and Health Forum, CAM was shown to be used most often to treat back or neck pain and joint pain or stiffness.[4] The Miami Urgent Care Center Medical Clinic in Miami, Florida, recognizes this trend, as reflected by this message on their website: "Other treatment modalities used at Miami Urgent Care Clinic include physical therapy, massage therapy, and pain medication when needed."

This trend suggests that CAM approaches to pain management are the first, not the last, step in the treatment of pain in many cases.

3   Ayers A. Riches in the niches: target demographics for urgent care. 2011. Available from: http://www.alanayersurgentcare.com/Linked_Files/UCAOA_Targeted_Marketing_2011_07_04.pdf. Accessed February 26, 2014.
4   Samueli Institute. 2010 Complementary and Alternative Medicine Survey of Hospitals. Alexandria, VA: Samueli Institute; 2011. Available from: http://www.samueliinstitute.org/file%20library/our%20research/ohe/cam_survey_2010_oct6.pdf. Accessed February 26, 2014.

UCR Health Centers in Chandler, Arizona, offer not only urgent care, occupational medicine, and rehabilitation services but also chiropractic care, acupuncture, and medical massage therapy, presenting a good example of how urgent care can reach out to specific demographic groups. Recognition of this growing market segment can also be seen in the way centers are implementing their intake processes, such as the Integrative Medicine Assessment Questions tool used at Lake Oconee Urgent & Specialty Care Center in Georgia. Of note are the instructions to the assessment tool:

> Please read each question carefully and answer to the best of your abilities. It is our hope that these questions will help us better understand you; your mind, body, spirit, emotions, and your beliefs about illness and health. This assessment allows us to offer the best recommendations for your emotional, physical, spiritual, and intellectual wellbeing. Because at Lake Oconee Urgent Care our aim is to keep you healthy![5]

Clearly, there is a growing market for CAM, not only to promote health but also to treat illness and disease, including pain, anxiety, and depression. All three urgent care centers featured here thus far—Miami Urgent Care Center Medical Clinic, UCR Health Centers, and Lake Oconee Urgent & Specialty Care Center—are knowingly or unknowingly attracting the lifestyles of health and sustainability (LOHAS) market. In a *New York Times* article in 2003, Amy Cortese described this market as "…a growing opportunity for products and services that appeal to a certain type of consumer."[6] Cortese further tied the LOHAS market to "cultural creatives," meaning that segment in Western society that has, according to sociologist Paul H. Ray and psychologist Sherry Ruth Anderson (in their book *The Cultural Creatives: How 50 Million People Are Changing the World*, Three Rivers Press), developed beyond standard paradigms of "Modernists or Progressives versus Traditionalists or Conservatives." Ray and Anderson claim that as of 2000, this group of adult Americans was 50 million strong, and Astin has found that cultural creatives are more likely to use CAM.[7]

The LOHAS CAM market, including the niches of personal health and integrative health care, is currently estimated to represent $117 billion, and its market size is estimated at between 13% and 19% of the US adult population.[8]

Of course, urgent care centers are not necessarily located in areas with high concentrations of highly educated women in higher socioeconomic groups

---

5   Lake Oconee Urgent & Specialty Care Center. Integrative medicine assessment questions. © 2011. Eatonton, GA: Lake Oconee Urgent & Specialty Care Center. http://lakeoconeeurgentcare.com/forms/LakeOconee_IntegrativeMed_assessment.pdf. Accessed February 26, 2014.
6   Cortese A. They care about the world (and they shop, too). *New York Times*. July 20, 2003. Available from: http://lib.store.yahoo.net/lib/underthecanopy/NYTLOHAS.pdf. Accessed February 26, 2014.
7   Astin JA. Why patients use alternative medicine: results of a national study. *JAMA*. 1998;279:1548–53.
8   LOHAS online. About. © 2010 Lohas. Louisville, CO: LOHAS Forum. Available from: http://www.lohas.com/about. Accessed February 26, 2014.

who likely embrace the LOHAS and culturally creative lifestyle. CAM integration may still be a good option, however, even in urban settings where the profile may be at the other end of the spectrum. In fact, in 2004 Rolniak and colleagues found that almost half (47%) of urban ED patients were using CAM, and that the four top modalities of choice (in order) were prayer, spirituality, music therapy, and meditation.[9] The answer to our question of whether there is a growing market for CAM, therefore, is that it is not only growing but is also becoming more and more socioeconomically and demographically diverse.

First-mover advantage is a concept emphasized in strategic marketing. If you are one of the first to recognize and meet the needs of an emerging market, then you stand to benefit so long as that market is sustainable. If traditional urgent care centers stay still and wait, they run the risk of being forced to imitate other first movers. One example is Seattle Homeopathy, a center with two locations, in Seattle and Bellevue, Washington, run by Jennifer White, ND, CCH, FHANP. White describes her business as "naturopathic and homeopathic," but also as one that addresses acute problems and urgent care needs, as follows: "For 24/7 acute/urgent homeopathic or naturopathic care, call the doctor at (206) 854-8111. There is a $30 minimum charge for the acute/urgent care phone. After the first five minutes, $2/minute will be charged."

Seattle Homeopathy is operated by a naturopathic physician, not a medical doctor or a doctor of osteopathy, proving that licensed CAM practitioners from professions other than allopathic and osteopathic medicine are now entering the urgent care business, and there is no indication that this trend will stop. Is your urgent care practice growing with this market?

Is There a Way to Make Sustainable Revenue From This Service?

The goal of any business is to generate a profit. In 1993, Eisenberg and colleagues found that nearly half of the US population (42%) spent $27 billion out of pocket on CAM services.[10] Furthermore, US adults spent nearly $34 billion out-of-pocket dollars on CAM in 2007, accounting for 1.5% of the total US health-care expenditures and 11.2% of the total out-of-pocket health expenditures. Of these out-of-pocket CAM dollars, one-third, or $11.9 billion, was spent on visits to CAM practitioners.[11] Premier Urgent Care Center in Melbourne, Florida, is taking advantage of this market with transparent pricing of its massage therapy services, priced at $25 for a 30-minute visit and $45 for a 60-minute visit. The center also offers gift certificates.

Given that the vast majority of individuals who use CAM pay cash, this revenue stream is more predictable, depending on the pricing and overhead models

9 Rolniak S, Browning L, MacLeod BA, Cockley P. Complementary and alternative medicine use among urban ED patients: prevalence and patterns. *J Emerg Nurs.* 2004;30:318–24.
10 Eisenberg DM, Kessler RC, Foster C, et al. Unconventional medicine in the United States—prevalence, costs, and patterns of use. *N Engl J Med.* 1993;328:264–52.
11 Nahin R, Dahlhamer J, Stussman B. Health need and the use of alternative medicine among adults who do not use conventional medicine. *BMC Health Serv Res.* 2010;10:220.

of your urgent care center. For example, a basic exam performed by a naturopathic physician in Portland, Oregon, at Renewal Centers Urgent Care is priced at $75. Among acupuncturists, it is not uncommon for a single acupuncturist to work with two patients at the same time in two different rooms in a staggered fashion, creating a concrete opportunity to increase revenue by increasing productivity. The Healthy Rewards programs of the health-care insurer Cigna have also made strides in this direction, offering coverage for CAM using affinity and discount initiatives. Alternative medicine is one of the covered services under this program, and is described as follows:

> Healthy Rewards is a discount program. Some Healthy Rewards programs are not available in all states. If your CIGNA plan includes coverage for any of these services, this program is in addition to, not instead of, your plan benefits. Healthy Rewards programs are separate from your medical benefits. A discount program is NOT insurance, and the member must pay the entire discounted charge.[12]

Discount programs offered by most of the major health insurance plans allow participating providers to attract more patients and benefit financially by receiving payment in cash.

In 2005, updates to the Current Procedural Terminology (CPT) were made, including the following codes for acupuncture:

- *97810*   Acupuncture, one or more needles, without electrical stimulation, initial 15 minutes of personal one-on-one contact with the patient
- *97811*   Each additional 15 minutes of personal one-on-one contact with the patient, with reinsertion of needles
- *97813*   Acupuncture, one or more needles, with electrical stimulation, initial 15 minutes of personal one-on-one contact with the patient
- *97814*   Each additional 15 minutes of personal one-on-one contact with the patient, with reinsertion of needles

In summary, CAM represents another source of primarily cash revenue.

Is There a Way to Differentiate Your Business From Others in the Same Industry?

The three basic competitive strategies for any business are low cost, differentiation, and niche.

Integrating CAM within an urgent care center is a move that reflects one type of differentiation strategy. The key message in targeting specific demographics to

---

12   Cigna. Improving health has many rewards. Bloomfield, CT: Cigna. © 2012 Cigna. Available from: http://www.cigna.com/sites/prudential/pdf/2013prudentialHealthyRewards.pdf. Accessed February 26, 2014.

support this strategy is that your urgent care center is distinct from others in a way that the individuals in those groups will value.

To adopt such a differentiation approach, you must first make the decision to provide CAM services for those seeking wellness and health promotion or those seeking CAM as part of their treatment regimen for disease or illness (or both groups). Davis et al found that nearly one-third (27.4%) of individuals who use CAM do so for wellness and health promotion and nearly one-fifth (17.4%) use CAM as a treatment modality.[13] Again, Premier Urgent Care Center in Melbourne is a good example of a facility that has initiated a differentiation strategy by opening its Premier Back Center, staffed by both a chiropractor and a licensed massage therapist. Their services are described as follows on their website:

> For both your Chiropractic care and Massage Therapy, you will be treated in our spa-like atmosphere, surrounded by therapeutic sounds and scents, which promote relaxation and healing.[14]

It is evident by this description that Premier Urgent Care Center is seeking to differentiate itself by appealing to individuals interested in wellness and health promotion in combination with a uniquely tailored treatment approach.

Another example is Bozeman Urgent Care Center in Bozeman, Montana. Staffed by a naturopathic physician, the center both differentiates and positions itself as a family-care and primary-care facility, as indicated on its website:

> We offer the same services as a family or primary care physician. To help us provide this service we offer general medical care, occupational medicine, labs, school and sports physicals, and limited on site non-medicinal prescriptions. The Bozeman Holistic Urgent Care is especially convenient when you cannot wait for an appointment, or your doctor is on vacation.[15]

A more discreet way to differentiate your center from competing urgent care centers is by highlighting the credentials of your clinical team as opposed to your services and products. For instance, Dr. Clarice Moussalli's biographic profile on the website of Sentara Healthcare in Williamsburg, Virginia, showcases the fact that this physician is double-boarded in emergency medicine and integrated holistic medicine.[16]

Yet another approach to differentiate your urgent care center without providing CAM services is to adopt the approach of Carolinas HealthCare System

---

13   Davis MA, West AN, Weeks WB, Sirovich BE. Health behaviors and utilization among users of complementary and alternative medicine for treatment versus health promotion. *Health Serv Res.* 2011;46:1402–16.

14   Premier Urgent Care. Premier Back Center. Melbourne, FL: Premier Urgent Care. © 2012 Premier Urgent Care. Available from: http://premierurgentcare.com/chiropractic/. Accessed February 26, 2014.

15   Available from: http://www.bozemanurgentcare.com/.

16   Sentara Healthcare. Physician profile: Clarice Moussalli, MD. Williamsburg, VA: Sentara HealthCare. ©2014 Sentara Healthcare. Available from: http://www.sentara.com/Doctors/Urgent-Care-Physician-Clarice-Moussalli-MD/Doctor-ID/467637. Accessed February 26, 2014.

Urgent Care in the Charlotte, North Carolina, metropolitan area. When this book was written, the center provided free access to educational materials in its "101 Complementary and Alternative Medicine" article collection. The content, consisting of articles like "What Is Homeopathy?" was developed and disseminated by Healthwise, a patient education company. Sarah Holdon, author of "Urgent Care Centers," an article appearing in the *Lehigh Valley Marketplace*, writes, "A few [centers] even offer massage therapy or chiropractic care."[17] In this article, Holdon profiled Coordinated Health in Bethlehem, Pennsylvania. A visit to Coordinated Health's website showcases a smoking cessation program and massage therapy services as well as treatment for anxiety and depression.[18]

All of these approaches are good ways to begin your entry into the CAM market, even if your center is not quite ready to begin offering direct-care services to patients. In brief, CAM is a wise way to differentiate your urgent care center from your competitors' centers.

Are There Any Risks to Providing or Not Providing This Service?

The focus on patient safety and quality will continue in all settings, including those in urgent care. Thus providers need to know what CAM therapies patients have used, so that they can obtain comprehensive medical histories and conduct thorough physical examinations. In far too many cases, patients and providers adopt a "don't ask, don't tell" approach to CAM use. This lack of both telling and asking about CAM use has potential complications, including those that arise from side effects and herb–drug interactions.[19] To avoid this possibility and minimize risk, be sure to include questions about CAM use in all forms to be completed by patients and as a routine part of your assessments.

INTEGRATING COMPLEMENTARY AND ALTERNATIVE MEDICINE: TWO STRATEGIES

Addressing each of the four questions in the preceding section may cause you to reach one of the following conclusions:

- ▶ CAM does not fit within your existing business model.

- ▶ More information is required before you can make the decision about integrating CAM into your existing model, while being wary of the "analysis paralysis" trap.

- ▶ CAM is currently in alignment with your existing business model.

---

17 Hodon S. Urgent care centers. *Lehigh Valley Marketplace*. Available from: http://www.lehighvalleymarketplace.com/departments/health-watch/urgent-care-centers/. Accessed February 26, 2014.
18 Coordinated Health. Rehabilitation services. Bethlehem, PA. Available from: http://www.coordinatedhealth.com/Services/Rehabilitation/Rehabilitation-Services.aspx. Accessed February 26, 2014.
19 Rogers EA, Gough JE, Brewer KL. Are emergency department patients at risk for drug-herb interactions? *Acad Emerg Med*. 2001;8:932–4.

Assuming you reach the third conclusion—that CAM is aligned with your business model—you are now ready to explore two strategies for integrating CAM into your urgent care center. The first way to integrate CAM into your facility is through the provision of clinical care. The second method is through the payment for CAM services rendered.

Provision of Clinical Care: The Complementary and Alternative Medicine Connection

Because it has already been established through the business planning process that there is a growing market for CAM and that you can differentiate your urgent care center by providing CAM services, we will focus on those specific modalities that are likely to meet the needs of your patients. Dillard and Knapp reported that pain is one of the more common complaints among ED patients and urgent care patients. The researchers, therefore, made the following recommendation to integrate CAM when working with patients complaining of pain:

> Adding nondrug therapies of physical therapy, cognitive-behavioral therapy, TENS, hypnosis, biofeedback, psychoanalysis, and others can complete the conventional picture. Armed with understanding of pain dynamics and treatments, practitioners can better meet patient needs, avoid serious side effects, and improve care when addressing pain management in the emergency department.[20]

In addition to the specific services you offer, the environment of your center has a clinical impact on your patients and a customer service impact on those waiting in the waiting room. Your facilities should be designed in such a way that *positive distraction*, or what is called an optimal healing environment, is built in. Ulrich has listed many ways to promote positive distractions, including but not limited to caring, laughter, natural views, smiling human faces, and even animals.[21] Natural views are particularly powerful not only because they enhance the patient's waiting-room experience but also because they boost the staff's overall job satisfaction, as evidenced by lowered self-reported stress and improved health status.[22] The benefits of purposeful environmental design are too many and varied to list here—or for you to ignore. If for some reason your facility is without building options, then decorate with natural art or art that meets these criteria from Schweitzer et al: "All visual art (paintings, prints, photographs) displayed in patient areas should have unambiguously positive subject matter and convey a sense of security and safety."[23]

---

20 Dillard JN, Knapp S. Complementary and alternative pain therapy in the emergency department. *Emerg Med Clin North Am.* 2005;23:529–49.
21 Ulrich RS. Effects of gardens on health outcomes: theory and research. In: Marcus CC, Barnes M, eds. *Healing Gardens: Therapeutic Benefits and Design Recommendations.* New York: John Wiley & Sons, 1999;27–86.
22 Leather P, Pyrgas M, Beale D, Lawrence C. Windows in the workplace: sunlight, view, and occupational stress. *Environment and Behavior.* 1997;30:739–62.
23 Schweitzer M, Gilpin L, Frampton S. Healing spaces: elements of environmental design that make an impact on health. *J Altern Complement Med.* 2004;10(Suppl 1):S71–83.

The bottom line is that attention to your center's physical plan is more than a facilities management decision; it is also a clinical one, as demonstrated by Ulrich: "…[I]t is encouraging that the report indicated that an impressively high percentage (80%) of the most rigorous studies found positive links between environmental characteristics and patient health outcomes."[24]

For those patients presenting with pain while they are waiting to be seen by a provider, researchers recommend offering simple comfort measures, such as positioning options, a warm blanket, yoga, music, massage, imagery, and breathing techniques.[25] Interventions like these have two benefits: reducing pain in a way that meets the Joint Commission accreditation guidelines and achieving enhanced customer service and offering the patient a way to be more relaxed when it is time to interact with the provider in the examination or procedure room. A viable urgent care center must offer services that meet the needs of a growing patient base but do it in a way that the center does more than break even. The goal? To generate a sustainable profit.

Payment for Complementary and Alternative Medicine Services: The Cash Connection

Most patients pay for CAM with cash. Cash business is good for cash flow and tends to make income statements healthier, assuming that expenses do not exceed income. Rarely, CAM treatments are covered by the patient's health insurance, generally as part of a large self-insured employer's discount program. Health Net of California, Inc. is an example of one of the relatively few health insurance companies that cover acupuncture and chiropractic services, including "…emergencies and urgent care visits and referral visits to non-participating acupuncturists."[26]

One of the more successful CAM health plans is American Specialty Health Incorporated, founded in 1987. It had $183 million in revenue in 2011. It has more than 900 employees and serves more than 18 million members in its benefit programs, 91 million in its discount program, 5.5 million in its prevention and wellness program, and 1.2 million in its fitness and exercise programs. From the provider side, nearly 28,000 CAM practitioners are part of the plan's network.

If your urgent care centers see workers' compensation and Medicaid patients, check with your state about reimbursement for CAM. Washington State, for example, mandates that all health insurance plans include naturopathic physicians as primary-care providers.

---

24 Ulrich RS. Evidence based environmental design for improving medical outcomes. Proceedings of the Healing by Design: Building for Health Care in the 21st Century Conference. Montreal, Quebec, Canada, March 1–10, 2000.
25 Hogan SL. Patient satisfaction with pain management in the emergency department. *Top Emerg Med*. 2005;27:284–94.
26 Health Net. Health Net's starting line-up (SLU) portfolio. 2010 benefit grids. Available from: http://www.rbgsocal.com/MIDSIZE_Quote/MM_Plan_Guides/HN%20SLU%20benefitgrids_broker%202010.pdf. Accessed February 26, 2014.

The Affordable Care Act forbids health insurance providers from discriminating "…against any health care provider who is acting within the scope of that provider's license or certification under applicable State law."[27] This provides a historic opportunity to consider whether and how CAM should be broadly integrated into US health insurance plans.

FROM STRATEGIC DECISION TO STRATEGIC IMPLEMENTATION

The case has been made that the integration of CAM into health-care settings, both inpatient and outpatient, is a movement that is here to stay and ever-evolving. Given its retail orientation, it seems only natural that CAM will be integrated into urgent care settings as a way to address the clinical challenges confronting such centers, as well as to offer services in a way that meets or exceeds the changing expectations and demands of patients. To begin or strengthen the integration of CAM in your urgent care center, follow these six strategic recommendations:

- ▶ Administer a survey among your providers, staff members, patients, and referral sources to determine the frequency with which these four stakeholder groups currently use CAM.
- ▶ On the basis of the survey results, conduct a gap analysis exposing how far what you currently offer is from what your stakeholders are currently using.
- ▶ On the basis of the gap analysis, formulate concrete plans to close the gap by providing education and training and developing policies and procedures to make sure that the gap remains closed.
- ▶ Consider in your facility's planning efforts how to create an optimal healing environment that recognizes the benefits for your patients, their families, and your team.
- ▶ Decide whether offering CAM is a point of differentiation within the market that you can leverage to attract more patients, referral sources, and high-quality talent to work in your urgent care center.
- ▶ Reflect on whether offering CAM fits with the personal and professional belief system of your center's board and senior leadership, and then whether it is aligned with the center's vision, mission, and strategies.

KEY POINTS

1. On a global level, far more individuals use CAM and IM than conventional medicine.
2. Most patients use both CAM or IM and conventional medicine.

---

27 42 US Code § 300gg-5, Non-discrimination in health care, section 27062010.

3. Insurance companies are increasingly covering CAM and IM services.
4. Not all conventional medical procedures are based on randomized controlled trials. Therefore, what is the rationale for holding CAM and IM services to a different standard?
5. Consumers are demanding that health-care organizations offer CAM and IM services.
6. Consumers are willing to pay cash for CAM and IM services.
7. Consumers are seeking a holistic orientation to treatment.
8. Urgent care centers can differentiate themselves from competitors by offering CAM and IM services.
9. Urgent care centers should assess CAM and IM use and interest among their current and prospective patients.
10. Urgent care centers should consider incorporating CAM and IM services into their own worksite health-promotion programs to increase retention, enhance performance, and improve the health status of the physicians as well as employees.

CHAPTER 45

Pediatric Urgent Care

Gary Gerlacher

A TEARFUL CAREGIVER WALKS INTO the clinic at 9:00 PM carrying a bleeding 5-year-old with a chin laceration, and you are the only provider available. Either your heart rate increases and you feel nauseated with dread or you are thinking about the most effective way to calm the caregiver and child and to repair the laceration with no more tears. If your plan is just to restrain the child and repair the laceration while the child screams, you are practicing medicine. If your plan is to engage the patient, to help the child talk about anything other than the injury, and to repair it while the child sits on the caregiver's lap laughing, then you are practicing pediatric urgent care.

Like all of the practice of medicine, pediatric urgent care is an art form that requires the right combination of resources and skills to perform effectively. Infants cannot talk; toddlers do not cooperate; grade-school kids will not quietly sit still; and teenagers will not acknowledge your existence, because they already know everything. Every child is different, and you have no idea when you walk into the room if the child will be cooperative, disruptive, terrified, endearing, indifferent, or hyperactive. To succeed in pediatric urgent care you must be able to adapt your skills quickly to whatever state of chaos your patient presents.

The patient is only half of your problem. You also have to treat the caregivers. Unlike adult patients, who are usually able to understand and explain their problems, children rely on caregivers to provide a medical history. The fears and concerns of caregivers (Will my child have brain damage from a concussion?) are different from the fears of the child (Will I miss *SpongeBob SquarePants* tonight?). In addition to diagnosing and treating the child correctly with as little drama as possible, you must understand and address the fears and concerns of caregivers.

If it sounds like treating children is more complicated than treating adults in some ways, you are correct. So why bother? Moving beyond the obvious rewards of helping children feel better and caregivers sleep soundly, you have an enormous business opportunity in pediatric urgent care. Each of the 75 million children in the United States is a certified germ-dispersal unit, coughing, sneezing, nose-picking, spitting, and vomiting multiple times per year. School-age children tend to be sick several times per year, whereas most adults are sick only occasionally. To these millions, add visits for injuries, when courageous children decide to challenge the laws of gravity. When you include consultations for caregiver concerns about potential problems or questions, pediatric urgent care includes hundreds of millions of visits per year.

Currently in the United States, approximately 9,000 urgent care clinics see both adult and pediatric patients. These clinics vary in their comfort levels with pediatrics, which is based on the health-care providers' training. Generally, the comfort of the provider with delivering care decreases with the age of the patient. Some clinics even refuse to treat patients below a certain age. In this void, fewer than 300 pediatric urgent care clinics have emerged in the United States. Generally, these clinics see patients up to age 18 and are usually staffed by a pediatrician. The use of pediatric nurse practitioners as either primary or secondary providers is increasing in popularity. What sets these clinics apart is their commitment to providing not only high-quality medical care for children but also an environment comfortable for the child, reflecting a commitment to ensuring that the experience of the visit meets the expectations of families. If you are involved in the operation of any urgent care center, pediatric patients will be a significant percentage of your business. How you treat children and their families will ultimately determine the clinic's level of success.

PEDIATRIC URGENT CARE MODEL

Exclusively pediatric urgent care clinics in the United States have some unique features compared to the general urgent care model. Most pediatric urgent care centers are open only in the evenings during the week and during the day on weekends. Very few pediatric centers are open during traditional working hours, because kids are in school or day care, and if they are sick, many of them have access to their pediatricians during these regular hours. Most of the models complement the hours of local pediatricians rather than compete with them. General urgent care clinics can supplement income during daytime hours with preemployment screening, drug testing, workers' compensation cases, and even rehabilitation for injuries in some cases. None of these services are available for pediatric urgent care clinics to supplement income during the day. Most pediatric urgent care centers are staffed full time with a pediatrician, although the use of pediatric nurse practitioners is becoming more popular. The pediatric urgent care clinic is also more likely than a general urgent care to have a registered nurse (as opposed to a medical assistant or technician) delivering care, because of the complexities of evaluating and caring for patients of different ages.

With the exception of flu shots, very few pediatric urgent care clinics provide vaccinations. Most owners believe in the importance of each child having a medical home with comprehensive well-child care. With the complexity of the current vaccine schedule, the cost of inventory and storage of the vaccines, and the increasing number of families on alternative vaccine schedules, the administration of vaccines in a pediatric urgent care center is neither good medicine nor good business practice.

Most importantly, 100% of staff members should be comfortable treating children. It does not matter how much clinical experience or education a person has if they do not enjoy working with pediatric patients. When interviewing potential employees, consider attitude and personality more than work experience. You can teach them skills, but it is hard to change someone's personality. An energetic, inexperienced employee with a great attitude about kids is more likely to become a star employee than an experienced employee with a chronically bad attitude. Your staff will create the culture of your business—make sure it is a kid-friendly culture.

DESIGN AND SUPPLIES

Kids are not big fans of visiting any medical office. They fear shots and other painful procedures. A child who walks into a new place will instantly decide if it is a fun place or a scary place. This initial impression sets the tone for the remainder of the visit. If a child can walk into the clinic and see an area with toys, books, murals, and a familiar TV show in the waiting room, it will feel like a comfortable and familiar environment. Most children try to break away from their caregivers and head straight for the play area. Although space is at a premium in retail medicine, everyone has to have a waiting room. Dedicating an area of the waiting room to a child-friendly experience will help set a positive tone for the visit. In any urgent care clinic, all public spaces should be kid-friendly. Remember that kids spend the majority of their time looking at the world from a height of less than 4 feet. A few murals placed low on the walls may not be very noticeable to the adults but will make a world of difference to the children. Design considerations include your staff members' uniforms. Colorful T-shirts with friendly logos or bright scrubs are much less intimidating than button-down shirts and slacks. And though you may like the way you look in a white coat, I can assure you that the pediatric patient does not feel the same way.

When designing a clinic for children, remember two rules: If they see it, they will try to pick it up; and if it can break, they will break it. There is no way to slow the fundamental force of childhood curiosity, so design your clinics with these rules in mind to increase the safety of the clinic for your pediatric patients, as well as to decrease your repair and replacement costs.

Have nothing below a height of 4 feet in the exam rooms, other than the seat and exam table. Exam rooms in the clinic should have built-in beds that are lower than a traditional hospital bed, as well as a seat attached that the child can use to climb up and down into the bed safely. The bed should be positioned so that the child can be seen from the hallway when the door is open. All of the trash cans should be in closed, lockable cabinets with holes at the top to dispose of trash, to avoid awkward moments like a 3-year-old digging through the trash to see what brand of diaper the previous patient was wearing.

The TV should be mounted high on the wall where only an adult can reach it, although kids will try to form a human pyramid to reach the controls despite the presence of a remote on the counter. Make sure the TV is tuned to an appropriate channel, and remember that many of the cartoon channels change to adult themes at night. Provide a convenient channel guide for the caregivers, remembering that the family or other caregivers may choose to watch sports or news instead of cartoons. Lighting should be subtle, with the ability to dim the lights if a child wants to rest while receiving intravenous fluids or breathing treatments.

Some fixtures in traditional exam rooms should not be included in pediatric rooms. Sinks should be in common areas of the halls, with hand sanitizer in every room. A child in a small room with a sink will eventually play in it and design a new version of the Bellagio fountains right there in your exam room. Although most caregivers discourage these activities, a surprising number do not mind the small floods their children create. Sinks in exam rooms are expensive, occupy valuable space, and can create a huge mess with children around.

Keep very little equipment in the exam rooms. Cabinets should contain basic supplies for wound care and vomit cleanup, ear speculums, and tongue blades. Instead of leaving an otoscope and ophthalmoscope in the room, providers should carry one to each room and recharge them, between visits with patients, in the physicians' area. It does not matter how high you mount the otoscope on the wall—the kids will eventually get to it.

Children like to wander and explore, so all entrances and exits should be easily visible to staff members to prevent kids from slipping outside unnoticed. And staff members should always have a clear view of the waiting room. If a child seizes, vomits, or develops respiratory distress, they should immediately be able to identify the problem and aid the family.

Finally, many caregivers forget the diaper bag in a rush to bring their child to the clinic. A supply of wipes and diapers in all sizes as well as Pedialyte and formula should be readily available for caregivers. Keep crackers and juice boxes available for older children as well.

CUSTOMER SERVICE

Customer service is one of the most important determinants of success in any retail medicine endeavor, but especially in pediatric urgent care. In theory, every clinic should be able to diagnose and prescribe the correct medicine for a child with strep throat. Getting the diagnosis and treatment correct is the purpose of the business, but doing so does not earn bonus points with patients. They expect you to get it right every time. To gain loyalty, focus not only on what you are doing but also on how you do it. You have experienced great customer service in retail settings, where the staff went above and beyond to meet your needs. There is no reason why your staff should not provide the same experience for your patients.

In pediatric urgent care, service focused on the child should begin the moment they enter the door. Have you ever watched a caregiver get a sick kid, a 3-year-old, and a newborn situated in a clinic and fill out paperwork? It should be an Olympic sport. To solve these difficulties, the position of a greeter can be created. A greeter is usually a high school student who works full time in the waiting room and welcomes people to the clinic. The greeter helps families get through the door and check in, distracts children while the caregiver completes paperwork, and helps them in any way they need. Kids need juice boxes? The caregiver needs someone to watch a child while the adult goes to the restroom? Need a TV channel changed? Need a diaper? Need help carrying the kids back to the car? A small financial investment in a greeter tells caregivers that your clinic focuses on meeting their needs on their schedule.

The next step is how to address the child. Most caregivers write the formal name on the paperwork (Charles), but not what the child prefers to be called (Chuck). Frequently, children are called by their given name only when they are in trouble: "Charles! Were you playing with Super Glue and the cat again?" If you spend the next 10 minutes calling him Charles, he is going to think he is in big trouble. If the child is old enough, simply ask them what they like to be called. If not, check with the caregivers. Make sure to document the correct name on the chart so that other staff members can address the child correctly during the visit and through any follow-up phone calls.

Engage the child in something that has nothing to do with medicine. Ask how old they are, what grade they are in, what job they will have when they grow up, or who their favorite sports star is. Ask questions they know the answers to and are comfortable talking about to engage them. Once they are comfortable talking with you about sports, talking with you about medicine will not be as scary. If they are holding a stuffed animal, ask the child to tell you the name and story behind the animal. Almost every child will talk incessantly about their favorite animal. Finally, seal the friendship by asking them for a high five or knuckles. Once they have made the initial physical contact of a high five, it is not as scary to have a stethoscope or otoscope touch them. I go for a high five or knuckles on every patient old enough to understand the idea.

For the history, always clarify who all of the adults are in the room. Never assume that a man and a woman in the room are the parents. Most of the time parents are there, but occasionally aunts, uncles, stepparents, ex-wives and ex-husbands, or the worst possible combination—dad, current girlfriend, and ex-wife—arrives. Get the information accurately from the primary caregiver and avoid any distracting drama. The visit is about the child, and the adults can work on their issues on their own time. Occasionally, a friendly reminder of this fact is necessary to refocus the adults.

For the pediatric exam, distraction and comfort are the best allies. If the patient is nervous, ask the child to sit on a caregiver's lap. Try to get them talking about something, reading a book with a caregiver, or watching TV. Focus them on anything but you. Move slowly, and let them know what you are doing at each step. Do the simple things first, such as listening to the heart and lungs, and save the ears and throat for last. Involve the child throughout the exam. If the child is nervous, have them look for treasure in your ear with the otoscope before you look in the child's ear for treasure. In the majority of cases, if you make the exam interactive and converse with the child it can be a positive experience for them.

Remember to gain as much information as possible by observation before you approach the child.

Children are more likely than adults to be seen early on in an illness. Even though a caregiver might suffer at home with flu for 5 days before making an appointment for themselves, the same caregiver will bring their child to a clinic 5 minutes after the onset of fever. I always warn the caregivers that the child will do one of three things over the next 24 hours: improve, stay the same, or worsen. Although only two of these outcomes are acceptable, it is important to remind the caregiver that the child's condition may worsen and that the plan for follow-up may change. Many of these children who present early on may fall in the category of initially well but brought in by worried caregivers, but will develop worsening symptoms over the next day. Good communication with caregivers is essential to prevent their anger when the child's condition worsens.

Discharge is an important aspect of the visit in terms of customer satisfaction. All of the work examining and diagnosing the child correctly is useless if the caregiver does not understand or agree with the treatment plan. Take time to explain everything and answer every question. Never let a caregiver look confused or upset and leave the clinic with unanswered questions. One mother became tearful when I explained that her child had bronchitis and needed an antibiotic. Reluctant to talk about it until pressed on the issue, she finally revealed that her niece had recently been given an initial diagnosis of bronchitis, only to find out a few days later that she had leukemia. The tearful mom was concerned that her child might have leukemia too. We talked about it, and I answered all of her questions. Instead of spending a sleepless night worrying about childhood cancer, the mom headed home with a smile. Remember that an upset caregiver can wield the power of Facebook, Twitter, and message boards to share a bad experience at your clinic with thousands of people before leaving the parking lot. Answer the caregiver's questions and address their concerns appropriately, and they can positively advertise your clinic to those same thousands.

Make sure that your health-care providers and staff members exude confidence when speaking with caregivers. Pediatric urgent care is as much about reassuring the caregivers as it is about diagnosing diseases and treating the children. Listen to what caregivers have to say about your business. Although their feedback can be crazy at times ("You should have a separate waiting room for every child"), many of their ideas are easily implemented improvements. Many of the best ideas, including the position of a greeter discussed earlier, come from caregiver feedback on surveys.

Finally, no pediatric urgent care discharge is complete without stickers, lollipops, and flavored-ice treats. Each child may not need all three, but have them in the clinic. There is nothing better than seeing kids who arrived in tears laugh as they excitedly sort through the sticker basket to find just the right one. These small amenities cost pennies but mean much more to the children and ultimately to the caregivers, who appreciate anything that makes their kids smile again.

SAFETY

Patients' safety is always a priority, and pediatric patients require special considerations. Although adults have a wide range of weights, most of the dosing for medications is standard for any adult. For pediatric patients, dosages can vary by a factor of 10 depending on weight. Correct dosage of medication begins with an accurate weight, which should be documented on the chart in kilograms. In addition to a normal adult scale, the clinic should have an appropriate-size scale to weigh infants and toddlers. Unless you are unable to weigh a patient because of injury, do not accept a caregiver's word on how much the patient weighs. In winter, the staff members should ask caregivers to remove the child's coat, boots, and scarf before the child is weighed. Clothing can double the weight of some pediatric patients. Keep a simple chart for converting kilograms to pounds available for caregivers, but never document a weight in pounds on the chart.

Most pediatric medications are dosed on a milligram-per-kilogram basis. Providers should write the dosage in milligrams only, and staff members should administer the medication only after confirmation that the dose is within an appropriate range of milligrams per kilogram. Staff members should never administer a medicine with an order based on volume, such as 1 teaspoon of Benadryl. Most—but not all—concentrations are standardized. This has been particularly problematic when dosing Tylenol. In general, oral orders should be avoided because they make it more likely that there will be a mistake.

Keep only one concentration of each medicine on hand when possible. If you have ceftriaxone (Rocephin) in 250-mg, 500-mg, and 1000-mg concentrations, the likelihood of a reconstitution error increases. Oral steroids can be similarly problematic, because some health-care providers prefer Orapred (15 mg/5 mL) and some want Veripred (20 mg/mL). To decrease the possibility of medication errors, choose one as the only oral steroid liquid in the clinic.

Discharge prescriptions are another area where mistakes can be made, especially during a busy shift with pressure to discharge patients quickly. Many discharge software and electronic health record systems are programmed to warn the provider if the dose is outside the recommended range for the patient's weight. A chart with all of the common antibiotics detailing the dosages by each 5-kg increment in patient weight is a handy reference for the provider writing the prescription, and the discharging staff can double-check the written prescription against the chart. Review the prescription with the caregiver. All of the work to get the prescription correct is wasted if the caregiver cannot understand the dosing instructions.

Desk staff members should be trained to recognize obvious signs of severe illness in arriving children. All nonmedical staff members should immediately be able to recognize the basic signs of respiratory distress (flaring, grunting, retractions, tachypnea) and of altered mental status, and should be trained to notify a nurse or other health-care provider if any of these symptoms is identified. Nonmedical personnel should know to notify the nurse or provider immediately of any high-risk situations, such as child abuse, neonatal fever, or significant bleeding. Desk staff members should look for these situations with every child who enters the clinic.

Another unfortunate but inevitable concern in pediatric urgent care is child neglect or intentional injury. Many of these children will be taken to urgent care centers or emergency departments as opposed to a regular provider, who is better positioned to notice patterns of abuse and neglect. These children may be brought into the clinic by the abuser or by another adult who may also be a victim of the abuser. Evaluate the medical history relative to the injury to decide whether the explanation makes sense. If the child is old enough, ask the patient how the injury occurred. If the child's story or presentation seems amiss, pursue it further. Remember that you are an advocate for your child patient. If you believe that the child has sustained an intentional injury, document the information, contact the proper authorities, and ensure that the child leaves to a safe environment. All 50 states in the United States have mandatory reporting laws for cases of suspected child abuse, and this information should be readily available to your staff members. When abuse is a possibility, the appropriate government agency and the child's pediatrician should be contacted, and the child should be transferred to a local children's hospital for further evaluation. Obtaining the detailed social history necessary to determine a safe disposition for the child is beyond the scope of an urgent care center. If there is any concern at all that the family members in the room may have been involved in the injury, notify emergency medical services (EMS) and the police to ensure that the child is safe during transport. Never leave a shift wondering if you should have done something more for that child.

EMERGENCY PREPAREDNESS

Hopefully, you will never need to open a crash cart for a pediatric patient, but if you are in business long enough, you will. The most important piece of emergency equipment is the phone. Make sure a staff member is dialing 911 if someone is opening the crash cart. Do not assume that the staff member has notified EMS in a panic situation. In most suburban areas, EMS will have a response time of less than 5 minutes to a clinic and you will have time for only the initial stabilization of the patient (airway, breathing, circulation [the ABCs]) in preparation for transport to a definitive treatment facility. In more rural settings, you must be prepared for prolonged resuscitation of the patient because of longer EMS response times.

An excellent resource is the American Academy of Pediatrics policy statement "Pediatric Care Recommendations for Freestanding Urgent Care Facilities."[1] The policy recommends emergency equipment and supplies for the clinic, and it clarifies the role of the health-care provider in a pediatric emergency. Table 1 outlines suggested emergency equipment and supplies, and Table 2 outlines the emergency medications your clinic should have available. This is the most definitive

---

1   American Academy of Pediatrics. Pediatric care recommendations for freestanding urgent care facilities. *Pediatrics.* 2005;116:258–60.

Table 1. Prioritizing Office Emergency Equipment and Supplies

Equipment and Supplies	Priority
Airway management	
• Bag-valve-mask (450 and 1000 mL)	E
• Clear oxygen masks, breather and nonrebreather, with reservoirs (infant, child, adult)	E
• Endotracheal tubes (uncuffed 2.5–5.5 mm; cuffed 6.0–8.0 mm)	S
• Esophageal intubation detector or end-tidal carbon dioxide detector	S
• Laryngoscope blades (straight 0–4; curved 2–3)	S
• Laryngoscope handle (pediatric, adult) with extra batteries, bulbs	S
• Magill forceps (pediatric, adult)	S
• Nasogastric tubes (sizes 6–14F)	S
• Nasopharyngeal airways (sizes 12–30F)	S
• Nebulizer (or metered-dose inhaler with spacer/mask)	E
• Oropharyngeal airways (sizes 00–5)	E
• Oxygen-delivery system	E
• Pulse oximeter	E
• Stylets (pediatric, adult)	S
• Suction catheters (sizes 5–16F) and Yankauer suction tip	S
• Suction device, tonsil tip, bulb syringe	E
Vascular access and fluid management	
• Arm boards, tape, tourniquet	S
• Automated external defibrillator with pediatric capabilities	E
• Butterfly needles (19- to 25-gauge)	S
• Cardiac arrest board/backboard	E
• Catheter-over-needle device (14- to 24-gauge)	S
• Color-coded tape or preprinted drug doses	E
• Heating source (overhead warmer/infrared lamp)	S
• Intraosseous needles (16-gauge, 18-gauge)	S
• Intravenous tubing, microdrip	S
Miscellaneous equipment and supplies	
• Sphygmomanometer (infant, child, adult, thigh cuffs)	E
• Splints, sterile dressings	E
• Spot glucose test	S
• Stiff neck collars (small/large)	S

E, essential; S, strongly suggested (essential if emergency medical services response time is >10 minutes).

Table 2. Office Emergency Drugs

Drugs and Fluids	Priority
Drugs	
• Activated charcoal	S
• Albuterol for inhalation[a]	E
• Antibiotics	S
• Anticonvulsants (diazepam, lorazepam)	S
• Atropine sulfate (0.1 mg/mL)	S
• Corticosteroids (parenteral/oral)	S
• Dextrose (25%)	S
• Diphenhydramine (parenteral, 50 mg/mL)	S
• Epinephrine (1:1000)	E
• Epinephrine (1:10,000)	S
• Naloxone (0.4 mg/mL)	S
• Oxygen	E
• Sodium bicarbonate (4.2%)	S
Fluids	
• 5% dextrose, 0.45 normal saline (500-mL bags)	S
• Normal saline solution or lactated Ringer's solution (500-mL bags)	S

[a]Metered-dose inhaler with spacer or mask may be substituted.
E, essential; S, strongly suggested (essential if emergency medical services response time is >10 minutes).

statement on the care of critically ill pediatric patients in urgent care settings, and anyone involved in urgent care should review the article.

The Broselow Pediatric Resuscitation System is another option to provide emergency pediatric equipment for your clinic. Equipment and medications are in packets that are color-coded according to the child's weight. Even if the weight is unknown, there is a Broselow tape color-coded to the correct patient equipment. The Broselow system is easy to use and well organized for an emergency. The complete package costs about $2000 and requires regular checking of medications for expiration and renewal.

Another excellent resource is smart phone applications for pediatric emergencies. Many are on the market, but I use palmPEDi (available for iOS and Android). The application costs $1.99, and with one touch on an entry for the patient's weight, standard medication dosages and equipment sizes are quickly accessible. Encourage providers to have a similar application on their phones, and hope that they never need to use it.

At a minimum, all health-care providers and staff members caring for children should be certified in Pediatric Advanced Life Support or take an equivalent course. Although this is not mandatory for desk personnel and greeters, it is still highly recommended that they take the course. I recommend that all nurses achieve certification via the Certified Pediatric Emergency Nurse exam as well. Trauma certifications such as Advanced Trauma Life Support focus on skills beyond the scope of urgent care centers and are generally not necessary for staff members to attain.

Regardless of the equipment you have in the clinic, nothing will work unless staff members know where the equipment is and how to use it. When there is downtime at the clinic, open the cart and go over the equipment and medications with staff members. Show them how equipment for an infant is markedly different from equipment for a 10-year-old child. Practice different scenarios with them to get them comfortable using the equipment on the cart. Make sure that batteries and expiration dates are checked regularly and all equipment is in working order. If you open the crash cart only during a true emergency, things are not going to go smoothly.

KEY POINTS

1. Patient safety comes first. Make sure your staff members have the right equipment, training, and resources to diagnose and treat pediatric patients effectively.

2. The physical environment of your clinic should be kid-friendly, with toys, books, stickers, and appropriate TV shows easily accessible.

3. The patient and the family will have different fears and concerns. To have a successful business, you must successfully communicate with both the patient and the family at the appropriate level.

4. Practice emergency procedures with your staff to maximize efficiency of care in stressful situations.

5. The pediatric urgent care market is a large potential opportunity for your business, generating hundreds of millions of visits nationally each year.

6. A greeter in your waiting room adds an extraordinary customer service advantage for a very small cost.

7. Customer service is one of the most important determinants of success in any retail medicine endeavor, but especially in pediatric urgent care.

8. Take your time explaining the discharge diagnoses and follow-up plans to patients and caregivers. Answering all of the questions before they leave the clinic is good medicine and good customer service.

9. Train your nonmedical staff to identify the common signs of respiratory distress, altered mental status, and high-risk diagnoses such as neonatal fever and child abuse.
10. If you approach pediatric patients with the expectation that they are going to cry and hate you, then your expectations will probably be met. Challenge yourself to make each child smile and laugh, and you will find your practice much more rewarding and successful.

CHAPTER 46

Urgent Care Center Financing

Glenn Dean

THE FINANCIAL PLAN

For any phase of the business cycle, the primary and fundamental step in identifying the capital needed for funding the business is the creation of a detailed and integrated financial plan. As discussed in other chapters, a pro forma income statement is insufficient for projection of capital requirements primarily because of capital expenditures and the timing of cash flows. Instead, an integrated balance sheet and statement of cash flows is preferred for determining capital requirements.

The working capital equation is a commonly used method for evaluation of capital needs of an organization. Working capital is a measure of operational efficiency and financial liquidity, and an indication of a company's ability to satisfy short-term obligations and generate free cash flow. Positive working capital predicts capability of funding continuing operations without the need for raising capital through issuing equity or incurring debt. Conversely, negative working capital exposes the likely requirement for a funding source. This is the formula:

$$\text{Working capital} = [\text{Current assets}] - [\text{Current liabilities}]$$

For urgent care center businesses, this equation translates to cash and accounts receivable minus accounts payable and accrued expenses. Calculating and managing working capital as a predictor of future cash needs has some drawbacks. The equation does not take the timing of cash flow into account. The accounts receivable collection cycle is usually longer than accounts payable terms. Salaries, benefits, medical supplies, rent, utilities, technology, insurance, and pay-per-click advertising initiatives cannot be paid with accounts receivables. Although working capital is a measure of liquidity, the cash-flow statement is a better predictor of cash available to satisfy obligations.

One of the fundamental functions of pro forma financial statements is to determine cash requirements for the business. The integrated income statement, balance sheet, and statement of cash flows is a more accurate predictor of cash requirements than a working capital calculation.

The statement of cash flows, also called the "sources and uses of cash," presents important specific details about the level of cash required and how the capital resources will be deployed. The uses of cash are identified below in four distinct but not exclusive phases in the business cycle:

- Development (cash needed before opening the doors)—needs for cash include the following:
  - Site selection, lease negotiation, architecture, and construction
  - Recruiting, health-care providers, and staff training
  - Contract negotiation and provider credentialing
  - Purchase of equipment and supplies
  - Pre-opening marketing initiatives

- Working capital (operations funding)—needs for cash include the following:
  - Salaries and fringe benefits
  - Rent, utilities, communication, and insurance
  - Business development
  - To prevent negative cash flow from growing patient volume and delayed receivables collection

- Expansion (i.e., developing and operating additional locations)—needs for cash include the following:
  - Selling the business

Cash typically comes from two types of investment instruments, debt and equity. With debt financing, an additional burden of interest expense increases the level of cash required. Equity financing does not (in most cases) require interest payments, but investors receive ownership in the business. The integrated financial plan shows the income statement and balance sheet differences in debt and equity financing for a given level of required capital.

Debt Financing

Funding with a debt instrument is borrowing money that must be repaid over time. The principal and interest are known amounts, and therefore planning for the monthly payments is straightforward; interest is tax deductible in most cases. The major disadvantage of debt as funding is the obligation created and the negative impact on cash flow. Debt financing can leave a business vulnerable to economic and business-specific downturns, which in turn inhibits growth by contributing to depletion of cash reserves that would otherwise be deployed for business-development initiatives.

Equity Financing

Funding through an equity investment, meaning an exchange of capital for a share of ownership in the business, is less risky than debt financing because there is typically no obligation to pay the money back, and use of this instrument does not drain working capital. The risk is transferred to the investor in return for a share of operating profits and percentage of proceeds of any future acquisition equal to the relative ownership percentage. Equity is often an expensive form of corporate currency; giving up ownership in return for capital investment may seem more attractive, but the relative decrease in ownership preserved may require returns that are in excess of the interest rate for debt financing.

SOURCES OF CAPITAL

Access to various sources of capital is dependent on several factors, including the current phase of the business cycle, sophistication of business and financial plans, profitability, experience and management track record, length of time in business, competitive advantage, and status of competition. Generally speaking, businesses in the early stages of development are funded by friends and family members, as well as by bank financing, including loans from the US Small Business Administration (SBA). Management teams with a history of success and a proven business model may have access to angel investors and more sophisticated private equity (PE) funds.

Regulation D

Investments in companies are securities and trigger state and federal securities laws. Therefore, companies selling securities must be aware of the provisions of Rules 504, 505, and 506 of Regulation D of the US Securities and Exchange Commission (SEC). For exemption from registration requirements, these rules are differentiated by the cumulative dollar amount of securities offered and the level of investor sophistication. Generally speaking, for exemption from registration requirements, companies may sell only "restricted" securities to "accredited" investors.

Rule 504 of Regulation D is for most companies that offer to sell up to $1 million of their securities in any 12-month period. This rule exempts the company from registration requirements, provided that the organization is not a "blank check company" (no specific business plan or purpose) and investors receive "restricted" securities that cannot be sold without registration or an applicable exemption. The most common exemption is Rule 144 of the Securities Act of 1933, which allows public resale of restricted and controlled securities if a number of conditions are met.

Legal Entities and Investment

There are three main types of small business entities: C-corporation, S-corporation (corporation with a subchapter S election), and limited liability company (abbreviated as C-corp, S-corp, and LLC, respectively). C-corps and S-corps issue shares to shareholders, and the LLC issues units to members. The S-corp and LLC structures are flow-through entities, meaning the net income (or loss) is not taxed at the entity level but flows through to the shareholders or to members' personal tax returns via schedule K-1 of Form 1041; a taxable benefit accrues to the equity owners in the start-up phase when company losses accumulate and offset future taxable income. Structuring a new entity as an LLC provides a balance between tax benefits for the members and funding flexibility for investors. C-corps are taxed at the entity level, and although losses are carried forward, there is no tax benefit to the shareholders.

C-corps can have multiple classes of securities, and LLCs can have multiple classes of units, but only one class of stock is permissible for S-corps. All shareholders have equal rights when there is only one class of stock. Sophisticated investors may require a conversion to a C-corp or LLC before making an investment, because of liquidation preferences apportioned to classes of preferred stock, typically their favored security instrument.

If the future objective is to become a C-corp, converting from an S-corp is straightforward—just terminate the S election. Conversion from an LLC is a bit more involved; usually a separate entity is created as a C-corp and the LLC is then merged into the new entity to preserve existing contracts and other relationships.

Friends and Family

No matter how you look at it, seeking investment capital from friends and family integrates money and relationships, which is not always optimal. To mitigate the risk of losing more than just invested capital, create a formal term sheet, which provides a clear understanding of the offering. Although most investors understand they are taking a risk, and friends and family may have altruistic intentions and want to help the company get off the ground, it is advisable to create an arm's-length agreement from the term sheet that clearly discloses risk of the investment and includes a precise definition of the security instrument. There are three types of investment vehicles most common to friends and family investors: equity, debt, and convertible debt.

Equity investments are a lower risk to the company but a higher risk to the investor. Issuing equity requires the company, at an early stage of business development, to place a value on each unit or share of stock or to assign a percentage of the company given up in exchange for the investment. To complicate matters, liquidity is an important factor; closely held entities in the start-up phase are subject to a marketability discount because the value of a minority interest in a company whose securities are restricted from sale is significantly less than a liquid investment with the same risk profile.

In the early stage of company development, a debt offering may be perceived as a lower-risk option than offering equity, especially when you have little history and uncertain methodologies for setting valuation and equity percentages. A convertible note, which may be converted into equity at the closing of a subsequent round of financing, will provide a more realistic valuation, but it requires a subsequent priced round of financing to fulfill its function. Value is created when the convertible-note investor receives a discount on the conversion to equity based on a future valuation tied to the subsequent round of funding. Preferred stock may be a better option because it serves as a fixed income security until it is converted to common stock, and includes a liquidation preference for dissolution or acquisition. The disadvantage of preferred stock is that transactions are complicated and require an attorney for preparation and execution of documents, creating even more expenses for start-up businesses with scarce capital resources.

A straightforward approach to valuing the company is to use the integrated financial statements to forecast the cash requirements and free cash flow generated by operations. First, calculate the net present value (NPV) of the future free cash flow using a discount rate appropriate for the risk of executing the forecast and achieving cash-flow objectives, probably higher than 20%. Calculation of the "per share" or unit price, a pre-money valuation for the entity, is accomplished by dividing the number of outstanding shares or units by the value of the entity. For an LLC, the price per unit defines the ownership exchanged for an equity investment.

Term Sheet

A term sheet is a nonbinding agreement that clearly defines the basic terms and conditions of an investment and lays the groundwork to ensure that the parties involved in the transaction are in agreement on important details. The term sheet lists the issuer, the pre-investment valuation of the company, the amount of investment requested, and an explanation of the security offered. In the case already described, the security would be the same class of LLC units held by the founders of the company. Because the term sheet is nonbinding, it is simply the basis for a formal agreement between the company and the investor, typically a subscription agreement.

Subscription Agreement

A subscription agreement is used by private companies to raise capital from private investors by selling ownership in the company without registering with the SEC. It is a binding contract that exchanges an investment in the company for a specific level of ownership. The terms of the agreement are defined in the term sheet, and the agreement acts as a limited partnership to significantly lower the risk to the investor who does not participate in the management of the business.

Bank Financing

Traditional bank financing for a small business is not available for most start-up businesses unless the owner has a track record of success, a strong personal credit history, and significant collateral. The application process can be lengthy, and personal guarantees are almost certainly required. For a business in the early stages of development, a better option may be to seek a government-guaranteed loan through the SBA.

For businesses with positive cash flow and a strong balance sheet, short-term business loans may be available for funding growth. A strong balance sheet will serve as collateral for the loan, but expect the remainder to be collateralized by a personal guarantee. In addition, the lending institution will use loan covenants that require the borrower to maintain certain conditions, such as liquidity ratios, debt-to-equity percentages, and income levels, to keep the loan in good standing. If any of the loan covenants default, an acceleration clause may require that the outstanding balance be due and payable immediately. These covenants are designed to protect the bank and to convince companies not to undertake activities and precipitate circumstances that potentially put the loan proceeds at risk.

Government-Guaranteed Loans

Although the SBA has several loan programs, the most common government-guaranteed loan is an SBA 7(a) general small-business loan. The SBA does not lend money; instead, it provides loan guarantees to significantly decrease the risk to lending institutions that participate in the programs as regular, certified, or preferred lenders. Basic eligibility requirements for SBA loan programs include a good personal credit history, industry experience, significant contributions to the business, and collateral and predicted ability to repay the loan from cash generated by the business. In most cases, the SBA requires a personal guarantee.

The following documents are required for SBA loan applications:

- SBA 7(a) business loan application
- Personal history and personal financial statement
- Business plan, including historical and projected financial statements
- Business license
- Lease agreement for the business location
- Personal and business federal tax returns for the last 3 years

For entrepreneurs starting a business for the first time, or for those without a substantial track record of success, an SBA loan may be an attractive funding source. Through the SBA, the federal government encourages the growth of small business by providing access to capital. The requirements for equity and collateral are less stringent than those used by commercial lenders, and the proven success and operational experience of the management team are less important than PE investors require.

To qualify for an SBA 7(a) loan, a business must be operated for profit and have, in general, less than $7 million in annual revenue and fewer than 500 employees, have reasonable invested equity, demonstrate the need for loan proceeds, and use the funds for a sound business purpose by establishing a new business or assisting in the acquisition of one or expanding an existing business.

The typical 7(a) small business loan has a term of 7 to 10 years with a variable interest rate of prime plus 2.25% to 2.75%. Monthly payments include principal and interest and are amortized over the life of the loan, with one main exception: Interest-only payments may be requested during the start-up phase.

The SBA normally guarantees 75% of loans greater than $150,000 and charges a 3% fee that is based only on the amount guaranteed. There is an additional 0.5% and 0.25% fee on loans greater than $750,000 and $1 million, respectively, because higher guaranteed amounts entail higher risk and thus result in larger fees.

Angel Investors

An angel investor is a high-net-worth individual who invests capital for businesses in the early stages of development. Angels are accredited investors and therefore meet the standard for exemption from some securities laws per Regulation D; these investors are sufficiently experienced to make such investment decisions without additional protections from the SEC. Angels sometimes form groups or networks to spread the risk so that they can invest in several companies.

Angel investment fills the gap between investment from friends and family and PE; angel investment is typically seen when businesses are beyond the start-up phase but need additional capital to fund operations or develop and execute business development strategies while they gain traction in the marketplace. Angels invest their own capital and typically expect high rates of return to balance the risk of early-stage investment. These securities are usually structured as equity ownership or convertible debt with the potential to return several times the original investment. The most common exit strategies are initial public offering and strategic acquisition; angels usually demand a clear pathway to an exit before considering an investment. For small urgent care operations, acquisition is the likely exit strategy.

Angels look for strong management teams with experience and a proven track record in industries with high growth potential. The process is straightforward:

1. Submission of an application (usually accompanied by an executive summary)

2. Screening by the management team: An angel group often selects a champion to investigate the opportunity.

3. Investment meeting:

    a. The key principals present the business plan and financials to the angel group.

    b. There is a concluding question-and-answer session.

4. Due diligence, performed by a selected champion and key members of the group: Members of the angel group are more likely to write checks if the selected champion and other key members of the due diligence team invest in the company too.

    a. Validation of management's representation of the business plan and historical results

b. Assessment of the market opportunity and the capability to execute the business plan
5. Term sheet negotiation, in preparation for development of investment agreements

Private Equity

PE funds are generally created for investment by accredited investors and institutions with access to risk capital for the purpose of acquiring equity positions in companies that have high growth potential or can be aggregated into larger operations. PE firms raise capital and manage the funds to yield attractive returns to investors. The amount of capital raised correlates to the track record and experience of the PE firm's principals who spread the risk by investing in multiple companies within a sector. Each equity investment has a timeline, typically between 4 and 7 years, for return on investment; limited PE partners (investors) expect a higher-than-average return for taking the risk.

PE firms usually acquire a platform company in a particular industry and then seek to add additional companies to the platform through acquisition. These add-ons may be competitors of the original platform company or may be businesses with one or more links to it, but they are added with the goal of increasing overall revenues and earnings of the platform investment and achieving scale in the market. PE investors also look for equity investments in a particular type of company, one that fits the profile of the PE portfolio companies and has a management team willing to run the company's day-to-day operations after the closing; it is imperative that the team be willing to continue running the company and manage the expansion. Ideally, the company seeking funding will partner with the PE firm to implement its strategy for growth and eventual exit.

Two main reasons for considering PE financing are expansion of operations and planning for an exit from the business. Whether you are considering expansion or selling the business, assessing the operation will be similar in scope. The PE firm will undertake a formal due diligence process for evaluating and documenting the opportunity to determine whether to make an investment. To shorten the time required to complete the assessment and maximize the value of the organization, it is crucial to be fully prepared for this process.

Cash Requirements

To expand operations with PE funding, a successful track record is required. PE firms are more likely to invest in a proven management team with a successful and profitable operating platform to develop additional locations. A formal business plan is essential if PE funding will be used to expand operations. The plan describes the opportunity, profiles the management team and advisors, defines the strategy, presents a thorough market assessment and analysis of the competition, and specifies cash requirements as part of an integrated financial plan.

A financial plan created to secure funding for initial development and business growth contains the benchmark for measuring performance. Key drivers of the forecast are of course updated using historical results, and variance analysis is used to predict future performance of each category. Measuring and updating the forecast for the primary location serves as a historical reference for creation of a reasonable and repeatable forecast for subsequent locations. The integrated financial plan predicts working-capital requirements to fund development as well as operations and business-development strategies to increase patient volume, which then leads to greater profitability.

PREPARING THE COMPANY

The main objective of preparation for acquisition or investment is to maximize entity valuation through improvements in profitability and efficiency of the operation. From a financial perspective, the goal is to maximize earnings before interest, taxes, depreciation, and amortization (EBITDA) over the last 12 months. To increase EBITDA, the company grows revenue or decreases expenses.

Growing revenue involves increasing the number of patients or collecting more cash. In the short term, the payer mix and contracts are fixed; therefore, increasing collections suggests improving the efficiency of front-desk operations. Collection of fees that the patient is responsible for at time of service is paramount to a competent and effective billing and collection process. Bad debt expense consists primarily of unpaid patient responsibility; collecting this amount equates to an increase in revenue and EBITDA and is, in other words, net income right to the bottom line.

The most common valuation formula is to multiply the trailing 12-month (TTM) EBITDA by a multiple.

$$\text{Entity value} = \text{TTM EBITDA} \times \text{EBITDA multiple}$$

EBITDA is a calculated value based on generally accepted accounting principles (GAAP) accrual accounting; therefore, the variable in the valuation equation is the multiple itself. For a given EBITDA calculation, entity values can vary widely on the basis of a number of factors, including rate of growth, level of debt, age and quality of capital assets, terms of the lease, and changing demographics of the surrounding area. In principle, the EBITDA valuation method is a straightforward calculation designed to approximate the NPV of future cash flows. The method works reasonably well for a stable and profitable business when industry average multiples are used but may result in undervaluation with a high growth rate unless a premium is added to the multiple to account for the expected future earnings growth. The EBITDA method is problematic for a new business that has not yet achieved profitability. In such case other valuation methods would be employed such as cost plus a premium or NPV of forecasted future cash flows.

THE PRIVATE EQUITY PROCESS

Engaging With a Firm
PE firms are continuously looking for potential investments in a particular sector to enhance their portfolio. Sourcing investment opportunities is challenging and involves networking, research, and cold-calling desirable companies. Introductions of management teams to PE firm executives are often facilitated by brokers or dealers, who are usually paid a percentage of the deal.

Once an introduction has been made and a threshold of interest has been reached, a nondisclosure agreement is executed. This document creates a confidential relationship between the parties to protect the company's confidential and proprietary information. The next step is performance of initial due diligence and evaluation of the management team. The PE firm will perform industry research, examine management's representation of the business opportunity, and create a preliminary financial model that quantifies the investment and potential returns. If the prospective investment is approved by the investment committee (if required by the firm), a nonbinding letter of intent will be drafted.

Letter of Intent—Term Sheet
The letter of intent is a nonbinding proposal usually sent from the PE firm to an acquisition or funding target indicating a strong interest in proceeding with a transaction. The document is usually crafted and sent after completing the preliminary due diligence process, meeting with management, and performing an internal financial analysis of current operations and the potential impact of growing or expanding operations or consolidating with a larger group. Key provisions of the letter of intent include investment or purchase price, timing, and exclusivity for a period of time, which covers the formal due diligence process.

Due Diligence
Before engaging with a PE firm, it is advisable to prepare the company for the PE inspection. Following is a minimal list of documents, contracts, and statements that are typically requested as part of the due diligence process:

- Entity-formation documents:
  - LLC
    - Articles of organization
    - Operating agreement
    - Membership table
  - Corporation (most commonly subchapter S)
    - Articles of incorporation
    - Bylaws
    - Board of directors and corporate officers
    - Capitalization table (shareholders)
    - Shareholder agreement

- Historical financial statements:
  - Income statement—monthly over the last 2 years at a minimum
  - Balance sheet—monthly to track account changes over time
  - Statement of cash flows—sources and uses of cash
  - Revenue cycle data
    - Billing and collection statements
    - Practice-management reports

- Financial projections:
  - Integrated income statement, balance sheet, and cash-flow statement
  - Patient volume and average reimbursement rates and totals
  - Revenue cycle statistics
    - Net realizable revenue (billed charges minus contractual adjustments)
    - Collection schedule (timing of cash payments and days receivables outstanding)
    - Bad debt percentage
  - Business-development strategy and marketing plan

- Staffing model and organizational chart:
  - Employment agreements

- Lease agreement

- Contracts

- Proof of insurance:
  - Malpractice
  - General liability
  - Errors and omissions for directors and officers

- Vendor invoices for random inspection

- Bank statements and reconciliations

- Manual of policies and procedures

- Detailed information about settled lawsuits and pending litigation

Once the on-site due diligence process is complete, the PE team will assemble for purposes of creating a formal report. The report will detail the operation, assess the competitive landscape, evaluate the management team, identify the business risk, and quantify the opportunity. In essence, the report will confirm or challenge the preliminary assessment that led to the letter of intent.

Selection

After the due diligence report is drafted, the team will build a detailed financial model that identifies key revenue and cost drivers of the business and expected financial performance based on the level of capital invested. This model results in a quantifiable return on investment based on a specific exit strategy and timeline.

If the PE firm decides to make an offer, it will write an investment memorandum that summarizes the investment opportunity and recommends investing in or acquiring the company at a specific valuation.

Challenges of Private Equity Funding

Unless they are acquisitions, PE transactions are typically structured with preferred shares. As the name suggests, preferred shares are treated preferentially, compared with common shares; this includes liquidation preferences. In the event of liquidation, fully participating preferred shareholders have the right to be paid the stock's purchase price before any proceeds are distributed to common shareholders and may have the right to receive a pro rata share of all remaining proceeds that the common shareholders receive. Conversely, nonparticipating preferred shareholders have the right to receive their original investment or convert to common shares and receive their pro rata distribution, but not both.

Some preferred shares are sweetened with warrants, a security that allows the holder to buy the underlying stock at a fixed exercise price up to the expiration date. If the exercise price is below the value of the underlying share, it has a dilutive effect on the value of common stock and may trigger an expense to the income statement, putting some loan covenants at risk of default.

If the PE investment results in a minority position, there may be some triggers in the agreement that transfer control to the PE firm if certain predetermined performance measures are not met. By transferring control, the owners put their positions with the company at risk and may ultimately suffer from declining percentage of ownership through subsequent offerings and dilution, which they no longer control.

HIRING CONSULTANTS

Hiring consultants is perhaps the most overlooked part of the entire financing process. Chances are good that you are not an expert in entity structures, business and financial planning, business valuation, structuring funding deals, legal document creation, navigation through the due diligence process, and closing transactions. Money spent for experts will significantly shorten the timeline and prevent costly mistakes. In most cases, the capital spent to improve efficiency, maximize valuation, and structure the deal that is right for your organization will yield a return on investment that will pay back the cost many times over.

CONCLUSION

Preparation is the key to securing funding for the business at any point in its life cycle. There are fundamental documents and processes that have historically attracted investment capital; therefore, learning from those who have done it before is a clever shortcut. Create the financial plan, identify uses of funds to support the required investment, and clearly identify the opportunity with a cogent business plan that assesses the competitive landscape and quantifies potential returns. A proven business model and an experienced management team with a successful track record will be necessary to secure investment capital from PE firms for business expansion or positioning for acquisition. Diligent preparation for these processes provides the best opportunity for an above-average return on investment in companies with similar risk profiles.

KEY POINTS

1. An integrated financial plan with an income statement, balance sheet, and cash flow statement is necessary when seeking funding for a business.

2. Debt financing adds additional cash-flow burden to the operation but preserves equity.

3. Equity financing limits risks of debt obligations but decreases ownership percentage.

4. The management team must pay close attention to securities laws when structuring any offer to sell securities; specifically, Regulation D of the Securities Act of 1933 must be considered to ensure that the company is exempt from registering with the SEC.

5. Legal structure of the entity dictates taxation regulations and the types of securities that can be offered.

6. Friends and family investment carries the additional burden of complications for relationships; to mitigate risk, treat the investment as an arm's-length transaction by using documentation for any third-party investment.

7. There are two main reasons for considering PE financing: expansion of operations and exiting the business.

8. Expansion of operations requires an experienced management team with a proven track record. For expansion, create a formal business plan that describes the opportunity, profiles the management team and advisors, defines the strategy, assesses the market, presents a competitive analysis and specifies cash requirements, and includes an integrated financial plan.

9. There is a direct correlation between efficiency of the operation and company value; be fully prepared for the due diligence process before it begins.

10. PE funding is a long and grueling process; such funds are used for expanding operations or for an acquisition, not for short-term growth capital or bridge funding.

11. Hire consultants. The increased efficiency and valuation will pay back the cost many times over.

CHAPTER 47

The Future of Urgent Care

John Shufeldt

The urgent care industry has gone through at least one life cycle and is likely at the tail end of its second life cycle. It may be at the beginning of the third cycle as a result of the coming changes in health-care reimbursement methodology and consolidation in the post–Accountable Care Act (ACA) phase of our health-care system.

In contradistinction to when the industry was at the end of the first life cycle in the late 1980s, urgent care is now an integral component of the care-on-demand provider network that we enjoy in the United States and is thus here to stay, provided the industry continues to adapt to changes, adopts evidence-based quality standards, and remains adept at navigating through turbulent times.

THE FIRST LIFE CYCLE

Most agree that the first urgent care centers were started in the mid-1970s by entrepreneurial physicians who saw the need for on-demand care resources for minor injuries and illnesses. These were sometimes called, maybe derisively, docs-in-the-box and were heralded at the time as a stopgap to offload busy emergency departments and compensate for the lack of primary-care providers.

Regina Herzlinger, in her excellent book *Market-Driven Health Care: Who Wins, Who Loses in the Transformation of America's Largest Service Industry*, details the story of one urgent care chain in the first cycle called Health Stop. Health Stop, during the mid- and late 1980s, was ahead of its time. They were backed by the venerable venture capital firm Hambrecht & Quist and offered the same value proposition and conveniences urgent care centers offer today.

Unfortunately, Health Stop failed. According to Professor Herzlinger, Health Stop failed because of its lack of efficiency, not appropriately incentivizing providers, lack of shared information technology systems, and lack of consumer loyalty. Health Stop and many of its contemporaries precipitously disappeared in the late 1980s and early 1990s.

THE SECOND LIFE CYCLE

Whether these early failures represent the end of the first life cycle or simply a 15-year false or slow start is up for debate. No matter which school of thought you adhere to, it is clear that today we are at some point on the curve of the next phase of urgent care medicine, which has lasted approximately 20 years.

Most centers have overcome the challenges that forced Health Stop out of business. As an industry, we have better practice-management systems, professional managers, and improved patient queuing and have figured out best practices to appropriately incentivize health-care providers. As an industry, we share best practices at national meetings, and many of our industry leaders speak and write regularly about best practices.

In the first decade of the 21st century, many worried that retail clinics might be the beginning of the end of our current phase. Retail clinics offered inexpensive care-on-demand services in high-traffic areas for many of the bread-and-butter complaints treated in urgent care centers. Moreover, managed-care organizations jumped on the bandwagon, and the two largest retail pharmacy chains snapped up the two industry leaders. What started as a cash business for private operators quickly morphed into a co-pay–waving value proposition unabashedly promoted by insurers and marketed heavily by their retail owners.

The retail clinic model as the next evolution of urgent care has largely failed to fill the on-demand niche. These clinics, given their small footprint and reduced staffing, suffer from some of the same patient-queuing challenges faced by Health Stop. This is not to say they don't provide excellent care—they do. But these clinics cannot manage to see enough patients in their current configuration to make much of a dent in the highly competitive urgent care environment.

Our industry now faces an entirely new set of challenges, marking the end of our second life cycle. As an industry, we are coming under enormous pressure to consolidate. This is driven by two forces:

- ▶ Health-care reform and the ACA—driving changes in payment methodology and forcing patients to find a medical home and stay in network, resulting in the consolidation of health systems and the acquisition of points of entry
- ▶ Private equity—there remains a land grab for high-quality, well-positioned urgent care centers in the United States

These forces are acting together to drive not only urgent care centers but most retail health-delivery models into larger, more scalable groups that can contract en masse with payers and suppliers.

THE THIRD LIFE CYCLE

The third urgent care life cycle will be marked by three distinct changes in the current environment:

- ▶ Consolidation in our industry
- ▶ Changes in payment methodology that reward improved patient outcomes and cost savings
- ▶ The adoption and integration of telemedicine

By my count there are approximately 5,880 centers in the United States that meet the definition of an urgent care center (open 7 days a week, health-care provider always on-site, x-ray on-site, no appointment necessary, able to perform basic laboratory tests and procedures).

According to figures from the Urgent Care Association of America and from my own research, only about 20% of these centers are in groups of 5 or more sites. The majority of the centers in the United States still have fewer than 5 sites dispersed in a fairly narrow geographic area.

These numbers demonstrate that we remain a highly fragmented industry, which means that from a managed-care organization's perspective we are easy to divide and conquer. If one center does not accept the health plan's fee schedule, the one down the street will. This separate-and-conquer negotiation style is being played out across the United States. This is unfortunate. With the relative paucity of primary-care providers in the system and pipeline, we, as an industry, should be in great shape vis-à-vis the supply–demand curve to drive reimbursement and access points upward.

Post-ACA, many sectors in the health-care space are moving away from a pure fee-for-service methodology. Primary-care providers are being shifted into population-management, outcome-based payment schemes that reward better health outcomes by following nationally recognized best practices.

Given that urgent care does not fit into this mold, how, then, will centers be compensated in the future? Generally speaking, urgent care centers, unless they are part of a large specialty network or part of an accountable care organization or health system, will not necessarily play in the population-health payment methodology unless the particular center provides care for a given population of primary-care patients. We will, however, remain an integral component of cost shifting as more patients are encouraged to leave or are forced out of emergency departments into more economical outlets for care.

In the near future, the avenue for on-demand care sought by consumers will be largely dictated by regional health systems. Patients will be incentivized financially to remain in network. Thus, contracting the urgent care centers with a network (which should also serve as an aggregator of various health plans) will be essential.

The good news is that in the post-ACA phase the urgent care industry will see an influx of patients with pent-up health-care needs who will be able to access care because they now have some form of health insurance. Judging by the past, it will take a number of months to a few years before these patients are assimilated into the health-care system; during that time, the urgent care industry will fill the gap by acting as an entry point. Once these patients are assimilated, there likely will still not be enough primary-care providers to fill the gap for on-demand care. It is predicted that by 2020 there will be a need for 45,000 more primary-care providers.

The need for more primary-care points of access is also driving entirely new ways to treat patients. Thanks to remote monitoring, point-of-care testing, and the availability of high-speed Internet and cloud-based architecture, telemedicine as a new delivery model is here to stay.

Telemedicine offers patients, employers, and health plans a convenient and low-cost way for managed-care patients to be treated for minor conditions without ever leaving their home or office. Many health plans now have options for telemedicine, and more than 15 states have enacted parity statutes that mandate that telemedicine be compensated at the same rate as an in-person examination.

Urgent care providers can access this space in a number of ways. The only caution is that whatever telemedicine provider you choose, that provider must be using an information technology platform that complies with the Health Insurance Portability and Accountability Act (HIPAA) and not be simply seeing patients via popular video-calling platforms.

No matter which HIPAA-compliant modality is chosen by the urgent care center operatror, telemedicine offers wide access to a large number of patients who would not otherwise be exposed to the center's service offering, because these patients would otherwise be outside the center's catchment area.

CONCLUSION

Urgent care is entering its third life cycle, which will be marked by not only sector-wide but also industry-wide changes to the health-care landscape. Urgent care center operators are innovators and early adopters. The current changes in health care will create opportunities that expand our patient base; do not significantly detract from our revenue, at least in the aggregate; and further solidify our once-nascent industry.

Index

Note: Page numbers followed by *f* refer to a figure. Page numbers followed by *t* refer to a table.

A

AABB, CLIA accreditation, 417
AAUCM. *See* American Academy of Urgent Care Medicine
absenteeism of workers, and occupational medicine, 539
abuse. *See* compliance program
AC Group, Inc., 323, 332, 334, 337
accessories in urgent care center, 74–75, 553–556, 601–602
accountable care organizations (ACOs), 463–473
   described and types of, 463–464
   reasons for ACOs to align with urgent care centers, 9, 465–467
   reasons for urgent care centers to work with ACOs, 467–468
   strategic options for urgent care centers, 468–472, 472*t*
accounting methods: cash vs. accrual, 157–158
accounts payable (A/P), 174, 177, 187, 188*t*
accounts receivable (A/R), 172, 173*t*, 191–193, 199
Accreditation Association for Ambulatory Health Care (AAAHC), 145, 147
accreditation of urgent care center, 145–155
   American Academy of Urgent Care Medicine (AAUCM), 145–146, 147, 150–152
   background and overview, 145–147
   Evidence of Standards Compliance (ESC), 149, 150
   Joint Commission, 145–146, 147–150
   Measures of Success forms, 149
   types of accreditation, 149
   Urgent Care Association of America (UCAOA), 146, 152–153
accredited, defined, 149
accrual accounting, 157–158
accrued salaries, 174, 177
ACOs. *See* accountable care organizations
acupuncture, 592, 596
additional services in urgent care, 575–585
   business strategy elements, 575–578
      outlooks, changing, 577–578
      vision and values, 575–577
   creative ideas for, 575, 582–584
      aesthetic services and products, 583
      alternative services, 583
      chronic pain management services, 584
      orthopedic services, 583–584
      pain-management services, 583–584
      rehabilitative services, 583
      wellness services and products, 583
   financial structure, 581–582
   management structure, 580–581
   research and planning, 578–580
Advance Trauma Life Support, 609
advertising and promotion expense, 164–165
advertising plan, 356–358
aesthetic services and products, 583
aesthetics inside urgent care center, 74–75, 553–556
affiliates, in health plan contract, 309
Affordable Care Act (ACA, 2010)
   audits and health-care fraud recoveries, 512
   and compliance program, 499
   effect on physician shortage, 247, 263, 276
   employee vs. independent contractor, 290–291
   future of urgent care, 625–627
   and health insurance coverage, 6–7, 8–9
   on health insurance plans and CAM, 597
   and HITECH Act, 320
   and virtual care, 488
aging by payer, 199–200
aging reports, in accounts payable, 188*t*, 192–193, 192*t*
Alexa, 399
Alignment: Using the Balanced Scorecard to Create Corporate Synergies (Kaplan & Norton), 404
alternative medicine. *See* integrative medicine
alternative services, 583
A.M. Best rating, 116, 125

629

American Academy of Family Physicians, 263, 319
American Academy of Pediatrics, 606
American Academy of Urgent Care Medicine (AAUCM), 145–146, 147, 150–152
American Board of Medical Specialties, 551
American Board of Preventive Medicine, 535
American Board of Radiology, 482
American College of Emergency Physicians, 8
American Institute of Architects (AIA), 52, 53
American Journal of Medical Quality, study on social networks, 398
American Journal of Public Health, on lack of health insurance, 7
American Medical Association (AMA)
  disruptive provider definition, 270
  E&M coding and documentation, 561, 562
  objectives in provider compensation agreement, 294
  on physician ownership and employment, 107
American Medical Group Association, 550
American Osteopathic Association, 417
American Recovery and Reinvestment Act, 320
American Red Cross, 395
American Society of Histocompatibility and Immunogenetics, 417
American Specialty Health Inc., 596
American Taxpayer Relief Act (2012), 96
American Telemedicine Association, 496, 497
Americans with Disabilities Act (ADA), 59, 76, 218–219, 280
amortization schedule, 175–176, 175t, 177
analyzers and test equipment
  contracts for reagent and analyzer, 438
  delivery, training, and validation for clinical laboratory, 439–441
  selecting for clinical laboratory, 425, 436
ancillary agreements, in sale of urgent care company, 94–95
Anderson, Mark, 323
angel investors, 617–618
Anthem Blue Cross and Blue Shield, 466
anti-kickback statute
  about regulations and employment contracts, 299
  due diligence on material contracts, 92
  and electronic health records, 330
  statute and regulation number, 504
anti-sandbagging provision, 90
application service provider (ASP) of EHR, 331
arbitration clause, in health plan contract, 309–310
architect for urgent care center, 51, 56, 57

architectural program, 66–74
  See also floor plan of urgent care center
archiving images with PACS, 476, 479–480
Arizona
  state regulations, 578–579
  UCR Health Centers, Chandler, 590
Articles of Incorporation, 78
Articles of Organization, 78
artwork on walls, 60, 553, 595, 601
as-built drawings for construction, 58
asset acquisitions in sale of urgent care company, 97–99
assets, current, in working capital, 193–194
assets, on balance sheet, 172–173, 173t, 174t, 195, 198t
assignment and assumption agreement, 94–95
Association for Cooperative Operations Research and Development certificates, 122–123
Association of American Medical Colleges (AAMC), 263
audiometry equipment, 538
auditing in compliance program, 507–508, 517
audits by managed-care organizations and regulatory agencies, 511–520
  audit types, 513–516
    by commercial payers, 512, 513
    by government payers, 511–512, 513–515
    financial risk, 517–518
    Medicaid claims audits, 515
    Medicare claims audits, 512, 513–515
    by Office of Inspector General (OIG) and Department of Justice (DOJ), 515–516
  preparation for, 516–517
  responding to, 517–519
    commercial-payer and government-payer audits, 517–518
    criminal investigations and subpoenas from OIG, 518–519
auto coverage, non-owned and hired, business insurance, 122
aviation medical examiner (AME), 543

B

back office. *See* staffing mix, clinical back office
background investigations, 509
bad debt, 172, 190–193, 619
balance sheet, 168–177, 170t–171t
  assets, 172–173
    cash and cash equivalents, 172
    inventory, 173
    net property, plant, and equipment (PP&E), 173, 174t

patient accounts receivable, 172, 173*t*
prepaid expenses, 173
variance calculations for, 195, 198*t*
equity, 176–177
membership interest, 176–177
retained earnings, 177
liabilities, 174–176 (*See also* liability considerations)
accounts payable (A/P), 174
accrued salaries, 174
capital lease obligations, 174–176
long-term debt, 176
other current liabilities, 174
variance calculations for, 195, 198*t*
variance calculations for asset and liability categories, 195, 198*t*
balanced scorecard, 404
The Balanced Scorecard (Kaplan & Norton), 404
balancing report for heating and cooling system, 58
bank financing, 615–616
barriers, artificial and natural, in site selection, 25
behavior-based performance goals, 284
beneficiary assignment, and ACOs, 464
benefits, employee, 93, 164, 284–286
best practices, 626
beta test site, 142
bidding
to build urgent care center, 53
with general contractor, 51–52, 56
standard bidding form and comparison, 53, 54*f*, 55*f*
bilingual staff members, 14
bill of sale, 94
billed charges revenue recognition, 189–190
billing
for additional services, 582
and claims in revenue cycle process, 343–344
and collection, 186
in employment agreements, 292–293
E&O insurance, 125, 167
expense, 168
functions and duties of reception and billing staff, 234–236
biometric screening in wellness programs, 493, 540
biometric time clock, 186
biopsychosocial model, 588
Bitly, 400
blogging in social media
for brand development, 399

for consumer decision-making, 368, 369
for crisis management, 390
Blue Cross, 395
bonding requirements in contract with general contractor, 55
bonus compensation, variable component, for provider, 295–296
Boston University, study of pharmacy use, 30
brand development, 393–401
benefits of branding, 393
brand experience, 397
brand identity, 393–394
brand personality, 396–397
online branding, 397–399
company blog, 399
directories, 398
social networks, 398–399
tools of the trade, 399–400
visual identity, 394–396
brand promise, 354
brand standards guide, 358
branded messages, 278, 279*f*
Brandify, 399
break-even point of additional services, 582
break room, in design of floor plan, 73–74
breath alcohol testing, 538
Broselow Pediatric Resuscitation System, 608
budget allocation process, for marketing budget, 355
building out the urgent care center, 49–61
clinical laboratory
patient draw site, 443, 445, 446*t*–447*t*
physical site completion, 439
construction manager, decision on, 49
construction process, 57–60
as-built drawings, 58
certificate of occupancy or completion, 58
closeout book, 58–59
construction meetings, 57, 61
noncontractor items, 59–60
pay applications, 57
punch lists, 57–58
substantial completion, 58
tenant improvement reimbursement, 59
design and specification approvals, 50
design-build or design-bid-build?, 50–51
floor plan (*See* floor plan of urgent care center)
general contractors, bidding and contracting, 51–56, 60, 61
lenders, 56
length of time to open, 49–50

permitting, 56–57
site selection (*See* site selection of urgent care center)
Bush, George W., 320
business analysis, 353–354
business formation, 77–86
    entity types and characteristics of corporations and LLCs, 77–79
    liability and tax considerations
        of corporations, 80–82
        of general and limited partnerships, 82
        of LLCs, 82–84
        of professional entities, 84–85
    See also additional services in urgent care; corporations; LLCs (limited liability companies)
business insurance, 121–124
    See also insurance requirements for urgent care center
business plan, 11–21
    basic layout, 12
    company description, 13
    competitor analysis, 14–15
    cover page, 12–13
    executive summary, 13
    financial plan, 18
    implementation strategy, 16–17, 18–19
    industry analysis, 13
    informational resources, 11–12
    for integrating complementary and alternative medicine, 588–594
    management plan, 17
    market analysis, 13–14
    marketing strategy, 15–16
    mistakes, 18–19
    online premade plans, 19
    products and services description, 15
buying and decision-making timeline, 366–369, 367*f*, 384, 397
bylaws, 78

C

C-corporations, 80–81
    and asset acquisitions, 97
    investments and capital, 613–614
CAD (computer-aided design) drawings, 58
California
    and corporate practice of medicine, 107, 109–110, 113
    cost reductions of urgent care centers, 466
    Fair Employment and Housing Act, 218
    Family Rights Act, 217
    Health Net of California, Inc., 596
    Labor Code, social media privacy protection, 227
    laboratory licensure and regulations, 429*t*
    on misclassification of employees as ICs, 229
    Pregnancy Discrimination Act, 217
    Supreme Court, *Brinker Restaurant Corporation v. Superior Ct.,* 220
callbacks to patients, 532
CAM (complementary and alternative medicine). *See* integrative medicine
capital call, 79
capital lease obligations, 174–176, 180
capital sources, 613–619
    See also financing an urgent care center
capital transactions, 96
capitation
    California cost reductions, 466
    and carve-outs in health plan contract, 310
    in HMO plan, 307
captive PC structure, 109
Carnegie, Dale, 371–374
carpet in urgent care center, 75, 553
carve-outs in health plan contract, 310
cash
    CAM payments, 596
    and cash equivalents, assets, on balance sheet, 172
    and internal controls, 184, 185*t*
    provider compensation, 293–294
    requirements in financing urgent care center, 618–619
cash-basis accounting, 157, 167
cash-basis revenue recognition, 189
cash-flow statement, 177–180, 178*t*–179*t*
catastrophic loss insurance, 123
causes of action with physician extenders, 248–249
Center for Telehealth and e-Health Law, 496, 497
Centers for Disease Control and Prevention, laboratory regulations, 415
Centers for Medicare & Medicaid Services (CMS)
    and ACOs, 465
    on audits and fraud recoveries, 511–512
    E&M coding and medical documentation, 561, 569–570
    EMTALA enforcement, 451–452
    laboratory regulations, 415
        accreditation organizations, 417
        applying for licensure, 428
        quality system approach, for laboratory testing, 422

surveys of laboratories, 418
websites, 416*t*
published guidance on compliance programs, 501–502
surveys of patient satisfaction, 549–550
certificate of completion, 58
Certificate of Formation, 78, 91
Certificate of Incorporation, 78, 91
certificate of occupancy, 52, 57, 58
certificate types under CLIA, 417–418
Certification Commission for Healthcare Information Technology (CCHIT), 330, 337
certified coder, 574
certified medical examiners, 543
Certified Pediatric Emergency Nurse, 609
chain of command in management plan, 17
charter of corporation, 78
check-out area, improving patient satisfaction, 554, 556
check requests, 189
child abuse, 527, 606
chiropractic care, 593, 596
chronic pain management services, 584
Cigna, Healthy Rewards program, 592
Civil Rights Act. *See* Title VII of Civil Rights Act
claims
auditing in compliance program, 508
clean claims and claims provisions, in health plan contract, 310–311
and E&M issues, 561, 568, 572
in revenue cycle process, billing, denials and unpaid claims, 343–344
claims-made insurance, 117–118
CLIA regulations. *See* Clinical Laboratory Improvement Amendments (CLIA)
client server model of EHR, 331
clinic acquisitions, on cash-flow statement, 180
clinic manager, functions and duties of, 243–245
clinical back office. *See* staffing mix, clinical back office
clinical consultant, laboratory personnel, 422–423, 436, 437*t*, 438
Clinical Laboratory Improvement Amendments (CLIA). *See* laboratory overview
clinical laboratory, moderate-complexity, 427–449
three months out
analyzers, test systems, and test kit selection, 436
insurance contract negotiation, 428
laboratory equipment and supply distributor, 428, 433
license application, 428, 429*t*–432*t*
technical consultant, 433
test menu selection, 433, 434*t*–435*t*
two months out
laboratory information systems, 439
personnel and laboratory support staff, 436, 437*t*, 438
physical site completion, 439
reagent and analyzer contracts, 438
one month out
analyzers delivery, training, and validation, 439–441
hire personnel, 439
inspection preparation, 445, 447–448
laboratory information system integration, 441
patient draw site setup, 443, 445, 446*t*–447*t*
policies and procedures, 441–442
proficiency testing, 442–443, 443*t*–445*t*
quality-assessment plan, 442
See also laboratory overview
closeout book, in construction process, 58–59
closing date, 98
closing transactions in sale of urgent care company, 98
cloud-based system for EHR, 331
CMS. *See* Centers for Medicare & Medicaid Services
co-pays and deductibles, 342
COA. *See* nonwaived testing, moderate (COA or COC)
COC. *See* nonwaived testing, moderate (COA or COC)
coding, E&M. *See* evaluation and management (E&M) of coding
COLA, and Clinical Laboratory Improvement Amendments, 239, 417
collateral formats, 359–360
collection, 186, 342
collective bargaining, 225
College of American Pathologists, CLIA accreditation, 417
colors and visual identity of brand, 394–395
colors inside urgent care center, 74–75, 555–556
commercialization of practice of medicine, and CPOM, 107–108
Commission on Office Laboratory Accreditation (COLA), 239, 417
common area maintenance, 46

communication plan, for building urgent care center, 50
communications
   and marketing messages, 358–360
   open-door policy for compliance program, 507
   and patient satisfaction, 557
   in physician leadership, 211, 214
   telephone expense, 166
   what employers want, in occupational medicine, 540–541
company analysis, for marketing, 353–354
compensation
   and employee benefits, 93, 164, 284–286
   employee salaries and wages, 163
   of providers (*See* provider compensation)
competency of patients, and informed consent, 525, 527
competition inventory, in site selection, 26–29
competitive advantage, and strategic talent management, 275
competitor analysis, 14–15, 352–353
complementary and alternative medicine (CAM). *See* integrative medicine
Complementary and Alternative Medicine Survey of Hospitals, 589
compliance officer, 506, 516, 517
compliance program, 499–510
   in audit preparations, 516
   corrective action, 509
   enforcement, 508–509
   Health Care Reform (2010), 499–501
   monitoring and auditing, 507–508
   OIG list of key laws and resources, 504–505
   open lines of communication, 507
   published guidances, 501–503, 508–509
   risk assessment, 503
   seven fundamental elements of, 502–503
   training and education, 506–507
   written standards, policies, and procedures, 503, 505–506, 509
Compliance Program Guidance for Medicare Fee-for-Service Contractors, 501–502
Comprehensive Accreditation Manual for Ambulatory Care (CAMAC), 147
Comprehensive Error Rate Testing (CERT) program, 513–514, 516
computed radiography (CR), 140, 475, 476
computed tomography (CT), 140, 475, 478–479
computer hardware for EHR, 331, 333, 334
concerted activity, 225–226
conditional accreditation, defined, 149
conditions, covenants, and [deed] restrictions (CC&Rs), 64
conditions precedent to closing, 98
conditions to closing, 98
conference room, in design of floor plan, 74
confidential information, 88, 335–336
confidentiality and nondisclosure agreement (NDA), 88–89, 300, 620
Congressional Budget Office, on health insurance coverage, 7
Connecticut, laboratory licensure and regulations, 429*t*
consent. *See* informed consent
construction contracts, 53, 58
construction documents, during design phase, 49
construction manager, deciding on, 49
construction process, 57–60
   See also building out the urgent care center
construction schedule, 53, 55
Consumer Assessment of Healthcare Providers and Systems (CAHPS), 550–551
consumer-driven health plan designs, 489
consumers, informed on health care costs, 7–8, 489
contingency agreements, hiring providers from search firms, 268
contract for health plan. *See* health plan contracting
contractor to build urgent care center. *See* general contractor (GC)
contractual adjustments, 190–191
contractual agreements with vendors, 142–143
control
   in management-control process, 403
   in organizational hierarchy, 210
control principles for financial management, 183–184
convertible note, 614
corporate practice of medicine (CPOM), 105–114
   friendly professional corporation (PC) structure, 109–112
   health-care regulatory limitations, 299–300
   noncompliance penalties, 112–113
   professional entity statutes, 108–109
   theories underlying CPOM doctrine, 106–108
corporations, 80–82
   and asset acquisitions, 97
   characteristics of, compared with LLCs, 77–79
   legal liability, 80
   shareholders' (stockholders') agreement, 78, 91
   shareholders (stockholders) as owners, 77

tax considerations, 80–82
corrective action in compliance program, 509
CorVel, 539
cost-saving alternatives, in building urgent care center, 53
costs
   of electronic health record, 332–336
   informed consumers on health care costs, 7–8, 489
   to provide medical care, and health plan contract, 305
covered services, in health plan contract, 311
COW. *See* waived testing (COW)
CPOM. *See* corporate practice of medicine
CPT. *See* Current Procedural Terminology (CPT)
CR (computed radiography), 140, 475, 476
credentialing of providers, 119–121
criminal conduct, response to audits, 517, 518–519
   See also compliance program
crisis communications management, 385–392
   crisis defined, 385
   crisis-management plan, 387–388
   power of video, 390
   prevention, preparation, and response, 387, 390–391
   reputation repair, 386, 391–392
   social media in, 389–390
   spokesperson assigned to media, 388–389
   threat identification, 386
cross-marketing, 580
CT (computed tomography), 140, 475, 478–479
The Cultural Creatives: How 50 Million People Are Changing the World (Ray & Anderson), 590
culture, of urgent care center, 556
current assets, in working capital, 193–194
current liabilities, in working capital, 194
Current Procedural Terminology (CPT)
   acupuncture codes, 592
   auditing in compliance program, 508
   audits for health-care fraud recoveries, 512
   codes for levels of service, 565–568, 572
   E&M code definitions, 562
   in revenue and performance measurement, 189–190, 191, 344
customer analysis, for marketing, 351–352

D

data distribution, in metric-driven management, 407–408
data, electronically stored, and audit subpoenas, 519
data lines, in urgent care center, 60
data organization for site selection, 41–42
data room, 90
debt financing, 612
debt, long-term, 176, 180
dedicated emergency departments, EMTALA definition of, 453–454
deductibles and co-pays, 342
Defense of Marriage Act (DOMA), 225
deferred sign and close, 98
deferred submittal, 56
Deficit Reduction Act (2005), 515
delayed sign and close, 98
denial of accreditation, defined, 149
depreciation expense, 168, 169*t*, 177
design-build, compared with design-bid-build, 50–51
design plans for urgent care center, 50
designated health services, 298
DICOM (digital imaging and communications in medicine), 479, 481
dietary supplements, 587
digital imaging and communications in medicine (DICOM), 479, 481
digital PACS. *See* picture archiving and communication system (PACS)
digital radiography (DR), 140, 475, 476
direct mail campaign, 357
direct marketing, 372
directed care, 535–536
directories online, 398
directors and officers liability (D&O) insurance, 167
disability insurance, 124–125
disabled patients. *See* Americans with Disabilities Act (ADA)
disciplinary actions, in compliance program, 508–509
discipline and termination, in strategic talent management, 286
disclosures
   of appropriate information, and informed consent, 525–526
   prohibitions in sale of urgent care company, 88–89
   of protected health information in occupational medicine, 542–543
discrimination, Title VII: nondiscrimination policy, 220
dissenters' rights, 78
distributor sales representative for laboratory equipment, 428, 433

documentation
  in performance management, 284
  See also medical documentation
Doppler ultrasound, 478
DOT physicals for occupational medicine, 543–544
DR (digital radiography), 140, 475, 476
due diligence
  for angel investors, 617–618
  in private equity process, 620–621
  in sale of urgent care company, 89–93
durable medical equipment (DME), and vendor selection, 131
dyscompetent physicians, 271

E

The E-Myth Physician: Why Most Medical Practices Don't Work and What to Do About It (Gerber), 577
E-Verify, 225
e-visits, 485, 492
  See also virtual care
Early Survey Program (ESP), 151
earnings before interest, taxes, depreciation, and amortization (EBITDA), 158, 619
economic value added (EVA), 406
education. *See* training and education
EHR. *See* electronic health record (EHR) systems
Electronic Health Record Association, 337
electronic health record (EHR) systems, 319–338
  about studies, background, and benefits of, 319–321
  client server compared with application service provider, 331
  costs of, 332–336
  getting started on selection, 322–323
  in health plan contract follow-up, 317
  information technology expense, 165
  and laboratory information systems (LIS), 439, 441
  pitfalls and privacy issues, 336
  product demonstration, 331–332
  as revenue cycle management partner, 346
  site visits, 332
  solutions for your requirements, and common features of EHR solutions, 323, 324t–328t
  vendor selection and certification, 323, 329–330
electronic medical records (EMRs), compared with EHRs, 320
electronic remittance advice (ERA), 186

electronically stored data, and audit subpoenas, 519
eligibility and verification
  in health plan contract, 312
  of patient registration, 342
E&M. *See* evaluation and management of coding
emergency departments (EDs)
  and ACOs, reducing nonemergency visits, 465–466, 467
  belief systems about patients, differences from urgent care centers, 521
  cost of, overcrowding, and consumers, 5–8
  and patient anti-dumping act (*See* EMTALA [Emergency Medical Treatment and Active Labor Act])
  transfers, and metrics, 410
emergency medical conditions
  common subtle conditions presenting in urgent care, 522–524
    abdomen, 523
    chest, 523
    genitourinary, 524
    neurologic, 522–523
    others, 524
    vital signs, 522
  critical care events in urgent care center, 528–529
    back-office tasks, 528–529
    checklists and care paths, 529
    front-office tasks, 528
    provider tasks, 529
  EMTALA definition of, 457
  identifying extremis in triage, 236
  pediatric urgent care, 606–609
    certification of staff, 609
    drugs for, 608t
    equipment and supplies, 607t, 608
Emergency Medical Treatment and Active Labor Act. *See* EMTALA
emotional intelligence, 212
empathy, 213, 558
employee benefits, 93, 164, 284–286
employee duties, in employment agreements, 291–292
employee handbook, complying with Fair Labor Standards Act, 220
employee matters
  duties, in employment agreement, 291–292
  embezzlement, 183, 184, 187
  nonsolicitation provision, 89
  in sale of urgent care company, 92–93
Employee Retirement Income Security Act (ERISA, 1974), 225

employees
  bilingual, 14
  compared with independent contractors (*See* independent contractors)
  effectiveness of, 278
  metrics on experience of, 412*t*
  morale of, and finances, 18
  vested, and equity compensation, 296, 297
  See also employee matters; staff; staffing mix
employer-based health care, virtual care, 489, 492, 493
employer, defined for nondiscrimination policy, 220
employers and occupational medicine, 539, 540–541
employment contracts, 289–303
  employee vs. independent contractor, 289–291
    legal liability, 289
    tax consequences, 289–291
  health-care regulatory limitations, 298–302
    anti-kickback statute, 92, 299
    corporate practice of medicine doctrine, 299–300
    noncompetition provision, 300, 301–302
    nondisclosure provisions, 300
    nonsolicitation provisions, 301
    physician self-referral: Stark law (*See* Stark law [physician self-referral])
  provisions of employment agreements, 291–298
    billing and collection, 292–293
    employee duties, 291–292
    patient medical records, 293
    provider compensation (*See* provider compensation)
    provider qualifications and requirements, 292
    termination, 296–298
employment issues. *See* human resources overview, labor and employment issues
employment practices liability insurance (EPLI), 125
EMTALA (Emergency Medical Treatment and Active Labor Act), 451–461
  enforcement, 451–452, 460
  institutions applicable to, 452–455
    dedicated emergency department, 453–454, 460
    Medicare-participating hospitals, 452–453
  requirements for providers and institutions, 451, 455–459, 460

    medical screening exam, 455–457
    stabilization, 457–458
    transfers, 458–459
  urgent care centers, and compliance with, 238
Engel, George, 588
entity structuring. *See* business formation
Equal Employment Opportunity Commission, on retaliation in sexual harassment claims, 222
equipment
  analyzers (*See* analyzers and test equipment)
  audiometry equipment, 538
  choosing equipment vendors, 136–140, 142 (*See also* vendor selection for equipment and supply)
  computed radiography, 140, 475, 476
  computed tomography, 140, 475, 476
  digital radiography, 140, 475, 476
  durable medical equipment (DME), 131
  information technology and electronic equipment list, 138*t*
  laboratory equipment and supply distributor, 428, 433
  medical equipment and supplies list, 129*t*–130*t*
  office, equipment, and personnel lease agreement, 99
  pediatric emergency preparedness, equipment and supplies, 607*t*, 608
  picture archiving and communication system (PACS), 476, 479–480
  ultrasound equipment (*See* ultrasound equipment)
  x-ray equipment (*See* x-ray equipment)
equity acquisitions in sale of urgent care company, 95–97, 99
equity compensation for provider, 296
equity investments financing, 612–613, 614
equity issuance on cash-flow statement, 180
equity, on balance sheet, 176–177
equityholders' agreement, 79
escrow agreement, 95
Esri, 33
ethical conduct. *See* compliance program
evaluation and management (E&M) of coding, 561–574
  code definitions, 562–565
  levels of service, 565–568
    codes 99201 to 99205 and 99291, 565*t*, 566–568, 566*t*
    new patients and established patients, 565, 565*t*, 566*t*
    undercoding and overcoding, 572

medical documentation, 568–573
  CMS guidelines, 568–570
  coding specific to urgent care, 572–573
  key components of, 343
  in malpractice prevention, 532
  in revenue cycle process, 342–343
  tips on documentation, 570–572
medical necessity, 561–562, 568–569
Medicare audits, 512
evaluation of providers, 211–213
evergreen provisions
  in employment agreements, 297
  in health plan contract, 312
Every Door Direct Mail, 357
evidence-based human resources practices, 277–286
  See also strategic talent management
Evidence of Standards Compliance (ESC), 149, 150
examination rooms
  design for pediatrics, 601–602
  and patient satisfaction, 68–69, 554, 555
  supplies list, 131*t*
examinations, types of, 565
exit interviews, usefulness in compliance program, 508
exit transactions, sale of urgent care company, 87–103
  indemnification, 99–102
    indemnification baskets, 101–102
    indemnification cap, 102
    representations and warranties, 100
    survival period, 101
  mechanics of, 87–95
    ancillary agreements, 94–95
    confidentiality and nondisclosure agreement, 88–89
    due diligence, 89–93
    letter of intent, 93
    purchase agreement, 93–94
  stages of, 102
  transaction structure, 95–99
    asset acquisitions, 97–99
    equity acquisitions, 95–97
  See also financing an urgent care center
expectations, of strategic talent, 285
expeditors, 57
expense reports, 189
expenses, on income statement, 162–168
  advertising and promotion, 164–165
  billing, 168
  clinic staffing, 162–163, 162*t*
  clinical salaries and wages, 163
  communications, 166

depreciation, 168, 169*t*
employee benefits, 164 (*See also* benefits, employee)
information technology, 165
laboratory fees, 164
legal and professional, 165–166
management, 168
medical malpractice insurance, 166–167 (*See also* medical malpractice)
medical supplies, 164
medications, 164
operating expenses, 163*t*
other expenses, 167–168
other insurance, 167
purchased services, 166
radiology fees, 164
rent and lease expense, 167
selling, general, and administrative, 168
explanation of benefits (EOB), 186
extended reporting period coverage, 117–118
extra-expense coverage, in business insurance, 123–124
extrapolated leadership, 203

F

Facebook, and branding, 398
Fair Labor Standards Act (FLSA), 219–220
Family and Medical Leave Act (FMLA), 217–218
Federal Motor Carrier Safety Administration, 543
Federal Unemployment Tax, 289
Federation of State Medical Boards, 248
fee-splitting application, as management service fee, 110–111
fiduciary liability and fidelity protection, 125
financial impact
  of crisis management, 386
  of recruitment and selection, 281
financial management, 183–201
  evaluation, 195, 199–200
    accounts receivable, 199
    aging by payer, 199–200
    revenue, 199
  internal control, 183–189
    billing and collection, 186
    cash, 184, 185*t*
    check requests and expense reports, 189
    control principles, 183–184
    employee theft and embezzlement, 183, 184, 187
    payroll and independent contractors, 186–187
    petty cash, 186

purchasing and accounts payable, 187, 188*t*
performance measurement, 189–195 (*See also* performance measurement)
   accounts receivable, 191–193
   financial statements and variances, 195, 196*t*–197*t*, 198*t*
   revenue, 189–191
   variance analysis, 194–195
   working capital, 193–194
financial plan, 18, 611–613
financial statements
   and variance analysis, 195, 196*t*–197*t*, 198*t*
   See also pro forma financial statements
financing an urgent care center, 611–623
   financial plan, 611–613
   hiring consultants, 622
   preparing the company, 619
   private equity process, 620–622
   sources of capital, 613–619
      angel investors, 617–618
      bank financing, 615–616
      cash requirements, 618–619
      friends and family, 614–615
      government-guaranteed loans, 616–617
      legal entities and investment, 613–614
      private equity, 618
      Regulation D, 613, 617
      subscription agreement, 615
      term sheet, 615
   See also exit transactions, sale of urgent care company
fire alarms, 56
fire sprinklers, 56, 65
first-mover advantage, 591
fixed assets purchase, on cash-flow statement, 180
flood insurance, 123–124
floor plan of urgent care center, 63–76
   aesthetics, 74–75
   approval during site-procurement, 49
   architectural program, 66–74
      future growth, 67
      wish list, 66–67
   functions and spaces
      break room, 73–74
      conference and training rooms, 74
      exam rooms, 68–69
      front lobby and waiting area, 67
      laboratory, 70–71
      nurse station, 71–72
      offices, 71
      patient satisfaction improvements, 553–556
      pediatrics considerations, 601–602
      procedure room, 69
      reception area, 68
      restrooms, 72–73
      space for occupational medicine, 538
      storage and supplies, 73
      triage area, 68
      utilities, 73
      waiting area (*See* waiting area)
      x-ray room, 70
   site-selection checklist, 63–66
      parking, 64
      utilities, 64–66 (*See also* utilities, in site-selection checklist)
      zoning and building use, 63–64
Florida
   laboratory licensure and regulations, 429*t*
   Miami Urgent Care Center Medical Clinic, 589
   Premier Urgent Care Center, Melbourne, 591, 593
Flynn Brothers, Inc. v. First Medical Associates (1986), 112
Forrester Research, 337
The 4 Disciplines of Execution: Achieving Your Wildly Important Goals (McChesney, Covey, Huling), 406, 408
fraud, and audit recoveries, 512
   See also compliance program
friendly professional corporation (PC) structure, 109–112
friends and family, as source of capital, 614–615
front office. *See* staffing mix, front office
full accreditation, defined, 151
furniture
   and aesthetics in design of floor plan, 74–75
   and interior designer, 60
   list of, for lobby, 139*t*
   and patient satisfaction, 553–556
   for pediatrics, 601–602
future of urgent care, 625–628

G

Gates, Bill, 403
General Accounting Office, on electronic health record systems, 319
general contractor (GC), bidding and contracting, 51–56, 60, 61
general liability coverage, in business insurance, 122
general partnerships, 82
generally accepted accounting principles (GAAP), 167

Georgia, Lake Oconee Urgent & Specialty Care Center, 590
goals, behavior-based performance, 284
Google+, 398
Google Alerts, 389, 399
Google Analytics, 399
Google Caffeine, 374
Google Maps Engine Pro, 33
Google search engine, 381
governance rights of owners, 78–79
government-guaranteed loans, 616–617
governmental audits. *See* audits by managed-care organizations and regulatory agencies
greeter, in pediatrics urgent care, 602–603, 609
grocery stores, 29–30
gross lease, 46
group purchasing organization (GPO), 130–131

H

harassment. *See* sexual harassment under Title VII of Civil Rights Act
hardware, computer hardware for EHR, 331, 333, 334
Harvard Business Review, 3, 213
Hawaii, laboratory licensure and regulations, 430t
Health Care and Education Reconciliation Act (2010), 499
health-care providers. *See* providers
Health Care Reform (2010), 499–501
health-care regulatory limitations, 298–302
    anti-kickback statute, 299 (*See also* anti-kickback statute)
    corporate practice of medicine doctrine, 299–300 (*See also* corporate practice of medicine [CPOM])
    noncompetition provision, 300, 301–302
    nondisclosure provisions, 300
    nonsolicitation provisions, 301
    physician self-referral: Stark law, 298–299 (*See also* Stark law [physician self-referral])
    See also physicians
Health Information Technology for Economic and Clinical Health (HITECH) Act, 319, 320–321, 493, 494
health insurance
    audits (*See* audits by managed-care organizations and regulatory agencies)
    and CAM, 596–597
    consumer-driven health plan designs, 489
    contract negotiation for clinical laboratory, 428
    lack of coverage, 6–7
    reimbursement and contractual adjustments, 190–191
Health Insurance Portability and Accountability Act. *See* HIPAA
health maintenance organization (HMO), 307
Health Net of California, Inc., 596
health plan contracting, 305–318
    contract follow-up, 316–317
    contract review and action points, 308–315
        affiliates, 309
        arbitration, 309–310
        capitation and carve-outs, 310
        clean claims and claims provisions, 310–311
        covered services, 311
        credentialing of providers, 311–312
        eligibility and verification, 312
        evergreen and renewal provisions, 312
        indemnification and mutual liability, 312–313
        medically necessary, 313
        new plans and product lines, 313–314
        policies and procedures (P&Ps), and obligations, 314
        professional liability coverage, 314
        termination without cause, 314–315
        unilateral modifications, 315
    miscellaneous items in contracts
        audits and reviews, 513
        E&M coding and reimbursement guidelines, 572
        workers' compensation, networks, and silent PPOs, 537
    negotiation, 315–316
    preparation for contracting, 305–308
        center objectives and leverage, 307–308
        health plan reputation and payment methods, 306
        payment models, 306–307
        utilization and costs, 305
Health Stop, 625–626
Healthcare Effectiveness Data and Information Set (HEDIS), 550
Healthwise, 594
Healthy Rewards program, 592
heating, ventilation, and air-conditioning. *See* HVAC
Henry J. Kaiser Family Foundation, Employer Health Benefits Survey, 489, 490f
HIPAA (Health Insurance Portability and Accountability Act, 1996)
    in compliance program, for audits, 516

compliance with floor plan considerations, 71, 72, 76
and electronic health records (EHR), 331
on image and interpretation privacy, 482
and occupational medicine, 542–543
on patient draw station, 445
and revenue cycle management partner, 348
and virtual care, 10, 485, 493, 494, 628
hiring and managing medical providers, 263–273
   disruptive providers, 270–272
   hiring physician leader (*See* physician leadership)
   hiring quality providers, 264–265
   locum tenens, 121, 265–267
   physician shortage, 263–264
   post-hiring challenges, 270
   resources (websites) for finding providers, 269–270
   search firms, contingency agreements, 268
   search firms, retained agreements, 267–268
   word-of-mouth search, 268–269
hiring staff members
   and malpractice prevention, 532
   physician extenders, 249–250
   physician leader, 204–207
   positive staff, and patient satisfaction, 557–558
   See also staffing mix
HITECH (Health Information Technology for Economic and Clinical Health) Act, 319, 320–321, 493, 494
hold-harmless clauses, in health plan contract, 312
hospital-physician ACOs, 463
hospitals, EMTALA definition of, 452–453
hot assets, 97
How to Win Friends and Influence People (Carnegie), 371
human resources management. *See* strategic talent management
human resources overview, labor and employment issues, 217–231
   Americans with Disabilities Act (ADA), 218–219
   Defense of Marriage Act (DOMA), 225
   Fair Labor Standards Act (FLSA), 219–220
   Family and Medical Leave Act (FMLA), 217–218
   immigration issues, 225
   independent contractors (ICs), 228–230
   social media and technology in workplace, 225–228
   Title VII: nondiscrimination policy, 220
   Title VII: sexual harassment policy, 220–224
HVAC (heating, ventilation, and air-conditioning)
   balancing report for heating and cooling system, 58
   design-build decisions, 51
   utilities in site-selection checklist, 64–65
hybrid pay structures for physicians, 256

I

IBA/Kelsey study on buying, 397
IBISWorld report, on urgent care industry, 4
ICs. *See* independent contractors
Illinois, social media privacy protection, 227
IM. *See* integrative medicine
image viewers, 479
imaging and interpretation, 475–484
   about radiology and types of equipment, 475–476
   archiving images, 479–480
   choosing equipment vendors, 136–140
   computed tomography (CT) scanners, 475, 478–479
      conventional scanners, 478
      multislice scanners, 479
      spiral scanners, 479
   image interpretation, 480–482
      radiology overreads, 481
      radiology providers, choosing, 481–482
      types of, 480–481
   patient safety concerns
      laboratory and imaging follow-up, 527, 530
      missed radiology interpretations, 527
      radiology overreads, 524, 531
   radiation safety, 480
   ultrasound systems, 475, 476–478
      2-D ultrasound, 477
      3-D ultrasound, 477–478
      Doppler ultrasound, 478
   x-ray equipment, 475, 476 (*See also* x-ray room)
immigrant population, 14
immigration issues, and human resources, 225
in-service programs, 282
incentive-based pay-for-performance (P4P) compensation, 285–286
income statements, 158–168, 159*t*–161*t*
   expenses, 162–168 (*See also* expenses, on income statement)
   revenue, 158–162
   variance calculations for revenue and expense categories, 195, 196*t*–197*t*

indemnification and mutual liability, in health plan contract, 312–313
indemnification, in sale of urgent care company, 99–102
independent contractors (ICs)
  versus employees, 228–230, 280, 289–291
  and payroll, 186–187
independent medical examinations (IMEs), 544
independent public relations practitioner, 382–384
industry analysis, in business plan, 13
information processing, 184
information technology and electronic equipment list, 138t
information technology expense, 165
informed consent
  malpractice prevention, 531–532
  for patient safety, 525–526
  requirement in virtual care, 493–494
inpatients, and EMTALA, 453
insurance
  course of construction insurance, 55
  medical malpractice expense, 166–167
  other types, on income statement, 167
  workers' compensation (See workers' compensation)
  See also health insurance
insurance requirements for urgent care center, 115–126
  business insurance, 121–124
    considerations for, 124
    expense on income statement, 167
    extra-expense coverage, 123–124
    general liability coverage, 122
    loss-of-income coverage, 123–124
    non-owned and hired auto coverage, 122
    property coverage, 122–123
  life and disability, 124–125
  medical-professional liability insurance
    credentialing of providers (See also credentialing of providers)
  medical-professional liability insurance, 116–121
    business insurance coverage, 124
    credentialing of providers, 119–121
    insurers' financial condition, 116–117
    limit of liability, 119
    premium development, 118
    types of insurance products, 117–118
  other types of insurance, 125
  types of coverage, 115
  workers' compensation, 124

integrated financial plan, 611–612
integrative medicine (IM), 587–598
  about complementary and alternative medicine (CAM), 587
  business plan to integrate CAM, 588–594
    differentiation strategy, 592–594
    market analysis, 588–591, 589t
    risks to provide or not, 594
    sustainable revenue from, 591–592
  strategic implementation, 597
  strategies to integrate CAM, 594–597
Integrative Medicine Assessment Questions tool, 590
interest expense, 175–176
interior designer for urgent care center, 60
internal assessment for occupational medicine, 537–538
internal control, 183–189
  See also financial management, internal control
internal marketing, 580
Internal Revenue Service (IRS)
  20-point test, 280, 290
  and independent contractors (ICs), 228
International Statistical Classification of Diseases and Related Health Problems (ICD), 190, 191, 536
interpretation of images. See imaging and interpretation
interstate commerce, 219
interviews
  exit, usefulness in compliance program, 508
  interviewing candidates for physician leader, 206–207
  structured vs. unstructured, 279
inventory assets, 173, 177
IV supplies list, 132t

J

jail sentences, 106, 113
JAMA, on physician shortage, 263
job crafting, 282
job satisfaction, and work engagement, 287
Johnson & Johnson, 395
Joint Commission
  accreditation of urgent care center, 145–146, 147–150
  CLIA accreditation, 417
  code of conduct and disruptive providers, 271
Joint Commission on Accreditation of Hospitals, 145
Journal of Urgent Care Medicine, 128, 266

K

key drivers, 158, 162*t*
key performance indicators (KPIs), 184, 195, 403
KLAS, 337
knowledge pyramid, in metric-driven management, 404, 405*f*
Kotter, John P., 213

L

labor issues. *See* human resources overview, labor and employment issues
laboratory
   area, and patient satisfaction, 70–71, 554, 555
   defined, 415, 428
   equipment and supply distributor, 428, 433
   fees for overreads, 164
   moderate-complexity (*See* clinical laboratory, moderate-complexity)
   personnel (*See* laboratory personnel)
   results, follow-up for malpractice prevention, 530
   services, choosing vendor for new line of business, 141
laboratory director, 422–423, 436, 437*t*, 438
laboratory information systems (LIS), 439, 441
laboratory overview, 415–426
   Clinical Laboratory Improvement Amendments (CLIA)
      about laboratory regulations, 415–416
      applying for licensure, 428
      certificate and testing, 419–420
      certificate types, 417–418
      certification costs, 418–419
      change-of-ownership, 418, 419
      inspection preparation, 445, 447–448
      nonwaived testing, moderate (COA or COC), 417, 418, 421–423, 425
      provider-performed microscopy (PPM), 417, 418, 421
      surveys, 418
      waived testing (COW), 417, 418, 420–421, 425
      websites and links, 416*t*
   getting started, 425
   selecting tests to offer, 423–425
laboratory personnel
   clinical consultant, 422–423, 436, 437*t*, 438
   laboratory director, 422–423, 436, 437*t*, 438
   requirements and hiring, 436, 437*t*, 438, 439
   technical consultant, 422–423, 436, 437*t*, 438
   testing personnel, 419, 420, 421, 436, 437*t*, 438
land-use plan, 63

landlords, and business insurance, property coverage, 122–123
laws
   and CPOM, 105–106, 112–113
   obeying when interviewing, 280
   OIG list of key health care laws, 504
laws, federal
   Affordable Care Act (*See* Affordable Care Act)
   American Recovery and Reinvestment Act, 320
   American Taxpayer Relief Act, 96
   Americans with Disabilities Act (ADA), 59, 76, 218–219, 280
   Civil Rights Act (*See* Title VII of Civil Rights Act)
   Defense of Marriage Act (DOMA), 225
   Deficit Reduction Act, 515
   Emergency Medical Treatment and Active Labor Act (*See* EMTALA)
   Employee Retirement Income Security Act, 225
   Fair Labor Standards Act (FLSA), 219–220
   Family and Medical Leave Act (FMLA), 217–218
   Health Care and Education Reconciliation Act, 499
   Health Information Technology for Economic and Clinical Health (HI-TECH) Act, 319, 320–321, 493, 494
   Health Insurance Portability and Accountability Act (*See* HIPAA)
   Liability Risk Retention Act, 116
   Medicare Modernization Act, 514
   National Labor Relations Act, 225–226
   Social Networking Online Protection Act (SNOPA), 227, 231
   Tax Relief and Health Care Act, 514
lead-shielding requirements, 50, 70
leadership, defined, 207
   See also physician leadership
leading indicators, and metrics, 413
lease agreement, 95, 98–99
lease expense, 167
legal and professional expense, 165–166
legal entities and investment, 613–614
legal issues in nonphysician ownership. *See* corporate practice of medicine (CPOM)
legal liability
   of corporations, 80
   employees vs. independent contractor, 289
   of general and limited partnerships, 82
   of LLCs, 83

of professional entities, 84
See also liability considerations
lenders, in building urgent care center, 56, 60
letter of intent, 47, 93, 620
liabilities, current, in working capital, 194
liabilities, on balance sheet, 174–176, 195, 198*t*
liability considerations
    of asset acquisitions, 97–99
    of equity acquisitions, 96–97
    indemnification and mutual liability, in health plan contract, 312–313
    limit of liability, in insurance, 119
    professional liability coverage, in health plan contract, 314
    See also legal liability
Liability Risk Retention Act, 116
licensing
    for building urgent care center, 50
    and CPOM, 108
    information for exit transactions, 91
    See also permitting for building urgent care center
lien wavers, 56, 57, 61
life insurance, 124–125
life support, triage, and respiratory supplies list, 133*t*
lifestyles of health and sustainability (LOHAS) market, 590–591
lighting in urgent care center, 74–75, 553–556, 602
limited liability companies (LLCs). *See* LLCs (limited liability companies)
limited partnerships, 82
listening, 558, 604
litigation, information in sale of urgent care company, 93
LLC agreement, 79
LLCs (limited liability companies), 82–84
    and asset acquisitions, 97
    characteristics of, compared with corporations, 77–79
    formation mechanics, 78, 85
    governance of, 78–79, 83
    investments and capital, 613–614
    legal liability, 83
    tax considerations, 84
local marketing, and continual referral sources, 360–362
local mutual insurance companies, 116
lockbox, 186
locum tenens, hiring medical providers, 121, 265–267
logos, 396
LOI. *See* letter of intent
loss-of-income coverage, in business insurance, 123–124
Louisiana
    laboratory licensure and regulations, 430*t*
    on management service fees, 111

M

mail opening, 187
maintenance of urgent care center, 58, 61
    agreements and services from vendors, 139
malpractice. *See* medical malpractice
managed-care organizational audits. *See* audits by managed-care organizations and regulatory agencies
managed-care products for urgent care centers, 307
management
    clinic manager, functions and duties of, 243–245
    defined, 208
    of leadership culture, 207–213 (*See also* physician leadership)
    partner for revenue cycle management, 344–348
management company, expense on income statement, 168
management-control process, and metric-driven management, 403, 404–406
management plan, in business plan, 17
management review, in internal control, 184
management service fee, and CPOM, 110–112
management services agreement, 95, 98–99, 109, 111
management structure, for additional services, 580–581
market analysis
    on additional services, 578
    in business plan, 13–14
    for complementary and alternative medicine, 588–591, 589*t*
    in marketing analysis, 352
    occupational medicine, 536–537
market area definition for site selection, 23–25
market barriers, in site selection, 25
Market-Driven Health Care: Who Wins, Who Loses in the Transformation of America's Largest Service Industry (Herzlinger), 625
marketing metrics, 412*t*
marketing overview, 351–364
    compelling messages and communications, 358–360
    collateral, 359–360
    message-development goals, 359

promos, 360
signage, 360
customer relationships and loyalty, 362
local marketing and continual referral sources, 360–362
marketing analysis, 351–354
    company analysis, 353–354
    competitive analysis, 352–353
    customer analysis, 351–352
plans and guides, 355–358
    brand standards guide, 358
    budget for marketing, 355
    marketing and sales plans, 355–356
    media and advertising plan, 356–358
tracking results, 362–363
marketing plan, 355–358
    on additional services, 580
    and internal marketing, 580
    for occupational medicine, 544
marketing strategy
    in business plan, 15–16
    expenditures on income statement, 165
Maryland
    laboratory licensure and regulations, 430*t*
    social media privacy protection, 227
Massachusetts, laboratory licensure and regulations, 430*t*
massage therapy, 593
mean, defined, 47
Measures of Success forms, 149
media
    advertising plan, 356–358
    and crisis management, 387, 388–391
    and public relations, 378–380
median, defined, 47–48
Medica Choice, costs of emergency care, 6
Medicaid
    audits (*See* audits by managed-care organizations and regulatory agencies)
    and electronic health records, 320, 330
    and primary-care availability, 9
    virtual care reimbursement, 495
Medicaid integrity contractors (MICs), 515
Medicaid Integrity Program audits, 515
medical conditions. *See* emergency medical conditions
medical documentation, 568–573
    See also evaluation and management (E&M) of coding, medical documentation
medical equipment and supplies list, 129*t*–130*t*
    See also equipment; supplies
medical indications and tests, 434*t*–435*t*
medical malpractice
    EMTALA violations, 452

insurance, 166–167
prevention and patient safety, 530–532
utility of radiology overreads, 481, 531
and virtual care, 487, 494
medical necessity, 313, 561–562, 568–569
medical-professional liability insurance, 116–121, 124
    credentialing of providers (*See also* credentialing of providers)
medical providers. *See* providers
medical review officer, 538–539
medical screening exam, EMTALA requirement, 455–457
Medicare
    and ACOs, 463–465
    audits (*See* audits by managed-care organizations and regulatory agencies)
    and electronic health records, 320, 330
    and Medicaid anti-kickback statute, 92, 299
    physician shortage, 8–9, 263
    taxes from provider compensation, 289
Medicare administrative contractors (MACs), claims audits, 513–514
Medicare Modernization Act (2003), 514
Medicare-participating hospitals, EMTALA definition of, 452–453
Medicare Shared Savings Program (MSSP), 463, 471
medications
    dispensing, 141, 578, 580, 582
    expense, 164
    in pediatrics, 605, 608*t*
Megatrends (Naisbitt), 403
membership interest, 176–177
memorandum of understanding, 93
mentorship, 213
Mercer, 540
message-development goals, for marketing, 359
metric-driven management, 403–414
    balanced scorecard, 404
    corrective action, 409–410
    data distribution, 407–408
    knowledge pyramid, 404, 405*f*
    management-control process, 403, 404–406
    performance improvement, 408–409
    priority setting, 406–407
    selection of metrics, 410–413
metrics, 212, 403
metrics continuum, 408
minors and patient competency, and informed consent, 525, 527
moderate-complexity clinical laboratory. *See* clinical laboratory, moderate-complexity

modified claims-made insurance, 117–118
Mongan Institute for Health Policy, 9
Montana
    Bozeman Urgent Care Center, 593
    laboratory licensure and regulations, 430t
mutual liability and indemnification, in health plan contract, 312–313

N

National Center on Complementary and Alternative Medicine, 587
National Committee for Quality Assurance, 550
National Flood Insurance Program, 124
National Hospital Ambulatory Medical Care Survey, 8
National Institutes of Health, National Center on Complementary and Alternative Medicine, 587
National Labor Relations Act, 225–226
National Labor Relations Board
    on confidential investigations of sexual harassment, 224
    social media policies and concerted activity, 225–226
National Registry of Certified Medical Examiners, 543
National Safety Council, 395
natural products for alternative medicine, 587
NDAs (confidentiality and nondisclosure agreements), 88–89, 300, 620
negligent hiring, 249
negligent supervision cause of action, 249
negotiations on health plan contract, 306, 308, 315–316
net income, 158, 177
net lease, 46
net present value (NPV), 615
net property, plant, and equipment (PP&E), 168, 173, 174t
net realizable revenue, 191
net revenue, 158
net revenue per visit (NRPV), 158, 189
net working capital, 168
Nevada, laboratory licensure and regulations, 431t
New York state
    CMS laboratory exemption, 417
    and corporate practice of medicine, 110, 113
    laboratory licensure and regulations, 431t
news for media, 380
    See also public relations
NNN rental rate, 37

non-owned and hired auto coverage, in business insurance, 122
noncompetition agreements or provisions, 95, 300, 301–302
noncompliance penalties, in CPOM, 112–113
nondisclosure agreements or provisions, 88–89, 300, 620
nondiscrimination policy, Title VII of Civil Rights Act, 220
nonphysician ownership. See corporate practice of medicine (CPOM)
nonsolicitation provisions, 89, 301
nonwaived testing, moderate (COA or COC), 417, 418, 421–423, 425
North Carolina, Carolinas HealthCare System Urgent Care, Charlotte, 593–594
North Dakota, laboratory licensure and regulations, 431t
nose coverage insurance, 117
nurse practitioner
    functions and duties of, 242–243
    growth of profession, 247
    supervision of, 250–251
    See also physician extenders
nurse station, in design of floor plan, 71–72
nursing facilities, Health Care Reform and compliance programs, 499–501

O

Obama, Barack, 320
objectives of urgent care center, and leverage in health plan contracting, 307–308
occupational medicine (OM), 535–546
    DOT physicals, 543–544
    employer wants, 540–541
    HIPAA, 542–543
    internal assessment, 537–538
    market assessment, 536–537
        work-related injuries, 536
    marketing, 544
    on-site services, 540
    physical therapy, 539
    referrals, 542
    scope of care, 538–539
    wellness programs, 539–540
    workers' compensation, 124, 535–536, 542
Occupational Medicine Skills Assessment tool, 538
Occupational Safety and Health Administration, floor plan considerations, 76
occurrence insurance, 117–118
offer letter. See letter of intent
office, equipment, and personnel lease agreement, 99

Office of Inspector General (OIG)
    audits for health-care fraud recoveries, 512, 515–516, 518–519
    and compliance programs, 500–501
    seven fundamental elements of compliance program, 502–503
office supplies list, 139*t*
office supply vendors, choosing, 142
offices, in design of floor plan, 71
offsets (recoupment), in health plan contract, 311
OIG. *See* Office of Inspector General
OM. *See* occupational medicine
on-site services for occupational medicine, 540
on-site visits for accreditation, 146, 150, 153
onboarding, in strategic talent management, 281–282
online branding, 397–399
    company blog, 399
    directories, 398
    social networks, 398–399
    tools of the trade, 399–400
online diligence platform, 90
open-access POS plan, 307
operating agreement, of LLCs, 79
operating expenses, 46, 158, 163*t*
operational controls, in management plan, 17
operational net income, 158
operational paralysis, 16
operational staff, in organizational hierarchy, 209, 211*f*
operations manual, for urgent care center building, 58–59, 61
operations metrics, 411*t*–412*t*
optimal healing environment, 595–596
Oregon
    laboratory licensure and regulations, 431*t*
    Renewal Centers Urgent Care, 592
organizational goals, 208–209
organizational hierarchy, 209–211, 210*f*
organizational responsibility, 209–211
orientation and onboarding, in strategic talent management, 281–282
orthopedic services, 583–584
overreads of images
    in medical documentation, 571
    for patient safety, 524, 531
    utility for patient safety and quality assurance, 475, 481

P

pain-management services
    as additional service, 583–584
    in CAM, 589, 595

parking, 64
partnerships
    and asset acquisitions, 97
    general and limited, 82
    of revenue cycle management, 344–348
pass-through, 47
patient accounts receivable
    assets, on balance sheet, 172, 173*t*
    on cash-flow statement, 177
patient anti-dumping act, 451
patient compensation fund, 119
patient competency, and informed consent, 525, 527
patient data for marketing analysis, 352
patient draw site setup, 443, 445, 446*t*–447*t*
patient medical records, 293, 335–336
Patient Protection and Affordable Care Act. *See* Affordable Care Act
patient registration, and revenue cycle, 340–342
patient safety, 521–533
    differences between urgent care and emergency departments, 521
    emergency and subtle conditions presenting in urgent care, 522–524 (*See also* emergency medical conditions)
    emergency events and personnel tasks, 528–529
    informed consent, 525–526
        in common conditions presenting in urgent care, 522–524
        disclosure of appropriate information, 525–526
        patient competency, 525
        types of: general, specific, implied, 526
    laboratory and imaging follow-up, 527
    malpractice prevention, 530–532
        callbacks, 532
        care paths, and standing orders, 532
        discharge instructions, 530
        documentation, 532
        hiring practices, 532
        informed consent, 531–532
        laboratory and x-ray results follow-up, 530
        radiology overreads, 531
        service recovery, and happy patients, 531
    in pediatrics, 605–606
    radiological interpretations, 527
    right to refuse care, 526–527
patient satisfaction, 547–560
    improving, 553–558
        medical care areas and patient emotional experience, 555–556

medical treatment areas and patient physical experience, 553–554
maintaining, 558
measuring (*See* patient satisfaction surveys)
positive staff members, 556–558 (*See also* staff, and patient satisfaction)
patient satisfaction surveys
　data basics, 551–552
　　analysis, 552
　　questionnaires, 552
　　volume of patient surveys, 551–552
　structure and purpose of, 548–551
　　options for collecting data, 550
　value of, 547–548
patients
　anti-dumping act (*See* EMTALA)
　customer relationships and loyalty, 362
　identifying extremis in triage, 236
　improved satisfaction and ACOs, 466–467
　metrics on experience of, 412*t*–413*t*
　misidentification of, 148
　new compared with established, for E&M coding, 565, 565*t*, 566*t*
pay applications during construction, 56, 57
pay-for-performance (P4P) compensation, 285–286
pay structure for physicians. *See* provider compensation
Payment Error Rate Measurement (PERM) program, 515
payment methods and models for health plan contract, 306–307
payroll, and internal controls, 186–187
Pediatric Advanced Life Support, 609
pediatric urgent care, 599–610
　about certified germ-dispersal units and caregivers, 599–600
　customer service, 602–604
　design of facility for children, 601–602
　emergency preparedness, 606–609
　　certification of staff, 609
　　drugs for, 608*t*
　　equipment and supplies, 607*t*, 608
　model of urgent care, 600–601
　patient safety, 605–606
　supplies, 601–602
Pennsylvania
　Coordinated Health, Bethlehem, 594
　laboratory licensure and regulations, 431*t*
percentage-based service fees, 110
percentage-of-collection financial model of EHR, 333
performance-based provider compensation structures, 254, 256–257, 259

performance improvement with metrics, 408–409
performance management, of strategic talent, 282–284
performance measurement, 189–195
　defined, 212
　in internal control, 184
　revenue cycle analytics, 344
　See also financial management, performance measurement
performance measures of provider, 209
performance tools and metrics, in evaluation of providers, 212
permitting for building urgent care center
　about requirements, 56–57
　average length of time, 50
personnel groupings, 209–210, 211*f*
　See also staffing mix
petty cash, 186
phantom stock, 265
pharmaceutical supplies list, 137*t*
pharmacies, and site selection, 30
phone lines in urgent care center, 60
photographs of work in construction process, 57
physical therapy for occupational medicine, 539
physicals for truck and bus drivers, and aviation pilots, 543
physician assistant supervision, 251
physician extenders (physician assistant or nurse practitioner), 247–252
　about scope of services, 247
　causes of action with, 248–249
　functions and duties of, 242–243
　risk mitigation, 249–250
　state statutes on supervision, 250–251
Physician Insurers Association of America, 248
physician job boards, 269–270
physician leaders, 203
physician leadership, 203–216
　about organizational leadership, 203–204
　common pitfalls, 214
　interviewing and hiring the right leader, 206–207
　job criteria establishment, 204–206
　　health-care knowledge, 205
　　problem solving, 205–206
　　technical industry knowledge, 204–205
　management of leadership culture, 207–213
　　communicating effectively, 211
　　evaluating providers, 211–213
　　organizational goals setting, 208–209

organizational responsibility establishment, 209–211
physician-only ACOs, 463
physician ownership of urgent care center, compared with layperson ownership. *See* corporate practice of medicine (CPOM)
physician–patient relationship, and CPOM, 107
Physician Quality Reporting System, 550
physician self-referral. *See* Stark law (physician self-referral)
physicians
   employment of, and corporate practice of medicine, 106–107
   functions and duties of, 240–243
   shortage of, 8–9, 247, 263–264, 276
   tasks in critical care events, 529
   See also providers
Physicians Foundation, on physician shortage, 9, 264
picture archiving and communication system (PACS)
   archiving images, 476, 479–480
   choosing equipment vendors, 140
piggyback on networks, 307
Pitney Bowes, 14
plan, do, study, and act (PDSA), 408
point-of-care test kits, 424
point-of-care testing, 428. 431
point of service (POS) managed-care, 307
policies and procedures (P&Ps)
   for analyzers and test systems, 441–442
   for compliance program, 503, 505–506
   in health plan contracting, 314
   internal control in urgent care center, 183
population
   profile for site selection, 31–33
   statistics for site selection, 23–24
positive distraction, 595
PP&E (property, plant, and equipment). *See* net property, plant, and equipment
PPM (provider-performed microscopy), 417, 418, 421
practice management services, and CPOM, 109–110
preferred provider organization (PPO), 307
   silent PPOs, 537
preferred stock, 614–615, 622
preliminary denial of accreditation, defined, 149
premium development, for insurance, 118
prepaid expenses
   assets, on balance sheet, 173
   on cash-flow statement, 177

primary care
   in addition to urgent care, coding for, 573
   lack of availability, 8–9
prior acts coverage, 117
private equity process, 618, 620–622
pro forma financial statements, 157–182
   accounting methods: cash vs. accrual, 157–158
   balance sheet, 168–177, 170*t*–171*t* (*See also* balance sheet)
      assets, 172–173
      equity, 176–177
      liabilities, 174–176
   cash-flow statement, 177–180, 178*t*–179*t*
   income statement, 158–168, 159*t*–161*t*
      expenses, 162–168 (*See also* expenses, on income statement)
      revenue, 158–162
pro rata share, 47
procedure room, in design of floor plan, 69
professional associations, 84, 108
professional corporation (PC), 77, 84, 108, 109
professional entity statutes, and CPOM, 108–109
professional expense, 165–166
professional liability coverage, in health plan contract, 314
professional LLCs, 77, 84, 108, 109
proficiency testing (PT), 419, 423, 442–443, 443*t*–445*t*
profit-and-loss statement (P&L), 158
promos for marketing, 360
property coverage, in business insurance, 122–123
property, ideal, for site selection, 33–40
property, plant, and equipment (PP&E). *See* net property, plant, and equipment
protocols, for critical care events, 532
provider compensation, 253–261, 293–296
   and benefits for strategic talent, 284–286
   competitive compensation structure, 258
   consistency of compensation structure, 257–258
   in employment agreements, 293–296
      cash compensation, 293–294
      equity compensation, 296
      fixed component: salary, 294–295
      variable component: bonus compensation, 295–296
   hybrid structures, 256
   as management tool, 256–257
   measuring physician contributions, 258–259
   relative value units (RVUs), 254–256
   types of compensation structures, 254

performance-based, 254, 256–257, 259
straight hourly, 254, 259
provider performance measures, 209
provider-performed microscopy (PPM), 417, 418, 421
provider self-evaluation, 212–213
providers
   with blemished records, 120
   credentialing of, 119–121
   disruptive, 270–272
   evaluating, 211–213
   functions and duties of clinical back office, 240–243
   job boards, 269–270
   in organizational hierarchy, 209, 211f
   qualifications and requirements, in employment agreement, 292
   tasks in critical care events, 529
   See also physicians
provisional accreditation, defined, 149, 151
public relations, 377–384
   goals of, 377–378
   hungry media, 378–380
   positive patient experiences, 382
   selecting PR agency or independent practitioner, 382–384
   tactics, 380–382
public safety in crisis management, 386, 391
punch lists, in construction process, 56, 57–58
purchase agreement in sale of urgent care company, 93–94, 103
purchased services expense, 166
purchasing and accounts payable, 187, 188t

Q

QR (Quick Response) codes, 360
quality-assessment plan (QA plan) for clinical laboratory, 442
quality of care, and ACOs, 464, 469t, 470t
quality system approach, for laboratory testing, 422
Quantcast, 399
questionnaires on patient satisfaction, 552
   See also patient satisfaction surveys

R

radiation safety, 50, 480
radio advertising, 356, 366
radiography equipment, 140
radiologist, and overreads, 475, 481–482, 524, 531
radiology
   area, improving patient satisfaction, 554, 556
   departmental design, 475–476

fees for overreads, 164
sample vendor worksheet for, 128t
See also imaging and interpretation
radiology technician, 162–163, 239–240
radiology technologist, 475
reagent and analyzer contracts, for clinical laboratory, 438
real estate terminology, 44–48
realistic job preview, 279
reasonable accommodation, 218
reasonable patient standard, 525
reasonable physician standard, 525
reception area, 68, 234–236, 340–342
records, of financial statements, 184
recovery audit contractor (RAC) program, 512, 514, 515
recruitment and selection of strategic talent, 278–281
redemption option, 296
referral marketing, and social media networks, 369
referrals for occupational medicine, 542
registered agent, 78
registration area, improving patient satisfaction, 554, 555
registration staff
   patient registration and revenue cycle, 340–342
   pediatrics concerns, 605–606
   sample guidelines for, 341f
regulated analytes, 423
Regulation D, 613, 617
regulations
   considerations in ownership, 105–106, 112–113
   of laboratories (See laboratory overview)
regulatory research, for additional services, 578–580
rehabilitative services, 583
reimbursement
   insurance contractual adjustments, 190–191
   linked to medical necessity, 313, 561–562, 568–569
   for occupational medicine, 537
   tenant improvement reimbursement in construction process, 59
   for virtual care, 487, 495
reinsurance, 116–117
relative value units (RVUs), 254–256
   as bonus compensation, variable component, 295–296
   medical necessity and E&M, 562
renewal provisions, in health plan contract, 312
rent, 37, 46, 47, 167

representations and warranties, in sale of urgent care company, 100–101
reputation of urgent care center, in crisis management, 386, 391–392
reserve method of bad debt accounting, 192
resource-based relative value system (RBRVS), 562
resources
 for compliance programs, 504–505
 for considering virtual care, 496
 proficiency testing providers, 443t–445t
 referral sources in local marketing, 361
 reports on electronic health record systems, 337
 websites to find medical providers, 269–270
respondeat superior, 248
responsibility, defined, 209
restrooms, in design of floor plan, 72–73
retail clinics, 626
retail markets, and site selection, 29–31, 33
retained agreements, hiring providers from search firms, 267–268
retained earnings, on balance sheet, 177
retaliation in sexual harassment claims, 221–222
return on investment (ROI), and physician compensation, 253
revenue
 in evaluation of financial statements, 199
 on income statement, 158–162
 and performance measurement, 189–191
 sustainable, from CAM services, 591–592
revenue cycle, 339, 340f
revenue cycle management, 339–349
 choosing a management partner, 344–348
  electronic health record (EHR) service as, 346
 controlling the process, 339–344
  billing and claims, 343–344
  medical documentation, 342–343
  patient registration, 340–342
  revenue cycle analytics, 344
Rhode Island, laboratory licensure and regulations, 432t
right to refuse care, 526–527
risk assessment, in compliance program, 503
risk pool, in POS plan, 307
risk retention groups (RRGs), 116

S

S-corporations, 80–81, 613–614
safe harbors to anti-kickback statute, 299
safety of patients. See patient safety
safety requirements, in urgent care center, 59

salary, fixed component for provider compensation, 294–295
sale of urgent care company. See exit transactions, sale of urgent care company
sales plan, 355–356
same-sex domestic partners, 225
SBA. See Small Business Administration
scope of care
 for occupational medicine, 538–539
 scope of services for physician extenders, 247
 See also additional services in urgent care
SCORE, 12
scoreboards, 407
scorecard, balanced, 404
search firms, for hiring medical providers, 267–268
Section 7 activity, 225–226
seducing signal, 278, 279f
segregation of duties, 183, 184
self-evaluation of physician leader, 212–213
seller indemnification liability, 100
selling, general, and administrative (SG&A) expense, 166, 168
Service Corps of Retired Executives, 12
sexual harassment under Title VII of Civil Rights Act, 220–224
 policy provisions, 222–224
 Supreme Court decisions, 221–222
shell space, 63
shopping centers, 29–30, 33–39, 44–46
signage for urgent care center
 exterior, 39–40
 interior, 59–60
 in marketing and advertising plan, 357, 360
signing date, 98
site-selection checklist in floor plan design, 63–66
 parking, 64
 utilities, 64–66
 zoning and building use, 63–64
site selection of urgent care center, 23–48
 comparison of sites, 41–43
 competition inventory, 26–29
 general market area definition, 23–25
 ideal property identification, 33–40
  rental rates analysis, 37
  shopping center visibility, 37–39
  signage for visibility, 39–40
  traffic count determination, 33–36
 population profile, 31–33
 real estate terminology, 44–48
 retail markets and traffic flow, 29–31
Site To Do Business, 33

Small Business Administration (SBA), 12, 613, 615, 616–617
smartphone applications for pediatric emergencies, 608
social media
  and brand development, 398–399
  and crisis management, 389–390, 391
  and technology in workplace, 225–228
social media and consumer engagement, 365–376
  Carnegie's principles, 371–374
  consumer buying and decision-making timeline, 366–369, 367f
  consumer-generated content, 371–374
  evolution of interaction between providers and patients, 365–366
  long-term investment, 375
  narrowing the gap of communication, 366
  platforms of social media, 368
  positive patient experiences for public relations, 382
  referral marketing, 369
  search and social media link, 374–375
Social Networking Online Protection Act (SNOPA), 227, 231
Social Security tax, 289
social skill, 213
software-as-a-service (SaaS) model, 165
software for EHR, 331, 332–334
software licenses for EHR, 333
specialty supplies list, 135t–136t
specification approvals for urgent care center, 50
stabilization, EMTALA requirement, 457–458
staff
  expense on income statement, 162–163, 162t
  in organizational hierarchy, 209–210, 210f
  See also employee matters; employees
staff, and patient safety issues
  critical care events in urgent care center, 528–529
    back-office tasks, 528–529
    checklists and care paths, 529
    front-office tasks, 528
    provider tasks, 529
  hiring practices, and malpractice prevention, 532
staff, and patient satisfaction, 556–558
  attitude, 556–557
  communication, 557
  courtesy and respect, 557
  empathy, 558
  listening, 558, 604

positive culture, 556
  terminating negative staff, 557–558
staffing mix, 233–246
  clinic management, 243–245
  clinical back office, 238–243
    medical assistance, 238–239
    physician extenders, 242–243 (See also physician extenders)
    physicians, 240–242
    radiology, 239–240
    tasks in critical care events, 528–529
  front office, 234–238
    lobby and waiting area, 67–68
    patient registration and revenue cycle, 340–342
    reception and billing duties of staff, 234–236
    tasks in critical care events, 528
    triage, functions and duties of staff, 68, 236–238
  other roles and staff, 245
    certified coder, 574
    certified medical examiners, 543
    compliance officer, 506, 516, 517
    greeter, in pediatrics urgent care, 602–603, 609
    as internal marketers, 580
    laboratory personnel (See laboratory personnel)
    nurse practitioner (See nurse practitioner)
    radiologist, 475, 481–482, 524, 531
    radiology technician, 162–163, 239–240
    radiology technologist, 475
    registration (See registration staff)
  staff composition, 233–234
  staffing ratios, 245
standing orders, for critical care events, 532
Stark law (physician self-referral)
  about regulations and employment contracts, 298–299
  and additional services, 580
  due diligence on material contracts, 92
  and electronic health records, 330
  statute and regulation number, and resources, 504, 505
start-up costs, of additional services, 582
state requirements
  laboratory regulations, 415, 416t, 428, 429t–432t, 447
  social media and technology in workplace, 227
  for telehealth service reimbursements, 487, 495

stock options, 265, 296
storage and supplies, in design of floor plan, 73
strategic talent management, 275–287
    compensation and benefits, 284–286
    defined, 275
    discipline and termination, 286
    evidence-based human resources practices, 277
    learning and development, 282
    major functions of, 275, 276f
    orientation and onboarding, 281–282
    performance management, 282–284
    recruitment and selection, 278–281
        financial impact of, 281
        obeying the law, 280
    War for Talent, 275–277
    See also human resources overview, labor and employment issues
StrategicHealthSolutions, LLC, 514
strategy, and organizational goals, 209, 214
The Strategy-Focused Organization (Kaplan & Norton), 404
strengths, weaknesses, opportunities, and threats. See SWOT
strict liability statute, 298
subpoena for audit, 516, 518–519
subscription agreement, 615
substantial completion, 58
supervisor, defined for sexual harassment claims, 221
supplemental medical review contractor (SMRC) programs, 512, 514–515
supplies
    for clinical laboratory setup, 446t–447t
    laboratory equipment and supply distributor, 428, 433
    medical supplies expense, 164
    for pediatric emergency, 607t
    and storage in design of floor plan, 73
    See also vendor selection for equipment and supply
support services agreement, 99
surety bond, 53
survey for accreditation, 148–149, 151
    See also accreditation of urgent care center
survey of laboratory by CMS, 418
surveys of patient satisfaction. See patient satisfaction surveys
survival period, in sale of urgent care company, 101
SWOT analysis, in marketing plan, 355
SWOT matrix, on medication dispensing, 578, 579t

T

tail coverage insurance, 117–118, 119, 166
talent management. See strategic talent management
tax considerations
    of asset acquisitions, 97
    of corporations, 80–82
    of employee vs. independent contractor, 289–291
    of equity acquisitions, 96
    of general and limited partnerships, 82
    of LLCs, 84
    of professional entities, 85
tax identification number, 96, 98
Tax Relief and Health Care Act (2006), 514
technical consultant, laboratory personnel, 422–423, 433, 436, 437t, 438
telemedicine, as the future, 628
    See also virtual care
telephone expenses, 166
tenant improvement reimbursement, in construction process, 59
tenant improvements (TIs), 47, 63
Tennessee
    laboratory licensure and regulations, 432t
    on management service fees, 110–111
term sheet, 93, 614, 615
termination
    and discipline, of strategic talent, 286
    of health plan contract, without cause, 314–315
    of negative staff, and patient satisfaction, 557–558
    and patient medical records, 293
    as provision of employment agreement, 296–298
test kits, selection of, 436
test menu selection, for clinical laboratory, moderate-complexity, 433, 434t–435t
testing. See laboratory overview
testing personnel, in clinical laboratory, 419, 420, 421, 436, 437t, 438
Texas
    code on informed consent and telemedicine, 493–494
    Flynn Brothers, Inc. v. First Medical Associates (1986), 112
theory of successor liability, 99
third-year residents, 120
threshold deductible, 101
time clock, 186
Title VII of Civil Rights Act
    employee threshold, 280
    nondiscrimination policy, 220

sexual harassment policy, 220–224
tracking results of marketing, 360, 362–363
trademark protection of brand identity, 394
traffic flow, and site selection, 29–31, 33–36
training and education
    CME (continuing medical education) in laboratory testing, 416t
    for communication skills, 557
    for compliance program, 506–507
    learning and development, in strategic talent management, 282
training room, in design of floor plan, 74
transfers of patients
    CPT definition, 564
    EMTALA requirement, 458–459
triage
    area, and patient satisfaction, 68, 554, 555
    compared with medical screening exam, EMTALA requirement, 456–457
    functions and duties of staff in front office, 236–238
triple net basis, rental rate, 37, 167
truck and bus drivers, physical exams, 543
turn and burn mentality, 253, 266
typefaces and visual identity of brand, 394

U

UCR Health Centers, Chandler, Arizona, 590
ultrasound equipment, 475, 476–478
    2-D ultrasound system, 477
    3-D ultrasound system, 477–478
    choosing equipment vendors, 140
    Doppler ultrasound, 478
    See also imaging and interpretation
umbrella insurance policy, 167
unaccredited, defined, 151
unilateral modifications, in health plan contract, 315
unique selling proposition, 354
upselling, 580
urgent care
    defined, 3, 26
    future of, 625–628
Urgent Care Association of America (UCAOA)
    accreditation of urgent care center, 146, 152–153
    Benchmarking Survey, 4, 536
    Certified Urgent Care Center guidelines, 146
    definition of urgent care, 3, 26
    networking for vendors, 128
    numbers of urgent care centers, 627
    Occupational Medicine Skills Assessment tool, 538
urgent care centers
    Bozeman Urgent Care Center, Bozeman, Montana, 593
    Carolinas HealthCare System Urgent Care, Charlotte, North Carolina, 593–594
    Coordinated Health, Bethlehem, Pennsylvania, 594
    Lake Oconee Urgent & Specialty Care Center, Georgia, 590
    Miami Urgent Care Center Medical Clinic, Miami, Florida, 589
    Premier Urgent Care Center, Melbourne, Florida, 591, 593
    Renewal Centers Urgent Care, Oregon, 592
    Seattle Homeopathy, Washington, 591
    Sentara Healthcare, Williamsburg, Virginia, 593
    UCR Health Centers, Chandler, Arizona, 590
urgent care industry, 3–10
    consumers, informed, 7–8
    definition of urgent care, 3, 26
    emergency care costs, 5–6
    emergency department overcrowding, 5
    future of, 625–628
    growth of, 4–5
    industry life cycle, 3–4
    insurance coverage, 6–7
    primary-care availability, 8–9
    virtual care delivery, 10
Urgent Care Integrated Network, and vendor selection, 131
urinary drug screens (UDSs), 535, 537, 538
US Bureau of Labor Statistics (BLS)
    physicians and surgeons numbers, 271
    work-related injuries and absenteeism, 536, 539, 540
US Census Bureau, 6, 14, 33
US Department of Health and Human Services (HHS), 500, 512
    See also Office of Inspector General (OIG)
US Department of Homeland Security, 225
US Department of Justice (DOJ), 515–516
US Department of Labor, 219–220, 229, 535
US Department of Transportation (DOT), 537–539, 543
US Federal Sentencing Guidelines, 499, 501–502
US Food and Drug Administration, 479
US Health Care Financing Administration, 255
US Health Resources and Services Administration, 263
US News & World Report, 3
US Patent and Trademark Office, 394

US Postal Service, Every Door Direct Mail, 357
US Securities and Exchange Commission (SEC), Regulation D, 613, 617
US Social Security Administration, 225
US Supreme Court decisions
   Burlington Indus. v. Ellerth (1998), 221
   Faragher v. City of Boca Raton (1998), 221
   University of Texas Southwestern Medical Center v. Nassar (2013), 221–222
   Vance v. Ball State University (2013), 221
utilities, in site-selection checklist, 64–66
   electricity, 66
   HVAC system, 64–65
   physical space requirements, 73
   sewer, 66
   water for domestic use, 65
   water for fire-protection use, 65

V

vaccinations, 600
validation process of analyzers, 439–441
value engineering, in building urgent care center, 53, 61
value proposition, 354
variance analysis, 194–195, 196*t*–197*t*, 198*t*
vendor partnerships, 143
vendor selection for equipment and supply, 127–144
   contractual agreements, finalizing, 142–143
   costs to expect, 131, 139*t*
   equipment vendors, 136–140
   group purchasing organization (GPO), 130–131
   laboratory equipment and supply distributors, 428, 433
   medical supply vendors, 140–141
   for new line of business, 141
   office supply and equipment vendors, 142
   researching vendor companies, 128–130
   supply lists
      exam room supplies, 131*t*
      information technology and electronic equipment, 138*t*
      IV supplies, 132*t*
      life support, triage, and respiratory supplies, 133*t*
      medical equipment and supplies, 129*t*–130*t*
      office supplies and lobby furniture, 139*t*
      pharmaceutical supplies, 137*t*
      specialty supplies, 135*t*–136*t*
      wound care supplies, 134*t*
   vendor partnerships, 143
   vendor representatives, 132–133, 136

vendor services, verifying, 143
   worksheet to specify services needed, 127–128, 128*t*, 142
vendors, fictitious, 187
vendors for electronic health record systems, 323, 329–332
vicarious liability cause of action, 248–249
video chat and videoconference, 485, 490–491, 492
   See also virtual care
video, power of, in crisis management, 390
Virginia, Sentara Healthcare, Williamsburg, 593
virtual care, 440–498
   about evolving industry of, 10, 485, 486*f*
   considerations in planning to provide, 493–495
      cannibalization, 495
      HIPAA and HITECH compliance, 494
      informed consent requirement, 493–494
      malpractice coverage, 486, 487, 494
      reimbursement, 487, 495
      telehealth platform, 495
   key influences, 486–489
   process of setting up, 496–497
   telemedicine as the future, 628
   use cases, 489–493
      e-visits, 492
      follow-up care, 492
      worksite clinics and employer-based health care, 492
      worksite wellness, 493
visibility, in site selection, 36, 37–40
vision
   and organizational goals, 208
   and values, aligning in business strategy, 575–577
visual identity of brand, 394–396
volume-based compensation. *See* performance-based provider compensation structures

W

waiting area
   design for pediatrics, 601–602
   identifying patients in extremis in triage, 236
   optimal healing environment for CAM, 595–596
   and patient satisfaction, 67, 553–554, 555
waived testing (COW), 417, 418, 420–421, 425
War for Talent, 275–277
warranties
   for construction, 58, 61

in sale of urgent care company, 100–101
Washington state
  CMS laboratory exemption, 417
  on health insurance plans and CAM, 596
  laboratory licensure and regulations, 432t
  Seattle Homeopathy, 591
Watson Wyatt study, 492
websites
  for CMS, and links, 416t
  in crisis management, 389, 391
  to find providers, 269–270
  public relations use of, 381
  in social media plan, 367–369
wellness programs of companies
  and occupational medicine, 539–540
  and virtual care, 493
wellness services and products, 583
West Virginia, laboratory licensure and regulations, 432t
whirlwind, 408
wildly important goals (WIGs), 406–407, 408t
withhold of a percentage, 307
word-of-mouth marketing, 365
word-of-mouth search for providers, 268–269
work engagement, and job satisfaction, 287
workers' compensation
  insurance requirement, 124
  and occupational medicine, 535–536, 542
working capital, 193–194, 612
working capital equation, 611
working drawings, during design phase of building, 49
worksite clinics, 492, 540
worksite wellness, 493, 539
wound care supplies list, 134t

X

x-ray equipment, types of, 475, 476
  See also imaging and interpretation
x-ray room, 66, 70

Z

zone integrity program contractors (ZPICs), 514
zoning requirements for urgent care center, 50, 63–64

ADDITIONAL WORKS

Textbook of Urgent Care Medicine
www.urgentcareeducation.com
by Dr. Lee Resnick and Dr. John Shufeldt

Textbook of Urgent Care Procedures
www.urgentcareeducation.com
by Dr. Lee Resnick and Dr. John Shufeldt

Ingredients of Outliers: A Recipe for Personal Achievement
www.ingredientsofoutliers.com
by Dr. John Shufeldt

Courses for Continuing Medical Education (CME)

www.urgentcarecme.com

www.urgentcarenursing.com

Resources for urgent care centers

www.ucinet.org

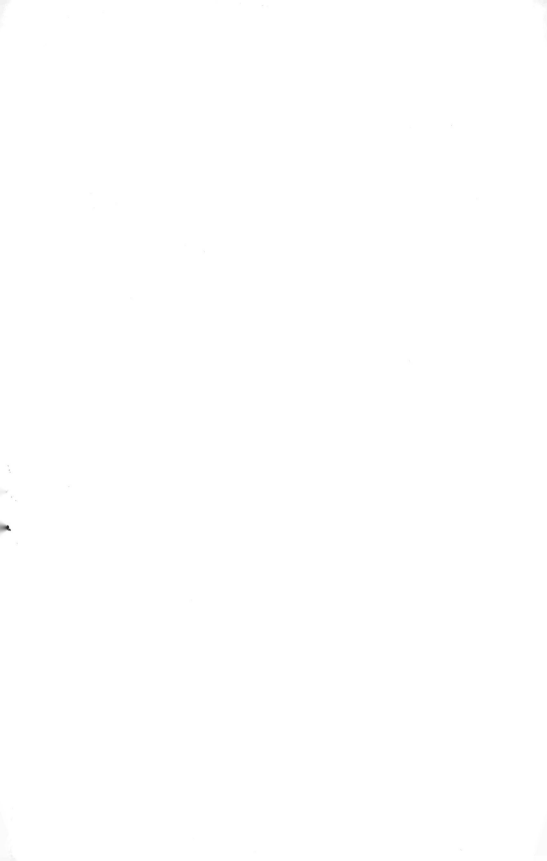